Handbook for Prescribing Medications During Pregnancy

Third Edition

Donald R. Coustan, M.D.

Professor and Chairman
Department of Obstetrics and Gynecology
Brown University School of Medicine;
Obstetrician and Gynecol
Women and Infants Hospital
Surgeon-in-Ch
Department of Gynecology
Rhode Island Hos
Providence, Rhode

Tara K. Mochizuki, PH

Attorney-at-Law
Formerly Assistant Clinical Profe
University of California, Sa
School of Pharmac
San Francisco, California;
Pediatric Pharmacist
University of California Medical Center
San Diego, California

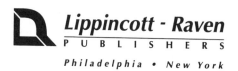

Lippincott - Raven
PUBLISHERS

Philadelphia • *New York*

Previous edition copyright © 1986 by Richard L. Berkowitz, Donald R. Coustan, and Tara K. Mochizuki.
First edition copyright © 1981 by Little, Brown and Company (Inc.).

Acquisitions Editor: Lisa McAllister
Developmental Editor: Rebecca Irwin Diehl
Manufacturing Manager: Kevin Watt
Production Manager: Robert Pancotti
Production Editor: Emily Harkavy
Cover Designer: Patricia Gast
Indexer: Dorothy Jahoda
Compositor: Compset
Printer: R.R. Donnelley

Printed in the United States of America

9 8 7 6 5 4 3 2 1

Library of Congress Cataloging-in-Publication Data

Handbook for prescribing medications during pregnancy / [edited by] Donald R. Coustan, Tara K. Mochizuki. — 3rd ed.
    p.   cm.
  Includes bibliographical references and index.
  ISBN 0-316-15826-7
  1. Obstetrical pharmacology—Handbooks, manuals, etc.
I. Coustan, Donald R. II. Mochizuki, Tara K.
  [DNLM: 1. Drug Therapy—in pregnancy handbooks.
2. Pharmacology handbooks.   WQ 39 H2355 1998]
RG528.H36 1998
615'.704—DC21
DNLM/DLC
for Library of Congress   98-17363
                                     CIP

To our children—
Tim and Elizabeth Chu,
and grown children—
Becky, Rachel, and David Coustan.

Contents

Contributors to the Third Edition

Marshall W. Carpenter, M.D.
Stephen R. Carr, M.D.
Donald R. Coustan, M.D.
Walter H. Gajewski, M.D.
Maureen P. Malee, M.D.
Tara K. Mochizuki, Pharm.D., J.D.
Helayne M. Silver, M.D.
Jami A. Star, M.D.

Research Assistants:
Larissa R. Graff, Pharm.D.
May A. Jue, Pharm.D.

Contributors to the Second Edition

Gaetano Bello, M.D.
Gertrud S. Berkowitz, Ph.D.
Richard L. Berkowitz, M.D., M.P.H.
Donald R. Coustan, M.D.
Jane E. Gordon, Ph.D.
Lauren Lynch, M.D.
Tara K. Mochizuki, Pharm.D., J.D.
Isabelle Wilkins, M.D.

Contributors to the First Edition

Richard L. Berkowitz, M.D.
Elizabeth A. Capriotti, R.Ph.
John R. Cote, Pharm.D.
Donald R. Coustan, M.D.
Ronald A. Cwik, M.D.
Alan H. DeCherney, M.D.
Greggory R. DeVore, M.D.
Allan D. DiCamillo, R.Ph.
Arnold J. Friedman, M.D.
Joel A. Giuditta, R.Ph.
Peter A. Grannum, M.D.
Robert J. Harrison, R.Ph.
Thomas K. Hazlet, Pharm.D.
Joyce M. Heineman, R.Ph.
Brian D. Hotchkiss, R.Ph.
David J. Iamkis, R.Ph.
Daniel J. Kazienko, R.Ph.
Phyllis C. Leppert, M.D.
Mark C. Malzer, M.D.
Mary Jane Minkin, M.D.
Tara K. Mochizuki, Pharm.D.
William O'Brien, M.D.
Phillip H. Radell, M.D.
Peter L. Ricupero, R.Ph.
Roberto J. Romero, M.D.
Paul J. Roszko, R.Ph.
Bonnie R. Saks, M.D.
C. Robert Sturwold, R.Ph.
Khalil Tabsh, M.D.
C. Edward Todd, R.Ph.
Ellen M. Todesca, R.Ph.
Cecily R. Victor, R.Ph.

Preface to the Third Edition

It has now been 17 years since the publication of the first edition of *Handbook for Prescribing Medications During Pregnancy,* and 12 years since the second edition. The book has been highly successful, and the publisher has urged the production of a new edition for a number of years. The long delay was due to reticence on the part of the authors to embark upon another large project. Drs. Coustan and Mochizuki have written the third edition, with the help of a number of contributors and editorial assistants whose names appear in the Contributors' list. Dr. Berkowitz has regrettably found it impossible to participate this time around, but his tremendous contributions in both organizing and editing the first two editions, as well the entries he wrote, stand as essential attributes of the project. We thank him for his previous participation and for the important influence he has had on both of us.

The goal of the third edition is no different from that of the previous two: To provide clinicians with an up-to-date desktop and portable reference on the use of drugs in pregnancy. A good deal of information has accrued since the last edition, with many new drugs on the market and many older drugs no longer widely prescribed. The format of the first two editions has been maintained, with the authors attempting to make a practical recommendation for each entry. All of the previous entries have been updated and, in many cases, extensively rewritten. There have been many new agents added to the book, and several have been deleted because their use is no longer prevalent. The previous appendix on antineoplastic agents has been expanded from 12 to 21 entries by Dr. Walter Gajewski, a highly gifted gynecologic oncologist at Brown University/Women and Infants Hospital of Rhode Island. The appendix on vitamins and minerals has been extensively updated. In the second edition, we added an appendix on industrial chemicals. In the interest of keeping the book compact, and because the topic is so broad and yet so bereft of credible information, that appendix was eliminated from the current edition.

Approximately one third of the entries were written, or rewritten, by members of the Division of Maternal Fetal Medicine and by Dr. Walter Gajewski of the Division of Gynecologic Oncology in the Department of Obstetrics and Gynecology at Brown University/Women and Infants Hospital of Rhode Island; Drs. Coustan and Mochizuki divided the remaining entries. In addition, invaluable research assistance was provided to Dr. Mochizuki by students at the University of California, San Francisco, School of Pharmacy. The authors wish to acknowledge the hard work and enthusiasm of their colleagues who played such an important role in the project.

As each of the authors took on other responsibilities both at home and in the workplace, the project took much longer than was initially anticipated. Our original publisher, the medical division of Little, Brown, was sold to Lippincott-Raven Publishers. We thank Nancy Chorpenning, our last editor at Little, Brown, and Lisa McAllister, our editor at Lippincott-Raven

Publishers, for their patience and their many kindnesses as the project dragged on. It would not have happened without their support.

We hope that the third edition of *Handbook for Prescribing Medications During Pregnancy* meets the needs of our readers, and is of benefit to their patients. We urge the reader to review the prefaces to the first two editions. As in the previous two editions, it should be noted that certain caveats still apply. Our recommendations are based on currently available information, and may require revision as more is learned. Some published data may have escaped our attention, despite our best efforts to be comprehensive. We welcome comments and suggestions from our readers, and would like to hear if anyone is aware of relevant data that were overlooked.

Donald R. Coustan, M.D.
Tara K. Mochizuki, Pharm.D., J.D.

Preface to the Second Edition

Our stated purpose for creating the first edition of *Handbook for Prescribing Medications During Pregnancy* was to provide clinicians with an up-to-date desktop reference on the use of drugs in pregnancy. The popular and critical success of that effort suggests that readers have found this handbook to be useful, and as a result, we have been encouraged to prepare a second edition. In order to remain relevant, this book must continue to incorporate the most currently available data. This, of course, means that periodic updating of the material is mandatory in order to add new information and maintain the validity of the recommendations being made.

The format used in the first edition has been preserved in the main body of the text. All of the original 140 entries have been reviewed, updated, and in many cases, substantially rewritten. Furthermore, 54 new drugs have been added. The appendix containing 17 vitamins and minerals has also been thoroughly updated. A new appendix containing 12 antineoplastic agents has been added. These drugs are discussed as a separate group because they all have the potential of being harmful to the developing fetus but sometimes must be administered for overriding maternal considerations. In that difficult setting, it is clearly beneficial to know which agent maximizes benefit to the mother while minimizing risk to her fetus. Finally, an appendix containing data on the effects of 30 industrial chemicals on obstetric patients has been added, as well as an appendix on immunization.

The authors have been responsible for the updating of all the material that appeared in the first edition and have written the new drug entries. Dr. Berkowitz was greatly assisted in this task by Dr. Gaetano Bello, Dr. Isabelle Wilkins, and Dr. Lauren Lynch, all of the Mount Sinai Medical Center. Dr. Coustan and Dr. Mochizuki worked alone. The extremely complex appendix on industrial chemicals was written by Dr. Gertrud S. Berkowitz and Dr. Jane E. Gordon.

The reader is encouraged to read the Preface to the First Edition because it describes the layout of each entry, the types of recommendations made, and the organization of the indexes. All of this remains relevant for the second edition. The only portion of the original preface that no longer applies is the last paragraph. All of the authors were at the Yale University School of Medicine when the first edition was published. Dr. Berkowitz and Dr. Coustan have since moved to New York City and Providence, Rhode Island, respectively, where they still function as practicing perinatologists. Dr. Mochizuki has moved to San Francisco and has obtained a law degree. She currently works at the interface of our legal system and the pharmaceutical industry. As in the first edition, however, each entry in this book has been reviewed by all three authors.

We sincerely hope that the second edition of *Handbook for Prescribing Medications During Pregnancy* proves to be of practical benefit to our readers and their patients. It must be noted, however, that the caveats in the Preface to the First Edition still apply. Our recommendations are based on currently available information, and they may require revision as more is learned. Furthermore, some published data may have escaped our attention despite our best efforts to be comprehensive. Many readers have contacted us with suggestions, questions, and comments regarding the first edition. We request that this continue and stress that if anyone is aware of relevant data that have been overlooked, he or she should not hesitate to contact us so that appropriate additions can be made in future editions.

Finally, the authors thank the contributors mentioned above as well as the outstanding staff at Little, Brown and Company for helping to make this book possible. It truly could not have been done without them.

R.L.B.
D.R.C.
T.K.M.

Preface to the First Edition

This book was inspired by the frequent phone calls received by each of the editors regarding the administering of drugs to pregnant women. Its purpose is to provide clinicians with an up-to-date desktop reference on the use of drugs during pregnancy. The publication of new data in multiple journals makes it very difficult to stay abreast of current work in this dynamic field. Furthermore, no major reference work has been devoted specifically to this subject. Since the pharmacological actions of drugs administered during pregnancy may have effects that reach far beyond the therapeutic intent for which they were prescribed, few areas of information have more practical importance.

Because of the bewildering variety of pharmacological preparations currently available in the United States, we have made no attempt to be comprehensive. Instead we have tried to select widely available and frequently prescribed preparations as well as those specifically indicated for uncommon conditions that can affect obstetrical patients. We have also included discussions of some drugs that are not indicated during pregnancy because they might be inadvertently taken before conception has been confirmed.

This book is not intended to rival standard pharmacological textbooks in terms of detailed descriptions of mechanisms of action, metabolic degradation pathways, stoichiometric parameters, and the like. It is a synopsis of the most current relevant information about the effects of individual drugs on the pregnant woman. In addition, we have attempted to present data concerning both the mutagenic and teratogenic potential of each agent on the developing fetus. Each entry begins with the indications for use of that particular drug and the author's specific recommendations. If the drug is absolutely contraindicated during pregnancy, or relatively contraindicated because other therapeutic agents are preferable, this is stated and explained. Drugs that do not fall into these categories are divided into those that are (1) safe for use during pregnancy, (2) indicated only for specific conditions, or (3) the subject of ongoing controversy. In any of these cases a further discussion ensues. A section on special considerations during pregnancy discusses effects that are specifically related to the pregnancy. These include sequelae to both mother and fetus as well as the impact on breastfeeding infants. Appropriate dosages are then presented, followed by a listing of potential general adverse effects. The drug's pharmacological properties are next described in terms of major mechanisms of action, and its absorption and biotransformation are summarized. Finally, each entry concludes with a few relevant recommended readings.

The problems of studying the effects on the fetus of drugs administered to the mother are formidable. In many cases this information is simply not known. Many pharmacological agents have been released by the FDA without specific approval for use during pregnancy. The *Physicians' Desk Reference* frequently offers the familiar caveat: "The safety of _____ in human pregnancy has not been established. The use of the drug in pregnancy requires that the expected therapeutic benefit be weighed against possible hazard to mother and infant." This is not terribly helpful. Obviously, pharmacological agents should not be given during the first trimester, when embryogenesis is occurring, unless absolutely necessary. Another important principle, however, is that medically indicated drug therapy should not be withheld from pregnant women. We have offered specific recommendations about the advisability of utilizing particular drugs with the understanding that they never should be administered frivolously during pregnancy. Our suggestions are based on currently available information, and they may need revision as more is learned. Furthermore, despite our efforts to be thorough, it is certainly possible that some published reports may have escaped our attention. We plan to continue to maintain an active surveillance of the literature and hope to update the material with subsequent editions. If a reader is aware of any data that have been overlooked, he or she should not hesitate to contact the editors so that appropriate additions can be made in the future.

Our approach has been to consider each drug individually. We have not tried to write a manual of therapeutics. Consequently, this book is not particularly intended for the reader who is attempting to formulate a treatment plan for a specific complex problem, such as asthma or hypertension. If, however, the reader is interested in knowing whether a particular drug, such as ephedrine, should be prescribed for the pregnant asthmatic, this can quickly be determined. If a drug is not recommended because another one is considered preferable, the preferred alternative is cited.

The entries are arranged alphabetically by generic name. Some of the more common brand names are also presented with each drug. A general index includes both generic and trade names, while a classification index subdivides the drugs into functional groups by generic name only. Groups of related drugs, such as the penicillins, are sometimes presented in a single entry. The individual constituents of these families, however, are listed separately in the general index and are also considered independently within the entry when this is warranted. Over-the-counter (OTC) preparations are listed according to their major generic ingredients. Tobacco, alcohol (ethyl), and marijuana are separate entries. Vitamin and mineral requirements during pregnancy are discussed in the Appendix.

The individual entries were prepared by house staff and faculty members in the Department of Obstetrics and Gynecology of the Yale University School of Medicine and staff members of the Department of Pharmacy Services of the Yale-New Haven Medical Center. (The author's initials can be found in parentheses following each entry.) All entries were reviewed by the three editors, two of whom are practicing perinatologists, while the third is a clinical pharmacist. Some recommendations concerning drug preference, dosage schedules, and routes of administration reflect approaches that are utilized on the obstetric service of the Yale-New Haven Medical Center, in preference to other acceptable alternatives. Whenever this is the case, it has been so stated in the text.

R.L.B.
D.R.C.
T.K.M.

Handbook for Prescribing Medications During Pregnancy

Acarbose (Precose®)

INDICATIONS AND RECOMMENDATIONS

Acarbose is relatively contraindicated during pregnancy because other therapeutic agents, in particular insulin, are preferable. Acarbose is an α-glucosidase inhibitor that is used to treat type 2 diabetes by reducing the intestinal absorption of starches, dextrin, and disaccharides. By delaying absorption of these carbohydrates, postprandial glycemia is diminished. No information was available in the literature regarding the use of acarbose during pregnancy. Acarbose is not well absorbed from the gastrointestinal tract. Side effects include primarily gastrointestinal symptoms such as flatulence, abdominal pain, and diarrhea, presumably due to the delayed carbohydrate absorption. Elevated liver enzymes were found in approximately 15% of treated patients taking acarbose for up to 12 months. These transaminase elevations were dose-related and were reversible. Because of the lack of data regarding acarbose use in pregnancy, insulin is still considered the treatment of choice for diabetes during pregnancy.

RECOMMENDED READING

Bayer Corporation. Precose. Entry in *Physicians Desk Reference* (52nd ed.). Montvale, NJ: Medical Economics, 1998. Pp. 628–631.

Davis, S.N., and Granner, D.K. Insulin, oral hypoglycemic agents, and the pharmacology of the endocrine pancreas. Chapter 60 in *Goodman and Gilman's The Pharmacological Basis of Therapeutics* (9th ed.), J.G. Hardman and L.E. Limbird, eds. New York: McGraw-Hill, 1996. Pp. 1510–1511.

Angiotensin-Converting Enzyme (ACE) Inhibitors: Benazepril (Lotensin®), Captopril (Capoten®), Enalapril (Vasotec®), Fosinopril (Monopril®), Lisinopril (Prinivil®), Quinapril (Accupril®), Ramipril (Altace®)

INDICATIONS AND RECOMMENDATIONS

The ACE inhibitors are contraindicated during pregnancy. These are orally active inhibitors of angiotensin-converting enzyme, the enzyme responsible for conversion of inactive angiotensin I to the potent pressor peptide angiotensin II. All of these agents have similar mechanisms of action, indications, adverse effect profiles, and contraindications. They differ primarily in chemical formula, potency, and pharmacokinetics. In nonpregnant patients, these drugs are primarily used for the treatment of severe or resistant hypertension.

Administration of ACE inhibitors during the second and third trimesters can cause oligohydramnios, fetal calvaria hypoplasia, fetal pulmonary hypoplasia, fetal growth retardation, fetal death, neonatal anuria, and neonatal death. These effects may be due in part to fetal hypotension. Therefore, once pregnancy is diagnosed it is imperative that ACE inhibitor therapy be discontinued as soon as possible.

While data have shown definite fetotoxic effects of ACE inhibitors administered during the second and third trimesters, reported cases describing bony malformations, limb contractures, facial abnormalities, and lung hypoplasia have been associated with ACE inhibitor exposure throughout pregnancy. Therefore, complete safety of exposure to ACE inhibitors during the first trimester cannot be assured.

Several of these agents, including captopril, enalapril, and lisinopril, are known to cross the placenta and inhibit ACE activity in the human fetus. No data are available for the other agents. Small amounts of captopril are excreted in the breast milk of lactating mothers.

Since better-studied antihypertensive agents are effective in controlling maternal blood pressure in the overwhelming majority of cases, ACE inhibitor therapy cannot be recommended for use during pregnancy.

RECOMMENDED READING

Barr, M., Jr. Teratogen update: angiotensin-converting enzyme inhibitors. *Teratology* 60:399, 1994.

Bhatt-Mehta, V., and Deluga, K.S. Fetal exposure to lisinopril: neonatal manifestations and management. *Pharmacotherapy* 13:515, 1993.

Boutroy, M.J., et al. Captopril administration in pregnancy impairs fetal angiotensin converting enzyme activity and neonatal adaptation. *Lancet* 2:935, 1984.

Devlin, R.G., and Fleiss, P.M. Selective resistance to the passage of captopril into human milk. *Clin. Pharmacol. Ther.* 27:250, 1980.

Fiocchi, R., et al. Captopril during pregnancy. *Lancet* 2:1153, 1984.

Martin, R.A., et al. Effect of ACE inhibition on the fetal kidney: decreased renal blood flow. *Teratology* 46:317, 1992.

Oates, J.A. Antihypertensive agents and the drug therapy of hypertension. Chapter 33 in *Goodman and Gilman's The Pharmacological Basis of Therapeutics* (9th ed.), J.G. Hardman and L.E. Limbird, eds. New York: McGraw-Hill, 1996. Pp. 743–751.

Piper, J.M., Ray, W.A., and Rosa, F.W. Pregnancy outcome following exposure to angiotensin-converting enzyme inhibitors. *Obstet. Gynecol.* 80:429, 1992.

Pryde, P.G., et al. Angiotensin-converting enzyme inhibitor fetopathy. *J. Am. Soc. Nephrol.* 3:1575, 1993.

Shotan, A., et al. Risks of angiotensin-converting enzyme inhibition during pregnancy: experimental and clinical evidence, potential mechanisms, and recommendations for use. *Am. J. Med.* 96:451, 1994.

Thorpe-Beeston, J.G., et al. Pregnancy and ACE inhibitors. *Br. J. Obstet. Gynaecol.* 100:692, 1993.

Acetaminophen (Tempra®, Tylenol®, and in many combinations)

INDICATIONS AND RECOMMENDATIONS

Acetaminophen is safe to use during pregnancy in therapeutic dosages. Maternal overusage may cause significant sequelae, including hepatic necrosis. Although this compound does cross the placenta, available evidence suggests that congenital malformations are not associated with maternal use. The use of large dosages by a pregnant woman, however, has been anecdotally reported to result in fetal renal changes similar to those seen in adults. Because of concern about the fetal effects of therapeutic doses of aspirin, acetaminophen is the analgesic and antipyretic of choice during pregnancy. Acetaminophen is deemed compatible with breast-feeding according to the American Academy of Pediatrics.

SPECIAL CONSIDERATIONS IN PREGNANCY

There are no unique maternal problems when acetaminophen is taken in recommended dosages during pregnancy. Although it crosses the placenta, no teratogenic effects on the fetus have been reported. Fetal hemolytic anemia and methemoglobinemia are theoretical possibilities but are unlikely because a single 2-g dose converts less than 3% of the total circulating hemoglobin to methemoglobin, a level of methemoglobin of little clinical significance. Renal abnormalities were noted in a newborn whose mother ingested 1.3 g acetaminophen daily throughout the pregnancy. In a case-control series of 76 cases of gastroschisis and 2142 controls, mothers of infants with gastroschisis demonstrated a relative risk of 1.7 (CI 1.0–2.9) for recalling having taken acetaminophen during the first trimester. Relative risks for a number of other drugs, including pseudoephedrine and salicylates, were also significant. Clearly, no causal relationship has been established and the authors considered the associations to be tentative, postulating that an underlying maternal illness rather than the medications may have been responsible.

In a case series of 60 pregnancies in which acetaminophen overdose occurred, among the 24 cases in which toxic levels of acetaminophen were documented, there was a significant correlation between the time elapsed prior to administering the loading dose of N-acetylcysteine (the antidote) and the likelihood of spontaneous abortion or stillbirth. The authors recommend early treatment with N-acetylcysteine when toxic levels of acetaminophen are suspected in a pregnant woman.

DOSAGE

The usual dose of acetaminophen is 325–650 mg every 4 hours, with a maximum dosage of 4 g/day. The drug is available in tablets and suppositories (120, 325, and 650 mg) and in elixir and syrup (120 mg/5 ml).

ADVERSE EFFECTS

A variety of central nervous system (CNS) symptoms have been attributed to acetaminophen, including relaxation and drowsiness as well as stimulation and euphoria. Patients occasionally complain of lightheadedness, dizziness, and a sense of unreality and detachment. An erythematous or urticarial skin rash associated with a drug fever can occur. Idiosyncratic responses include neutropenia, leukopenia, pancytopenia, and thrombocytopenia. Methemoglobinemia and hemolytic anemia may occur as acute toxic reactions, but they are usually seen in association with chronic overdosage. Hepatic necrosis may occur with overdosage. Nephrotoxicity secondary to papillary necrosis and chronic interstitial nephritis have been described in chronic abusers. Excessive ingestion can also cause hypoglycemic coma and myocardial damage.

MECHANISM OF ACTION

Acetaminophen is an active metabolite of phenacetin. Both the antipyretic and analgesic actions of acetaminophen seem to be due to a direct hypothalamic effect. The effect of endogenous pyrogens on CNS heat regulatory centers is inhibited, which results in peripheral vasodilatation with subsequent loss of body heat. The analgesic actions are less well understood. In one randomized, double-blind crossover study of third-trimester gravidas, a single dose of 1000 mg of acetaminophen resulted in a significant diminution of urinary excretion of prostacyclin metabolites, but not thromboxane metabolites, compared to placebo. The same investigators found that acetaminophen reduced the production of prostacyclin, but not thromboxane, in vitro in human umbilical cord endothelial cells. These effects are opposite to those observed with low-dose aspirin administration and in theory might adversely impact on hypertensive disorders of pregnancy. Acetaminophen is a relatively weak antiinflammatory drug.

ABSORPTION AND BIOTRANSFORMATION

Acetaminophen is rapidly absorbed from the gastrointestinal tract and reaches peak plasma concentrations in 0.5–1.0 hour. It becomes evenly distributed among all body fluids. The plasma half-life is 1–3 hours, but may exceed 12 hours in an overdose. Approximately 3% is excreted unchanged in the urine whereas 80% is metabolized in the liver to inactive conjugates and to a hepatotoxic intermediate metabolite. The intermediate is detoxified by glutathione, and all metabolites are excreted by the kidneys. Absorption and disposition of acetaminophen do not appear to be changed by pregnancy.

RECOMMENDED READING

Collins, E. Maternal and fetal effects of acetaminophen and salicylates in pregnancy. *Obstet. Gynecol.* 58:57S, 1981.

Committee on Drugs of the American Academy of Pediatrics. The transfer of drugs and other chemicals into human milk. *Pediatrics* 93:137, 1994.

Insel, P.A. Analgesic-antipyretic and antiinflammatory agents and drugs employed in the treatment of gout. Chapter 27 in *Goodman* and Gilman's The Pharmacological Basis of Therapeutics (9th ed.), J.G. Hardman and L.E. Limbird, eds. New York: McGraw-Hill, 1996. Pp. 631–633.

Janes J., and Routledge, P.A. Recent developments in the management of paracetamol (acetaminophen) poisoning. Drug Safety 7:170–177, 1992.

Nelson, M.M., and Forfar, J.O. Associations between drugs administered during pregnancy and congenital abnormalities of the fetus. Br. Med. J. 1:523, 1971.

Niederhoff, H., and Zahradnik, H. Analgesics during pregnancy. Am. J. Med. 75:117, 1983.

O'Brien, W.F., Krammer, J., O'Leary, T.D., and Mastrogiannis, D.S. The effect of acetaminophen on prostacyclin production in pregnant women. Am. J. Obstet. Gynecol. 168:1164, 1993.

Rayburn, W., Shukla, U., Stetson, P., and Piehl, E. Acetaminophen pharmacokinetics: comparison between pregnant and nonpregnant women. Am. J. Obstet. Gynecol. 155:1353, 1986.

Riggs, B.S., Bronstein, A.C., Kulig, K., et al. Acute acetaminophen overdose during pregnancy. Obstet. Gynecol. 74:247, 1989.

Werler, M.M.J., Mitchell, A.A., and Shapiro, S. First trimester maternal medication use in relation to gastroschisis. Teratology 45:361, 1992.

Acetazolamide (Diamox®)

INDICATIONS AND RECOMMENDATIONS

The use of acetazolamide during pregnancy should be limited to adjunctive therapy for increased intraocular pressure as in open angle glaucoma and the treatment of increased intracranial pressure caused by pseudotumor cerebri. It may also be used in the prophylactic management of petit mal epilepsy in women whose seizures increase at the time of menstruation. Although animal data implicate the drug as a teratogen, no human data support this. Periodic monitoring of electrolyte balance is recommended when this drug is given during pregnancy.

SPECIAL CONSIDERATIONS IN PREGNANCY

Acetazolamide has been shown to cause forelimb malformations in some offspring of pregnant rats receiving doses of 200 mg/kg. This is greater than 10 times the usual adult human dosage. Ectrodactyly has also been seen in the offspring of golden hamsters and mice exposed to this drug in utero. Furthermore, prenatal exposure of the mouse to high doses of acetazolamide has caused posteriad extension of portions of one or both frontal bones. To date, retrospective data have not shown any significant incidence of malformations in infants whose mothers have received therapeutic doses of acetazolamide during pregnancy. There is, however, an isolated report of sacrococcygeal teratoma in a 27-week-old stillborn whose mother was treated with acetazolamide up to the nineteenth week of gestation. It is not known as to whether acetazolamide enters human breast milk.

Acetazolamide is also used in the prophylaxis and treatment of high-altitude sickness, a constellation of symptoms caused by rapid ascent to altitudes above 8000 feet. Because the cause of high-altitude sickness appears to be hypoxia, it would be preferable for pregnant women to avoid such rapid ascent.

The American Academy of Pediatrics Committee on Drugs found that the use of acetazolamide is usually compatible with breast-feeding.

DOSAGE

The recommended adult dose of acetazolamide for adjunctive treatment of open angle glaucoma is 250 mg taken orally qd-qid or a 500-mg sustained release capsule taken bid. For rapid lowering of intraocular pressure, 500 mg may be given parenterally. As an adjunct in the prophylactic management of epilepsy, the suggested dose is 8–30 mg/kg/day in divided doses in addition to other anticonvulsants.

ADVERSE EFFECTS

Serious side effects are rare. Most adverse reactions are dose-dependent and usually diminish in response to a decrease in the amount being administered or to withdrawal of the drug. Patients may experience drowsiness, temporary myopia, skin rashes, anorexia, and nausea. The most common side effects are changes in fluid and electrolyte balance, especially metabolic acidosis and hypokalemia. More serious, but rarer, adverse reactions include sulfonamide hypersensitivity reactions, bone marrow depression, and renal toxicity. Individuals allergic to sulfonamides may be allergic to acetazolamide.

MECHANISM OF ACTION

Acetazolamide is a sulfonamide that acts by a noncompetitive inhibition of carbonic anhydrase to reduce the formation of hydrogen ion and bicarbonate ion from carbon dioxide and water. This inhibition results in decreased production of aqueous humor, increased renal excretion of bicarbonate ion with alkalinization of the urine, and increased excretion of sodium and potassium with resultant diuresis. Plasma bicarbonate is decreased and plasma chloride increased.

The anticonvulsant activity of acetazolamide is thought to be due to the induced metabolic acidosis. Another postulated mechanism is a direct action on the brain by increased carbon dioxide tension, which has been shown to retard neuronal conduction. In addition, cerebrospinal fluid formation may be decreased.

ABSORPTION AND BIOTRANSFORMATION

Acetazolamide is readily absorbed from the gastrointestinal tract with peak plasma concentrations occurring within 2 hours. Onset of action after an oral dose is approximately 1 hour later, whereas its duration is 8–12 hours. A time release preparation is available, the duration of which is 18–24 hours. When given intravenously, onset of action occurs within 2 minutes, peak effect occurs at 15 minutes, and duration is 4–5 hours. Its major route of elimination is via the kidney, where it undergoes active tubular secretion.

RECOMMENDED READING

Beck, S.L. Another special effect of prenatal acetazolamide exposure in the mouse. *Teratology* 27:51, 1983.

Beck, S.L. Assessment of adult skeletons to detect prenatal exposure to acetazolamide in mice. *Teratology* 28:45, 1983.

Committee on Drugs of the American Academy of Pediatrics. The transfer of drugs and other chemicals into human milk. *Pediatrics* 93:137, 1994.

Heinonen, O.P., Slone, D., and Shapiro, S. *Birth Defects and Drugs in Pregnancy.* Littleton, MA: Wright-PSG, 1977. Pp. 372, 441, 495.

Jackson, E.K. Diuretics. Chapter 29 in *Goodman and Gilman's The Pharmacological Basis of Therapeutics* (9th ed.), J.G. Hardman and L.E. Limbird, eds. New York: McGraw-Hill, 1996. Pp. 691–695.

Layton, W., and Hallesy, D.W. Deformity of forelimb in rats: Association with high doses of acetazolamide. *Science* 149:306, 1965.

Nakatsuka, T., Komatsu, T., and Fujii, T. Axial skeletal malformations induced by acetazolamide in rabbits. *Teratology* 45:629, 1992.

Tsao, E. High-altitude sickness. *Emerg. Med. Clin. North Am.* 10:23, 1992.

Worsham, F., Jr., Beckman, E.N., and Mitchell, E.H. Sacrococcygeal teratoma in a neonate. Association with maternal use of acetazolamide. *J.A.M.A.* 240:251, 1978.

Acetylcysteine (Mucomyst®)

INDICATIONS AND RECOMMENDATIONS

Acetylcysteine may be administered to pregnant women for the treatment of acetaminophen poisoning. Acetylcysteine is a mucolytic agent that is used in nonpregnant individuals to decrease the viscosity of mucous secretion in chronic bronchopulmonary disease. Following acetaminophen overdose, it can reduce the extent of liver injury.

SPECIAL CONSIDERATIONS IN PREGNANCY

There is no information regarding the use of acetylcysteine as a mucolytic in pregnant women. In the treatment of acetaminophen toxicity there appears to be a statistically significant correlation between the time to loading dose of acetylcysteine and pregnancy outcome, with an increase in the incidence of spontaneous abortion or fetal death when treatment is begun more than 10 hours after acetaminophen ingestion. Acetaminophen crosses the placenta and appears to achieve therapeutic blood levels in the fetus. There is no evidence that acetylcysteine administration is teratogenic.

DOSAGE

In acetaminophen overdose, acetylcysteine must be administered immediately if less than 24 hours has elapsed from the time of ingestion. A loading dose of 140 mg/kg should be given orally after lavage or emesis, and without the presence of activated charcoal. The maintenance dose of 70 mg/kg is given 4 hours later and at 4-hour intervals for a total of 17 doses unless the acetaminophen assay reveals a nontoxic level.

ADVERSE EFFECTS

Large doses of oral acetylcysteine may result in nausea and vomiting. Rash, mild fever, pruritis, angioedema, bronchospasms, tachycardia, hypotension, and hypertension have occurred.

MECHANISM OF ACTION

In the treatment of acetaminophen overdose, acetylcysteine may protect the liver by maintaining or restoring glutathione levels, or by acting as an alternate substrate for conjugation of the reactive metabolite of acetaminophen.

ABSORPTION AND BIOTRANSFORMATION

Following an oral dose, peak plasma concentrations are achieved within 1–2 hours. Protein binding is approximately 50%. The half-life of reduced acetylcysteine is 6.25 hours. The primary method of elimination is nonrenal.

RECOMMENDED READING

Horowitz, R.S., et al. Placental transfer of *N*-acetylcysteine following human maternal acetaminophen toxicity. *J. Toxicol.* 35:447–451, 1997.

Insel, P.A. Analgesic-antipyretic and antiinflammatory agents and drugs employed in the treatment of gout. Chapter 27 in *Goodman and Gilman's The Pharmacological Basis of Therapeutics* (9th ed.), J.G. Hardman and L.E. Limbird, eds. New York: McGraw-Hill, 1996. Pp. 632–633.

Janes, J., and Routledge, P.A. Recent developments in the management of paracetamol (acetaminophen) poisoning. *Drug Safety* 7: 170–177, 1992.

Riggs, B.S., et al. Acute acetaminophen overdose during pregnancy. *Obstet. Gynecol.* 74:247–253, 1989.

Acyclovir (Zovirax®)

INDICATIONS AND RECOMMENDATIONS

Acyclovir may be administered to pregnant women for the treatment of disseminated herpes simplex virus (HSV) or varicella pneumonia. Its use for the treatment of genital herpes recurrences during pregnancy in an attempt to decrease the need for cesarean section appears promising; however, more studies are required before its use in this situation can be recommended.

SPECIAL CONSIDERATIONS IN PREGNANCY

Animal studies indicate that acyclovir is not a significant teratogen. Acyclovir crosses the placenta, and at term maternal-to-cord plasma ratios range from 1.07 to 1.90. Amniotic fluid levels of acyclovir are 2–8 times those in maternal plasma; placental levels are 1.5–4 times those of maternal plasma; and newborn plasma levels are similar to maternal plasma levels.

Acyclovir appears to be well tolerated in pregnancy and its use has not been associated with fetal malformation. An Acyclovir in Pregnancy Registry has been established by a manufacturer to gather data regarding its use in this circumstance. No significant risk to mother or fetus has been reported, but the number of patients treated is still too small to support any unequivocal conclusions.

Acyclovir has been used in pregnant women with life-threatening disease secondary to disseminated HSV. These infections usually have a high mortality rate for both infant and mother. It is generally accepted that acyclovir therapy in this setting is warranted.

Varicella pneumonia during the first trimester is associated with the fetal varicella syndrome, which includes limb atrophy, skin scarring, cataracts, and CNS involvement. A child who survives will usually have significant neurologic impairment. Chicken pox during the second and third trimesters is associated with an increased incidence of varicella pneumonitis with a maternal mortality rate of up to 40%. Although it is best to prevent chicken pox in the mother by vaccination, preventing exposure, or administering zoster immune globulin, should varicella pneumonitis occur during pregnancy acyclovir can attenuate the life-threatening maternal infection and perhaps decrease the incidence of congenital varicella. In one retrospective review of 21 cases of varicella pneumonitis of pregnancy during the second or third trimester, only three of the treated women (14%) died of uncontrolled infections or complications. Two infants died, one was stillborn at 34 weeks, and one succumbed to complications of prematurity at 26 weeks. No infants were born with features of congenital varicella.

Acyclovir is currently being studied to see if its use will decrease the need for cesarean sections in women with recurrent genital HSV. In one study of 300 women with culture-positive HSV, those on a regimen of 400 mg PO tid begun at 38 weeks gestation had no cesarean sections compared to the placebo group, which had a 26% incidence. No treated infant developed neonatal HSV and no toxicities were reported. In a second randomized placebo-controlled prospective study of women whose initial genital herpes diagnosis occurred during pregnancy, no patient treated with acyclovir starting at 36 weeks gestation had a recurrence at delivery, whereas 36% of the patients treated with placebo had recurrences.

Acyclovir is secreted in breast milk. At a maternal dose of 200 mg 5 times daily, the breast milk concentration was 3.24 times higher than the maternal serum level. The investigators estimated the exposure of the nursing child to be less than 1 mg/day, presenting a low theoretical risk if the infant has normal renal function.

DOSAGE

The intravenous dosage for acyclovir is 5–10 mg/kg infused at a constant rate over 1 hour every 8 hours for 7 days. Oral therapy for an initial case of genital herpes is 200 mg every 4 hours, 5 times daily for 10 days. For chronic suppressive therapy, the dose is 400 mg bid for up to 12 months. Doses must be decreased if renal function is impaired.

ADVERSE REACTIONS

Acyclovir is generally well tolerated. With oral use, it is known to cause nausea, diarrhea, rash, and, rarely, renal insufficiency and neurotoxicity. With intravenous use, acyclovir is known to cause renal insufficiency and neurotoxicity. High-dose bolus injection can cause crystallization of the drug in the renal tubules with a reversible increase in serum creatinine or, rarely, acute tubular necrosis.

MECHANISM OF ACTION

Acyclovir is a synthetic purine nucleoside, which is taken up by and activated within the viral cell to form the active agent acyclovir triphosphate (acyclovir TP). Acyclovir TP competitively inhibits viral DNA polymerases and is incorporated into viral DNA where it acts as chain terminator. Acyclovir is much less toxic to normal, uninfected cells because it is preferentially taken up and converted to the active form by HSV-infected cells.

ABSORPTION AND BIOTRANSFORMATION

Ten percent to 30% of an orally administered dose is bioavailable. Acyclovir distributes widely into body fluids and is concentrated in breast milk, amniotic fluids, and the placenta. Its half-life is 1.5–6 hours. Renal excretion is the primary route of elimination with 85% being excreted unchanged in the urine. Fifteen percent is excreted as metabolites.

RECOMMENDED READING

Andrews, E.B., et al. Acyclovir in pregnancy registry: six years experience. The Acyclovir in Pregnancy Registry Advisory Committee. *Obstet. Gynecol.* 79:7, 1992.

Broussard, R.C., Payne, D.K., and George, R.B. Treatment with acyclovir of varicella pneumonia in pregnancy. *Chest* 99:1045, 1991.

Hayen, F.G. Antimicrobial agents: antiviral agents. Chapter 50 in *Goodman and Gilman's The Pharmacological Basis of Therapeutics* (9th ed.), J.G. Hardman and L.E. Limbird, eds. New York: McGraw-Hill, 1996. Pp 1193–1204.

Henderson, G.I., et al. Acyclovir transport by the human placenta. *J. Lab. Clin. Med.* 120:885, 1992.

Myer, L.J., et al. Acyclovir in human breast milk. *Am. J. Obstet. Gynecol.* 158:586, 1988.

Pregnancy outcomes following systemic prenatal acyclovir exposure June 1, 1984–June 30, 1993. *M.M.W.R.* 42:806, 1993.

Scott, L.L., et al. Acyclovir suppression to prevent cesarean delivery after first-episode-genital herpes. *Obstet. Gynecol.* 87:69, 1996.

Scott, L.L. Perinatal herpes: current status and obstetric management strategies. *Pediatr. Infect. Dis. J.* 14:827, 1995.

Smego, Jr., R.A., and Asperilla, M.O. Use of acyclovir for varicella pneumonia during pregnancy. *Obstet. Gynecol.* 78:1112, 1991.

Wagstaff, A.J., Faulds, D., and Goa, K.L. Aciclovir. A reappraisal of its antiviral activity, pharmacokinetic properties and therapeutic efficacy. *Drugs* 47:153, 1994.

Watts, D.H. Antiviral agents. *Obstet. Gynecol. Clin. North Am.* 19: 563, 1992.

Albumin (Albuminar®, Albutein®, Buminate®)

INDICATIONS AND RECOMMENDATIONS

The use of albumin during pregnancy should be limited to the treatment of acute oliguria secondary to hypovolemia. It can also be used as a temporary plasma expander during hypovolemic states secondary to hemorrhage if blood is not immediately available. Central venous pressure should be carefully monitored when albumin is administered during pregnancy.

SPECIAL CONSIDERATIONS IN PREGNANCY

Albumin does not cross the placenta. Pregnancy is generally accompanied by an increase in maternal intravascular volume; in severe pregnancy-induced hypertension, however, hypovolemia often occurs. In this situation, albumin may occasionally be used to increase oncotic pressure and improve renal perfusion. If albumin is given, central pressures should be monitored to document hypovolemia and to prevent the development of heart failure due to secondary intravascular overload.

DOSAGE

Albumin is supplied in 5% and 25% solutions, with 50 ml of the 25% solution containing 12.5 g albumin and 100 ml containing 25 g. The onset of action is immediate because it is given intravenously. The albumen is harvested from pooled human venous plasma by the Cohn method of fractionation and is heated for 10 hours at 60°C in order to inactivate infectious agents such as the hepatitis virus.

ADVERSE EFFECTS

Albumin is inert. The major side effect is intravascular overload, especially in the patient with compromised cardiovascular status; congestive heart failure may occur in this setting.

MECHANISM OF ACTION

The intravenous administration of albumin raises the oncotic pressure of the intravascular space. Extracellular fluid is thus drawn into the intravascular compartment. Hypotension is improved, and renal perfusion is increased, with a resultant increase in urinary output.

RECOMMENDED READING

Berkowitz, R.L., ed. The management of hypertensive crises during pregnancy. In *Critical Care of the Obstetric Patient.* New York: Churchill Livingstone, 1983. P. 299.

Gifford, R.W., Jr. A guide to the practical use of diuretics. *J.A.M.A.* 235:1890, 1976.

Alcohol, Ethyl (Ethanol)

INDICATIONS AND RECOMMENDATIONS

The chronic use of ethanol in large doses [more than 2.2 g absolute alcohol (AA) per kilogram of body weight per day] has been associated with a constellation of fetal anomalies, known as the fetal alcohol syndrome (FAS). Therefore, chronic ingestion of greater than 2.2 g/kg AA per day throughout pregnancy is absolutely contraindicated. Not enough data are available, however, to determine whether an occasional social drink (less than 1 ounce AA per day) is harmful to the fetus; and no recommendation can be made regarding social drinking during pregnancy. Although ethanol has been used for the treatment of premature labor, a β-mimetic agent or $MgSO_4$ is preferred in this situation.

SPECIAL CONSIDERATIONS IN PREGNANCY

Chronic ethanol ingestion during pregnancy has been associated with FAS. According to criteria developed by the Fetal Alcohol Study Group of the Research Society on Alcoholism in 1980, FAS is diagnosed when there are abnormalities in each of the following three categories: (1) prenatal or postnatal growth retardation; (2) central nervous system (CNS) (neurologic abnormality, developmental delay, or intellectual impairment); and (3) characteristic facial dysmorphology with at least two of the following three signs: (a) microcephaly, (b) microphthalmia or short palpebral fissures, and (c) poorly developed philtrum, thin upper lip, or flattening of the maxillary area.

It is not clear as to whether alcohol itself, its metabolite acetaldehyde, or both together produce the abnormalities. Both substances cross the placenta, and in animal studies both affect somites, deforming the brain and spinal cord and producing severe growth retardation. Furthermore, the quantity and regularity of alcohol consumption around the time of conception and during various stages of pregnancy have different effects. Studies indicate that heavy regular drinking during the first trimester has the greatest effect on fetal maldevelopment, whereas excessive alcohol consumption later in pregnancy may have greater impact on fetal nutrition and size as well as later neurobehavioral deficits. However, data are difficult to interpret due to inconsistent exposures with differing amounts, trimesters, simultaneous risk factors, and chronicities. In addition, genetic factors may account for differences in fetal susceptibility to alcohol exposure.

Studies have shown that chronic alcohol ingestion of greater than 2.2 g/kg/day AA increases the incidence of abnormalities associated with FAS. For the average pregnant woman, this quantity is approximately equivalent to 4.5 ounces of pure alcohol, 9 ounces of 100 proof liquor, nine 4-ounce portions of 12% table wine, or nine 12-ounce containers of beer per day. Estimates of the incidence of FAS among offspring of alcoholic mothers range from a high of 40% (in a series of case reports) to as low as 2.5% to 10.0% in the few prospective series available. In addition to those children with full-blown FAS, there are evidently a large number who have "fetal alcohol effects" but who do not satisfy all of the criteria for the syndrome. It is most difficult to estimate the incidence of these problems because many of the manifestations (most notably growth retardation) are not specific to alcohol.

In a large prospective study of 31,604 pregnancies, the consumption of at least one to two drinks daily was associated with a substantially increased risk of producing growth retardation and the reduction in mean birth weight was dose-related. In this study, the consumption of less than one drink daily had no demonstrable effect on birth weight. Thus, although it would be very difficult to establish the daily alcohol consumption below which there is no risk, the existing data do not warrant advising pregnant women that they must drink no alcohol at all or, more particularly, instilling a sense of guilt over past alcohol use.

In a blinded study, the infants of eight mothers who drank a mean of 21 ounces AA per week were compared with the infants of 29 mothers who never drank and of 15 mothers who drank but stopped in the second trimester. Neurobehavioral examinations on the third day of life showed significantly more tremors, hypertonia, restlessness, excessive mouthing movements, inconsolable crying, and reflex abnormalities among the infants of mothers who drank throughout pregnancy compared to those in the two control groups. None of these infants had FAS. The authors conclude that there may be neonatal withdrawal from alcohol among non-FAS infants of those who drink "moderately" throughout pregnancy.

Early reports indicated an increased miscarriage rate among moderate but frequent drinkers; however, later studies show no significant risk of abortion with low-level alcohol consumption during pregnancy.

Ethanol has been used in the treatment of premature labor in the third trimester, although β-mimetic agents or $MgSO_4$ are preferred in this situation.

ADVERSE EFFECTS

Side effects of alcohol consumption include nausea and vomiting (with the potential for aspiration pneumonia), hypoglycemia, CNS depression, and mild hypotension. These effects are seen whether the alcohol is taken orally or intravenously (as in the treatment of premature labor). The complications of excessive consumption include increased blood lactate, hyperlipemia, and fatty liver. The continued use of large amounts of alcohol can lead to alcoholic hepatitis and cirrhosis. There are, however, individual differences in response to alcohol; in particular, not all heavy drinkers develop hepatitis and cirrhosis.

MECHANISM OF ACTION

The CNS is most markedly affected with the social ingestion of alcohol. Ethanol is a primary and continuous depressant of the CNS. The apparent stimulation gained from social drinking results from the unrestrained activity of parts of the brain when inhibitory control mechanisms for those parts are depressed. It is this "stimulation" that gives ethanol-containing products their high potential for abuse. Other physiologic effects include vasodilatation, stimulation of gastric secretions, and diuresis due to inhibition of the antidiuretic hormone.

Ethanol inhibits release of the neurohypophyseal hormones oxytocin and vasopressin from the posterior pituitary gland. Intravenous or oral administration in early premature labor (with intact membranes) will postpone labor in two-thirds of cases. This is somewhat better than results in women in control groups who were given intravenous glucose. It is assumed that the effect of alcohol on labor is due to inhibition of oxytocin release.

ABSORPTION AND BIOTRANSFORMATION

Ethyl alcohol is absorbed from the stomach, small intestine, and colon. Absorption from the small intestine is rapid and complete. In the liver, ethanol is metabolized to acetaldehyde at a rate of 10 ml/hour. Acetaldehyde is then normally oxidized to acetyl coenzyme A, which in turn is metabolized in the citric acid cycle.

RECOMMENDED READING

American College of Obstetricians and Gynecologists (A.C.O.G.). *Alcohol and Your Unborn Baby* (patient information booklet). Washington, DC, 1982.

Hanson, J.W., Jones, K.L., and Smith, D.W. Fetal alcohol syndrome. *J.A.M.A.* 235:1458,1976.

Jacobson, J.L., et al. Teratogenic effects of alcohol on infant development. *Alcoholism Clin. Exp. Res.* 17:174, 1993.

Kline, J., et al. Drinking during pregnancy and spontaneous abortion. *Lancet.* 2:176, 1980.

Laroque, B., et al. Effects of birthweight of alcohol and caffeine consumption during pregnancy. *Am. J. Epidemiol.* 137:941, 1993.

Mills, J.L., et al. Maternal alcohol consumption and birth weight: how much drinking during pregnancy is safe? *J.A.M.A.* 252: 1875, 1984.

Ouellette, E., et al. Adverse effects on offspring of maternal alcohol abuse during pregnancy. *N. Engl. J. Med.* 297:528, 1977.

Rosett, H.L., et al. Patterns of alcohol consumption and fetal development. *Obstet. Gynecol.* 61:539, 1983.

Rosett, H.L., and Weiner, L. *Alcohol and the Fetus.* New York: Oxford University Press, 1984.

Shu, X.O., et al. Maternal smoking, alcohol drinking and caffeine consumption, and fetal growth: results from a prospective study. *Epidemiology.* 6:115, 1995

Sisenwein, F.E., et al. Effects of maternal ethanol administration during pregnancy on the growth and development of children at four to seven years of age. *Am. J. Obstet. Gynecol.* 147:52, 1983.

Sokol, R.J., et al. The Cleveland NIAAA prospective alcohol-in-pregnancy study: the first year. *Neurobehav. Toxicol. Teratol.* 3:203, 1981.

Streissguth, A.P., et al. Drinking during pregnancy decreases word attack and arithmetic scores on standardized tests: adolescent data from a population-based prospective study. *Alcoholism Clin. Exp. Res.* 18:248, 1994.

Zervoudakis, I.A., et al. Infants of mothers treated with ethanol for premature labor. *Am. J. Obstet. Gynecol.* 137:713, 1980.

Allopurinol (Zyloprim®)

INDICATIONS AND RECOMMENDATIONS

The use of allopurinol is relatively contraindicated during pregnancy because other therapeutic agents are preferable (e.g., probenecid). It is used for the treatment of both the primary hyperuricemia of gout and hyperuricemia secondary to hematologic disorders and antineoplastic therapy.

Allopurinol and its metabolite, alloxanthine, inhibit xanthine oxidase, the enzyme that catalyzes the conversion of hypoxanthine to xanthine and xanthine to uric acid. Thus, serum and urine levels of uric acid are decreased whereas levels of the more soluble oxypurine precursors are increased. The decrease in serum urate levels occurs during the first 1–3 weeks of therapy.

Attacks of gout may occur more frequently during the initial months of therapy. Hypersensitivity reactions, predominantly erythematous, pruritic, or maculopapular cutaneous eruptions, may occur. Occasionally these lesions may be exfoliative, urticarial, or purpuric. Fever, malaise, and muscle aches may also become manifest. Transient leukopenia, leukocytosis, and eosinophilia are rare reactions but may require cessation of therapy. Headache, drowsiness, nausea and vomiting, diarrhea, and gastric irritation occur occasionally.

Allopurinol has been associated with induction of facial clefts and minor skeletal abnormalities in mice but is not teratogenic in rats or rabbits. Due to its structural similarity to purines, there is a theoretical possibility that this drug or one of its metabolites may be incorporated into nucleic acids. It has been shown, however, that neither allopurinol nor alloxanthine is incorporated into DNA during any stage of replication and that neither produces any mutagenic effect. Allopurinol's effects on the human fetus are unknown. Treatment with allopurinol can inhibit ovulation induction in rabbits, but this has not been confirmed in humans.

Gout is uncommon in women and is rarely seen before menopause. Elevated serum uric acid is common in toxemia but rarely requires therapy. Probenecid has been safely used and is indicated for treatment of hyperuricemia in pregnancy.

Allopurinol and oxypurinol have been detected in breast milk only in small amounts in one lactating mother. No side effects were seen in the neonate. If allopurinol use is necessary in the puerperium, the American Academy of Pediatrics considers allopurinol use to be acceptable during breast-feeding.

RECOMMENDED READING

Committee on Drugs, American Academy of Pediatrics. The transfer of drugs and other chemicals into human milk. *Pediatrics.* 93:137, 1994

Kamilli, I., and Gresser, U. Allopurinol and oxypurinol in human breast milk. *Clin. Invest.* 71:161, 1993.

Miyazaki, T., Kuo, T.-C., Dharmarajan, A.M., Atlas, S.J., and Wallach, E.E. In vivo administration of allopurinol affects ovulation and early embryonic development in rabbits. *Am. J. Obstet. Gynecol.* 161:1709, 1989.

Stevenson, A.C., Silcock, S.R., and Scott, J.T. Absence of chromosome damage in human lymphocytes exposed to allopurinol and oxipurinol. *Ann. Rheum. Dis.* 35:143, TAG1976.

Alpha$_2$ Adrenergic Agonists: Clonidine (Catapres®), Guanfacine (Tenex®), Guanabenz (Wytensin®)

INDICATIONS AND RECOMMENDATIONS

Experience with use of clonidine and other alpha$_2$ agonists in pregnancy has been limited in comparison to that of the closely related antihypertensive drug, methyldopa. Therefore they are rarely used as the drug of choice for treatment of hypertension in pregnancy. While the use of clonidine for treatment of narcotic withdrawal symptoms has been well described in nonpregnant individuals, use in pregnancy for this indication has not been described and therefore cannot be recommended. Recently, use of epidural clonidine combined with bupivicaine has been reported to enhance the analgesic effect of local anesthetic in laboring patients, however this use of clonidine is currently investigational. Clonidine is an imidazoline derivative with a relatively rapid onset of action, used in the treatment of both chronic hypertension and hypertensive emergency as well as to block withdrawal symptoms from heroin or cocaine. Guanabenz and guanfacine are closely related phenylacetylguanidine derivatives used to treat hypertension.

SPECIAL CONSIDERATIONS IN PREGNANCY

There have been several small series describing clonidine use in pregnancy. In 5 pregnancies chronically exposed to clonidine, follow-up of the neonates revealed significant hypertension between 12 and 24 hours of life, lasting for 24 hours, in 4 cases. There were no apparent sequelae, and at one year of life all 5 had normal development. This experience raises the possibility of rebound hypertension caused by withdrawal of the maternal source of drug. In contrast, in a report of 47 pregnant hypertensive patients receiving clonidine as part of a randomized trial comparing its use to that of methyldopa, rebound hypertension was not seen in the neonates. The difference in the two reports may explained by a difference in the frequency of blood pressure monitoring in the neonates. In the smaller study, blood pressure was measured every 6 hour; in the larger study, blood pressure was measured only twice during the first 24 hours of life.

A case has been reported of a neonate with Roberts syndrome born to a hypertensive mother who was treated with clonidine, 0.3 mg/day, throughout her pregnancy. This syndrome, which includes tetraphocomelia, cleft lip and palate, and dysmorphia, could be due to a disturbance in development before the seventh week of gestation. While the syndrome may be a genetic disorder transmitted in an autosomal recessive pattern, the question of a relationship between this infant's abnormalities and the mother's use of clonidine during the early first trimester should be considered.

Animal studies have demonstrated decreases in fetal breathing, alterations in fetal electrocortical activity and suppression of REM sleep. While the clinical significance of these findings is uncertain, there is one human study suggesting clonidine may be a behavioral teratogen. On long term follow-up of 22 children exposed to clonidine in utero, there was an excess of sleep disturbances such as somnambulism and night terrors noted in comparison to children of hypertensive mothers not treated with medication.

No information could be located describing the pregnancy effects of guanabenz or guanfacine.

DOSAGE

For treatment of chronic hypertension the usual starting dose of clonidine is 0.1 mg orally twice daily, increasing by 0.1 mg daily to a usual maximum dose of 0.6 to 1.2 mg per day as needed. For treatment of hypertensive emergency, the usual initial dose is 0.1 mg orally, repeated hourly as needed. The usual dose of guanfacine is 1 mg daily at bedtime to minimize somnolence.

ADVERSE EFFECTS

Side effects include postural hypotension, fluid and sodium retention, drowsiness, and bowel disturbances. Occasionally a weakly positive Coombs' test will result, and an acute hypertensive crisis may accompany abrupt withdrawal of the drug after prolonged therapy.

MECHANISM OF ACTION

Alpha₂ agonists reduce blood pressure primarily by stimulating alpha-adrenergic receptor sites in the hypothalamus and other vasomotor centers in the central nervous system. They stimulate presynaptic alpha₂-adrenoreceptors, reducing the release of norepinephrine peripherally, leading to a decrease in sympathetic tone. They cause vagal stimulation, leading to slowing of heart rate. If two drug therapy is required, a desirable feature of clonidine is that it will block the reflex tachycardia caused by vasodilator therapy. It also suppresses the release of renal renin, leading to increased fluid retention, which may limit the antihypertensive effect without concomitant diuretic use.

ABSORPTION AND BIOTRANSFORMATION

The onset of action of orally administered clonidine is relatively rapid, with onset in 30 to 60 minutes, and maximum effect at 2 to 4 hours. The half life ranges from 12 to 16 hours. 50% of the drug is metabolized in the liver, the rest excreted unchanged in the urine. Clonidine readily crosses the placenta with concentrations in cord serum equal to maternal blood levels. Clonidine is concentrated in breast milk, with concentrations reaching up to four times that of maternal serum. The other alpha₂ agonists have similar profiles.

RECOMMENDED READING

Bamford, O.S., Hawkins, R.L., Blanco, C.E. Effects of clonidine on breathing movements and electrocortical activity in the fetal lamb. *Am. J. Obstet. Gynecol.* 163:662–668, 1990.

Boutroy, M.J., Gisonna, C.R., Legagneur, M. Clonidine: placental transfer and neonatal adaption. *Early Human Dev.* 17:275, 1988.

Cigari, I., Kaba, A., Bonnet, F., Brohon, E., Dutz, F., Damas, F., Hans, P. Epidural Clonidine combined with Bupivicaine for analgesia in labor. Effects on mother and neonate. *Regional Anesth.* 20(2): 113, 1995.

Frohlich, E.D. The sympathetic depressant anti-hypertensives. *Drug Ther.* 5:24, 1975.

Hartikainen-Sorri, A.L., Heikkinen, J.E., Koivisto, M. Pharmacokinetics of Clonidine during pregnancy and nursing. *Obstet. Gynecol.* 69:598, 1987.

Hoffman, B.B., Lefkowitz, R.J. Catecholamines, sympathomimetic drugs, and adrenergic receptor antagonists. Chapter 10 in *Goodman and Gilman's The Pharmacological Basis of Therapeutics* (9th ed.) J.G. Hardman and L.E. Limbird eds. New York: McGraw-Hill, 1996. Pp. 217–219.

Horvath, J.S., Phippard, A., Korda, A., Henderson-Smart, D.J., Child, A., Tiller, J. Clonidine Hydrochloride- a safe and effective antihypertensive agent in pregnancy. *Obstet. Gynecol.* 66:634, 1985.

Huisjes, H.J., Hadders-Algra, M., Touwen, B.C.L. Is clonidine a behavioural teratogen in the human? *Early Human Dev.* 14:43, 1986.

Johnson, C.I., and Aickin, D.R. The control of high blood pressure during labour with clonidine (Catapres). *Med. J. Aust.* 2:132, 1971.

Kelly, J.V. Drugs used in the management of toxemia of pregnancy. *Clin. Obstet. Gynecol.* 20:395, 1977.

Martin, J.D. A critical survey of drugs used in the treatment of hypertensive crises of pregnancy. *Med. J. Aust.* 2:252, 1974.

Stoll, C., Levy, J.M., and Beshara, D. Robert's syndrome and clonidine. *J. Med. Genet.* 16:486, 1979.

Tuimala, R., Punnonen, R., Kauppil, E. Clonidine in the treatment of hypertension during pregnancy. *Ann. Chirurg. Gynaecol.* 74, Suppl. 197:47, 1985.

Yudkin, J.S. Withdrawal of clonidine. *Lancet.* 1:546, 1977.

Alprostadil (Prostaglandin E_1, Caverject®, Muse®, Prostin VR®)

Alprostadil (prostaglandin E_1) is contraindicated in pregnancy. It is approved for use for the treatment of erectile dysfunction in impotent males and for palliative therapy to temporarily maintain the patency of the ductus arteriosus in neonates who have certain ductus-dependent congenital heart defects. Prostaglandins of the E series stimulate uterine activity. The related autacoid prostaglandin $E_{2\alpha}$ is used therapeutically in early pregnancy as an abortifacient and at or near term for cervical ripening. Because alprostadil has no indicated use in adult women and could induce labor, it should not be used during pregnancy.

REFERENCES

Hammerman, C. Patent ductus arteriosus. Clinical relevance of prostaglandins and prostaglandin inhibitors in PDA pathophysiology and treatment. *Clin. Perinatol.* 22:457, 1995.

Lea, A.P., Bryson, H.M., and Balfour, J.A. Intracavernous alprostadil. A review of its pharmacodynamic and pharmacokinetic properties and therapeutic potential in erectile dysfunction. *Drugs and Aging.* 8:56, 1996.

Amantadine (Symmetrel®)

INDICATIONS AND RECOMMENDATIONS

The use of amantadine is relatively contraindicated in pregnancy because other therapeutic agents are preferable. It is an antiviral agent used in the prevention and symptomatic treatment of influenza A respiratory tract illness in patients who, because of underlying disease (e.g., cardiovascular, pulmonary, metabolic, neuromuscular), are at high risk for complications and dangerous sequelae of viral infections. In addition, it is occasionally used in the treatment of Parkinson's disease and drug-induced extrapyramidal reactions, and has recently been used to limit relapses in patients with multiple sclerosis and juvenile rheumatoid arthritis.

Its antiviral activity, specific to influenza A virus, includes inhibition of an early step in viral replication. In Parkinsonism, it is thought to release dopamine from dopaminergic terminals, and it is less effective than levodopa.

No large-scale studies of amantadine use in pregnancy have been performed. Two case reports describe fetal cardiac malformations in association with first-trimester exposure to amantadine. In one case, its use was associated with the development of a complex cardiovascular lesion (single ventricle and pulmonary atresia); in the other case, the fetus was diagnosed with multiple cardiac lesions, including Tetralogy of Fallot and a large ventricular septal defect. This infant also had tibial hemimelia. Another report described four pregnant women receiving amantadine for Parkinson's disease, three of whom suffered complications of pregnancy. These included two miscarriages and one patient with preeclampsia who delivered an infant with an inguinal hernia. In two case reports of women receiving amantadine during two consecutive pregnancies (for multiple sclerosis and spasmodic torticollis), no anatomic abnormalities were noted in the four infants.

Amantadine is readily absorbed after oral administration and is present in breast milk. It is excreted in the urine without significant metabolism.

Because it is unlikely that women of childbearing age will suffer from a chronic disease that creates a high risk for influenza A, amantadine use during pregnancy for this indication will rarely be necessary. Occasionally, women with Parkinson's disease, multiple sclerosis, or rheumatoid arthritis may require treatment with amantadine. As its teratogenicity is undetermined, other safer agents are recommended as first-line therapies.

RECOMMENDED READING

Coulson, A.A. Amantadine and teratogenesis (letter). *Lancet.* 2:1044, 1975.

Hayden, F.G. Antimicrobial agents (antiviral agents). Chapter 50 in *Goodman and Gilman's The Pharmacological Basis of Therapeutics* (9th ed.), J.G. Hardman and L.E. Limbird, eds. New York: McGraw-Hill, 1996. Pp. 1209–1211.

Levy, M., Pastuszak, A., and Koren, G. Fetal outcome following intrauterine amantadine exposure. *Reprod. Toxicol.* 5: 79, 1991.

Monto, A.S. Prevention and drug treatment of influenza. *Am. Family Physician.* 28:165, 1983.

Nora, J.J., Nora, A.H., and Way, G.L. Cardiovascular maldevelopment associated with maternal exposure to amantadine (letter). *Lancet.* 2:607, 1975.

Pandit, P.B., et al. Tibial hemimelia and tetralogy of Fallot associated with first trimester exposure to amantadine. *Reprod. Toxicol.* 8:89, 1994.

ε-Aminocaproic Acid (Amicar®)

INDICATIONS AND RECOMMENDATIONS

The utility of ε-aminocaproic acid (EACA) in the pregnant patient is extremely limited. The use of EACA should be considered only when the condition being treated is serious and no other better studied option is available.

SPECIAL CONSIDERATIONS IN PREGNANCY

There is a single case report in which EACA was administered in the second trimester (no dosage reported) for several days before surgery in a patient with a subarachnoid hemorrhage and multiple aneurysms. This was not accompanied by apparent adverse fetal effects.

MECHANISM OF ACTION

As an inhibitor of fibrinolysis, EACA was introduced as a treatment for patients with hypofibrinogenemic hemorrhage. EACA competitively inhibits plasminogen activators and directly inhibits plasmin action. Inhibition of plasmin activity results in a diminished capacity to hydrolyze thrombus components. Because of complications encountered, EACA is rarely used in the treatment of disseminated intravascular coagulation (DIC) states.

EACA has also been used in the treatment of hereditary angioneurotic edema, an autosomal dominant state associated with the absence of functional C1 inhibitor. A diagnosis is suggested by family history, a lack of urticarial lesions, prominence of recurrent attacks of gastrointestinal colic, and episodic laryngeal edema. Attenuated androgens have been used in the treatment of this disease, as has EACA. Because angioedema in pregnancy is typically a mild disease, EACA use is not recommended.

DOSAGE, ABSORPTION, AND BIOTRANSFORMATION

EACA is available for both intravenous and oral administration. In either case, the initial dose is 5 g in the first hour and 1 g/h for 8 hours. Absorption is comparable for both routes, and renal excretion is the primary route of elimination. The majority of EACA is excreted unchanged in the urine.

ADVERSE EFFECTS

EACA use can be accompanied by nausea, diarrhea, crampy abdominal pain, headaches, skin rash, and decreased blood pressure. Myopathy with weakness and fatigue, and, very rarely, rhabdomyolysis has been reported. In the treatment of DIC states, serious complications, including thrombotic strokes, can be encountered.

RECOMMENDED READING

Austen, K.F. Disorders of immune-mediated injury. In *Harrison's Principles of Internal Medicine.* K.J. Isselbacher et al., eds. New York: McGraw-Hill, 1994. Pp. 1630–1643.

Bang, N.U. Diagnosis and management of thrombosis. In *Textbook of Critical Care.* W.C. Shoemaker et al., eds. Philadelphia: W.B. Saunders, 1989. Pp. 894–895.

Willoughby, J.S. Sodium nitroprusside, pregnancy and multiple intracranial aneurysms. *Anaesth. Intens. Care.* 12:358, 1984.

Aminoglycosides: Amikacin (Amikin®), Gentamicin (Garamycin®), Kanamycin (Kantrex®), Streptomycin, Tobramycin (Nebcin®), Neomycin, Netilmicin (Netromycin®), Paromomycin (Humatin®)

INDICATIONS AND RECOMMENDATIONS

The aminoglycosides should be given during pregnancy only when serious aerobic gram-negative infections are suspected. Streptomycin has been used to treat *Streptococcus viridans* endocarditis, plague, tularemia, and brucellosis. It may be required for treatment of drug-resistant *Mycobacterium tuberculosis.* Kanamycin is rarely used, although it may also be effective in treating tuberculosis. Gentamicin, tobramycin, amikacin, and netilmicin are used to treat aerobic gram-negative infections, including those caused by *Pseudomonas aeruginosa.* Species resistant to gentamicin or tobramycin may be susceptible to amikacin or netilmicin. Neomycin has a broad spectrum of coverage, including *Staphylococcus aureus;* however, *P. aeruginosa* is resistant. It also may be used topically or orally. Paromomycin has been used without adverse effect to treat intestinal amebiasis and giardiasis after the first trimester. In addition, aminoglycosides may be synergistic with a cell wall–active agent in the treatment of *Listeria monocytogenes,* enterococci, and streptococci.

In pregnancy, gentamicin is preferable to tobramycin, amikacin, or netilmicin because it has been more extensively studied. Tobramycin may be valuable in treating *Pseudomonas* infections in patients with cystic fibrosis.

SPECIAL CONSIDERATIONS IN PREGNANCY

There are no unusual effects on the mother during pregnancy, but serum aminoglycoside levels are usually lower in pregnant than in nonpregnant patients receiving equivalent doses. Thus, it is important to monitor levels frequently to prevent subtherapeutic dosing in patients who are not clinically responsive to treatment.

All of these drugs cross the placenta but have lower concentrations in fetal blood when tested at full term than in simultaneously obtained maternal samples.

Animal studies have raised concerns regarding fetal nephrotoxicity secondary to in utero aminoglycoside exposure, particularly gentamicin. Rats exposed to gentamicin during gestation had evidence of oligonephronia as well as permanent alterations in the glomerular basement membrane. This drug has also been associated with hypertension as well as kidney impairment in 1-year-old rats exposed in utero. One study comparing the effects of gentamicin, netilmicin, and amikacin in rats found gentamicin to be the most toxic with respect to ultrastructural changes in the renal tubules. Tobramycin has been shown to cause impaired renal development in rat pups when given at doses nephrotoxic to the dam.

Streptomycin and kanamycin have been associated with congenital deafness or hearing impairment in the offspring of mothers who took these drugs during pregnancy. Ototoxicity has been reported with doses as low as 1 g streptomycin biweekly for 8 weeks during the first trimester. They should therefore not be administered during the first trimester or in dosages exceeding a total of 20 g during the last half of pregnancy, and should be avoided unless there are no acceptable alternative therapies available. No other congenital anomalies have been reported in humans in association with aminoglycosides. High doses of netilmycin may be associated with poor fetal growth. Studies of effects of aminoglycoside administration during labor have not demonstrated toxicity to the fetus.

In general, aminoglycosides are felt to be compatible with breast-feeding, as they are poorly absorbed orally. One theoretical complication would be a change in infant bowel flora. The American Academy of Pediatrics lists kanamycin and streptomycin as compatible with breast-feeding. Gentamicin is transferred to breast milk. It may be detectable in the serum of 50% of nursing infants at low levels unlikely to cause clinical effect. Peak levels are attained 3 hours after a dose. Small amounts of streptomycin are present in breast milk, but no studies have been performed to assess toxicity. Limited information is available regarding the other drugs in this class.

DOSAGE

Drug	Route	Dose (mg/kg/day)*	Interval
Neomycin	IM	15	q6h
Streptomycin	IM	15–25	14q12h
Kanamycin	IM/IV	15	14q8–12h
Gentamicin	IM/IV	3–5	14q8h
Tobramycin	IM/IV	3–5	14q8h
Amikacin	IM/IV	15	14q8–12h
Paromomycin	PO	25–30	q6–8h
Netilmicin	IM/IV	3.0–6.5	q12h

*Dosage must be adjusted in the face of renal impairment.

Once-daily dosing of gentamicin has been used successfully in patients with postpartum endometritis (5 mg/kg). This regimen has not been studied in pregnancy regarding its toxicity or efficacy.

ADVERSE EFFECTS

General

Irreversible eighth nerve toxicity may occur secondary to the use of aminoglycosides. In addition, aminoglycosides may be nephrotoxic in 8% to 26% of patients due to accumulation of the drug in the proximal renal tubular cells. There may be a decrease in concentrating ability, as well as proteinuria and hyaline and granular casts. Several days following, the glomerular filtration rate may decrease. The most common clinical finding is a slightly increased plasma creatinine. The effects on the kidney are almost always reversible. Finally, the use of aminoglycosides may be associated with neuromuscular blockade as aminoglycosides decrease acetylcholine release at the presynaptic junction. This may result in exacerbation of muscle weakness in the setting of defects in cholinergic function or release, i.e., patients with myasthenia gravis, or those exposed to curariform drugs or magnesium sulfate.

Streptomycin

Permanent vestibular eighth nerve damage may occur, as already noted. Paresthesias, rash, fever, pruritus, renal damage, and anaphylaxis are occasionally noted. Rarely, blood dyscrasias, optic or peripheral neuritis, myocarditis, and hepatic necrosis may develop. Neuromuscular blockade and apnea have been reported with parenteral administration of the drug.

Nephrotoxicity may be increased when the drug is given with cephaloridine, cephalothin, or polymyxins. Ototoxicity may be increased by interaction with ethacrynic acid and neuromuscular blockade with curariform drugs.

Kanamycin

Occasionally, auditory eighth nerve damage will occur. This may remain undetected until after therapy has been stopped and can be irreversible. Renal damage, rash, and peripheral neuritis also have been noted. Parenteral or intraperitoneal administration may produce neuromuscular blockade or apnea.

Effects of drug interactions include increased nephrotoxicity with cephalosporins and polymyxins, ototoxicity with ethacrynic acid, and neuromuscular blockade with curariform drugs.

Gentamicin

Occasionally, vestibular eighth nerve damage, rash, and renal impairment may occur. Rarely, auditory damage has been noted. Neuromuscular blockade and apnea may develop.

Effects of drug interactions include increased nephrotoxicity with cephalosporins and polymyxins, ototoxicity with ethacrynic acid, and neuromuscular blockade with curariform drugs.

Other

Tobramycin and amikacin produce essentially the same side effects as gentamicin. They are newer drugs, however, and additional adverse sequelae may become evident in the future.

Netilmicin is believed to have less ototoxicity and nephrotoxicity than other aminoglycosides. No vestibular damage has been detected after use in neonates.

Neomycin may be associated with hypersensitivity reactions, i.e., skin rashes, as well as ototoxicity and nephrotoxicity. After oral administration, intestinal malabsorption or superinfection may occur.

Paromomycin has low toxicity when administered orally.

MECHANISM OF ACTION

Aminoglycosides are bactericidal, the rate of which is concentration-dependent. In addition, there is residual antibiotic effect that persists after the serum level has decreased below the minimum inhibitory concentration. However, a transient phenomenon known as adaptive resistance also occurs, in which initial aminoglycoside administration may decrease the effectiveness of subsequent doses for 6–16 hours. The aminoglycoside antibiotics penetrate the cell wall and cytoplasmic membrane of susceptible microorganisms and act on the bacterial ribosomes. They bind to the ribosomes and block initiation of protein synthesis, inhibit translation, and cause a misreading of the microorganism's genetic code, which leads to the production of abnormal proteins and, ultimately, cell death. Resistance to aminoglycosides may develop as a result of inactivation of the drug by microbial enzymes, inability of the drug to permeate the microorganism, or alterations in ribosomal structure that decrease binding affinity.

ABSORPTION AND BIOTRANSFORMATION

These antibiotics are polycations, and their polarity is believed to be responsible for the pharmacokinetic properties common to the entire group. These include poor absorption after oral administration, poor penetration into the cerebrospinal fluid, and rapid excretion by the normal kidney. The aminoglycosides do not bind well to plasma proteins. Because their clearance is related to the glomerular filtration rate, dosage must be readjusted in the face of abnormal renal function, particularly as the ototoxic and nephrotoxic effects are directly related to concentration.

Aminoglycosides can accumulate in fetal plasma and amniotic fluid. During pregnancy, there is decreased clearance of gentamicin. The pharmacokinetics of tobramycin also have been studied in pregnancy, and clearance is noted to be decreased after 28 weeks gestation, possibly related to drug accumulation in the fetus. A once-daily dose regimen may limit potential toxicities for mother and fetus. Tobramycin accumulates in the fetal spleen and kidney after maternal administration. The aminoglycosides are absorbed rapidly after intravenous or intramuscular administration, with peak concentrations seen after 30–90 minutes.

RECOMMENDED READING

American Academy of Pediatrics. The transfer of drugs and other chemicals into human milk. *Pediatrics.* 93:137, 1994.

Bourget, P., Fernandez, H., Delouis, C., and Taburet, A.-M. Pharmacokinetics of tobramycin in pregnant women; safety and efficacy of a once-daily dose regimen. *J. Clin. Pharm. Ther.* 16:167, 1991.

Chahoud, I., Stahlmann, R., Merker, H.-J., and Neubert, D. Hypertension and nephrotoxic lesions in rats 1 year after prenatal exposure to gentamicin. *Arch. Toxicol.* 62:274, 1988.

Chambers, H.F., and Sande, M.A. The aminoglycosides. Chapter 46 in *Goodman and Gilman's The Pharmacological Basis of Therapeutics* (9th ed.), J.G. Hardman and L.E. Limbird, eds. New York: McGraw-Hill, 1996. Pp. 1103–1121.

Del Priore, G., Jackson-Stone, M., Shim, E.K., Garfinkel, J., Eichmann, M.A., and Frederiksen, M.C. A comparison of once-daily and 8-hour gentamicin dosing in the treatment of postpartum endometritis. *Obstet. Gynecol.* 87:994, 1996.

Holdiness, M.R. Teratology of the antituberculosis drugs. *Early Hum. Dev.* 15:61, 1987.

Kreutner, A.K., Del Bene, V.E., and Amstey, M.S. Giardiasis in pregnancy. *Am. J. Obstet. Gynecol.* 140:895, 1981.

Mallie, J.-P., Coulon, G., Billerey, C., Faucourt, A., and Morin, J.-P. In utero aminoglycosides-induced nephrotoxicity in rat neonates. *Kidney Int.* 33:36, 1988.

Robinson, G.C., and Cambon, K.G. Hearing loss in infants of tuberculous mothers treated with streptomycin during pregnancy. *N. Engl. J. Med.* 271:949, 1964.

Smaoui, H., Mallie, J.-P., Schaeverbeke, M., Robert, A., and Schaeverbeke, J. Gentamicin administered during gestation alters glomerular basement membrane development. *Antimicrob. Ag. Chemother.* 37:1510, 1993.

Weinstein, A.J., Gibbs, R.S., and Gallagher, M. Placental transfer of clindamycin and gentamicin in term pregnancy. *Am. J. Obstet. Gynecol.* 124:688, 1976.

Zaske, D.E., et al. Rapid gentamicin elimination in obstetric patients. *Obstet. Gynecol.* 56:559, 1980.

Aminosalicylate Sodium (PAS, Paser® Granules)

INDICATIONS AND RECOMMENDATIONS

Aminosalicylate sodium (PAS) may be used during pregnancy for the treatment of tuberculosis that is not amenable to treatment with more effective antitubercular agents. It is, however, a second-line drug and has been largely replaced by other, better tolerated, and more effective agents.

SPECIAL CONSIDERATIONS IN PREGNANCY

Although not commonly used, PAS has been prescribed for the treatment of tuberculosis in pregnant women. In the Collaborative Perinatal Project, various malformations were present in 5 of 43 infants with first-trimester exposure. Retrospective reports do not suggest that it is teratogenic, but large-scale prospective studies are lacking.

Should PAS be prescribed during pregnancy, it is important to note that it may interfere with absorption of oral folic acid and vitamin B_{12}. Parenteral supplementation of these compounds may therefore be necessary.

Aminosalicylate sodium attains levels of approximately 70 mg/L in maternal serum. Simultaneously measured breast milk levels are 1.1 mg/L, and therefore the drug could be considered safe. Nevertheless, infants exposed to PAS through breast milk should be monitored for symptoms of toxicity.

DOSAGE

The usual adult dose is 10–12 g/day PO divided bid or tid. As PAS may inhibit the absorption of rifampin, the doses of each should be separated by 8–12 hours.

ADVERSE EFFECTS

The most common side effects are nausea, vomiting, diarrhea, and abdominal pain. Less common is hypersensitivity reaction, which may include fever, rashes, leukopenia, agranulocytosis, thrombocytopenia, and infectious mononucleosis-like symptoms. In addition, goiter, both with and without myxedema, has been reported.

MECHANISM OF ACTION

The mechanism of PAS as an antitubercular agent is believed to be through inhibition of folate biosynthesis, similar to that of sulfonamides. It is bacteriostatic to *Mycobacterium* tuberculosis and inhibits the onset of bacterial resistance to isoniazid and streptomycin.

ABSORPTION AND BIOTRANSFORMATION

Aminosalicylate sodium is readily absorbed from the gastrointestinal tract and widely distributed to all parts of the body. It is concentrated in pleural and caseous tissue. Its half-life is approximately 1 hour. It undergoes metabolism in the liver, and 80% is excreted in the urine as either metabolite or free acid. Excretion is diminished in the presence of renal dysfunction.

RECOMMENDED READING

de March, A.P. Tuberculosis and pregnancy. Five to ten year review of 215 patients in their fertile age. *Chest.* 68:800, 1975.

Good, J.T., et al. Tuberculosis in association with pregnancy. *Am. J. Obstet. Gynecol.* 140:492, 1981.

Heinonen, O.P., Slone, D., and Shapiro, S. *Birth Defects and Drugs in Pregnancy.* Littleton, MA: Wright-PSG, 1977. P. 299.

Holdiness, M.R. Antituberculosis drugs and breast feeding (letter). *Arch. Intern. Med.* 144:1888, 1984.

Lowe, C.R. Congenital defects among children born to women under supervision or treatment for pulmonary tuberculosis. *Br. J. Prev. Soc. Med.* 18:14, 1964.

Mandell, G.L., and Petri, W.A., Jr. Antimicrobial agents. Chapter 48 in *Goodman and Gilman's The Pharmacological Basis of Therapeutics* (9th ed.), J.G. Hardman and L.E. Limbard, eds. New York: McGraw-Hill, 1996. P. 1164.

Wilson, E.A., Thelin, T.J., and Dilts, P.V., Jr. Tuberculosis complicated by pregnancy. *Am. J. Obstet. Gynecol.* 115:526, 1973.

Ammonium Chloride

INDICATIONS AND RECOMMENDATIONS

Ammonium chloride should only be used during pregnancy as an acidifying agent in the treatment of significant maternal metabolic alkalosis and in initiating a forced acid diuresis in specific instances of drug intoxication (e.g., quinine or amphetamines). The ammonium ion is thought to exert an expectorant action and is contained in some cough syrups, but it should not be administered to obstetric patients for this purpose.

Data regarding the effects of ammonium chloride salts in pregnancy are limited. When experimentally administered orally for up to 24 days in pregnant women, a metabolic acidosis was produced that resulted in reduced fetal oxygen saturations and pH along with increased fetal PCO_2 values. The acute intravenous administration of ammonium chloride to pregnant women has been shown to cause fetal and subsequent neonatal hypoxemia despite relatively unchanged maternal concentrations of oxygen. The degree of the fetal and neonatal responses appears to be proportional to the severity of the maternal acidosis. Therefore, in view of the limited experience with this compound during pregnancy and the alterations in fetal acid–base status that it may cause, its use should be limited to life-threatening situations in which safer alternatives are not available.

RECOMMENDED READING

Blechner, J.N., et al. Oxygenation of the human fetus and newborn infant during maternal metabolic acidosis. *Am. J. Obstet. Gynecol.* 108:47, 1970.

Goodlin, R.C., and Kaiser, I.H. The effect of ammonium chloride induced maternal acidosis on the human fetus at term: I. pH, hemoglobin, blood gases. *Am. J. Med. Sci.* 233:662, 1957.

Amobarbital (Amytal®)

INDICATIONS AND RECOMMENDATIONS

Amobarbital is contraindicated for use during pregnancy because other therapeutic agents are preferable. It is most frequently used as a short-acting sedative-hypnotic in a similar fashion to phenobarbital. Twenty cases of amobarbital overdose during pregnancy have been identified. Two fetal deaths were reported, but there was no increase in the incidence of congenital anomalies. Two studies have examined the teratogenic potential of amobarbital. One, based on 12 cases, reported an increase in major anomalies, including anencephaly and congenital heart disease. Based on data from the Collaborative Perinatal Project, use of amobarbital in the first trimester of pregnancy might be associated with an increased incidence of cardiovascular malformations, polydactyly in black offspring, genitourinary problems other than hypospadias, inguinal hernia, and clubfoot. Both studies involved only small numbers of cases, and there was no clear pattern of malformations, raising the possibility that the findings were due to chance.

Amobarbital freely crosses the placenta with levels in cord serum being similar to those in the mother. Either single or multiple dosing of mothers near term, however, results in neonatal half-lives that are up to 2.5-fold those in the maternal serum. This phenomenon is attributable to the fact that fetal-neonatal liver hydroxylation is not induced by the drug and its elimination is prolonged in the neonate. This could lead to accumulation in the neonate with resultant sedation.

RECOMMENDED READING

Czeizel, A., Szentesi, I., Szekeres, I., et al. A study of adverse effects on the progeny after intoxication during pregnancy. *Arch. Toxicol.* 62:1, 1988.

Draffan, G.H., et al. Maternal and neonatal elimination of amobarbital after treatment of the mother with barbiturates during late pregnancy. *Clin. Pharmacol. Ther.* 19:271, 1976.

Heinonen, O.P., Slone, D., and Shapiro, S. *Birth Defects and Drugs in Pregnancy.* Littleton, MA: Wright-PSG, 1977. Pp. 336, 344, 438.

Kraver, B., et al. Elimination kinetics of amobarbital in mothers and newborn infants. *Clin. Pharmacol. Ther.* 14:442, 1973.

Nelson, M.M., and Forfar, J.O. Associations between drugs administered during pregnancy and congenital anomalies of the fetus. *Br. Med. J.* 1:523, 1971.

Amphetamines: Amphetamine Sulfate (Benzedrine®), Dextroamphetamine Sulfate (Dexedrine®)

INDICATIONS AND RECOMMENDATIONS

Amphetamines should not be used during pregnancy. These central sympathomimetic agents have been used as appetite suppressants, antifatigue agents, and in the treatment of narcolepsy. They are commonly ingested as illicit drugs. Although the data are conflicting, there are studies that show an increased incidence of cardiac defects and cleft palate after fetal exposure to amphetamine. Administration of methamphetamine to pregnant ewes resulted in maternal and fetal hypertension, decreased uterine blood flow, and significant reduction in fetal pO_2. There has been one report of fetal death following maternal intravenous amphetamine injection. A case of apparent eclampsia immediately following amphetamine use has also been reported. Ultrasonographic evidence of cerebral injury was noted in 37% of 24 newborns of amphetamine-ingesting mothers in one study. In a 10-year follow-up study of 65 children born to mothers taking amphetamines, poor psychometric test results and aggressive behavior were noted. At present, weight reduction and fatigue prevention are not valid indications for amphetamine therapy. Thus, narcolepsy is the only clinical situation in which these drugs might be considered in the pregnant woman, and methylphenidate is probably a better choice for this rare condition (see "Methylphenidate Hydrochloride"). Amphetamines are concentrated in breast milk. The American Academy of Pediatrics considers amphetamines to be drugs of abuse that are contraindicated during breast-feeding.

RECOMMENDED READING

Committee on Drugs of the American Academy of Pediatrics. The transfer of drugs and other chemicals into human milk. *Pediatrics.* 93:137, 1994.

Dearlove, J.C., Betteridge, T.J., and Henry, J.A. Stillbirth due to intravenous amphetamine. *Br. Med. J.* 304:548, 1992.

Dixon, S.D., and Bejar, R. Echoencephalographic findings in neonates associated with maternal cocaine and methamphetamine use: incidence and clinical correlates. *J. Pediatrics.* 115: 770, 1989.

Elliott, R.H., and Rees, G.B. Amphetamine ingestion presenting as eclampsia. *Can. J. Anaesth.* 37:130, 1990.

Eriksson, M., and Zetterström, R. Amphetamine addiction during pregnancy: 10-year follow-up. *Acta Paediatr.* (Suppl) 404: 27, 1994.

Hoffman B.B., and Lefkowitz R.J. Catecholamines, sympathomimetic drugs, and adrenergic receptor antagonists. Chapter 10 in *Goodman and Gilman's The Pharmacological Basis of Therapeutics* (9th ed.), J.G. Hardman and L.E. Limbird, eds. New York: McGraw-Hill, 1996. Pp. 219–221.

Milkovich, L., and van den Berg, B.J. Effects of antenatal exposure to anorectic drugs. *Am. J. Obstet. Gynecol.* 129:637, 1977.

Steiner, E., Villén, T., Hallberg, M., and Rane, A. Amphetamine secretion in breast milk. *Eur. J. Clin. Pharmacol.* 27:123, 1984.

Stek, A.M., Baker, R.S., Fisher, B.K., Lang, U., and Clark, K.E. Fetal responses to maternal and fetal methamphetamine administration in sheep. *Am. J. Obstet. Gynecol.* 173:1592, 1995.

Amphotericin B (Fungizone®)

INDICATIONS AND RECOMMENDATIONS

The use of amphotericin B during pregnancy should be limited to the treatment of life-threatening fungal infections such as cryptococcosis, blastomycosis, coccidiomycosis, histoplasmosis, mucormycosis, aspergillosis, and disseminated candidiasis. Patients receiving amphotericin B should be hospitalized and their renal function monitored at least once a week. The effective treatment of these serious maternal infections is of overwhelming importance in such cases; the benefits clearly outweigh potential risks.

SPECIAL CONSIDERATIONS IN PREGNANCY

Generally, the side effects of amphotericin B are no worse in the pregnant than in the nonpregnant woman. In pregnant patients, however, preexisting anemia may be exacerbated by the anemia caused by amphotericin B and may necessitate transfusion. Amphotericin B readily crosses the placenta, may be retained in the placenta or amniotic fluid, and cord levels can approach maternal levels. A study of teratogenic effects in mammals showed no developmental toxicity attributable to this drug. The literature contains several reports of mothers who received amphotericin B during all stages of pregnancy. While some births were uncomplicated, others were accompanied by spontaneous abortion, growth restriction, and prematurity. There does not seem to be a correlation between the trimester of treatment and outcome of the pregnancy.

DOSAGE

The recommended starting dose is 0.25 mg/kg/day, which is then gradually increased to 1 mg/kg/day as tolerance to the common side effects (chills and fever) develops. The maximum dose, given in severe infections, is 1.5 mg/kg/day. The usual duration of therapy is from 6 weeks to 4 months but may be shorter if adverse effects require discontinuation. The drug is administered intravenously in a concentration of 0.1 mg/ml over 4–6 hours. Because of the long plasma half-life, alternate day dosing is feasible.

ADVERSE EFFECTS

Chills, fever (up to 40°C), vomiting, anorexia, and headache are commonly observed in patients during the infusion period. With repeated infusions, thrombophlebitis, anemia, and nephrotoxicity frequently occur. The severity of renal impairment is dose-related, generally not reaching clinical significance unless the cumulative dose is 4 g. Mild manifestations are reversible with cessation of therapy. Hypersensitivity reactions have included anaphylaxis, thrombocytopenia, flushing, generalized pain, and convulsions.

ABSORPTION AND BIOTRANSFORMATION

Amphotericin B is poorly absorbed from the gastrointestinal tract and is therefore given intravenously for the treatment of systemic infections. The plasma half-life is 24 hours. A small fraction of the dose appears in the urine and is detectable for as long as 7–8 weeks after therapy has been discontinued. No abnormal accumulation is seen in patients with renal failure. The drug appears to be stored in the body, very slowly released, metabolized, and then slowly excreted by the kidneys. No specific metabolites have been identified.

RECOMMENDED READING

Bennett, J.E. Antimicrobial agents: antifungal agents. Chapter 49 in *Goodman and Gilman's The Pharmacological Basis of Therapeutics* (9th ed.), J.G. Hardman and L.E. Limbird, eds. New York: McGraw-Hill, 1996. Pp. 1176–1179.

Bindschadler, D.D., and Bennett, J.E. A pharmacologic guide to the clinical use of amphotericin B. *J. Infect. Dis.* 120:427, 1969.

Buhl, M.R., et al. Temporofacial zygomycosis in a pregnant woman. *Infection* 20: 230, 1992.

Curole, D.N. Cryptococcal meningitis in pregnancy. *J. Reprod. Med.* 26:317, 1981.

Dean, J.L., et al. Use of amphotericin B during pregnancy: case report and review. *Clin. Infect. Dis.* 18:364, 1994.

Gradoni, L., et al. Mediterranean visceral leishmaniasis in pregnancy. *Scand. J. Infect. Dis.* 26(5):627, 1994.

Ismail, M.A., and Lerner, S.A. Disseminated blastomycosis in a pregnant woman. Review of amphotericin B usage in pregnancy. *Am. Rev. Resp. Dis.* 126:350, 1982.

Potasman, I., et al. *Candida* sepsis in pregnancy and the postpartum period. *Rev. Infect. Dis.* 13: 146–9, 1991.

Ruo, P. A case of torulosis of the CNS during pregnancy. *Med. J. Aust.* 1:558, 1962.

Anorexiants: Benzphetamine (Didrex®), Dexfenfluramine (Redux®), Diethylpropion (Tenuate®), Fenfluramine (Pondimin®), Mazindol (Mazanor®, Sanorex®), Phendimetrazine (Boutril®, Plegine®, Prelu-2®), Phentermine (Ionamin®, Fastin®)

INDICATIONS AND RECOMMENDATIONS

The anorexiants are contraindicated during pregnancy. They are sympathomimetic amines that suppress the appetite and are indicated as short-term (8- to 12-week) adjuncts to a weight program for obese patients. Their anorectic effects are temporary and believed to be mediated through direct stimulation of the satiety center in the hypothalamic and limbic regions of the brain. Maternal side effects may include palpitations, elevation of blood pressure, and tachycardia.

Studies performed in weaning pups whose mothers were given phenmetrazine in pregnancy demonstrated a decrease in survival and growth rate. Cases of skeletal and visceral anomalies in infants whose mothers had taken phenmetrazine during pregnancy have been reported, but no causal relationship has been proved. In the Collaborative Perinatal Project, no increase was seen in birth defects in the children of 58 mothers who took phenmetrazine during the first 4 months of pregnancy. Similarly, in a study comparing 1824 women receiving anorectic drugs during pregnancy with 8989 who did not receive these drugs, there was no increase in congenital anomalies (diagnosed by 5 years of age) among the 55 infants exposed to phenmetrazine within 84 days of the last menstrual period.

One anecdotal report associates the use of diethylpropion in the first trimester with sacral agenesis and multiple anomalies of the lower body. A retrospective case-control study, comparing 1232 women who took the drug during pregnancy with an equal number of control subjects, reports no increased incidence of malformation.

Phentermine treatment of mice during the last 5 days of gestation caused no signs of toxicity, as evidenced by maintenance of body weight or neonatal death or phospholipidosis of the lungs of the neonates. Chlorphentermine administered during the same time frame caused development of phospholipidosis of the dams and in the neonatal lung in addition to significant decrease in newborn body weight as well as an 83% infant mortality rate.

Fenfluramine has been identified as a behavioral teratogen in rats. Fenfluramine administration to pregnant rats caused increased neonatal mortality and significant weight reduction before weaning and had behavioral effects that were revealed in tests of preweaning development. Fenfluramine decreased the rate of conception and survival rate for weaning in mice, rats, guinea pigs, rabbits, monkeys, dogs, and cats. In these animals it caused no gross congenital malformations.

Administration of dexfenfluramine to pregnant rats during the last week of gestation caused an attenuation of the weight gain by the dam without effect on the number or birth rate of offspring. Dexfenfluramine and fenfluramine are known to cause profound and prolonged depletions of brain serotonin. When given to pregnant rats, dams sustained large depletions of brain serotonin more than 3 weeks after giving birth, whereas neonatal brain serotonin was reduced only slightly on the day after birth in some of the offspring.

The combination of fenfluramine or dexfenfluramine and phentermine has been shown to cause serious heart problems in nearly one-third of users, mostly relatively young women. The combination is associated with aortic and mitral heart valve disorders as well as potentially fatal pulmonary hypertension. In addition, patients without symptoms have been found to have abnormal echocardiograms. After reports of these serious adverse reactions in 1997, the manufacturers and distributors of dexfenfluramine and fenfluramine have voluntarily withdrawn the drugs from the market.

Because it is not appropriate for pregnant women to participate in weight reduction programs, anorexiants have no role during pregnancy.

RECOMMENDED READING

Abraham, E. Sacral agenesis with associated anomalies (caudal regression syndrome): autopsy case report. *Clin. Orthop. Rel. Res.* 145:168, 1979.

Bunde, C.A., and Leyland, H.M. A controlled retrospective survey in evaluation of teratogenicity. *J. New Drugs* 5:193, 1965.

Butcher, R.E., and Vorhees, C.V. A preliminary test battery for the investigation of the behavioral teratology of selected psychotropic drugs. *Neurobehav. Toxicol.* 1:207, 1979.

Connolly, H.M., et al. Valvular heart disease associated with fenfluramine-phentermine. *N. Engl. J. Med.* 337:581, 1997.

Gilber, D.L., et al. Toxicologic studies of fenfluramine. *Toxicol. Appl. Pharmacol.* 19:705, 1971.

Heinonen, O.P., Slone, D., and Shapiro, S. *Birth Defects and Drugs in Pregnancy.* Littleton, MA: Wright-PSG, 1977. Pp. 346–347, 439.

Hoffman, B.B., and Lefkowitz, R.J. Catecholamines, sympathomimetic drugs, and adrenergic receptor antagonists. Chapter 27 in *Goodman and Gilman's The Pharmacological Basis of Therapeutics* (9th ed.), J.G. Hardman and L.E. Limbird, eds. New York: McGraw-Hill, 1996. P. 224.

Milkovich, L., and van den Berg, B.J. Effects of antenatal exposure to anorectic drugs. *Am. J. Obstet. Gynecol.* 129:637, 1977.

Roland, N.E., and Robertson, R.M. Administration of dexfenfluramine in pregnant rats: effect on brain serotonin parameters in offspring. *Pharmacol. Biochem. Behav.* 42:885, 1992.

Silverman, M., and Okun, R. The use of an appetite suppressant (diethylpropion hydrochloride) during pregnancy. *Curr. Ther. Res.* 13:648, 1971.

Thoma-Laurie, D., Walker, E.R., and Reasor, M.J. Neonatal toxicity in rats following in utero exposure to chlorphentermine or phentermine. *Toxicology* 24:85, 1982.

Vorhees, C.V., Brunner, R.L., and Butcher, R.E. Psychotropic drugs as behavioral teratogens. *Science* 205:1220, 1979.

Antacids (Over-the-Counter): Aluminum Compounds, Calcium Carbonate, Magnesium Compounds, Sodium Bicarbonate

Many over-the-counter (OTC) preparations include a combination of gastric antacids. The different components of these preparations are described separately.

One retrospective study suggested an association between the administration of aluminum hydroxide, calcium carbonate, and magnesium compound antacids during the first 56 days of gestation and the occurrence of major and minor congenital anomalies. It should be noted, however, that this was a heterogeneous group of anomalies. It was found that 5.9% of 458 mothers giving birth to anomalous babies took antacids during the first trimester, whereas 2.6% of 911 mothers of normal babies took these drugs. No causality can be inferred, and no substantiating data have followed.

ALUMINUM COMPOUNDS

Indications and Recommendations

Aluminum hydroxide, aluminum carbonate, aluminum phosphate, and aluminum aminoacetate are safe to use during the last two trimesters of pregnancy as long as chronic high doses and concurrent ingestion of citric, lactic, and ascorbic acid are avoided. They are used to neutralize gastric acid and to treat phosphate nephrolithiasis. Of these agents, aluminum hydroxide is the most potent buffer and is used most often.

Special Considerations in Pregnancy

Parenterally administered aluminum is fetotoxic in animals. In addition, high-dose oral aluminum when given concurrently with citric or lactic acid has been shown to be fetotoxic in mice. Although these effects have not been described in humans, it would be prudent to limit the dose of these agents. In addition, as lactic, citric, and ascorbic acids act to increase the absorption of aluminum from the gastrointestinal tract, foods containing these substances should not be taken simultaneously with aluminum antacids.

Dosage

Aluminum hydroxide comes in tablets containing 300–600 mg. A 600 mg dose will neutralize 2–10 mEq acid in 30 minutes.

Adverse Effects

The most common side effect of aluminum-containing antacids is constipation; they have also been reported to cause intestinal obstruction and fecal impaction. Except for the phosphate salt, they also cause transient hypophosphatemia and hypophosphaturia; phosphate depletion syndrome with chronic use; increased calcium absorption, possibly leading to hypercalcemia and hypercalciuria; and hypomagnesemia. Aluminum antacids decrease the absorption of tetracycline, chlorpromazine, acetylsalicylic acid, anticholinergic agents, pentobarbital, and sulfadiazine. The absorption of both penicillin and pseudoephedrine is increased, and there is a slight decrease in the absorption of amino acids, ascorbic acid, vitamin A, and glucose.

Mechanism of Action

Aluminum hydroxide reacts with hydrochloric acid in the stomach to form aluminum chloride and water. Nonabsorbed aluminum hydroxide is converted to insoluble aluminum phosphate in the gastrointestinal tract, making this a useful substance in the treatment of phosphate nephrolithiasis.

Absorption and Biotransformation

Between 17% and 31% of an oral dose of aluminum hydroxide may be recovered in the urine.

CALCIUM CARBONATE

Indications and Recommendations

Calcium carbonate is safe to use during pregnancy in the last two trimesters as long as chronic high doses are avoided. It is used to neutralize acid in the stomach.

Special Considerations in Pregnancy

Fetal hypomagnesemia, increased deep tendon reflexes, and increased muscle tone have been reported.

Dosage

The average dose of calcium carbonate is 1000 mg; this dose will neutralize 13 mEq acid in 30 minutes.

Adverse Effects

The most common side effects include constipation, nausea, and belching. In some patients, calcium carbonate may act as a laxative, increasing fecal bulk or causing diarrhea. Patients taking large doses (more than 20 g/day) or with impaired renal function are at risk for developing hypercalcemia. In predisposed persons, hypercalciuria with nephrolithiasis and azotemia may occur. Patients taking calcium carbonate for the treatment of ulcer disease may note "rebound" aggravation of their ulcer symptoms. Although clinically significant alkalosis usually does not develop, calcium carbonate may contribute to the development of milk-alkali syndrome. The condition is generally reversible after the calcium carbonate is discontinued.

Mechanism of Action

Calcium carbonate reacts with hydrochloric acid in the stomach to form calcium chloride, carbon dioxide, and water.

Absorption and Biotransformation

Calcium carbonate is absorbed at a rate of 10% to 15% by healthy individuals and 10% to 35% by persons with peptic ulcer disease. A transitory hypercalcemia is noted after an oral dose of calcium carbonate, but this effect is less marked if the substance is taken chronically by a person with normal renal function.

MAGNESIUM COMPOUNDS

Indications and Recommendations

Magnesium trisilicate, magnesium carbonate, and magnesium hydroxide are safe to use during pregnancy in the last two trimesters as long as chronic high doses are avoided. They are used to neutralize acid in the stomach.

Special Considerations in Pregnancy

Neonatal hypermagnesemia with drowsiness, decreased muscle tone, respiratory distress, and cardiovascular impairment have been reported in newborns exposed in utero to chronic high maternal magnesium levels. Silicaceous nephrolithiasis has also been reported in newborns whose mothers were chronic magnesium trisilicate takers.

Dosage

Magnesium salts are found in numerous OTC preparations in various concentrations, often in combination with other, constipating antacids. A 1000 mg dose of magnesium neutralizes 13–17 mEq acid in 30 minutes. A 5 ml dose of milk of magnesia, an 8% aqueous suspension of magnesium hydroxide, neutralizes about 13.5 mEq acid. When given in 15- to 30-ml doses, milk of magnesia is used as a cathartic.

Adverse Effects

The most commonly reported side effect of magnesium compounds is a dose-related diarrhea that may be severe enough to cause fluid and electrolyte imbalances. In patients with renal insufficiency, these agents may cause hypermagnesemia, with its associated muscle weakness and hypotonia, sedation, confusion, and, in some cases, cardiovascular effects such as complete heart block. These compounds also may augment the absorption of warfarin compounds but decrease the absorption of barbiturates, quinidine, and digoxin. Chronic ingestion of magnesium trisilicate has been reported to result in formation of silicaceous stones in the urinary tract.

Mechanism of Action

Magnesium hydroxide (milk of magnesia 8%) reacts with hydrochloric acid to form magnesium chloride. Magnesium carbonate reacts with hydrochloric acid to form carbon dioxide and magnesium chloride. Magnesium trisilicate reacts with hydrochloric acid to form silicon dioxide and magnesium. Silicon dioxide, a gelatinous compound, may provide an adherent coating to an ulcer crater.

Absorption and Biotransformation

Approximately 5% of the magnesium in magnesium trisilicate is absorbed. In both magnesium hydroxide and magnesium carbonate, 5% to 10% of the magnesium is absorbed.

SODIUM BICARBONATE

Indications and Recommendations

The use of sodium bicarbonate is relatively contraindicated during pregnancy because other therapeutic agents are preferable. It is used to neutralize stomach acid but is absorbed systemically (unlike most of the other antacid agents). The systemic absorption leads to a short duration of action, with a resultant rebound increase in symptoms. Chronic use also leads to systemic alkalosis. The sodium load that is absorbed can also cause edema and weight gain. For these reasons, it is recommended that other, less systemically active agents be used if antacid therapy is considered necessary.

An exception to this relative contraindication is the use of sodium citrate as a preoperative antacid for patients undergoing cesarean section. Sodium citrate, available in combination with citric acid, is metabolized to sodium bicarbonate and thus acts as a buffer. Because other antacids contain particulate matter, which may cause bronchopneumonia if aspirated, many anesthesiologists prefer to give a clear antacid, i.e., sodium citrate. Because this preparation is only used acutely, the problems listed in the previous paragraph are unlikely in this clinical situation.

RECOMMENDED READING

American Pharmaceutical Association. *Handbook of Nonprescription Drugs.* Washington, DC, 1996. Pp. 261–271.

American Pharmaceutical Association. *Nonprescription Products: Formulations and Features 96–97.* Washington, DC, 1996. Pp. 261–271.

Brunton, L.L. Agents for control of astric acidity and treatment of peptic ulcers. Chapter 27 in *Goodman and Gilman's The Pharmacological Basis of Therapeutics* (9th ed.), J.G. Hardman and L.E. Limbird, eds. New York: McGraw-Hill, 1996. Pp 910–913.

Colomina, M.T., et al. Lack of maternal and developmental toxicity in mice given high doses of aluminum hydroxide and ascorbic acid during gestation. *Pharmacol. Toxicol.* 74: 236, 1994.

Domingo, J.L. Reproductive and developmental toxicity of aluminum: a review. *Neurotoxicol. Teratol.* 17:515, 1995.

Gibbs, C.P., and Banner, T.C. Effectiveness of Bicitra as a preoperative antacid. *Anesthesiology* 61:97, 1984.

McElnay, J.C., et al. The interaction of digoxin with antacid constituents. *Br. Med. J.* 1:1554, 1978.

Nelson, M.M., and Forfar, J.O. Associations between drugs administered during pregnancy and congenital abnormalities of the fetus. *Br. Med. J.* 1:523, 1971.

Schenkel, B., and Vorherr, H. Non-prescription drugs during pregnancy: potential teratogenic and toxic effects upon embryo and fetus. *J. Reprod. Med.* 12:27, 1974.

Anticholinesterases: Ambenonium (Mytelase®), Edrophonium (Tensilon®), Neostigmine (Prostigmin®), Physostigmine (Eserine®), Pyridostigmine (Mestinon®)

INDICATIONS AND RECOMMENDATIONS

Neostigmine and pyridostigmine are safe to use for the treatment of myasthenia gravis in pregnancy. Reports of the use of ambenonium and edrophonium in obstetric patients are limited, and while these drugs are probably safe, they are relatively contraindicated because the other agents in this group have been used more extensively. It is preferable to avoid physostigmine for this indication because it has a greater theoretical propensity to cross the placenta.

These agents are reversible anticholinesterase compounds. By inhibiting acetylcholinesterase, they result in the accumulation of acetylcholine at cholinergic receptor sites and are therefore capable of causing effects that resemble excessive cholinergic stimulation throughout the central and peripheral nervous systems. These drugs are used therapeutically in the treatment of glaucoma, myasthenia gravis, atony of intestinal and bladder smooth muscle, and to terminate the effects of competitive neuromuscular blocking drugs.

SPECIAL CONSIDERATIONS IN PREGNANCY

Although the reversible cholinesterase inhibitors have been shown to cause vertebral malformations and leg muscle hypoplasia in quail and chick embryos, there is no evidence for their teratogenicity in humans to date. Furthermore, despite theoretical concerns that these agents might promote premature labor, there is no evidence that this occurs, even when the drugs are given parenterally.

No congenital defects were noted in one report of 22 first-trimester exposures to neostigmine. In another study, 27 gravidas were given small doses of neostigmine for 3 days before the 14th week of pregnancy. One patient miscarried, and the other 26 delivered at or near term without reported complications or anomalies. One case report, however, describes a transient, but significant, fetal bradycardia in association with neostigmine use during an orthopedic procedure during the third trimester.

Pyridostigmine has been associated with changes in neurotransmitter levels in the rat brain, but this effect has not been documented in humans. The findings of the Collaborative Perinatal Project did not describe any adverse pregnancy outcomes related to use of this drug.

Unlike neostigmine and pyridostigmine, which are quaternary compounds, physostigmine is a tertiary ammonium compound that easily crosses both the blood–brain and placental barriers. In one study, this drug was given intravenously to laboring patients to reverse scopolamine delirium. All of the 15 women in this series became cooperative and oriented within 3–5 minutes, and all of their infants had 5-minute Apgar scores of 8 or greater.

Cholinesterase inhibitors may affect the neonates of myasthenic mothers treated with these agents throughout pregnancy. From 15% to 20% of newborns born to myasthenic women develop transient muscular weakness, and some authors have postulated that the anticholinesterases may contribute to this short-lived phenomenon. It is more likely, however, that this effect is due to the placental transfer of acetylcholine receptor blocking antibodies. The onset of neonatal myasthenia gravis actually may be delayed secondary to in utero exposure to anticholinesterase agents.

The use of ester-type local anesthetics, such as chlorprocaine and tetracaine, is relatively contraindicated in patients receiving anticholinesterase medications, as there may be increased toxicity.

Contrary to an earlier report, as well as what would be predicted from physicochemical laws of membrane transport, pyridostigmine has been shown to enter breast milk. Postpartum milk concentrations have been found to approximate those found in maternal plasma. By the 60th postpartum day, milk concentrations were noted to be 40% of those in maternal plasma. The amount of drug ingested by this route is negligible, but these data demonstrate that presumably ionized quaternary ammonium compounds do enter breast milk and therefore may also traverse the placenta. No evidence of infant toxicity has been described in association with pyridostigmine, although colic is a potential side effect. Pyridostigmine is considered compatible with breast-feeding by the American Academy of Pediatrics.

DOSAGE

In the treatment of myasthenia gravis, the optimal single dose of an anticholinesterase is determined by observing the patient's response to graduated doses. After establishing baseline values of vital capacity and muscular strength, an oral dose of 7.5 mg neostigmine or 30 mg pyridostigmine is given. Improvements in muscular strength are noted at frequent intervals until there is a return to the basal state. One hour later, the drug is again given, with the dose increased by 50% over the initial amount, and the observational process is repeated. This sequence is continued with increasing increments of one-half the initial dose until an optimal effect is achieved. The ideal single oral dose may range from the initial doses cited to more than 10 times these amounts.

An alternate approach is to give successive low-dose intravenous injections of neostigmine (0.125 mg) or pyridostigmine (0.5 mg) at intervals of several minutes while monitoring muscle strength in the same fashion as described previously. If the parenteral approach is used, the patient should be premedicated with 0.4–0.6 mg atropine to prevent muscarinic side effects. When the maximally effective total intravenous dosage has been established, the optimal single oral dose is approximately 30 times that amount.

Neostigmine is available in 15-mg oral tablets, usually taken every 2–4 hours. Pyridostigmine is available for oral use in 60-mg tablets taken every 3–6 hours or in a 180 mg sustained release tablet for use at bedtime. Ambenonium is marketed in 10-mg tablets and is taken every 3–6 hours.

Physostigmine salicylate is available in various strengths as an ophthalmic solution either alone or in combination with pilocarpine nitrate.

ADVERSE EFFECTS

Anticholinesterase compounds cause multiple side effects at both nicotinic and muscarinic sites. At autonomic effectors, miosis, spasm of accommodation, reduction of intraocular pressure, decreased heart rate, dilatation of blood vessels, increased gastrointestinal motility and secretion, and stimulation of secretory glands can occur. Skeletal muscle shows increased strength of contraction and occasionally fibrillation. Patients may experience muscle cramps, fasciculations, and/or weakness. Central nervous system effects include confusion and ataxia. Overdosage may lead to death from respiratory failure. Cardiovascular effects include bradycardia. It is sometimes difficult to know whether a patient's weakness is due to her myasthenia or to overdosage with an anticholinesterase. In this situation a neurologist should be urgently consulted and asked to evaluate the patient. Edrophonium may be used to differentiate between these two conditions, but extreme caution must be exercised because this drug can cause a respiratory arrest if the weakness is cholinergic in origin.

MECHANISM OF ACTION

All of these agents reversibly inhibit acetylcholinesterase at the neuromuscular junction. Several of these drugs exert a direct effect on the skeletal muscle. Anticholinesterase agents also stimulate postganglionic parasympathetic neurons, thus accounting for their muscarinic effects. Physostigmine is a naturally occurring tertiary amine and neostigmine is a synthetic quaternary compound. Both have a carbamyl ester linkage and are hydrolyzed by acetylcholinesterase, but much more slowly than is acetylcholine. The duration of acetylcholinesterase inhibition by the carbamylating agents is 3–4 hours. Pyridostigmine is a close congener of neostigmine. Edrophonium is an analog of neostigmine that lacks the carbamyl group. It has a brief duration of action because of the reversibility of its binding to acetylcholinesterase and rapid elimination by the kidneys after systemic administration. Because of its short action, edrophonium is often used in the "Tensilon test" to diagnose or verify optimization of dosage in the treatment of myasthenia gravis. Ambenonium is a potent bis-quaternary compound that is also used in the treatment of myasthenia gravis.

ABSORPTION AND BIOTRANSFORMATION

Physostigmine is readily absorbed from the intestines, subcutaneous tissues, and mucous membranes. The conjunctival instillation of this drug may cause systemic effects if measures are not taken to prevent absorption from the nasal mucosa. Physostigmine is largely metabolized by hydrolytic cleavage at the ester linkage by cholinesterases, and renal excretion plays only a minor role in its disposal. A 1-mg dose injected subcutaneously is largely destroyed within 2 hours.

Neostigmine and the related quaternary ammonium compounds are absorbed poorly after oral administration, which is why much larger doses are necessary than when they are administered parenterally. Neostigmine is metabolized by plasma esterases and the quaternary alcohol and parent compound are excreted in the urine. Significant placental transfer would not be expected, as this drug is highly ionized. Pyridostigmine and its quaternary alcohol are also excreted by the kidneys. The concentration of pyridostigmine in fetal blood is equivalent to that in maternal blood.

RECOMMENDED READING

American Academy of Pediatrics. The transfer of drugs and other chemicals into human milk. *Pediatrics* 93:137, 1994.

Clark, R.B., Brown, M.A., and Lattin, D.L. Neostigmine, atropine and glycopyrrolate: does neostigmine cross the placenta? *Anesthesiology* 84:450, 1996.

Fennell D.F., and Ringel, S.P. Myasthenia gravis and pregnancy. *Obstet. Gynecol. Surv.* 41:414, 1987.

Landauer, W. Cholinomimetic teratogens: studies with chicken embryos. *Teratology* 12:125, 1975.

Meiniel, R. Neuromuscular blocking agents and axial teratogenesis in the avian embryo. Can axial morphogenetic disorders be explained by pharmacological action upon muscle tissue? *Teratology* 23:259, 1981.

Smiller, B.G., et al. Physostigmine reversal of scopolamine delirium in obstetric patients. *Am. J. Obstet. Gynecol.* 116: 326, 1973.

Taylor, P. Anticholinesterase agents. Chapter 8 in *Goodman and Gilman's The Pharmacological Basis of Therapeutics* (9th ed.), J.G. Hardman and L.E. Limbird, eds. New York: McGraw-Hill, 1996. Pp. 161–176.

Wise, G.A., and McQuillen, M.R. Transient myasthenia of the newborn. Clinical and electromyographic studies. *Trans. Am. Neurol. Assoc.* 94:100, 1969.

Antihistamines (Over-the-Counter): Brompheniramine, Chlorpheniramine, Cyclizine, Doxylamine, Meclizine, Phenindamine, Pheniramine, Pyrilamine

INDICATIONS AND RECOMMENDATIONS

The over-the-counter (OTC) antihistamines vary in their chemical composition but are similar in that they are generally antagonists of the H_1 receptor. Their use in pregnancy should be limited to the treatment of allergic symptoms, the prophylaxis of motion sickness, and as sedatives. They have no proven value in treating the common cold. The antihistamine compounds available in OTC preparations, with the exception of brompheniramine, have not been implicated as having deleterious effects in the pregnant woman or fetus. As with any drug, however, antihistamines should be used only when absolutely necessary during pregnancy. Chlorpheniramine does not appear to have teratogenic effects at recommended dosages; however, no prospective studies are available. These drugs are not recommended for use by lactating women because of the possibility of lactation inhibition.

SPECIAL CONSIDERATIONS IN PREGNANCY

A large-scale study of drugs that could possibly have a teratogenic effect if taken during pregnancy included the following antihistamines available in OTC preparations: chlorpheniramine, pheniramine, and brompheniramine. Of these, only with first-trimester exposure to brompheniramine was there a statistically significant increased risk of teratogenicity. A subsequent prospective cohort study failed to confirm such an association, however, and a meta-analysis of published studies revealed no significant increase in the relative risk for malformations when brompheniramine was ingested during the first trimester. Animal studies have implicated meclizine and cyclizine as teratogenic agents. Large-scale studies in humans, however, have not shown an increased incidence of death or malformations in children of women who used any of these drugs during pregnancy. When, as is usual, they are found in combination products, the potential effects of all ingredients must be considered. In a study of 3026 surviving infants with birth weights of less than 1750 g, an association was found between maternal antihistamine use within 2 weeks of delivery and the likelihood of retrolental fibroplasia. These findings have not been independently corroborated.

Due to its anticholinergic properties, chlorpheniramine may inhibit lactation. In addition, small amounts may be secreted into breast milk. This drug and all antihistamines, therefore, should be avoided by the lactating mother.

DOSAGE

The dosage amount of any of these antihistamines varies with the particular preparation in which it is found. They are often found combined with other ingredients.

ADVERSE EFFECTS

Side effects of antihistamines are most commonly anticholinergic in nature and include dryness of the mouth, difficulty in voiding, and, rarely, impotence. Dizziness, lassitude, incoordination, fatigue, blurred vision, and nervousness also occur. Digestive tract effects include anorexia, nausea, vomiting, constipation, and diarrhea, all of which may be avoided by taking the drug with meals. Leukopenia and agranulocytosis are rarely seen. Toxic doses result in hallucinations, ataxia, athetosis, and convulsions. Death may result from cardiorespiratory collapse.

MECHANISM OF ACTION

Antihistamines act by competitive antagonism to prevent histamine from exerting its vasodilatory and bronchoconstrictive effects. They are effective in suppressing the symptoms of seasonal rhinitis but are less effective in the treatment of perennial rhinitis. They may also be effective in the treatment of certain allergic dermatoses. Antihistamines also have central effects that account for their sedative properties and their efficacy in the prevention of motion sickness.

ABSORPTION AND BIOTRANSFORMATION

The pharmacokinetics of these drugs are not well known. They are well absorbed from the gastrointestinal tract. As a group, they seem to be metabolized in the liver with little if any being excreted unchanged in the urine.

RECOMMENDED READING

Babe, K.S., Jr., and Serafin, W.E. Histamine, bradykinin, and their antagonists. Chapter 25 in *Goodman and Gilman's The Pharma-*

cological Basis of Therapeutics (9th ed.), J.G. Hardman and L.E. Limbird, eds. New York: McGraw-Hill, 1996. Pp. 581–592.

Greenberger, P., and Patterson, R. Safety of therapy for allergic symptoms during pregnancy. *Ann. Intern. Med.* 89:234, 1978.

Heinonen, O.P., Slone, D., and Shapiro, S. *Birth Defects and Drugs in Pregnancy.* Littleton, MA: Wright-PSG, 1977. Pp. 322–334.

Seto A., Einarson T., and Koren, G. Evaluation of brompheniramine safety in pregnancy. *Reprod. Toxicol.* 7:393, 1993.

Zierler, S., and Purohit, D. Prenatal antihistamine exposure and retrolental fibroplasia. *Am. J. Epidemiol.* 123:192, 1986.

Antihistamines: Nonsedating Selective H₁ Antagonists: Astemizole (Hismanal®), Loratidine (Claritin®), Terfenadine (Seldane®)

INDICATIONS AND RECOMMENDATIONS

The piperidine antihistamines listed above are second-generation H_1 receptor antagonists, which have not been well evaluated during pregnancy. They are used in the symptomatic treatment of various immediate hypersensitivity reactions where there is rhinitis, urticaria, and/or conjunctivitis. They are commonly used to treat seasonal rhinitis and conjunctivitis. Both terfenadine and astemizole can cause torsade de pointes, a form of polymorphic ventricular tachycardia, when taken in excessive doses or in combination with certain other drugs such as macrolide antibiotics such as erythromycin, clarithromycin, or troleandomycin, or antifungal agents such as ketoconazole or itraconazole, or in situations of impaired hepatic function. The mechanism is inhibition of the specific cytochrome P_{450} enzyme that metabolizes the drug, leading to toxicity. Loratidine does not appear to share this property with the other two agents. Because there is a single cohort study that failed to find increased pregnancy risk with astemizole, this drug is probably the most reasonable to prescribe when a nonsedating, selective H_1 receptor antagonist is deemed necessary during pregnancy. Caution must be exercised to avoid coadministration of the other drugs listed above, to avoid excessive dosage, and to rule out significant hepatic impairment when astemizole is prescribed.

SPECIAL CONSIDERATIONS IN PREGNANCY

A single prospective cohort study of astemizole has been published by investigators in Toronto and Philadelphia. A total of 114 women who called pregnancy hotlines and reported astemizole use during the first trimester were registered and then followed up after delivery. Pregnancy outcomes were compared with those of a set of matched controls, consisting of the next woman calling the hotline and matching for age, smoking, and alcohol use, who inquired about exposure to nonteratogens. There were no significant differences in pregnancy outcomes, and the incidence of major congenital malformations was identical (1.9%) in exposed and control groups. In view of the fact that animal teratogenicity studies were also reassuring, the authors conclude that astemizole can be used safely during pregnancy when indicated.

DOSAGE

The piperidine second generation H_1 receptor antagonists are all administered orally, and all are relatively long acting. Astemizole and loratidine are given in a 10-mg dose every 24 hours, whereas terfenadine is given as 60 mg every 12 hours. Ventricular arrhythmias have been reported with single overdoses of terfenadine as low as 360 mg and of astemizole as low as 20–30 mg daily.

ADVERSE EFFECTS

Other than the above-mentioned ventricular arrhythmias in the circumstance of overdosage, concomitant administration of certain other drugs, or liver dysfunction, side effects of piperidine second generation H_1 receptor antagonists have been relatively uncommon. Unlike first-generation agents, they are not sedating. Weight gain, angioedema, asymptomatic liver enzyme elevations, and hypersensitivity have been reported.

MECHANISM OF ACTION

These drugs are highly selective for H_1 receptors. They inhibit the response to histamine in a number of areas, including respiratory smooth muscle, and particularly capillary permeability which leads to edema and wheal formation, and the "flare-and-itch" response of nerve endings. Because they do not penetrate the central nervous system to any great extent and have little anticholinergic activity, their side effect profile is quite favorable.

ABSORPTION AND BIOTRANSFORMATION

The piperidine second-generation H_1 receptor antagonists are well absorbed after oral administration. Absorption of astemizole is reduced significantly when the drug is taken with meals, whereas that of loratidine is enhanced. Terfenadine and astemizole are converted to their carboxy metabolites, which are the active forms of the drugs, in their first pass through the liver.

RECOMMENDED READING

Babe, K.S. Jr., and Serafin, W.E. Histamine, bradykinin, and their antagonists. Chapter 25 in *Goodman and Gilman's The Pharmacological Basis of Therapeutics* (9th ed.), J.G. Hardman and L.E. Limbird, eds. New York: McGraw-Hill, 1996. Pp. 586–592.

Hoechst Marion Roussel Company. Seldane (terfenadine). Entry in *Physicians Desk Reference* (52nd ed.). Montvale, NJ: Medical Economics, 1998. Pp. 1238–1244.

Janssen Pharmaceutica. Hismanal (astemiizole): Entry in *Physicians Desk Reference* (52nd ed.). Montvale, NJ: Medical Economics, 1998. Pp. 1303–1304.

Pastuszak, A., Schick, B., Alimonte, D., et al. The safety of astemizole in pregnancy. *J. Allergy Clin. Immunol.* 98:748, 1996.

Schering Company. Claritin (loratadine). Entry in *Physicians Desk Reference* (52nd ed.). Montvale, NJ: Medical Economics, 1998. Pp. 2613–2620.

Antiretroviral Agents

Although there are a number of different antiretroviral agents and their mechanisms of action vary considerably, such agents are considered together in this section because of certain features held in common:

1. All were relatively recently developed, and consequently there are no long-term data, and few short-term data, regarding their effects on the fetus and offspring when they are administered during pregnancy.
2. All are used in the treatment of acquired immune deficiency syndrome (AIDS), a condition that is uniformly fatal, and their use is considered life extending if not life saving.
3. Some are used prophylactically in order to prevent acquisition of human immunodeficiency virus (HIV) or vertical transmission of the agent. This use should be considered as potentially life saving.

Therefore, this is a group of drugs that might not be considered "safe in pregnancy" under more typical circumstances, but that are often prescribed in view of the lack of viable alternatives. In general, patients should be made aware of the uncertainties associated with the use of antiretroviral agents during pregnancy, but also should be made aware of the relative certainty of adverse consequences when no treatment is taken. When therapy is to be initiated or changed during pregnancy, consideration should be given to choosing agents for which the greatest amount of pregnancy experience has been accumulated, particularly during the period of organogenesis.

The antiretroviral drugs fall into three main categories: (a) nucleoside analog reverse transcriptase inhibitors, (b) nonnucleoside reverse transcriptase inhibitors, and (c) protease inhibitors. The reverse transcriptase inhibitors interfere with the functioning of an enzyme necessary for viral replication, whereas the protease inhibitors interfere with the production of precursors of structural proteins and enzymes necessary for viral function. In general, combinations of antiretroviral agents are preferable to single agents because of their ability to reduce the viral load to levels below current limits of detectability. Most regimens contain two nucleoside analog reverse transcriptase inhibitors plus a protease inhibitor with strong in vivo potency or a nonnucleoside reverse transcriptase inhibitor. Such strong viral suppression may delay the appearance of viral resistance to the various agents. The details of the various multiple drug regimens are beyond the scope of this book.

Until recently, antiretroviral therapy was recommended only for symptomatic individuals or asymptomatic individuals with CD4 cell counts under 500/μl. Current recommendations of the

International AIDS Society USA Panel are that antiretroviral therapy be initiated for any patient whose plasma HIV RNA concentration exceeds 5000–10,000 copies per milliliter of plasma. In addition, patients with HIV infection and any detectable plasma HIV RNA who request therapy, and are committed to lifelong adherence, should be considered for therapy. The panel recommends that antiretroviral therapy not be withheld because of pregnancy when indicated for the health of the mother. Because there are no data regarding the safety and efficacy of specific treatment regimens during pregnancy, the panel recommends continuation of ongoing therapy in patients already taking combination therapy who become pregnant; however, because of the demonstrated success of zidovudine in reducing vertical transmission, this drug should be included as a component of any antiretroviral regimen used during pregnancy whenever possible.

NUCLEOSIDE REVERSE TRANSCRIPTASE INHIBITORS

Zidovudine (AZT, Retrovir®)

Indications and Recommendations

Zidovudine is an exception to the statement about the relative lack of short-term data regarding the use of antiretroviral agents in pregnancy. A nucleoside reverse transcriptase inhibitor, it was the first antiretroviral agent to be approved by the FDA. This drug has been used extensively in the treatment of HIV infection and was the therapy used in the protocol of Pediatric AIDS Clinical Trials Study Group 076, a randomized, placebo-controlled trial that demonstrated a reduction of vertical transmission from 26% to 8% in infants of mothers with HIV infections and CD4+ T-lymphocyte counts above 200 cells per cubic centimeter, who had not previously received antiretroviral therapy. Because the 076 trial involved zidovudine treatment beginning only after the time of organogenesis, the fact that infants exposed to the drug had no greater likelihood of malformations than placebo-exposed offspring does not rule out the possibility of teratogenesis with earlier exposure. Follow-up for 2 years did not reveal neurodevelopmental problems in these offspring. Small case series have not noted an excess of congenital malformations in infants exposed to zidovudine in utero, but the possibility still exists.

Zidovudine has been shown to cross the placenta to the fetus. In baboons, zidovudine levels are higher in cordocentesis obtained fetal than maternal blood and highest in amniotic fluid. Pharmacokinetic studies in humans at term showed similar or higher levels in umbilical cord blood at birth compared to maternal blood, but the neonatal half-life was 10 times that of the mother.

Dosage

Zidovudine is available as 100 mg capsules, 300 mg tablets, and syrup containing 50 mg/5 ml. The usual recommended dosage of zidovudine is 500–600 mg/day in divided doses. For prevention of maternal–fetal transmission, the drug should continue to be administered intravenously when the mother is in labor. A loading dose of 2 mg/kg of total body weight should be given over 1 hour, followed by a continuous infusion of 1 mg/kg/hour until the clamping of the umbilical cord.

Adverse Effects

Zidovudine has a number of known toxicities, including granulocytopenia and anemia, complications that are dose-related but also tend to occur more often in sicker patients. Symptoms such as headache, nausea and vomiting, insomnia, and myalgias often occur when therapy is initiated. Nail pigmentation, myopathy, neurotoxicity, hepatitis, esophageal ulceration, and macular edema have also been reported.

A number of potential drug interactions have been described. Fluconazole can inhibit glucuronidation of zidovudine, and probenecid may decrease renal excretion; either agent may increase the risk of bone marrow suppression. Clarithromycin decreases absorption. Rifampin can decrease plasma concentration of zidovudine. Coadministration with ganciclovir may increase the risk of hematologic toxicity. Somnolence has been reported when zidovudine was given with acyclovir.

Mechanism of Action

Zidovudine is a thymidine analog reverse transcriptase inhibitor with activity against retroviruses. After entering cells, the drug is phosphorylated by thymidine kinase, converted to a diphosphate, and then converted to a triphosphate by thymidylate kinase. The triphosphate competetively inhibits reverse transcriptase, competing with thymidine triphosphate. This causes DNA chain termination. Zidovudine preferentially inhibits HIV reverse transcriptase compared to human DNA polymerases. The HIV virus is able to mutate into resistant strains, making zidovudine less effective with long-term use.

Absorption and Biotransformation

Studies in humans have suggested similar absorption and elimination during pregnancy as in nonpregnant individuals. Oral bioavailability is 60% to 70%. Peak plasma levels are reached 30–90 minutes after a single oral dose. The serum half-life is approximately 1.3 hours. Zidovudine is converted to an inactive glucuronide metabolite during a first pass through the liver. As noted above, there is evidence of preferential accumulation in the fetal compartment and amniotic fluid.

Didanosine (ddI, Videx®)

Indications and Recommendations

Didanosine is a purine nucleoside analog reverse transcriptase inhibitor with activity against retroviruses. It was first approved for treatment of advanced infection, particularly in patients who had failed a prolonged course of zidovudine. It is often used in combination with zidovudine and stavudine. There is little information available regarding its effects in pregnancy, although it has been shown to cross the placenta. Its mechanism of action is similar to that of zidovudine, and it is orally absorbed. Peripheral neuropathy, pancreatitis, and gastrointestinal disturbances are the major side effects. It is reasonable for patients who conceive while taking this drug to continue taking it during pregnancy, provided they are counseled appropriately regarding the dearth of information about its effect on pregnancy.

Zalcitabine (ddC, Hivid®)

Zalcitabine is a cytosine nucleoside analog reverse transcriptase inhibitor with activity against retroviruses. It may be used in combination with zidovudine but is said to be the least potent of the nucleoside analogs. There are no data regarding zalcitabine's use in human pregnancy. In one study of fetal rats, zalcitabine had a toxic effect on thymus cells, raising the possibility of adverse effects on neonatal immunity. For this reason, it would be best to use other agents in pregnancy, when possible.

Stavudine (d4T, Zerit®)

Stavudine is a thymidine nucleoside analog reverse transcriptase inhibitor with activity against retroviruses. It may be used in place of zidovudine in patients who have failed zidovudine-containing regimens or who cannot tolerate zidovudine. It should not be used in combination with zidovudine because the two drugs may be antagonistic. There are no data regarding the use of stavudine during human pregnancy. The primary side effect is sensory neuropathy, occurring in 15% to 20% of patients. It is reasonable for patients who conceive while taking this drug to continue taking it during pregnancy, provided they are counseled appropriately regarding the dearth of information about its effect on pregnancy.

Lamivudine (3TC, Epivir®)

Lamivudine is a cytidine nucleoside analog reverse transcriptase inhibitor with activity against retroviruses. It is also active against hepatitis B. It may be used together with zidovudine or stavudine to reduce viral load and prevent emergence of zidovudine resistance. Data on use in human pregnancy are lacking, but it is reasonable for patients who conceive while taking this drug to continue it during pregnancy, provided they are counseled appropriately.

NONNUCLEOSIDE REVERSE TRANSCRIPTASE INHIBITORS

Nonnucleoside reverse transcriptase inhibitors inhibit HIV replication by binding to viral reverse transcriptase, rather than by undergoing intracellular metabolism masquerading as nucleosides. Resistance may develop quickly due to point mutations in the binding sites on reverse transcriptase. Because of the likelihood of rapid resistance developing, these drugs are generally used in combination with two nucleoside reverse transcriptase inhibitors rather than as monoagent therapy.

Nevirapine (Viramune®)

Nevirapine was the first available nonnucleoside reverse transcriptase inhibitor. It acts synergistically with nucleoside reverse transcriptase inhibitors. It is used in triple-drug regimens, most often with zidovudine and didanosine, a strategy called "convergent combination therapy." No information regarding human pregnancy could be located. Rash, including Stevens-Johnson syndrome, fever, nausea, and headache are commonly reported side effects.

Delavirdine (Rescriptor®)

Delavirdine acts synergistically with both nucleoside reverse transcriptase inhibitors and protease inhibitors. Although delavirdine was teratogenic in rats at considerably higher doses than would be utilized clinically, human data are lacking. The primary side effect reported has been skin rash.

PROTEASE INHIBITORS

Aspartate protease is an enzyme of HIV viruses which cleaves precursor proteins into functional core proteins necessary for viral maturation and replication. The protease inhibitors bind to the protease enzyme and are highly active against HIV. Some are analogs of peptide substrates, whereas others utilize alternative mechanisms. The use of protease inhibitors has been associated with increased bleeding in patients with hemophilia, hyperglycemia, and new onset or worsening of preexisting diabetes. Adverse interactions with other drugs are common, so much so that a listing is beyond the scope of this book. Readers are referred to *The Medical Letter* (39:111, 1997) for a list of such potential drug interactions. The introduction of protease inhibitors has been associated with marked improvement in the clinical course of HIV infections. By and large, the protease inhibitors are so new that human pregnancy information is lacking. Whereas under ordinary circumstances it would be preferable to advise pregnant women to avoid such drugs, this class of antiretroviral agents has made such a tremendous clinical impact that discontinuance could pose a significant threat to the lives and health of the involved women.

Saquinavir (Invirase®, Fortovase®)

Saquinavir is synergistic with reverse transcriptase inhibitors. Invirase was not very well absorbed, which was probably a factor in resistance and clinical failure. It has been reformulated as Fortovase, a soft gel preparation that has greater bioavailability. It is generally combined with nucleoside reverse transcriptase inhibitors and also is more bioavailable when combined with ritonavir, another protease inhibitor. Although the drug was not teratogenic in tests on rats, no human data are available. The most significant side effects have been diarrhea, nausea, and abdominal discomfort.

Ritonavir (Norvir®)

Ritonavir has been highly effective in patients with advanced disease and previous treatment with antiretroviral agents. As with saquinavir, no data regarding human pregnancy are available. Adverse effects include nausea and vomiting, diarrhea, asthenia, paresthesias, altered taste, renal failure, liver enzyme elevations, and elevations in cholesterol and triglycerides.

Indinavir (Crixivan)

Indinavir is generally combined with two nucleoside reverse transcriptase inhibitors and has been highly effective in lowering HIV RNA levels to undetectable levels in small studies of patients with low CD4 counts. Side effects included hyperbilirubinemia in 10% of patients, hemolytic anemia and hepatitis, kidney stones and crystalluria. No human pregnancy information is available.

RECOMMENDED READING

American College of Obstetricians and Gynecologists. *Human Immunodeficiency Virus Infections in Pregnancy.* ACOG Educational Bulletin #232. Washington, DC, 1997.

Bawdon, R.E., Sobhi, S., and Dax, J. The transfer of antihuman immunodeficiency virus nucleoside compounds by the term human placenta. *Am. J. Obstet. Gynecol.* 167:1570, 1992.

Carpenter, C.J., Fischl, M.A., Hammer, S.M., et al. Antiretroviral therapy for HIV infection in 1997: updated recommendations of the International AIDS Society-USA Panel. *J.A.M.A.* 277:1962, 1997.

Connor, E.M., Sperling, R.S., Gelber, R., et al., for the Pediatric AIDS Clinical Trials Group Protocol 076 Study Group. Reduction of maternal-infant transmission of human immunodeficiency virus type 1 with zidovudine treatment. *N. Engl. J. Med.* 331:1173, 1994.

Connor, E.M., Sperling, R.S., Shapiro, D., et al. Long term effect of ZDV exposure among uninfected infants born to HIV-infected mothers in AIDS clinical trials group 076. In *Proceedings of the 35th Annual Meeting of the Interscience Conference on Antimicrobial Agents and Chemotherapy;* San Francisco, 1995.

Dienstag, J., Perrillo, R., Schiff, E., et al. A preliminary trial of lamivudine for chronic hepatitis B infection. *N. Engl. J. Med.* 333:1657, 1995.

Foerster, M., Kastner, U., and Neubert, R. Effect of six virustatic nucleoside analogs on the development of fetal rat thymus in organ culture. *Arch. Toxicol.* 66:688, 1992.

Hankins, G.D.V., Lowery, C.L., Jr., Scott, R.T., et al. Transplacental transfer of zidovudine in the near-term pregnant baboon. *Am. J. Obstet. Gynecol.* 163:728, 1990.

Hayden, F.G. Antimicrobial agents: antiviral agents. Chapter 50 in *Goodman and Gilman's The Pharmacological Basis of Therapeutics* (9th ed.), J.G. Hardman and L.E. Limbard, eds. New York: McGraw-Hill, 1996. Pp. 1191–1223.

Medical Letter, Inc. Drugs for HIV infection. *The Medical Letter on Drugs and Therapeutics* 39:111, 1997.

Minkoff, H., and Augenbraun, M. Antiretroviral therapy for pregnant women. *Am. J. Obstet. Gynecol.* 1776:478, 1997.

O'Sullivan, M.J., Boyer, P.J.J., Scott, G.B., et al. The pharmacokinetics and safety of zidovudine in the third trimester of pregnancy for women infected with human immunodeficiency virus and their infants: phase I Acquired Immunodeficiency Syndrome Clinical Trials Group study (protocol 082). *Am. J. Obstet. Gynecol.* 168:1510, 1993.

Pons, J.C., Borbon, M.C., Taburet, A.M., et al. Fetoplacental passage of 2',3'-dideoxyinosine. *Lancet* 337:732, 1991.

Sperling, R.S., Roboz, J., Dische, R., et al. Zidovudine pharmacokinetics during pregnancy. *Am. J. Perinatol.* 9:247, 1992.

Sperling, R.S., Stratton, P., O'Sullivan, M.J., et al. A survey of zidovudine use in pregnant women with Human Immunodeficiency Virus infection. *N. Engl. J. Med.* 326:857, 1992.

Watts, D.H., Brown, Z.A., Tartaglione, T., et al. Pharmacokinetic disposition of zidovudine during pregnancy. *J. Infect. Dis.* 163:226, 1991.

White, A., Andrews, E., Eldridge, R., et al. Birth outcomes following zidovudine therapy in pregnant women. *M.M.W.R.* 43:409, 1994.

Aspartame (Equal®, Nutrasweet®)

INDICATIONS AND RECOMMENDATIONS

Aspartame, a nonnutritive artificial sweetener that is a combination of aspartic acid and phenylalanine, is safe for use during pregnancy. The FDA has approved the use of aspartame by the general population, including pregnant and lactating women. As with all foods containing phenylalanine, pregnant women with phenylketonuria should avoid ingesting aspartame.

SPECIAL CONSIDERATIONS IN PREGNANCY

There is no evidence that this agent is teratogenic in animals. Persons with phenylketonuria (PKU) are unable to metabolize phenylalanine normally. Sustained high maternal serum levels of phenylalanine are associated with mental retardation and microcephaly in infants of PKU mothers who do not restrict their diets during pregnancy. Because aspartame contains phenylalanine, there has been concern that the ingestion of large amounts of this food additive by pregnant women may be harmful to the fetus. Maternal blood phenylalanine levels below 60 μmol/dl have not been associated with adverse fetal effects, whereas levels above 110 μmol/dl are usually associated with mental retardation. Clinical testing has shown that the average 60 kg adult would have to consume 600 aspartame tablets or 24 L of aspartame-sweetened beverage at a single sitting to reach 50 μmol/dl, the blood level set by the FDA as being toxic to pregnant women. Therefore, although fetal toxicity might be possible if a pregnant phenylketonuric woman were continuously to ingest large levels of aspartame, there is a substantial safety factor between the blood levels that could occur in a heavy aspartame user and the lowest known toxic level for PKU patients. It is unlikely that adverse effects would be caused by customary intake of aspartame by a pregnant woman who is unaffected by PKU.

Aspartic acid, the second component of aspartame, does not readily cross the placenta and should not adversely affect the fetus in the amounts that would normally be consumed by a pregnant woman.

If stored at high temperatures or for long periods, aspartame decomposes to form methanol and diketopiperazine (DKP).

Methanol, a common decomposition product of dietary constituents, is produced in relatively small quantities. A liter of fruit juice would yield almost 3 times the methanol of a liter of aspartame-sweetened beverage, even if all of the aspartame decomposed. No measurable increases in blood levels of methanol occurred until single administered doses substantially exceeded the 99th percentile of expected aspartame use (see "Dosage," below). DKP is an uncommon constituent of foods; therefore, numerous animal studies were carried out with this compound prior to FDA approval of aspartame. It appears to be nontoxic to adults and children nor teratogenic or mutagenic in animals.

In one study of six healthy lactating women given 50 mg/kg aspartame, there was no significant increase in mean aspartate, glutamate, or glutamine levels. The phenylalanine level increased to 4 times above fasting, but fell to baseline after 4 hours.

DOSAGE

Aspartame is available in granulated form. One packet of Equal® contains 35 mg and is equivalent in sweetness to 2 teaspoonfuls of sugar. It is also available in tablet form. Carbonated beverages made with aspartame contain approximately 200 mg per 12 oz. serving. A multitude of other foods are now available with aspartame as the sweetening agent. The projected 99th percentile of aspartame intake in the general population is 34 mg/kg/day, or approximately 1700 mg for a 50-kg individual. This amount is equal to 8.5 12-oz. servings of aspartame-sweetened beverage, or approximately 50 packets of aspartame.

ADVERSE EFFECTS

No adverse effects of aspartame have been confirmed to date. However, the Centers for Disease Control (CDC) investigated numerous consumer complaints, which included headaches, dizziness, mood alterations, gastrointestinal symptoms, and allergic and dermatologic manifestations. The CDC found that the symptoms did not fit any specific pattern and that they were generally mild and common complaints in the general population. It concluded that while some people many be unusually sensitive to aspartame, the known data do not provide evidence that aspartame causes serious, widespread adverse effects.

MECHANISM OF ACTION

Aspartame, the methyl ester of aspartyl phenylalanine, has a sweetening potential approximately 200 times that of sucrose.

ABSORPTION AND BIOTRANSFORMATION

Aspartame is rapidly and completely hydrolyzed to its individual constituents: phenylalanine, aspartic acid, and methanol. These components are digested in the same way as natural constituents of the diet would be. The methyl group is hydrolyzed by intestinal esterases to methanol, which is oxidized to CO_2. The resultant dipeptide is split at the mucosal surface of the intestine by dipeptidases and the free amino acids are absorbed. The aspartic acid moiety is mainly transformed to CO_2 via the tricarboxylic acid cycle, whereas phenylalanine is incorporated into body protein unchanged or as the major metabolite tyrosine.

RECOMMENDED READING

Centers for Disease Control. Evaluation of consumer complaints related to aspartame use. *M.M.W.R.* 33:605, 1984.

Food and Drug Administration. Food additives permitted for direct addition to food for human consumption; aspartame. *Fed. Reg.* 48:31376, 1983.

Franz, M. Is it safe to consume aspartame during pregnancy? A review. *Diabetes Educator* 12:145, 1986.

Hayes, A.H., Jr. Summary of Commissioner's Decision on Aspartame. Department of Health and Human Services, Public Health Service, Food and Drug Administration, Docket No. 75F-0355. July 15, 1981.

Lennon, H. D., et al. The biological properties of aspartame. IV. Effects on reproduction and lactation. *J. Environ. Pathol. Toxicol.* 3:375, 1980.

Oppermann, J.A., Muldoon, E., and Ranney, R.E. The metabolism of aspartame in monkeys. *J. Nutr.* 103:1454, 1973.

Ranney, R.E., et al. The phenylalanine and tyrosine content of maternal and fetal body fluids from rabbits fed aspartame. *Toxicol. Appl. Pharmacol.* 32:339, 1975.

Stegink, L.D., Filer, L.J., and Baker, G.L. Plasma, erythrocyte and human milk levels of free amino acids in lactating women administered aspartame or lactose. *J. Nutr.* 109:2173, 1979.

Stegink, L.D., and Filer, L.J. *Aspartame Physiology and Biochemistry.* New York: Marcel Dekker, 1984.

Sturtevant, F.M. Use of aspartame in pregnancy. *Int. J. Fertil.* 30:85, 1985.

Tschanz, C., et al. *The Clinical Evaluation of a Food Additive: Assessment of Aspartame.* Boca Raton, FL: CRC Press, 1996.

Atosiban (Antocin®)

INDICATIONS AND RECOMMENDATIONS

Atosiban is a new tocolytic agent that is a specific antagonist of the oxytocin receptor, representing a new mechanism for the treatment of premature labor. At the time of this writing, the FDA is considering atosiban for approval as a tocolytic agent. Clinical studies show efficacy equivalent to β-mimetic therapy but with fewer side effects. Therefore, if approved, consideration should be given to atosiban for first-line therapy for the treatment of idiopathic premature labor.

SPECIAL CONSIDERATIONS IN PREGNANCY

In a study of 302 patients with well-documented acute preterm labor, intravenous atosiban was equally efficacious in comparison to intravenous ritodrine. In a study of 531 patients in preterm labor randomized to intravenous atosiban or intravenous placebo there was a significant increase in the percentage of patients undelivered at 48 hours and 7 days in the group treated with atosiban. In a separate group of 513 patients with preterm labor, initially treated with intravenous atosiban for up to 48 hours and then randomized to subcutaneous atosiban or placebo by pump, there was a significant increase in time until the first recurrence of labor in the atosiban group.

DOSAGE

For treatment of an acute episode of premature labor, the recommended dose is an initial intravenous bolus of 6.75 mg followed by an infusion of 300 µg/min for 3 hours, decreasing to a dose of 100 µg/min until uterine quiescence is achieved. For maintenance therapy, a subcutaneous infusion delivered by pump at a dose of 30 µg/min is recommended.

ADVERSE EFFECTS

In a study comparing the efficacy and safety of atosiban to ritodrine in 302 patients with premature labor, drug discontinuation due to side effects occurred in 26% of patients treated with ritodrine and 0.4% of patients treated with atosiban. In a double-blinded study of intravenous atosiban versus placebo therapy of 501 patients with preterm labor, nausea occurred more frequently in the atosiban group. With subcutaneous maintenance therapy, injection reaction sites and constipation occurred more frequently in the group randomized to atosiban in comparison to the group randomized to saline placebo. Once FDA approval occurs, the package insert may list other side effects. At the time of this writing, infant follow-up data including neurologic and developmental studies at birth, 6, 12, and 24 months, are still in progress in more than 1000 pregnancies treated with atosiban during pregnancy. Preliminary results in the 302 patients randomized to atosiban versus ritodrine show equivalent results on testing of infants at 6 and 12 months.

MECHANISM OF ACTION

Atosiban is a synthetic analog of oxytocin that is a specific competitive antagonist for the oxytocin receptor. It inhibits oxytocin-mediated intracellular calcium release in a dose-dependent fashion. In vitro it reduces oxytocin-stimulated prostaglandin synthesis. Despite structural homologies with vasopressin it has no measurable cardiovascular or antidiuretic activity in humans at usual dosages.

ABSORPTION AND BIOTRANSFORMATION

Atosiban is a nonapeptide and therefore cannot be administered orally due to degradation. Intravenous and subcutaneous routes of delivery have been most completely studied, with limited information on intranasal administration. With use of an initial intravenous bolus, steady-state levels are achieved within 15 minutes, and the half-life is 18 minutes. Atosiban is well absorbed by subcutaneous injection, with 97% bioavailability. Following a single subcutaneous dose, peak levels are observed at 30 minutes. Atosiban does cross the placenta in humans. However, umbilical vein concentrations are only 12% of the concentration in maternal uterine vein.

RECOMMENDED READING

Goodwin T.M., Paul R., Silver H.M., Spellacy W., Parsons M., et al. The effect of the oxytocin antagonist atosiban on preterm uterine activity in the human. *Am. J. Obstet. Gynecol.* 170: 474, 1994.

Goodwin, T.M., Valenzuela, G.J., Silver, H., and Creasy, G. Dose ranging study of the oxytocin antagonist atosiban in the treatment of preterm labor. *Obstet. Gynecol.* 88:331, 1996.

Goodwin, T.M., Valenzuela, G., Silver, H., Hayashi, R., Creasy, G., et al. Treatment of preterm labor with the oxytocin antagonist atosiban. *Am. J. Perinatol.* 13:143, 1996.

Romero, R., Goncalves, L.F., Gomez, R., and Munoz, H. Atosiban: a new therapeutic choice, clinical experience and research needs. *Res. Clin. Forums* 16:171, 1994.

Romero, R., Sibai, B.M., Sanchez-Ramos, L., Valenzuela, G.J., Veille, J.C., et al. A randomized, double-blind, placebo-controlled trial of an oxytocin antagonist (atosiban) in the treatment of preterm labor. *Am. J. Obstet. Gynecol.,* in press.

Valenzuela, G.J., Craig, J., Bernhardt, M.D., and Holland, M.L. Placental passage of the oxytocin antagonist atosiban. *Am. J. Obstet. Gynecol.* 172:1304, 1995.

Valenzuela, G.J., Sanchez-Ramos, L., Romero, R., Silver, H.M., Koulton, W.D., et al. Maintenance treatment of preterm labor with the oxytocin antagonist atosiban. *Am. J. Obstet. Gynecol.,* in press.

Zeeman, G.G., Dawood, F.S., and Dawood, M.Y. Oxytocin and its receptor in pregnancy and parturition: current concepts and clinical implications. *Obstet. Gynecol.* 89:873, 1997.

Atropine

INDICATIONS AND RECOMMENDATIONS

During pregnancy, parenteral atropine should be limited to its use as a preanesthetic agent in surgical patients to reduce salivation and bronchial secretions. There is concern that atropine, when used as a premedication for cesarean section to decrease the "barrier" pressure of the lower cardioesophageal sphincter, might predispose the newborn to aspiration. This effect could occur after a single dose because transplacental passage is rapid.

Atropine can abolish or diminish variable decelerations, but its use for this indication is not recommended. The intrapartum administration of atropine for the treatment of fetal bradycardia is controversial, but most perinatologists believe that it currently has no role in this setting.

Ophthalmic solutions for topical administration may be used to produce mydriasis and cycloplegia for refraction and in the treatment of inflammatory conditions of the uveal tract. Systemic absorption can be minimized by compressing the lacrimal sac during and for 1 minute following instillation of the drops.

The use of belladonna alkaloids in over-the-counter preparations is discussed under "Belladonna Alkaloids."

SPECIAL CONSIDERATIONS IN PREGNANCY

Atropine crosses the placenta and is secreted in breast milk; 93% of the maternal serum concentration has been found in umbilical vein blood within 5 minutes of the time the drug was injected into the maternal circulation. Fetal lamb studies have shown that atropine inhibits fetal bradycardia and may increase carotid and cerebral blood flow. In the human fetus, atropine is known to diminish beat-to-beat variability and to mask early (type 1) and mild variable fetal heart rate decelerations. Although atropine can abolish variable deceleration, its use is not recommended because the deceleration is a physiologic adaptation to stress that reduces oxygen consumption. In studies using atropine to reduce gastric secretion in patients undergoing cesarean section, no statistically significant changes in fetal heart rate or variability have been noted.

DOSAGE

The usual parenteral dose is 0.5–1.0 mg. The ophthalmic dose is 12 drops of a 0.5%, 1%, 2%, or 3% solution instilled 1 hour before refraction or up to 3 times a day for treatment of uveitis.

ADVERSE EFFECTS

Annoying anticholinergic effects include dryness of mucous membranes, thirst, and constipation. In larger dosages, slurred speech and blurred vision may occur. Overdosage may produce ataxia, excitement, disorientation, hallucinations, delirium, coma, high fever, and antidiuresis.

MECHANISM OF ACTION

The principal action of atropine occurs as a result of competitive antagonism of acetylcholine at muscarinic sites. It also has a direct effect on the medulla and higher cerebral centers.

Atropine-induced parasympathetic block may be preceded by a transient phase of mild stimulation. This is probably a result of central vagal stimulation by dosages too small to block peripheral muscarinic receptors. With average clinical dosages, the heart rate may be minimally slowed. Larger dosages, however, cause progressively increasing tachycardia by blocking vagal effects on the pacemaker in the sinoatrial node. Atropine decreases intestinal motility by blocking extrinsic parasympathetic nervous control as well as that of intramural nerve plexuses. Mydriasis and cycloplegia occur because atropine blocks the responses of the sphincter muscle of the iris and the ciliary muscle of the lens to cholinergic stimulation. In addition, the secretory activity of exocrine glands is decreased.

ABSORPTION AND BIOTRANSFORMATION

Atropine is usually administered parenterally, but it is well absorbed from all mucosal surfaces. Only limited absorption occurs from the eye, but any portion of a dose that traverses the nasolacrimal duct into the pharynx will be absorbed. Atropine is primarily hydrolyzed in the liver. Most of the drug is excreted in the urine within the first 12 hours, 13% to 50% being unchanged and the remainder appearing as metabolites.

RECOMMENDED READING

Abboud, T., et al. Fetal and maternal cardiovascular effects of atropine and glycopyrrolate. *Anesth Analgesia* 62:426, 1983.

Brown, J.H., and Taylor, P. Muscarinic receptor agonists and antagonists. Chapter 7 in *Goodman and Gilman's The Pharmacological Basis of Therapeutics* (9th ed.), J.G. Hardman and L.E. Limbird, eds. New York: McGraw-Hill, 1996. Pp. 148–159.

Cohn, H.E., Piasecki, G.J., and Jackson, B.T. The effect of atropine blockade on the fetal cardiovascular response to hypoxemia. *Gynecol. Invest.* 7:57, 1976.

Goodlin, R.C. Inappropriate fetal bradycardia. *Obstet. Gynecol.* 48:117, 1976.

Goodlin, R.C., and Haesslein, H. Fetal reacting bradycardia. *Am. J. Obstet. Gynecol.* 129:845, 1977.

Ikenoue, T., Quilligan, E.J., and Murata, Y. Circulatory response to atropine in the human fetus. *Am. J. Obstet. Gynecol.* 126: 253, 1976.

Kanto, J. New aspects in the use of atropine. *Int. J. Clin. Pharmacol. Ther. Toxicol.* 21:92, 1983.

Kivado, I., and Saari Roski, S. Placental transmission of atropine at full term pregnancy. *Br. J. Anaesth.* 49:1017, 1977.

Parer, J.T. The effect of atropine on heart rate and oxygen consumption of the hypoxic fetus. *Am. J. Obstet. Gynecol.* 148:1118, 1984.

Parer, J.T. Reply to Dr. Brand (letter). *Am. J. Obstet. Gynecol.* 151:142, 1985.

Scott, J.R., et al., eds. *Danforth's Obstetrics and Gynecology.* Philadelphia: J.B. Lippincott, 1990. P. 325.

Azathioprine (Imuran®)

INDICATIONS AND RECOMMENDATIONS

The administration of azathioprine to pregnant women should be limited to the treatment of serious, life-threatening conditions. This drug is an immunosuppressive agent approved for the treatment of transplant recipients (to prevent rejection) and adults with severe, active rheumatoid arthritis that has been shown to be unresponsive to conventional management. It has also been used for the treatment of other diseases presumed to have an autoimmune cause, including systemic lupus erythematosus and autoimmune thrombocytopenic purpura, when unresponsive to conventional therapy. Because of unresolved concerns about fetal effects, great caution should be taken in prescribing this drug during pregnancy. The package insert warns that the drug should not be used for treating rheumatoid arthritis in pregnant women.

SPECIAL CONSIDERATIONS IN PREGNANCY

Azathioprine and its metabolites, 6-mercaptopurine and thiouric acid, cross the placenta and appear in fetal blood, placenta, and amniotic fluid within 150 minutes of maternal oral administration in the late first and early second trimesters.

Azathioprine has been found to be teratogenic in some laboratory animals but not in others. Many human pregnancies have occurred in renal transplant recipients, most of whom have been treated with both azathioprine and prednisone. Although reports of this experience have largely been anecdotal, most exposed infants have been free of structural anomalies. There is a single case report of preaxial polydactyly, as well as one of pulmonic stenosis. There has been an increased frequency of small-for-gestational-age infants born to mothers receiving azathioprine, but it has been impossible to distinguish the effects of the drug from the effects of the underlying maternal disease.

There is a report of a child with two apparent de novo chromosomal aberrations, born to a mother taking azathioprine and prednisone before and during pregnancy. An increased percentage of chromosomal abnormalities (gaps, breaks, deletions, fragments) has been noted in lymphocytes of renal transplant recipients treated with azathioprine and also in their offspring. These chromosomal aberrations have generally disappeared from the children's bloodstreams by the age of 2–3 years and have not been associated with clinical problems. Some studies have failed to verify these chromosomal abnormalities.

Normal immunoglobulin levels have been demonstrated in seven neonates whose mothers were treated with azathioprine throughout pregnancy, but transient immunosuppression has been observed in one such infant whose mother received both azathioprine and prednisone. Another infant, exposed to azathioprine and prednisone throughout pregnancy, was lymphopenic at birth, had reduced immunoglobulin (Ig) M and G levels, and an absent thymic shadow on x-ray. This child had a cytomegalovirus (CMV) infection and persistently shed virus, but otherwise appeared immunologically normal at the age of 1 year. There is a second case report of a neonate with brain damage from intrauterine CMV infection whose mother took azathioprine and prednisone for lupus erythematosus. There is a single case report of a neonatal death secondary to profound immunosuppression after the mother had been treated with azathioprine 125 mg/day plus prednisone. Neonatal B-cell depletion was demonstrated in six infants born to mothers being treated with cyclosporine, azathioprine, and methylprednisolone because of renal transplants. It is not possible to distinguish the relative contributions, if any, of the three drugs. Another case series showed accelerated maturation of T cells in healthy children who had been exposed to azathioprine, but not cyclosporine, in utero. A series of 10 pregnancies in 8 renal allograft recipients receiving azathioprine demonstrated a direct correlation between maternal and blood leukocyte counts. The clinical significance of these findings is not known. Because there appears to be a correlation between maternal leukopenia and neonatal immunosuppression, a reduction in dosage to avoid leukopenia in the third trimester has been advised.

The risks to infants of nursing mothers who take azathioprine are not clear at present. Normal IgA levels have been found in the milk of one such mother, and in another report two nursing infants whose mothers took azathioprine grew normally, had normal blood cell counts, and had no increased infection rate.

Two cases of pregnancy occurring in renal transplant recipients who used intrauterine devices while taking azathioprine and prednisone have raised the possibility that immunosuppressive therapy may interfere with the effectiveness of this form of contraception. No incidence figures are available.

DOSAGE

Azathioprine is available in 50-mg tablets and as a solution for intravenous injection (100 mg/20 ml). For transplant recipients, the drug is initiated at 3–10 mg/kg/day in a single intravenous or oral dose. It is usually possible to reduce the dose to 1–3 mg/kg/day. For severe, resistant adult rheumatoid arthritis, the drug is initiated at 1 mg/kg/day (50 or 100 mg), and increased after 6–8 weeks if necessary. The dosage should be increased no more frequently than every 4 weeks, in steps of 0.5 mg/kg/day. The maximum dose used is 2.5 mg/kg/day. Once a therapeutic response has been demonstrated, the dosage should be reduced if possible, in steps of 0.5 mg/kg/day every 4 weeks. The lowest possible dosage should be used for maintenance. Patients with renal dysfunction may require lower dosages.

ADVERSE EFFECTS

Severe toxicities include leukopenia, thrombocytopenia, macrocytic anemia, and bone marrow depression. These problems are dose-related. It is recommended that complete blood counts be obtained weekly during the first month of therapy, twice monthly for the next 2 months, and monthly thereafter. Evidence of significant bone marrow suppression dictates immediate reduction in dosage or discontinuation of the drug. Serious infections may occur in patients receiving immunosuppressive agents and may be fatal.

There is evidence for an increased risk of solid tumors and lymphomas in patients treated with azathioprine. This appears to be especially true for transplant recipients, but cases have also been reported among patients with rheumatoid arthritis.

Gastric disturbances, including nausea and vomiting, are common among patients treated with this drug, especially during the first few months of therapy. These side effects are often ameliorated by administering the drug in divided doses and after meals. Hypersensitivity pancreatitis, toxic hepatitis with biliary stasis, skin rashes, alopecia, fever, arthralgias, diarrhea, and steatorrhea have also been reported. Two cases of cholestatic jaundice during pregnancy in heart transplant recipients taking azathioprine have been reported; both responded to discontinuation of the drug.

MECHANISM OF ACTION

Azathioprine is a prodrug of 6-mercaptopurine, a purine analog. It was synthesized in order to act as a "prodrug," which slowly liberates 6-mercaptopurine. It is believed that the intracellular accumulation of purine analogs can produce major metabolic disruptions, with subsequent cytotoxicity. Lymphocytes appear to be especially sensitive to such effects.

This drug suppresses cell-mediated hypersensitivity and alters antibody production. Suppression of T-cell effects is dependent on the drug being administered before the antigenic stimulus has been presented. Although transplant recipients taking azathioprine have subnormal responses to vaccines, low numbers of T cells, and abnormal phagocytosis by peripheral blood cells, their serum immunoglobulin levels and secondary antibody responses are usually normal. The mechanism by which azathioprine acts against autoimmune diseases is poorly understood.

ABSORPTION AND BIOTRANSFORMATION

Azathioprine is rapidly absorbed after oral administration with peak levels at 1–2 hours and is slowly converted to 6-mercaptopurine. Both compounds are excreted primarily in the urine, so that reduction in dosage is recommended for patients with reduced renal function. Tissue levels are not well correlated with blood levels, and the biological effect appears to be much longer than the serum half-life of approximately 5 hours.

RECOMMENDED READING

Cederqvist, L.L., Merkatz, I.R., and Litwin, S.D. Fetal immunoglobulin synthesis following maternal immunosuppression. *Am. J. Obstet. Gynecol.* 129:687, 1977.

Cote, C.J., Meuwissen, H.J., and Pickering, R.J. Effects on the neonate of prednisone and azathioprine administered to the mother during pregnancy. *J. Pediatrics* 85:324, 1974.

Coulam, C.B., et al. Breast-feeding after renal transplantation. *Transplant Proc.* 13:605, 1982.

Davison, J.M., Dellagrammatikas, H., and Parkin, J.M. Maternal azathioprine therapy and depressed haemopoiesis in the babies of renal allograft patients. *Br. J. Obstet. Gynaecol.* 92:233, 1985.

DeWitte, D.B., Buick, M.K., Cyran, S.E., et al. Neonatal pancytopenia and severe combined immunodeficiency associated with antenatal administration of azathioprine and prednisone. *J. Pediatrics* 105:625, 1984.

Diasio, R.B., and LoBuglio, A.F. Immunomodulators: immunosuppressive agents and immunostimulants. Chapter 52 in *Goodman and Gilman's The Pharmacological Basis of Therapeutics* (9th ed.), J.G. Hardman and L.E. Limbird, eds. New York: McGraw-Hill, 1996. Pp. 1300–1301.

Gebhardt, D.O.E. Azathioprine teratogenicity: review of the literature and case report. *Obstet. Gynecol.* 61:270, 1983.

Grekas, D.M., Vasiliou, S.S., and Lazarides, A.N. Immunosuppressive therapy and breast-feeding after renal transplantation. *Nephron* 37:68, 1984.

Hayes, K., Symington, G., and Mackay, I.R. Maternal immunosuppression and cytomegalovirus infection of the fetus. *Aust. N. Z. J. Med.* 9:430, 1979.

Laifer, S.A. Pregnancy after transplantation. Chapter 1 in *Current Obstetric Medicine,* Vol. 2, R.V. Lee, W.M. Barron, D.B. Cotton, and D.R. Coustan, eds. St. Louis: Mosby–Year Book, 1993. Pp. 1–23.

McGeown, M.G., and Nevin, N.C. Cytogenetic analysis on children born of parents treated with immunosuppressive drugs. *Proc. Eur. Dial. Transplant Assoc.* 15:384, 1978.

Imoran. Monograph in *Physicians Desk Reference* (52nd ed.). Montvale, NJ: Medical Economics, 1998. P. 1040.

Ostrer, J., Stamberg, J., and Perinchief, P. Two chromosome aberrations in the child of a woman with systemic lupus erythematosus treated with azathioprine and prednisone. *Am. J. Med. Genet.* 17:627, 1984.

Pilarski L.M., Yacyshyn, B.R., and Lazarovits, A.I. Analysis of peripheral blood lymphocyte populations and immune function from children exposed to cyclosporine or to azathioprine in utero. *Transplantation* 57:133, 1994.

Pirson, Y., et al. Retardation of fetal growth in patients receiving immunosuppressive therapy. *N. Engl. J. Med.* 313:328, 1985.

Price, H.V., et al. Immunosuppressive drugs and the foetus, *Transplantation* 21:294, 1976.

Rosenkrantz, J.G., et al. Azathioprine (Imuran) and pregnancy. *Am. J. Obstet. Gynecol.* 97:387, 1967.

Saarikoski, S., and Seppala, M. Immunosuppression during pregnancy: transmission of azathioprine and its metabolites from the mother to the fetus. *Am. J. Obstet. Gynecol.* 115:1100, 1973.

Schmid, B.P. Monitoring of organ formation in rat embryos after in vitro exposure to azathioprine, mercaptopurine, methotrexate or cyclosporin A. *Toxicology* 31:9, 1984.

Scott, J.R. Fetal growth retardation associated with maternal administration of immunosuppressive drugs. *Am. J. Obstet. Gynecol.* 128:668, 1977.

Sharon, E., et al. Pregnancy and azathioprine in systemic lupus erythematosus. *Am. J. Obstet. Gynecol.* 118:25, 1974.

Takahashi, N., Nishida, H., and Hoshi, J. Severe B cell depletion in newborns from renal transplant mothers taking immunosuppressive agents. *Transplantation* 57:1617, 1994.

Wagoner, L.E., Taylor, D.O., Olsen, S.L. et al. Immunosuppressive therapy, management, and outcome of heart transplant recipients during pregnancy. *J. Heart Lung Transplant* 13:993, 1994.

Williamson, R.A., and Karp, L.E. Azathioprine teratogenicity: review of the literature and case report. *Obstet. Gynecol.* 58:247, 1981.

Zerner, J., et al. Intrauterine contraceptive device failures in renal transplant patients. *J. Reprod. Med.* 26:99, 1981.

Azithromycin (Zithromax®)

INDICATIONS AND RECOMMENDATIONS

Azithromycin is relatively contraindicated in pregnancy because other agents are preferable. Azithromycin is a relatively new macrolide antibiotic with an extended spectrum of activity and prolonged half-life that allows once-daily dosing after an initial loading dose. It is active against gram-positive cocci, some gram-negative rods, many anaerobes, *Chlamydia trachomatis,* and *Mycobacterium avium* complex (MAC).

Reproductive studies with azithromycin in rats at doses equivalent to 2–4 times a normal human dose of 500 mg demonstrated no evidence of fetal harm or impaired fertility. There are no studies documenting the safety of azithromycin use in human pregnancy.

Although azithromycin is considered the drug of choice for treatment of chlamydia, the Centers for Disease Control does not recommend its use during pregnancy and instead recommends alternative treatment with erythromycin or amoxicillin. One study, in which azithromycin was compared to erythromycin for treatment of cervical *Chlamydia* infections in pregnant women, showed that azithromycin had equivalent efficacy and significant fewer gastrointestinal side effects, allowing increased compliance.

Azithromycin has caused reversible liver enzyme elevations during clinical trials; whether this effect would be increased among pregnant women (as with erythromycin estolate) is unknown.

Because infections with organisms sensitive to azithromycin are usually amendable to treatment with other antibiotics that have been better studied during pregnancy, azithromycin treatment should be used only for treatment of maternal infections if there is no safer alternative.

RECOMMENDED READING

Amsden, G.W. Erythromycin, clarithromycin, and azithromycin: are the differences real? *Clin. Ther.* 18:56, 1996.

Bush, M.R., and Rosa, C. Azithromycin and erythromycin in the treatment of cervical chlamydial infection during pregnancy. *Obstet. Gynecol.* 84:61, 1994.

Centers for Disease Control and Prevention. Sexually transmitted diseases treatment guidelines. *M.M.W.R.* (RR-14):50, 1993.

Clarithromycin and azithromycin. *Med. Lett. Drugs Ther.* 34:45, 1992.

Kapusnic-Uner, J.E., Sande, M.A., and Chambers, H.F. Antimicrobial agents: tetracyclines, chloramphenicol, erythromycin and miscellaneous antibacterial agents. Chapter 47 in *Goodman and Gilman's The Pharmacological Basis of Therapeutics* (9th ed.), J.G. Hardman and L.E. Limbird, eds. New York: McGraw-Hill, 1996. Pp. 1135–1140.

Beclomethasone Aerosol (Beclovent®, Vanceril®) and Nasal Spray (Beconase®)

INDICATIONS AND RECOMMENDATIONS

Beclomethasone is an aerosol gluococorticoid compound that may be used for the treatment of chronic bronchial asthma in pregnant women. Inhaled glucocorticoids are currently recommended as a first-line therapy in the treatment of asthma, especially for those patients who require more than one daily dose of a β_2-adrenergic agonist. It should be appreciated that the effect of beclomethasone on the fetus is presently unknown. Beclomethasone is also available as a nasal spray, used to treat seasonal or perennial rhinitis. Because of its unknown fetal effects and the availability of other agents for the above condition, beclomethasone nasal spray should be used for rhinitis only when other means of therapy are not effective.

SPECIAL CONSIDERATIONS IN PREGNANCY

Although no well-controlled studies of fetal risk with beclomethasone have been published, the authors of one survey of 45 pregnancies in 40 steroid-dependent asthmatics taking beclomethasone throughout pregnancy reported the incidence of congenital anomalies to be 2.3%. This rate is similar to what is seen in the general population. One additional study, looking at the outcome of 56 pregnancies in 51 women with severe asthma, requiring prednisone and/or beclomethasone, described a slightly increased risk of preterm delivery and low birth weight infants; no malformations were reported. It is unknown if the drug crosses the human placenta or is secreted into breast milk. Animal studies involving systemic glucocorticosteroids have suggested an increase in early fetal loss, cleft palate, and other malformations.

DOSAGE

The recommended dose is two inhalations (50 µg per inhalation) every 6–8 hours, with the maximum recommended dose 1000 µg/day. This dosage did not produce suppression of early morning cortisol concentration in adult volunteers. A therapeutic effect is usually present within a week of drug initiation. If a patient is to be switched from chronic oral systemic corticosteroids to beclomethasone, the aerosol should be used along with the systemic steroid while the dose of systemic steroid is tapered.

ADVERSE EFFECTS

Unlike systemic steroids, inhaled beclomethasone has minimal systemic effects. In conventional dosages, it produces little or no suppression of the pituitary-adrenal axis. Side effects include hoarseness, oral candidiasis (which may be reduced with the use of a spacer device), an increased incidence of pulmonary infection, possible bone resorption, skin thinning, and purpura.

MECHANISM OF ACTION

Although the mode of action of steroids in asthma remains unclear, their effects are probably multiple and are mediated mainly through their antiinflammatory effect as well as their ability to decrease airway responsiveness. In controlled trials, inhaled beclomethasone has been shown to be as effective as oral prednisone in controlling the symptoms of mild to moderate asthma in those asthmatics who require long-term corticosteroid therapy. The drug is not useful in an acute asthmatic attack because bronchospasm may prevent its distribution to more distal airways.

ABSORPTION AND BIOTRANSFORMATION

Beclomethasone is administered by a metered-dose oral unit. The drug is deposited in the mouth, nasal mucosa, trachea, bronchi, and lung tissue; approximately 10% to 25% enters the respiratory tract, and a significant amount is swallowed. Systemic absorption does occur, but the drug is highly protein-bound, thus limiting systemic effects. The drug is hydrolyzed to its monopropionate analog. Both the parent compound and its metabolite are absorbed into the general circulation and are transformed into an inactive form in the liver. The principal route of elimination of the drug and its metabolites is via the feces. Hypersensitivity to the drug and its propellant (trichlorofluoromethane and dichlorofluoromethane) has been reported.

BREAST-FEEDING

Beclomethasone is considered compatible with breast-feeding by the American Academy of Pediatrics.

RECOMMENDED READING

Barnes, P.J. Inhaled gluococorticoids for asthma. *N. Engl. J. Med.* 332:868, 1995.

Choo-Kang, Y.F.J., et al. Beclomethasone dipropionate by inhalation in the treatment of airways obstruction. *Br. J. Dis. Chest* 66:101, 1972.

Clark, T.J.H. Effect of beclomethasone dipropionate delivered by aerosol in patients with asthma. *Lancet* 1:1361, 1972.

Fitzsimmons, R., Greenberger, M.D., and Patterson, R. Outcome of pregnancy in women requiring corticosteroids for severe asthma. *J. Allergy Clin. Immunol.* 78:349, 1986.

Greenberger, P.A., and Patterson, R. Beclomethasone dipropionate for severe asthma during pregnancy. *Ann. Intern. Med.* 98:478, 1983.

Martin, L.E., et al. Absorption and metabolism of orally administered beclomethasone dipropionate. *Clin. Pharmacol. Ther.* 15:267, 1974.

Serafin, W.E. Drugs used in the treatment of asthma. Chapter 28 in *Goodman and Gilman's The Pharmacological Basis of Therapeutics* (9th ed.), J.G. Hardman and L.E. Limbird, eds. New York: McGraw-Hill, 1996. Pp. 659–682.

Belladonna Alkaloids (Over-the-Counter): Atropine, Homatropine, Scopolamine

INDICATIONS AND RECOMMENDATIONS

Belladonna alkaloids and their quaternary ammonium derivatives are present in a variety of over-the-counter (OTC) antidiarrheal and sedative products. They are usually combined with adsorbents for the treatment of diarrhea and antihistamines and analgesics for use as sedatives. As the belladonna alkaloids are not present in recognized therapeutic doses in OTC antidiarrheal preparations and because other nonabsorbable agents are available, their use for this purpose during pregnancy is not necessary. Products containing scopolamine in therapeutic dosages appear to be safe when used in the treatment of insomnia in pregnancy before the onset of labor. There is one report of two cases of sialorrhea (excessive salivation) in pregnancy, treated successfully with a combination of phenothiazine and belladonna alkaloids. The use of parenteral and ophthalmic solutions of atropine and of parenteral scopolamine is discussed in separate sections of this book.

SPECIAL CONSIDERATIONS IN PREGNANCY

The Collaborative Perinatal Project found no association between first-trimester exposure to atropine, homatropine, or scopolamine and congenital malformations. The use of both atropine and scopolamine near term has been associated with decreased beat-to-beat heart rate variability in the fetus. This phenomenon has been seen primarily with large-dose parenteral use. Small amounts of atropine are secreted in breast milk. When bromides are also contained in compounds, acneiform rash, hypotonia and lethargy, irritability, high-pitched cry, and difficulty in feeding have been reported in the newborn. The American Academy of Pediatrics considers atropine and scopolamine to be usually compatible with breast-feeding.

DOSAGE

The usual dosages of the belladonna alkaloids available in OTC medications are quite small. Scopolamine is found in doses of 0.083–0.500 mg in combination with other ingredients in OTC sedatives. The total dose of all belladonna alkaloids in the usual antidiarrheal compound is about 0.13 mg/30 ml.

ADVERSE EFFECTS

The most common side effect of these agents is dryness of the mouth and throat. Other anticholinergic effects such as blurred vision, photophobia, and urinary retention are uncommon at the dosage provided in OTC preparations. Scopolamine may disrupt the sleep cycle by decreasing rapid eye movement (REM) time. When it is discontinued after several days of use, a rebound in REM occurs, resulting in nightmares, insomnia, and the feeling of having slept badly. This effect is not usual at the doses present in most OTC preparations, but it may be experienced by patients who use these preparations chronically or who exceed recommended dosages.

The belladonna alkaloids are rapidly absorbed into the bloodstream and are distributed throughout the body. Elimination varies with the individual agent. The majority of the compounds are metabolized, but 13% to 50% of atropine and 1% of scopolamine are excreted in the urine unchanged.

MECHANISM OF ACTION

These antimuscarinic agents competitively inhibit acetylcholine at the receptor site of the effector organ. When used in doses equivalent to 0.6–1.0 mg atropine sulfate, belladonna alkaloids are effective in the treatment of diarrhea due to increased intestinal tone and peristalsis. However, most OTC antidiarrheal agents containing belladonna alkaloids contain less than this recognized effective dose.

When a sedative effect is the primary one required, scopolamine is the agent used. It acts as a hypnotic by depressing the cerebral cortex. Therapeutic dosages produce drowsiness, euphoria, fatigue, and dreamless sleep.

RECOMMENDED READING

Brown, J.H., and Taylor, P. Muscarinic receptor agonists and antagonists. Chapter 7 in *Goodman and Gilman's The Pharmacological Basis of Therapeutics* (9th ed.), J.G. Hardman and L.E. Limbird, eds. New York: McGraw-Hill, 1996. Pp. 149–154.

Committee on Drugs of the American Academy of Pediatrics. The transfer of drugs and other chemicals into human milk. *Pediatrics* 93:137–150, 1994.

Freeman, J.J., Altieri, R.H., Baptiste, H.J., et al. Evaluation and management of sialorrhea of pregnancy with concomitant hyperemesis. *J. Natl. Med. Assoc.* 86:704–708, 1994.

Heinonen, O.P., Slone, D., and Shapiro, S. *Birth Defects and Drugs in Pregnancy*. Littleton, MA: Wright-PSG, 1977. Pp. 346–353, 439.

Nelson, M.M., and Forfar, J.O. Associations between drugs administered during pregnancy and congenital abnormalities of the fetus. *Br. Med. J.* 1:523, 1971.

Schenkel, B., and Vorherr, H. Non-prescription drugs during pregnancy: potential teratogenic and toxic effects upon embryo and fetus. *J. Reprod. Med.* 12:27, 1974.

Benzamide Gastric Prokinetic Agents: Metoclopramide (Reglan®), Cisapride (Propulsid®)

INDICATIONS AND RECOMMENDATIONS

Metoclopramide appears to be safe to use in pregnancy. Approved indications include symptomatic gastroesophageal reflux, diabetic gastric stasis, the prevention of nausea and vomiting associated with cancer chemotherapy, and the facilitation of small bowel intubation and radiologic examination. Metoclopramide has been used as an antiemetic, as a preanesthetic medication to reduce gastric volume, and as a lactation-enhancing agent, although it has not been specifically approved for these indications. Cisapride is used to stimulate gastric motility in gastroesophageal reflux and diabetic gastric stasis. It is not an effective antiemetic. Because there has been less experience with cisapride in pregnancy, metoclopramide is preferable.

SPECIAL CONSIDERATIONS IN PREGNANCY

Animal studies have not documented teratogenicity for metoclopramide; similarly, there are no reports suggesting human teratogenicity. Cisapride was not teratogenic in rat and rabbit studies, but in very high doses was embryotoxic in both of these species. No human data regarding cisapride could be located.

Metoclopramide crosses the placenta in humans at term, with fetal plasma concentrations approximately half of maternal levels. Neonates exposed to this drug during labor did not exhibit differences in Apgar scores or cardiovascular or neurobehavioral effects when compared with placebo-treated control subjects. Studies in the first and third trimesters have demonstrated a rapid and significant increase in maternal serum prolactin, but not in growth hormone, levels after intravenous administration of metoclopramide. During the first trimester, the administration of this drug did not change maternal levels of progesterone, estradiol, human chorionic gonadotropin (HCG), or human placental lactogen (HPL). Fetal prolactin levels were not increased when laboring mothers were given the drug. Physiologic studies in all three trimesters have demonstrated a significant reduction in maternal gastric volume when metoclopramide was administered.

Metoclopramide administered prophylactically prior to epidural or spinal anesthesia for cesarean section reduces perioperative nausea and vomiting without causing side effects in the neonate.

Metoclopramide has been advocated for improvement of "defective lactation" in nursing mothers and has been shown to increase milk volume. However, one study has demonstrated milk/plasma ratios greater than 1:1 in five of seven mothers tested during the first 2 weeks post partum, with detectable levels of the drug in the plasma of two infants. The estimated infants' doses derived from mothers' milk were as high as 24 µg/kg/day in some instances. The recommended therapeutic dose in children is 500 µg/kg/day. Of greatest concern was the finding that four in seven newborns had serum prolactin levels above the highest seen in untreated control infants. More information is needed before the safety of metoclopramide in lactating mothers can be determined.

DOSAGE

Metoclopramide is available as a tablet containing 10 mg, a syrup containing 5 mg/5 ml, and an intravenous solution containing 5 mg/ml. The oral dose is 5–15 mg, up to 4 times daily, 15–30 minutes before meals. This may be continued for up to 12 weeks. An intravenous dose of 10–20 mg given over 2 minutes is administered when prevention of nausea and vomiting during chemotherapy is desired. The dose usually employed for improving milk production is 10 mg PO, 2–3 times daily. In studies of gastric volume reduction, the usual dose is 10 mg IV.

Cisapride is available in 10-mg and 20-mg tablets, and as a suspension containing 1 mg/ml. The usual dose is 10 mg 4 times daily taken at least 15 minutes before meals and at bedtime.

ADVERSE EFFECTS

The principal side effect of metoclopramide is sedation. However, dystonic-dyskinetic head and neck movements have been reported in two pregnant patients who took metoclopramide as an antiemetic. These extrapyramidal effects seem to be most common in young females, and the reactions resemble oculogyric crisis. These have been reported to occur in approximately 0.2% of patients taking doses greater than 30–40 mg/day. Diazepam or diphenhydramine (25–50 mg intravenously) can be used to reverse these problems.

Other side effects include occasional agitation, excitability, seizures, constipation or diarrhea, rash, and dry mouth. Methemoglobinemia and edema of the mouth, tongue, or orbital areas have occurred. There has been a case report of a postpartum patient developing supraventricular tachycardia immediately after intravenous metoclopramide administration.

Metoclopramide should not be used in patients with pheochromocytoma, as hypertensive crisis may be precipitated. It is also contraindicated in epileptics and in patients with gastrointestinal obstruction.

Cisapride has been associated with transient abdominal cramping and diarrhea. It may increase the absorption of diazepam and alcohol. Cardiac arrhythmias have been rarely reported.

MECHANISM OF ACTION

Metoclopramide relieves nausea and vomiting by blocking dopaminergic stimuli at the chemoreceptor trigger zone. Peripherally, it acts as a cholinergic agonist to increase tone in the esophageal sphincter, increase the tone and amplitude of gastric contractions, relax the pyloric sphincter and duodenal bulb, and increase peristalsis in the duodenum and jejunum. Gastric emptying and intestinal transit time are diminished. As was previously mentioned, prolactin release is potentiated. Additionally, there is a transient rise in aldosterone levels, which may be associated with fluid retention. Cisapride does not have antidopaminergic activity.

ABSORPTION AND BIOTRANSFORMATION

The onset of action of metoclopramide is 1–3 minutes after an intravenous dose and 30–60 minutes following an oral dose. Pharmacologic effects persist for 1–2 hours, with a plasma half-life of about 3 hours. The drug is metabolized by the liver. Approximately 85% of an orally administered dose (or its metabolites) appears in the urine within 72 hours. Cisapride is 30% to 40% bioavailable, and peak blood levels occur about 2 hours after oral dosing. Absorption is more complete when the drug is taken with food.

RECOMMENDED READING

Bevacqua, B.K. Supraventricular tachycardia associated with postpartum metoclopramide administration. *Anesthesiology* 68:124–5, 1988.

Bohnet, H.G., and Kato, A.K. Prolactin secretion during pregnancy and puerperium: Response to metoclopramide and interactions with placental hormones. *Obstet. Gynecol.* 65:789, 1985.

Brock-Utne, J.G., et al. The effect of metoclopramide on the lower oesophageal sphincter in late pregnancy. *Anaesth. Intensive Care* 6:26, 1978.

Brunton, L.L. Agents affecting gastrointestinal water flux and motility; emesis and antiemetics; bile acids and pancreatic enzymes. Chapter 38 in *Goodman and Gilman's The Pharmacological Basis of Therapeutics* (9th ed.), J.G. Hardman and L.E. Limbird, eds. New York: McGraw-Hill, 1996. Pp. 932– 933.

Bylsma-Howell, M., et al. Placental transport of metoclopramide: assessment of maternal and neonatal effects. *Can. Anaesth. Soc. J.* 30:487, 1983.

Cohen, S.E., et al. Does metoclopramide decrease the volume of gastric contents in patients undergoing cesarean section? *Anesthesiology* 61:604, 1984.

Janssen Pharmaceutical. Propulsid (cisapride). Entry in *Physicians Desk Reference* (52nd ed.). Montvale, NJ: Medical Economics, 1998. Pp. 1308–1309.

Kauppila, A., Kivinen, S., and Ylikorkala, O. A dose–response relation between improved lactation and metoclopramide. *Lancet* 1:1175, 1981.

Kauppila, A., et al. Metoclopramide and breast feeding: transfer into milk and the newborn. *Eur. J. Pharmacol.* 25:819, 1983.

Lussos, S.A., Bader, A.M., Thornhill, M.L., and Datta, S. The antiemetic efficacy and safety of prophylactic metoclopramide for elective cesarean delivery during spinal anesthesia. *Regional Anesth* 17:126, 1992.

Benzodiazepines: Alprazolam (Xanax®), Chlordiazepoxide (Librium®), Clonazepam (Klonopin®), Clorazepate (Tranxene®), Diazepam (Valium®), Lorazepam (Ativan®), Midazolam (Versed®), Oxazepam (Serax®), Prazepam (Centrax®), Temazepam (Restoril®), Triazolam (Halcion®) and others

INDICATIONS AND RECOMMENDATIONS

The use of benzodiazepines during pregnancy should be limited to the control of status epilepticus and the intermittent treatment of anxiety. Diazepam is the most widely used of these agents, and so the greatest amount of information about usage in pregnancy is available for this drug. Benzodiazepines are widely used in nonpregnant patients as sedatives, as hypnotics in sleep disorders, for the anxiety associated with depressive disorders, as preanesthetic medications, and in the management of opiate or alcohol withdrawal. Diazepam (and perhaps lorazepam) is the drug of choice for the treatment of status epilepticus but is not useful in the chronic management of epilepsy. It has been used to control eclamptic seizures, although magnesium sulfate is the drug of choice prior to delivery. Clonazepam is used in the treatment of absence seizures and myoclonic seizures in children but is rarely indicated in women of reproductive age. Chronic use of diazepam during pregnancy may be associated with significant adverse effects in the neonate and is therefore not recommended.

The use of other benzodiazepines in pregnancy has not been well studied. At least two studies of lorazepam used as a labor medication suggest that neonatal depression is likely to be associated with the use of this drug.

SPECIAL CONSIDERATIONS IN PREGNANCY

Diazepam (and presumably other benzodiazepines) rapidly crosses the placental barrier with fetal–maternal equilibrium being reached within 1 hour in humans. Benzodiazepine concentrations in cord blood have been reported to exceed the levels in maternal blood. This may be due to their marked lipid solubility and delayed metabolism by the immature fetal liver.

The intravenous injection of 5–10 mg diazepam into pregnant ewes has been associated with an immediate cessation of fetal breathing activity. In humans, loss of beat-to-beat fetal heart rate variability has been reported within 2 minutes of the intravenous administration of 20 mg diazepam. This effect lasts for approximately 60 minutes and does not affect fetal pH or Apgar scores. In addition, intravenous diazepam has been associated with a decrease in the frequency (but not amplitude) of uterine contractions during labor.

The data are inconsistent regarding teratogenicity and postnatal development following in utero exposure to benzodiazepines. A study performed in the early 1960s reported major congenital anomalies in 4 in 35 infants born to mothers taking chlordiazepoxide during the first 42 days of gestation (11.4%). Only 2 in 77 infants whose mothers were diagnosed as having minor psychoneurotic complaints but who were not medicated during this time period in pregnancy were found to have major congenital anomalies (2.6%). This finding has not been corroborated.

A number of epidemiologic studies have suggested a relationship between diazepam use and various birth defects. The strongest association appears to be with cleft lip or palate, but the actual risk is at most 0.2% for cleft palate and 0.4% for cleft lip with or without cleft palate. Parents of 611 infants with oral clefts and of 2498 control infants with other birth defects were interviewed via a structured questionnaire about drug use in pregnancy. Among the controls, 2.2% recalled taking diazepam during the first 4 months of pregnancy. Similarly, 2.2% of parents with pregnancies producing a baby with cleft lip and 1.8% of those with pregnancies producing cleft palate recalled taking diazepam during the first 4 months. Prospective data on 32,395 pregnancies were analyzed by investigators at the National Institutes of Health and revealed no significant increase in relative risk for oral clefts among first-trimester users of diazepam. On the other hand, a Swedish study of 10,646 gravidae indicated a strong association between first-trimester benzodiazepine use and congenital malformations (cleft lip and cleft palate, genitourinary anomalies). No specific pattern of malformations has been reported in association with alprazolam, lorazepam, or midazolam use in pregnancy. There is the possibility that benzodiazepine use may increase the teratogenic potential of valproic acid, and that the combination of benzodiazepines and alcohol or other drugs may increase may increase the incidence of congenital malformations. Ambiguity regarding benzodiazepine use in pregnancy continues, and it is probably best to avoid them during the first trimester unless the indications for their use are compelling.

Neonatal diazepam withdrawal symptoms have been reported after second- and third-trimester maternal ingestion, generally in doses of 15–20 mg/day for at least 12 weeks. It should be noted, however, that in one report only 10 mg every other day was taken for 16 weeks. The symptoms were similar to those seen in neonatal narcotic withdrawal. Severe neonatal respiratory depression can occur when diazepam is used in high dosages for control of eclampsia. Neonatal hypothermia is also commonly reported. In addition, hyperbilirubinemia in the neonate is believed to be potentiated by benzodiazepines, probably due to delayed bilirubin metabolism.

The benzodiazepines and their metabolite N-demethyldiazepam are secreted into human breast milk. Lethargy, sedation, and weight loss have been reported in nursing infants whose mothers took diazepam; their use by the lactating mother is not recommended. Because N-demethyldiazepam has a long half-life and is metabolized in the liver, it is not unexpected that neonates might be susceptible to such effects.

DOSAGE

Agent	How supplied	Usual dose
Alprazolam	0.25, 0.5, 1.0, and 2.0 mg tabs	0.75–4.0 mg/day
Chlordiazepoxide	5, 10, and 25 mg tabs and caps; 100 mg/2 ml ampules	15–60 mg/day
Clonazepam	0.5, 1.0, and 2.0 mg tabs	1.5–20 mg/day in 3 doses
Clorazepate	3.75, 7.5, 11.25, and 22.5 mg tabs	15–60 mg/day
Diazepam	2, 5, and 10 mg tabs; 5 mg/ml ampules	2–10 mg 2–4 times daily
Lorazepam	0.5, 1.0, and 2.0 mg tablets; 2 and 4 mg/ml ampules	2–6 mg/day in divided doses
Midazolam	1 and 5 mg/ml ampules	0.3–0.35 mg/kg over 20–30 sec for in duction of anes thesia
Oxazepam	10, 15, and 30 mg caps and tabs	10–15 mg tid or qid
Temazepam	7.5, 15, and 30 mg caps	15 mg q HS
Triazolam	0.125 and 0.25 mg tabs	0.125–0.25 mg/day

ADVERSE EFFECTS

Side effects most commonly encountered are drowsiness, excessive somnolence, lethargy, impairment of intellectual function, ataxia, and memory impairment. Paradoxic effects such as increased hostility or anxiety have been reported. Excessive intravenous administration or intravenous therapy in the presence of other central nervous system depressants can produce significant respiratory depression. The therapeutic index is high, and fatal benzodiazepine overdosage in the absence of other drugs is distinctly uncommon. Chronic administration can lead to drug dependence, and true physiologic addiction has been documented.

MECHANISM OF ACTION

The presence of specific benzodiazepine receptors in the central nervous system has been well documented, and these drugs bind to their receptors with high affinity. The ultimate effect of the benzodiazepine–receptor interaction is to enhance the inhibitory neuronal properties of τ-aminobutyric acid (GABA). The receptors are most abundant in the cortex and in limbic-forebrain areas. Although the presence of specific receptors suggests the existence of a corresponding natural neurotransmitter, such a compound has not yet been identified. Antagonists to benzodiazepines exist, and behavior reminiscent of fear and anxiety has been produced by their administration to animals.

ABSORPTION AND BIOTRANSFORMATION

The differences in the various compounds lie mainly in their lipid solubility. More lipid-soluble drugs cross the blood-brain barrier rapidly and thus have a rapid onset of action after a single intravenous dose, but their duration of action is limited by redistribution to lipid depots around the body. Conversely, less lipid-soluble forms have a slower onset of action but a longer duration. After oral dosing, gastrointestinal absorption is the rate-limiting factor. Diazepam is very rapidly absorbed, reaching peak concentrations in about 1 hour, as is its metabolite, N-demethyldiazepam. Some of the compounds with slower onset (i.e., prazepam) are limited by the rate of their conversion to N-demethyldiazepam, which is then immediately absorbed. Chlordiazepoxide and oxazepam are much more slowly absorbed, reaching peaks in several hours. The kinetics of these drugs are quite complex and a detailed discussion is beyond the scope of this book. Although absorption may be rapid, the elimination half-lives can be prolonged (more than 24 hours), and secondary peaks in blood levels may occur, presumably due to enterohepatic recirculation. Thus, the drugs may accumulate with increasing blood levels until a steady state is achieved, usually after the drug has been taken for 4–5 times the elimination half-life.

The benzodiazepines are cleared by the liver, either through oxidation or conjugation. Different compounds are differentially cleared by these two pathways. The clinical importance of this difference among compounds is not yet clearly established.

RECOMMENDED READING

Baldessarini, R.J. Drugs and the treatment of psychiatric disorders. Psychosis and anxiety. In *Goodman and Gilman's The Pharmacologic Basis of Therapeutics* (9th ed.), J.G. Hardman and L.E. Limbird, eds. New York: McGraw-Hill, 1996. Pp. 421–424.

Cole, A.P., and Hailey, D.M. Diazepam and active metabolites in breast milk and their transfer to the neonate. *Arch. Dis. Child.* 50:741, 1975.

Erkkola, R., and Kanto, J. Diazepam and breast feeding. *Lancet* 1:1235, 1972.

Erkkola, R., Kangas, L., and Pekkarinen, A. The transfer of diazepam across the placenta during labor. *Acta Obstet. Gynecol. Scand.* 52:165, 1973.

Greenblatt, D.J., and Shader, R.I., and Abernethy, D.R. Current status of benzodiazepines, parts 1 and 2. *N. Engl. J. Med.* 309:354, 410, 1983.

Laegreid, L., Olegard, R., Conradi, N., Hagberg, G., Wahlstrom J., and Abrahamsson L. Congenital malformations and maternal consumption of benzodiazepines: a case control study. *Dev. Med. Child. Neurol.* 32:432, 1990.

Laegreid, L., Kyllerman, M., Hedner, T., Hagberg, B., and Viggedahl, G. Benzodiazepine amplification of valproate teratogenic effects in children of mothers with absence epilepsy. *Neuropediatrics* 24:88, 1993.

McElhatton, P.R. The effect of benzodiazepine use during pregnancy and lactation. *Reprod. Toxicol.* 8:461, 1994.

Milkovich, L., and van den Berg, B.J. Effects of prenatal meprobamate and chlordiazepoxide hydrochloride on human embryonic and fetal development. *N. Engl. J. Med.* 291:1268, 1974.

Mofid, M., Brinkman, C.R., and Assali, N.S. Effects of diazepam on uteroplacental and fetal hemodynamic metabolism. *Obstet. Gynecol.* 41:364, 1973.

Patrick, M.J., Tilstone, W.J., and Reavey, P. Diazepam and breast feeding. *Lancet* 1:542, 1972.

Rosenberg, L., et al. Lack of relation of oral clefts to diazepam use during pregnancy. *N. Engl. J. Med.* 309:1282, 1983.

Safra M.J., and Oakley G.P. Valium: an oral cleft teratogen? *Cleft Palate J.* 13:198, 1976

Shepard, T.H. *Catalog of Teratogenic Agents* (6th ed.). Baltimore: Johns Hopkins University Press, 1989. Pp. 203–206.

Shiono, P.H., and Mills, J.L. Oral clefts and diazepam use during pregnancy. *N. Engl. J. Med.* 311:919, 1984.

St. Clair, S.M., and Schirmer R.G. First trimester exposure to alprazolam. *Obstet. Gynecol.* 80:843, 1992.

β-Adrenergic Blocking Agents: Acebutalol (ProSom®), Atenolol (Tenormin®), Esmolol (Brevibloc®), Labetolol (Normodyne ®, Trandate®), Metoprolol (Lopressor®), Nadolol (Corgard®), Pindolol (Visken®), Propranolol (Inderal®), Timolol (Blocadren®)

INDICATIONS AND RECOMMENDATIONS

Beta blockers may be used during pregnancy for treatment of specific conditions including hypertension, therapy of thyroid storm, reduction of cardiac afterload in patients at risk of aortic aneurysm dissection, control of β-adrenergic side effects of intravenous hydralazine therapy for an acute hypertensive episode, idiopathic hypertrophic subaortic stenosis, and any other condition that requires β-adrenergic blockade. One study of 104 gravidas with pregnancy- induced hypertension found that use of labetolol resulted in fewer women developing proteinuria compared to women treated with methyldopa, but this has not been confirmed by other controlled trials. There is a substantial body of literature indicating that β-adrenergic blockers may be safely used during pregnancy.

SPECIAL CONSIDERATIONS IN PREGNANCY

These drugs easily cross the placenta and are also secreted into breast milk, albeit in small amounts. There have been no reports of congenital malformations ascribed to beta blockers, although published experience during pregnancy with the newer agents is limited.

Intravenous administration of propranolol during dysfunctional labor has been reported to increase coordinated contraction patterns without an appreciable concomitant elevation in resting tonus. Clinical trials in which beta blockers have been used for other indications do not reveal an increased risk of premature labor, but one study reported cervical ripening in association with labetolol use near term.

There is a measurable reduction in uterine artery blood flow in rats and baboons following intravenous propranolol administration, but not in sheep. Umbilical blood flow was decreased in the sheep model, but was not affected in the rat model following intravenous propranolol administration.

Propranolol administered during pregnancy has been thought to cause intrauterine growth restriction (IUGR), but a definitive association has not been proved. Most of the studies involving propranolol in pregnant women have been retrospective and contain small numbers of patients. Randomized trials of atenolol and labetolol have found no clear association between beta blocker use in pregnancy and an increase in IUGR, suggesting that the differences seen in other studies were probably the result of differing degrees of hypertension.

Persistent beta blockade in the newborn period has been noted in association with the maternal use of atenolol, acebutolol, and nadolol in small case series. Neonatal hypoglycemia has been reported with maternal propranolol administration, but not with atenolol or acebutolol. When beta blockers are administered during labor, both mother and fetus should have continuous cardiac monitoring, especially if general anesthesia is used. Neonates of mothers given intravenous propranolol immediately before cesarean section have had difficulty in establishing spontaneous respiratory activity. Propranolol can cause nonreactivity of non–stress tests, which become reactive once the drug is discontinued. However, no adverse effects on fetal heart rate patterns in labor have been reported with atenolol.

β-Adrenergic blocking agents are concentrated in breast milk with breast milk/maternal serum concentration ratios of 2–4 reported. This notwithstanding, the amount of drug available to a nursing infant is probably not significant, and the American Academy of Pediatrics considers β-adrenergic blockade agent use to be compatible with breast-feeding. The infant should be observed carefully for evidence of beta blockade.

DOSAGE

TABLE 1. Pharmacology of β-adrenergic blocking agents

Drug	B₁ Selectivity	T½ (h)	Absorption[a] (%)	Elimination	Usual Daily oral dose (mg)
Acebutalol	+	6	70	Renal	200–400
Atenolol	+	6–9	50	Renal	50–100
Esmolol	+	0.15	NA	Serum esterase	IV only
Labetalol	+	3–4	>90	Hepatic	100–400
Metoprolol	+	3–4	90	Hepatic	50–300
Nadolol	-	14–24	30	Renal	40–320
Pindolol	-	5–12	>90	Renal	2.5–30
Propranolol	-	3–6	>90	Hepatic	20–120
Timolol	-	3–5	50	Hepatic	20–40

[a]Absorption may not reflect bioavailability due to rapid first-pass metabolism in some agents.

ADVERSE EFFECTS

Numerous side effects may occur with the use of beta blockers. These include sinus bradycardia in most patients and congestive heart failure in those with poor cardiac reserve who cannot tolerate a reduction in cardiac output. Bronchospasm occurs in 2% to 10% of patients who take nonselective beta blockers. A history of asthma is therefore a contraindication to the use of propranolol. Compromised peripheral circulation may be worsened, and beta blockers are contraindicated in patients with Raynaud's phenomenon. Central nervous system effects include insomnia, nightmares, hallucinations, depression, paresthesias, ataxia, and dizziness. Nausea, diarrhea, abdominal discomfort, constipation, and hyperglycemia are noted in some patients. Acute hypertensive episodes have been reported in patients with pheochromocytoma or when propranolol is given with methyldopa. It is hypothesized that α-methylnorepinephrine, a metabolite of methyldopa, becomes a potent pressor agent in the presence of β-adrenergic blockade.

MECHANISM OF ACTION

The β-adrenergic receptors of various tissues can be differentiated pharmacologically as being β_1 (lipolysis and cardiostimulation) and β_2 (bronchodilatation and vasodilatation) (Table 2). Blockers of these receptors are classified as being selective or nonselective according to their activity at relatively low dosage levels. When administered in usual therapeutic regimens, β_1 selective blocking agents, such as atenolol, primarily inhibit cardiac β-adrenergic receptors and have less of an effect on the β_2 receptors in the bronchi and vasculature. In higher dosages, however, β_1 selective agents will also block β_2 receptors.

β_1-Adrenergic blockade causes decreased cardiac output, slowing of the heart rate, and prolonged mechanical systole; β_2 blockade inhibits the release of renin by the kidney, and blood

TABLE 2.   Effects of β-adrenergic blocking agents

System	Receptor	Effect of blockade
Heart	β_1	Decreased rate of SA node discharge; decreased myocardial contractility; decreased atrial, AV node and ventricular conduction velocity; decreased ventricular automaticity
Blood vessels	β_1	Arteriolar constriction, especially in skeletal muscle
Lungs	β_2	Bronchoconstriction
Fat cells	β_1	Inhibition of lipolysis
Pancreas	β_2	Decreased insulin release
Liver	β_2	Decreased glycogenolysis and gluconeogenesis
Kidney	β_2	Decreased renin release

pressure is lowered further by direct action on the central nervous system.

Intravenous administration of nonselective beta blockers causes a rapid fall in heart rate and cardiac output by directly decreasing the force and frequency of myocardial contractions. Initially there is a rise in peripheral vascular resistance and no change or a slight decrease in blood pressure. An antihypertensive effect begins several hours after administration, especially in patients with elevated plasma renin activity. This effect occurs because of the persistent decrease in cardiac output as well as a fall in peripheral resistance back to or below control levels. The latter may be due to the central action of the drugs or to their inhibition of the release of renal renin.

Respiratory airway resistance is consistently increased by nonselective beta blockers. Insulin release is mediated by β-adrenergic mechanisms, and nonselective beta blockers blunt the normal response to an elevation in blood glucose. These drugs also block the adrenergic signs and symptoms of severe thyrotoxicosis.

ABSORPTION AND BIOTRANSFORMATION

Most beta blockers are readily absorbed from the gastrointestinal tract except for atenolol and nadolol, which are less lipid-soluble. Information regarding the absorption and biotransformation of various other beta blockers may be found in Table 1.

Renal insufficiency has very little effect on the metabolism of propranolol and metoprolol, and their dosage regimen need not be changed in patients with compromised renal function. The less lipid-soluble beta blockers nadolol and atenolol achieve lower brain concentrations than do propranolol, metoprolol, and timolol, and therefore may result in fewer central nervous system side effects.

Phenobarbital increases the clearance and decreases the half-life of the drugs metabolized by the liver, so that higher dosages may be required if these agents are administered concurrently.

RECOMMENDED READING

Committee on Drugs, American Academy of Pediatrics. The transfer of drugs and other chemicals into human milk. *Pediatrics* 93:137, 1994.

Cruikshank, D.J., Robertson, A.A., Campbell, D.M., and MacGillivray, I. Does labetolol influence the development of proteinuria in pregnancy-induced hypertension? A randomized controlled study. *Eur. J. Obstet. Gynecol.* 45:47, 1992.

Dubois, D., et al. Beta blocker therapy in 125 cases of hypertension during pregnancy. *Clin. Exp. Hypertens.* 2:41, 1983.

Dumez, Y., Tchobroutsky, C., Hornych, H., and Amiel-Tison, C. Neonatal Effects of maternal administration of acebutalol. *Br. Med. J.* 283:1077–9, 1981.

El-Qarmalawi, A.M., Morsy, A.H., al-Fadly, A., Obeid, A., and Hashem, M. Labetolol vs methyldopa in the treatment of pregnancy-induced hypertension. *Int. J. Gynecol. Obstet.* 49:125, 1995.

Fabregues, G., Alvarz, L., Varas Juri, P., Drisaldi, S., Cerrato, C., Moschettoni, C., Pituelo, D., Baglivo, H.P., and Esper, R.J. Effectiveness of atenolol in the treatment of hypertension during pregnancy. *Hypertension* 19(Suppl. 2):29, 1992.

Frishman, W.H., and Chesner, M. Beta-adrenergic blockers in pregnancy. *Am. Heart J.* 115:147, 1988.

Frishman, W.H. Beta-adrenergic blockers. *Med. Clin. North Am.* 72:37, 1988.

Margulis, E., Binder, D., and Cohen, A.W. The effect of propranolol on the non-stress test. *Am. J. Obstet. Gynecol.* 148:340, 1984.

Morgan, M.A., Silavin, S.L., Dormer, K.J., Fishburne, B.C., and Fishburne, J.I., Jr. Effects of labetolol on uterine blood flow and cardiovascular hemodynamics in the hypertensive gravid baboon. *Am. J. Obstet. Gynecol.* 168:1574, 1993.

Pickles, C.J., Symonds, E.M., Pipkin, F.B. The fetal outcome in a randomized double-blind controlled trial of labetolol versus placebo in pregnancy-induced hypertension. *Br. J. Obstet. Gynaecol.* 96:38, 1989.

Rubin, P.C. Beta blockers in pregnancy. *Br. J. Obstet. Gynaecol.* 94:292, 1987.

Rubin, P.C., et al. Obstetric aspects of the use in pregnancy-associated hypertension of the ß-adrenoceptor antagonist atenolol. *Am. J. Obstet. Gynecol.* 150:389, 1984.

Rubin, P.C., et al. Placebo-controlled trial of atenolol in treatment of pregnancy associated hypertension. *Lancet* 1:431, 1983.

Schneider, H., and Proegler, M. Placental transfer of beta-adrenergic antagonists studied in an in vitro perfusion system of human placental tissue. *Am. J. Obstet. Gynecol.* 159: 42–7, 1988.

Thornley, K.J., McAinsh, J., and Cruckshank, J.M. Atenolol in the treatment of pregnancy-induced hypertension. *Br. J. Clin. Pharmacol.* 12:725, 1981.

β₂-Adrenergic Agonists: Terbutaline (Brethine®), Albuterol (Proventil®, Ventolin®), Salmetrol (Seravent®), Pirbuterol (MaxAir®)

INDICATIONS AND RECOMMENDATIONS

β₂-Adrenergic agonists may be administered by metered dose inhaler or nebulizer to treat acute episodes of bronchial asthma. Terbutaline is also used subcutaneously as a second-line agent in the acute treatment of bronchial asthma. β₂-adrenergic agonists by metered dose inhalers are commonly used in the ambulatory management of chronic asthma as well.

Terbutaline is also extensively used to arrest premature labor. It is not approved by the FDA for this purpose. Ritodrine, another β₂-adrenergic agonist with apparent equal effectiveness, is the only drug currently approved as a tocolytic agent.

SPECIAL CONSIDERATIONS IN PREGNANCY

There are no published reports of teratogenesis in humans who use terbutaline or other such agents, although controlled studies establishing its safety early in gestation are not available.

The effectiveness of terbutaline in inhibiting premature labor has been demonstrated in several clinical trials. One double-blind controlled study found that 80% of patients' premature labor was arrested with terbutaline as compared to 20% in the control group. In addition, this drug has been shown to decrease both spontaneous and oxytocin-stimulated labor at full term. This effect was seen even in the second stage of labor. Terbutaline may also be used to treat acute intrapartum fetal distress by decreasing uterine activity.

A distinction must be made between a tocolytic agent's ability to acutely stop uterine contractions and its ability to prevent preterm birth. There exists an ongoing controversy regarding the efficacy of β$_2$-adrenergic agonists, or of any tocolytic agents, in preventing preterm delivery. A small randomized trial published in 1986 found that ritodrine was effective in delaying delivery for 24 hours but not in modifying the ultimate perinatal consequences of preterm labor. In 1992, the Canadian Preterm Labor Investigators Group published the results of a larger randomized, double-blind, placebo-controlled trial of ritodrine in preterm labor. Again, although ritodrine-treated patients were significantly less likely to deliver within 48 hours (21% versus 35%, $p < 0.001$) and perhaps 1 week (38% versus 47%, $p < 0.05$), differences in delivery before 32 weeks and before 37 weeks were not significant, nor were neonatal mortality or morbidities. Large randomized trials such as those cited above have not been carried out with terbutaline, but there is no reason to believe that the results would be any different. Perhaps the greatest proven benefit from tocolytics should be considered the delay of delivery for 48 hours in order to administer glucocorticoids, when appropriate, to enhance fetal pulmonic maturation.

Oral terbutaline has been commonly used as maintenance therapy in patients whose preterm labor was arrested by various tocolytic agents. Available data do not support a benefit from such maintenance therapy. In addition, the subcutaneous infusion of terbutaline by a portable infusion pump for long-term tocolysis has been described and is widely commercially available. The rationale is that lower dosages of terbutaline can be used, leading to less downregulation of receptors. This form of treatment is expensive, and large-scale randomized trials to show efficacy would be helpful. Patients requiring continuous parenteral tocolysis may be managed outside the hospital with continuous subcutaneous terbutaline infusion.

Various β-sympathomimetic agents, including ritodrine and terbutaline, have been reported to cause pulmonary edema when used in the treatment of premature labor. The precise mechanism for this adverse effect is in dispute. Katz et al., in a retrospective analysis of 160 patients, found an incidence of severe cardiovascular complications of 5% when intravenous terbutaline was used to treat premature labor. The most common problems encountered were pulmonary edema and/or electrocardiographic changes indicative of myocardial ischemia. All of these incidents occurred after at least 24 hours of terbutaline infusion, and the majority of patients had pulse rates in excess of 140 beats/min. Administration of corticosteroids and the presence of a multiple gestation increased the risk of complications, although pulmonary edema did occur in three patients who did not receive steroids.

On the other hand, Ingemarsson and Bengtsson, in an analysis of 330 patients treated with intravenous terbutaline as a tocolytic agent, found no cases of pulmonary edema or any other serious cardiovascular complication. Sixty-five of these patients also were given corticosteroids. In this study, however, intravenous fluid administration was carefully monitored, dextrose in water was used instead of normal saline, and the infusion rate of the drug was not increased further if the maternal pulse exceeded 120 beats/min. Only 2.7% of the patients developed side effects that led to discontinuation of terbutaline therapy. The most common problems in this small group were nausea, vomiting, and tachycardia. It therefore seems that terbutaline can be used safely in the treatment of premature labor if careful attention is paid to the amount of fluid infused and the maternal pulse rate. In addition, maternal potassium and glucose levels should be monitored and a baseline ECG obtained. In one series of 15 gravidas with peripartum cardiomyopathy, 4 had received long-term oral terbutaline tocolysis. All 4 had complete recoveries, compared to only 7 of the remaining 11 patients. While not proving an association, these data raise the possibility that agents such as terbutaline might trigger peripartum heart failure in some individuals. A review of over 8000 women treated with terbutaline administered by subcutaneous pump over a 6-year interval reported that pulmonary edema developed in 0.32% of patients and other cardiovascular problems in 0.2% of patients.

Diabetic mothers who take this drug may need increased dosages of insulin to maintain adequate diabetic control. A number of studies have demonstrated worsening glucose tolerance in normal pregnant women taking terbutaline in various forms, and some have shown an increased likelihood of gestational diabetes with this drug.

Wagner and coworkers studied pregnant patients with echocardiography during terbutaline administration and found increased chronotropic and inotropic activity. This was evidenced by increased heart rate, ejection fraction, and cardiac output as well as decreased end-systolic volume. In addition, terbutaline caused a decrease in systemic vascular resistance.

Terbutaline has been reported to cross the placenta readily after a single injection before delivery. Average cord blood–maternal vein concentration ratios range between 0.36 and 0.64. An increase in fetal heart rate has been observed after parenteral administration of the drug to pregnant women. One study utilized Doppler velocimetry to show no significant effect of oral terbutaline on fetal umbilical artery impedance at 26–32 weeks. The same authors demonstrated a 78% increase in fetal breathing movements after 5 mg of terbutaline was taken orally. Follow-up study of infants exposed to terbutaline in the second half of pregnancy reveals a modest rise in the incidence of postnatal hypoglycemia. Therefore, newborns exposed to this drug in utero should be observed for hypoglycemia. In one retrospective study of 2827 deliveries between 25 and 36 weeks, newborns who were exposed to β-sympathomimetic agents in utero had a greater likelihood of intraventricular hemorrhage (odds ratio = 2.47, CI = 1.34–4.56) compared to infants exposed to either magnesium sulfate or no tocolysis. This could be related to a risk of agents such as terbutaline, or to a protective effect of magnesium sulfate, as has been postulated by some investigators. A number of other neonatal problems have been described, including case reports of myocardial necrosis and of cardiovascular decompensation after long-term, and possibly high-dose, terbutaline pump therapy. No causal relationship has been documented.

The breast milk concentrations of terbutaline in a small number of nursing mothers treated for asthma were found to be similar or higher than maternal plasma concentrations. However, the drug was not detectable in the nursing infants' plasma, and no symptoms of β-adrenoreceptor stimulation could be found in any of the babies.

DOSAGE

For acute treatment of asthma in pregnancy, the dose of inhaled albuterol is 2.5 mg (0.5 ml of a 0.5% solution, diluted with 2–3 ml of normal saline)) and of metaproterenol is 15 mg (0.3 ml of a 5% solution, diluted with 2–3 ml of normal saline). The subcutaneous dose of terbutaline is 0.25 mg every 20–30 minutes for up to three doses. The onset of action of subcutaneous terbutaline is about 15 minutes, peak effect occurs in 30–60 minutes, and the duration of action is 1.5–4.0 hours.

Terbutaline has not been approved by the FDA for the treatment of premature labor, but because of the extensive experience in Europe and the United States, many centers do use it for this purpose. The usual intravenous dose is 10—25 μg/min. The subcutaneous dose is 0.25 mg q6h for as long as 3 days. When terbutaline is used to treat acute intrapartum "fetal distress," in patients without contraindications such as cardiovascular disease, tachycardia, thyrotoxicosis, fluid overload, or other conditions, the usual dose is 0.25 mg given either subcutaneously or as an intravenous bolus. Generally speaking, preparations are being made for expeditious vaginal delivery or cesarean section when this form of intrauterine resuscitation is utilized.

ADVERSE EFFECTS

Side effects include tachycardia, palpitations, headache, nausea, vomiting, anxiety, sweating, tremor, and tinnitus. These side effects are generally transient and do not require treatment.

Other common sequelae include maternal hyperglycemia, hypokalemia, mild anemia, increased free fatty acids and glycerol, and fetal tachycardia. Hypokalemia is generally believed to be secondary to the hyperglycemia and hyperinsulinemia that drive serum potassium into the cells. Since there is no loss of potassium from the body, serum levels quickly return to baseline values after terbutaline is discontinued. When present, the hypokalemia is usually asymptomatic and rarely requires treatment. Cerebral ischemia has been reported in two pregnant patients, each with a history of migraine, who were being treated with terbutaline for asthma or for preterm labor.

MECHANISM OF ACTION

Terbutaline is a sympathomimetic agent with predominantly β_2 activity. It is believed that sympathomimetics work by stimulating adenyl cyclase, the enzyme that catalyzes the conversion of adenosine triphosphate to cyclic AMP.

Terbutaline produces significant bronchodilatation, which may result in an increased vital capacity, forced expiratory volume in 1 second (FEV_1), peak expiratory flow (PEF), and maximum expiratory flow (MEF) in asthmatic patients. It is also effective in decreasing uterine activity during the second and third trimesters. In pregnant ewes and baboons, uterine blood flow is not decreased by the dosages required to inhibit premature labor.

ABSORPTION AND BIOTRANSFORMATION

Approximately 30% to 55% of an oral dose is absorbed from the gastrointestinal tract. Terbutaline is metabolized in the liver, primarily to an inactive sulfated conjugate, and after being metabolized is excreted in the urine. Only 1% of a subcutaneously administered dose is recovered from bile, indicating the absence of a significant enterohepatic circulation. Excretion of the drug and its metabolites is essentially complete within 72–96 hours after the administration of a single parenteral or oral dose.

RECOMMENDED READING

American College of Obstetricians and Gynecologists. *Preterm labor.* ACOG Technical Bulletin #206. Washington, DC, 1995.

American College of Obstetricians and Gynecologists. *Pulmonary disease in pregnancy.* ACOG Technical Bulletin #224. Washington, DC, 1996.

Andersson, K.E., et al. The relaxing effect of terbutaline on the human uterus during term labor. *Am. J. Obstet. Gynecol.* 121: 602, 1975.

Andersson, K.E., Bengtsson, L.P., and Ingemarsson, I. Terbutaline inhibition of midtrimester uterine activity induced by prostaglandin F₂ and hypertonic saline. *Br. J. Obstet. Gynaecol.* 82:745, 1975.

Angel, J.L., O'Brien, W.F., Knuppel, R.A., et al: Carbohydrate intolerance in patients receiving oral tocolytics. *Am. J. Obstet. Gynecol.* 159:762, 1988.

Arner, B. A comparative clinical trial of different subcutaneous doses of terbutaline and orciprenaline in bronchial asthma. *Acta Med. Scand.* 512 (Suppl.):45, 1970.

Arner, B., et al. Circulatory effects of orciprenaline, adrenaline and a new sympathomimetic β-receptor-stimulating agent, terbutaline, in normal human subjects. *Acta Med. Scand.* 512 (Suppl.):25, 1970.

Carlstrom, S., and Westling, H. Metabolic, circulatory and respiratory effects of a new sympathomimetic β-receptor-stimulating agent, terbutaline, compared with those of orciprenaline. *Acta Med. Scand.* 512 (Suppl.):33, 1970.

Canadian Preterm Labor Investigators Group. Treatment of preterm labor with the beta-adrenergic agonist ritodrine. *N. Engl. J. Med.* 327:308, 1992.

Fletcher, S.E., Fyfe, D.A., Case, C.L., et al. Myocardial necrosis in a newborn after long-term maternal subcutaneous terbutaline infusion for suppression of preterm labor. *Am. J. Obstet. Gynecol.* 165:1401, 1991.

Foley, M.R., Landon, M.B., Gabbe, S.G., et al. Effect of prolonged oral terbutaline therapy on glucose tolerance in pregnancy. *Am. J. Obstet. Gynecol.* 168:100, 1993.

Groome, L.J., Goldenberg, R.L., Cliver, S.P., et al. Neonatal periventricular-intraventricular hemorrhage after maternal-sympathomimetic tocolysis. *Am. J. Obstet. Gynecol.* 167:873, 1992.

Hallack, M., Moise, K.J.Jr., Smith, E.O. et al. The effects of indomethacin and terbutaline on human fetal umbilical artery velocimetry: a randomized, double-blind study. *Am. J. Obstet. Gynecol.* 168:865, 1993.

Hallack, M., Moise, K.J., Jr., Lira, N. The effect of tocolytic agents (indomethacin and terbutaline) on fetal breathing and body movements: a prospective, randomized, double-blind, placebo-controlled clinical trial. *Am. J. Obstet. Gynecol.* 167: 1059, 1992.

Hoffman, B.B., and Lefkowitz, R.J. Catecholamines, sympathomimetic drugs, and adrenergic receptor antagonists. Chapter 10 in *Goodman and Gilman's The Pharmacological Basis of Therapeutics* (9th ed.), J.G. Hardman and L.E. Limbird, eds. New York: McGraw-Hill, 1996. Pp. 213–216.

How, H.Y., Hughes, S.A., Vogel, R.L., et al. Oral terbutaline in the outpatient management of preterm labor. *Am. J. Obstet. Gynecol.* 173:1518, 1995.

Ingemarsson, I. Effects of terbutaline on premature labor. A double-blind placebo-controlled study. *Am. J. Obstet. Gynecol.* 125:520, 1976.

Ingemarsson, I., and Bengtsson, B. A five-year experience with terbutaline for preterm labor: low rate of severe side effects. *Obstet. Gynecol.* 66:176, 1985.

Katz, M., Robertson, P.A., and Creasy, R.K. Cardiovascular complications associated with terbutaline treatment for preterm labor. *Am. J. Obstet. Gynecol.* 139:605, 1981.

King, J.F., Grant, A., Keirse, M.J.N.C., et al. Betamimetics in preterm labour: an overview of the randomized controlled trials. *Br. J. Obstet. Gynaecol.* 95:211, 1988.

Lam, F., Gill, P., Smith, M., et al: Use of the subcutaneous terbutaline pump for long-term tocolysis. *Obstet. Gynecol.* 72:810, 1988.

Lampert, M.B., Hibbard, J., Weinert, L., et al. Peripartum heart failure associated with prolonged tocolytic therapy. *Am. J. Obstet. Gynecol.* 168:493, 1993.

Lindenbaum, C., Ludmir, J., Teplick, F.B., et al. Maternal glucose intolerance and the subcutaneous terbutaline pump. *Am. J. Obstet. Gynecol.* 166:925, 1992.

Macones, G.A., Berlin, M., and Berlin, J.A. Efficacy of oral beta-agonist maintenance therapy in preterm labor: a meta-analysis. *Obstet. Gynecol.* 85:313, 1995.

National Asthma Education Program. Report of the Working Group on Asthma in Pregnancy. *Management of Asthma During Pregnancy.* Bethesda, Maryland: Department of Health and Human Services, 1993; NIH publication #93–3279.

Parilla, B.V., Dooley, S.L., Minogue, J.P., et al. The efficacy of oral terbutaline after intravenous tocolysis. *Am. J. Obstet. Gynecol.* 169:965, 1993.

Patriarco, M.S., Viechnicki, B.M., Hutchinson, T.A., et al. A study on intrauterine fetal resuscitation with terbutaline. *Am. J. Obstet. Gynecol.* 157:384, 1987.

Perry, K.G.Jr., Morrison, J.C., Rust, O.A., et al. Incidence of adverse cardiopulmonary effects with low-dose continuous terbutaline infusion. *Am. J. Obstet. Gynecol.* 173:1273, 1995.

Regenstein, A.C., Belluomini, J., and Katz, M. Terbutaline tocolysis and glucose intolerance. *Obstet. Gynecol.* 81:739, 1993.

Rosene, K.A., Featherstone, H.J., and Benedetti, T.J. Cerebral ischemia associated with parenteral terbutaline use in pregnant migraine patients. *Am. J. Obstet. Gynecol.* 143:405, 1982.

Sackner, M.A., et al. Hemodynamic effects of epinephrine and terbutaline in normal man. *Chest* 68:616, 1975.

Shekarloo, A., Mendez-Bauer, C., Cook, V., et al. Terbutaline (intravenous bolus) for the treatment of acute intrapartum fetal distress. *Am. J. Obstet. Gynecol.* 160:615, 1989.

Svenningsen, N.W. Followup studies on preterm infants after maternal beta receptor agonist treatment. *Acta Obstet. Gynecol. Scand.* 108:67, 1982.

Thorkelsson, T., and Loughead, J.L. Long-term subcutaneous terbutaline tocolysis: report of possible neonatal toxicity. *J. Perinatol.* 11:235, 1991.

Wagner, J.M., et al. Terbutaline and maternal cardiac function. *J.A.M.A.* 246:2697, 1981.

Biguanide Hypoglycemic Agents: Metformin: (Glucophage®)

INDICATIONS AND RECOMMENDATIONS

Metformin is relatively contraindicated during pregnancy because other therapeutic agents, in particular insulin, are preferable. Metformin is used to treat type 2 diabetes and acts by inhibiting hepatic gluconeogenesis, thus decreasing hepatic glucose output, as well as by enhancing peripheral insulin action. It does not increase insulin production or release, and does not cause hypoglycemia. Used for many years in Europe, metformin was approved for use in the United States in 1995. Metformin rarely can cause lactic acidosis, particularly when there is preexisting renal impairment.

In an in vitro study of single human placental cotyledons, metformin had no significant effect on placental glucose uptake or transport. In a series of 60 pregnancies in patients with type 2 diabetes treated with metformin during the second and third trimesters in South Africa in the 1970s, perinatal mortality rates were similar to those treated with insulin and there was a high incidence of neonatal jaundice. Other than the South African experience, there is not much published information regarding the effects of metformin on fetus or mother during pregnancy. Because the pregnancy effects of metformin are not well understood, and because insulin crosses the placenta in small quantities if at all and is known to be effective in treating diabetes during pregnancy, insulin should be considered the drug of choice for such patients.

RECOMMENDED READING

Bailey, C.J., and Turner, R.C. Metformin. *N. Engl. J. Med.* 334: 574, 1996.

Coetzee, E.J., and Jackson, W.P.U. Metformin in management of pregnant insulin-independent diabetics. *Diabetologia* 16:241, 1979.

Davis, S.N., and Granner, D.K. Insulin, oral hypoglycemic agents, and the pharmacology of the endocrine pancreas. Chapter 60 in *Goodman and Gilman's The Pharmacological Basis of Therapeutics* (9th ed.), J.G. Hardman and L.E. Limbard, eds. New York: McGraw-Hill, 1996. P. 1510.

DeFronzo, R.A., Goodman, A.M., and the Multicenter Metformin Study Group: Efficacy of metformin in patients with non-insulin-dependent diabetes mellitus. *N. Engl. J. Med.* 333: 541, 1995.

Elliott, B.D., Langer, O., and Schuessling, F. Human placental glucose uptake and transport are not altered by the oral antihyperglycemic agent metformin. *Am. J. Obstet. Gynecol.* 176:527, 1997.

Bile Acid Sequestrants: Cholestyramine (Prevalite®, Questran®), Colestipol (Colestid®)

INDICATIONS AND RECOMMENDATIONS

Cholestyramine is safe to use for symptomatic relief of pruritus secondary to cholestasis of pregnancy. It is a bile acid sequestrant that in the nonpregnant patient is primarily used for the treatment of hyperlipoproteinemia that is not responsive to diet. The patient's prothrombin time should be monitored and fat-soluble vitamins supplemented when this drug is administered. Clinical experience with colestipol, a similar agent, during pregnancy is lacking, and therefore it should be used only when cholestyramine cannot be used.

SPECIAL CONSIDERATIONS IN PREGNANCY

Cholestyramine is often prescribed for symptomatic relief of the pruritus associated with cholestasis of pregnancy. It must be administered for several days before clear benefit is seen and provides no improvement in laboratory abnormalities. Cholestyramine is not absorbed, and the major problem associated with its administration is related to fat-soluble vitamin deficiency or interactions with other drugs.

One case report documents severe fetal intracranial hemorrhage during treatment with cholestyramine for intrahepatic cholestasis of pregnancy. The mother received cholestyramine 8 g/day from week 19 to 22 and 16 g/day thereafter. At 27 weeks, she delivered a 1660-g infant who died 15 minutes after birth. The infant had bilateral subdural hematomas, an enlarged liver, and bilateral plural effusions. The hemorrhage was thought to be a result of maternal vitamin K deficiency which in turn caused fetal vitamin K deficiency and fetal coagulopathy. The author hypothesized that supplementation of vitamin K to the mother might have prevented the fetal effects.

Cholestyramine has been used successfully in the treatment of primary sclerosing cholangitis during pregnancy. In this case, the one reported adverse effect was a mild increase in maternal prothrombin time, which returned to normal after oral vitamin K therapy.

DOSAGE

The usual dose of cholestyramine is 4 g qd or bid. The dose may be gradually increased to a maximum of 24 g/day in divided doses. Pruritus often recurs 1–2 days after withdrawal of the drug. Colestipol is given in either tablet or granule form in a dose of up to 16 g/day.

ADVERSE EFFECTS

Because these drugs are not absorbed from the gastrointestinal tract, most side effects are digestive. These include constipation, abdominal discomfort and distention, flatulence, nausea, vomiting, diarrhea, heartburn, anorexia, and steatorrhea. Deficiencies of fat-soluble vitamins can occur. Cholestyramine also is described by most patients as having an unpleasant taste.

MECHANISM OF ACTION

Cholestyramine and colestipol are resins that combine with bile acids in the intestine to form insoluble complexes that are excreted in the feces. As a result, bile acids are partially removed from the enterohepatic circulation. This may reduce the systemic circulating bile acid concentration, thereby reducing skin levels of bile acids and decreasing pruritus.

RECOMMENDED READING

Landon, M.B., Soloway, R.D., Freedman, L.J., and Gabbe, S.G. Primary sclerosing cholangitis and pregnancy. *Obstet. Gynecol.* 69:457, 1987.

Reyes, H. The spectrum of liver and gastrointestinal disease seen in cholestasis of pregnancy. *Gastroenterol. Clin. North Am.* 24:905, 1992.

Sadler, L.C., Lane, M., and North, R. Severe fetal intracranial haemorrhage during treatment with cholestyramine for intrahepatic cholestasis of pregnancy. *Br. J. Obstet. Gynaecol.* 102:169, 1995.

Shaw, D., et al. A prospective study of 18 patients with cholestasis of pregnancy. *Am. J. Obstet. Gynecol.* 142:621, 1982.

Witzham, J.L. Drugs used in the treatment of hyperlipoproteinemias. Chapter 36 in *Goodman and Gilman's The Pharmacological Basis of Therapeutics* (9th ed.), J.G. Hardman and L.E. Limbird, eds. New York: McGraw-Hill, 1996. Pp. 888–889.

Bromocriptine (Parlodel®)

INDICATIONS AND RECOMMENDATIONS

Most women with amenorrhea/galactorrhea syndromes who undergo ovulation induction with bromocriptine are advised to discontinue the medication once conception has occurred. Some clinicians continue therapy throughout pregnancy in order to prevent neurologic complications, and others use the drug selectively for pregnant women with macroadenomas or for those who develop neurologic complications during pregnancy. The manufacturer suggests that the drug be discontinued once pregnancy has been diagnosed. This recommendation is apparently based on the complications described below, seen in postpartum women taking the drug for suppression of lactation. The reported experience with the use of this drug during pregnancy to date suggests that fetal risk is not appreciable.

Although bromocriptine was formerly used to suppress postpartum lactation in women who chose not to nurse their babies, this indication was withdrawn by the manufacturer in 1994 because of reports of cardiovascular and neurologic complications occurring in postpartum women taking the drug. While no causal relationship was clearly established, the possible risks were believed to exceed the benefits when the drug was used for lactation suppression.

SPECIAL CONSIDERATIONS IN PREGNANCY

Most patients who have taken bromocriptine during pregnancy have done so inadvertently, after successful ovulation induction. Sandoz, the company that markets the drug, collected information on 2587 pregnancies in 2437 women who took bromocriptine at some time during pregnancy. Follow-up examinations were available for 988 infants. Rates of spontaneous abortion and congenital malformations were not increased above background levels. There were no obvious adverse effects discerned at neonatal follow-up, although the report did not include a control group. The dosage and duration of exposure to bromocriptine did not differ between the pregnancies producing anomalous and normal babies. A case report describing a neonate with trisomy 13, who had been exposed to bromocriptine for the first 20 days in utero, has not been supported in large series. A case-control study of 31 exposed children and 31 nonexposed controls showed no increase in karyotypic abnormalities in lymphocyte cultures taken at a median age of 40 months.

In a series reported from Paris, eight women with grade II and III prolactinomas were treated with bromocriptine at a dose (5–20 mg/day) sufficient to suppress the prolactin level below 20 ng/ml continuously throughout pregnancy. None had tumor-related neurologic complications. Two additional patients, not known to be pregnant, had their bromocriptine discontinued after 2–3 weeks of treatment. Both developed bitemporal hemianopia during the second trimester (at serum prolactin levels around 50 ng/ml), and the symptoms responded to bromocriptine in both cases. The authors believe that bromocriptine treatment should be continued throughout pregnancy in patients with prolactinoma. It should be pointed out, however, that prolactin levels in normal women generally exceed 100 ng/ml during pregnancy, and so there is no evidence that maintaining tumor patients at levels below 20 ng/ml is appropriate. In addition, most authors report a lower rate of neurologic complications in pregnant women with prolactinomas than the 2 in 2 (100%) noted in the untreated patients in the above study. A subsequent case series of 10 pregnancies in 4 individuals reported no neurologic sequelae after discontinuation of bromocriptine in early pregnancy. Thus, the prophylactic use of bromocriptine throughout pregnancy in such women remains controversial.

There are reports of pituitary macroadenomas responding to bromocriptine during pregnancy. A number of patients with excessive breast enlargement (gigantomastia) have been successfully treated with this drug during pregnancy.

DOSAGE

Bromocriptine is available as a 2.5 mg tablet and a 5 mg capsule. When bromocriptine is used to treat amenorrhea-galactorrhea, the starting dose is generally 1.25 or 2.5 mg at bedtime with a snack, increasing to bid after 3–7 days. The usual therapeutic dose ranges from 5 to 7.5 mg/day. Bromocriptine is also used, in much higher dosage, to treat acromegaly and Parkinson's disease. These diagnoses, however, are quite unusual among women in the reproductive age group.

ADVERSE EFFECTS

Side effects occur in the majority of treated patients. Nausea has been reported in more than 50%, with headaches, dizziness, fatigue, abdominal cramps, vomiting, nasal congestion, constipation, and diarrhea being somewhat less common. Faintness, believed to be due to orthostatic hypotension, is commonly reported, particularly when therapy is first initiated. Rarely, neurologic symptoms, including hallucinations, occur. When bromocriptine was used to suppress postpartum lactation, there were a number of cases reported to the manufacturers and to the FDA of hypertension, myocardial infarctions, strokes, and seizures, prompting the FDA and manufacturers to agree that this indication should be removed. Nevertheless, a Dutch study in which prescription records and hospital records were linked found no cases of hospitalization for hypertension, heart attack, or stroke among 2130 women prescribed the drug for lactation suppression, suggesting that the magnitude of any presumed relationship would be small. Much higher dosages have been used to treat patients with Parkinson's disease, with more severe side effects reported.

MECHANISM OF ACTION

Bromocriptine is an ergot derivative that activates lactotrope dopamine receptors, thus inhibiting the release of prolactin. The side effects of bromocriptine are also ascribed to its dopamine-like action.

ABSORPTION AND BIOTRANSFORMATION

Approximately 28% of an oral dose is absorbed from the gastrointestinal tract, and peak plasma levels are reached within 2 hours. The drug is highly protein-bound. It is completely metabolized, and excretion is in bile. Almost all of an orally administered dose is excreted in the feces over 120 hours.

RECOMMENDED READING

Ahmed, M., Al-Dossary, E., and Woodhouse, N.J. Macroprolactinomas with suprasellar extension: effect of bromocriptine withdrawal during one or more pregnancies. *Fertil. Steril.* 58:492, 1992.

Ascoli, M., and Segaloff, D.L. Adenohypophyseal hormones and their hypothalamic releasing factors. Chapter 55 in *Goodman and Gilman's The Pharmacological Basis of Therapeutics* (9th ed.), J.G. Hardman and L.E. Limbird, eds. New York: McGraw-Hill, 1996. Pp. 1371–1372.

Czeizel, A., Kiss, R., Ráz, K., Mohori, K., and Gláz, E. Case-control cytogenetic study in offspring of mothers treated with bromocriptine during early pregnancy. *Mutat. Res.* 210:23, 1989.

Eben, F., Cameron, M.D., and Lowy, C. Successful treatment of mammary hyperplasia in pregnancy with bromocriptine. *Br. J. Obstet. Gynaecol.* 100:95, 1993.

Hedberg, K., Karlsson, K., and Lindstedt, G. Gigantomastia during pregnancy: effect of a dopamine agonist. *Am. J. Obstet. Gynecol. 133:928, 1979.*

Herings, R.M.C., and Stricker, B.H.C. Bromocriptine and suppression of postpartum lactation: the incidence of adverse cardiovascular effects in women of child-bearing age. *Pharm. World Sci.* 17:133, 1995.

Imai, T., Yasuda, K., Ohta, T., and Miura, K. 13 trisomy born to a mother treated with bromocriptine: incidental or not? *Tohoku J. Exp. Med.* 153:233, 1987.

Konopka, P., et al. Continuous administration of bromocriptine in the prevention of neurological complications in pregnant women with prolactinomas. *Am. J. Obstet. Gynecol.* 146:935, 1983.

Krupp, P., and Monka, C. Bromocriptine in pregnancy: safety aspects. *Klin. Wochenschrift* 65:823, 1987.

Maeda, T., et al. Effective bromocriptine treatment of a pituitary macroadenoma during pregnancy. *Obstet. Gynecol.* 61: 117, 1983.

Turkalj, I., Braun, P., and Krupp, P. Surveillance of bromocriptine in pregnancy. *J.A.M.A.* 247:1589, 1982.

Yap A.S., Clouston, W.M., Mortimer, R.H., and Drake, R.F. Acromegaly first diagnosed in pregnancy: the role of bromocriptine therapy. *Am. J. Obstet. Gynecol.* 163:477, 1990.

Bulk-Forming Agents (Over-the-Counter): Agar, Bran, Methylcellulose, Psyllium, Tragacanth, Polycarbophil

INDICATIONS AND RECOMMENDATIONS

Bulk-forming agents are safe to use during pregnancy. While increasing dietary fiber is the first intervention that should be suggested, the over-the-counter (OTC) drugs listed above are used as stool softeners in people with constipation, hemorrhoids, anorectal disorders, hernias, and cardiovascular disease.

SPECIAL CONSIDERATIONS IN PREGNANCY

There are no maternal effects unique to pregnancy.

DOSAGE

Methylcellulose and carboxymethylcellulose are supplied as a 500 mg powder, tablet, or capsule. The dose is 1–6 g/day taken 1–4 times a day, each dose taken with one to two glasses of water. Onset of action is 1–2 days.

Psyllium preparations from the plantain seed are powders. One to two teaspoons of powder is mixed in water and taken 1–3 times a day.

Agar is usually mixed with psyllium or cathartics and 4–16 g is taken daily.

Tragacanth is available in many preparations in a variety of dosages.

Bran contains 20% indigestible cellulose and is generally taken with cereal.

ADVERSE EFFECTS

With the exception of the psyllium preparations, none of these bulk-forming laxatives is significantly absorbed, and thus no systemic effects occur. Psyllium preparations are absorbed to some degree and have been shown to decrease plasma cholesterol levels by interfering with absorption of bile acids. Calcium polycarbophil may release calcium into the gastrointestinal tract and so should be avoided in patients whose calcium intake is restricted. Carboxymethylcellulose and psyllium contain sodium, which may be absorbed. They should be avoided in patients on sodium-restricted diets. Because some of these laxatives may bind concomitantly administered medications, they should be taken at a separate time from other medications. Bulk-forming laxatives may increase flatulence and, if taken with inadequate water, intestinal obstruction may occur.

MECHANISM OF ACTION

These agents, which include methylcellulose and carboxymethylcellulose, psyllium preparations, agar, tragacanth, and bran, all swell when in contact with water, forming a mass that promotes peristalsis, decreases transit time, and keeps the feces soft.

RECOMMENDED READING

Brunton, L.L. Agents affecting gastrointestinal water flux and motility. Chapter 38 in *Goodman and Gilman's The Pharmacological Basis of Therapeutics* (9th ed.), J.G. Hardman and L.E. Limbird, eds. New York: McGraw-Hill, 1996. Pp. 920–921.

Nelson, M.M., and Forfar, J.O. Associations between drugs administered during pregnancy and congenital abnormalities of the fetus. *Br. Med. J.* 1:523, 1971.

Schenkel, B., and Vorherr, H. Non-prescription drugs during pregnancy: potential teratogenic and toxic effects upon embryo and fetus. *J. Reprod. Med.* 12:27, 1974.

Buspirone (Buspar®)

INDICATIONS AND RECOMMENDATIONS

Buspirone should only be used in pregnancy if other agents are not effective and the condition is serious enough to warrant use of a drug that has not been well studied and whose effects on the pregnant mother and her fetus are unknown. It is an antianxiety agent that is relatively unique in structure, and it is used for treatment of chronic anxiety disorders or for short-term relief of anxiety.

SPECIAL CONSIDERATIONS IN PREGNANCY

Studies of buspirone in rats and rabbits have shown no increase in infertility or congenital malformations. High doses in rats were associated with an increase in stillbirths. There are no well-controlled studies in humans. One case report described buspirone use during a pregnancy that was electively terminated at 12 weeks gestation. Examination of the fetus and placenta did not reveal any abnormalities. Buspirone is excreted in the breast milk of rats, but its presence in human milk is undocumented. Its use should be avoided in lactating mothers if possible.

DOSAGE

The recommended initial dose is 7.5 mg twice daily. This dosage may be increased by 5 mg/day, at 2- to 3-day intervals, until a therapeutic response is achieved, usually at 20–30 mg/day. The maximum daily dose is 60 mg.

ADVERSE EFFECTS

The most common side effects include nausea, headache, dizziness, nervousness, and excitement. Other common complaints include nonspecific chest pain, dream disturbances, sore throat, nasal congestion, and tinnitus. Rare allergic or dystonic reactions may occur.

MECHANISM OF ACTION

Buspirone belongs to a class of drugs known as azapirones. It is a partial serotonin agonist and has affinity for brain D_2-dopamine receptors. It may result in increased plasma prolactin levels. The exact mechanism of action of buspirone is unknown. It is structurally different than benzodiazepines and other anxiolytics, and it does not have anticonvulsant, muscle relaxant, or sedative effects. It does not show cross-tolerance with benzodiazepines.

ABSORPTION AND BIOTRANSFORMATION

Buspirone is rapidly absorbed and undergoes significant first-pass metabolism. Peak plasma levels (1–6 ng/ml) may be seen 40–90 minutes after a single oral dose of 20 mg. Most of the drug is protein-bound. The half-life is approximately 2–3 hours. The majority of drug is excreted as metabolites through the urine.

RECOMMENDED READING

Baldessarini, R.J. Drugs and the treatment of psychiatric disorders.
In Chapter 18 of *Goodman and Gilman's The Pharmacological
Basis of Therapeutics* (9th ed.), J.G. Hardman and L.E. Limbird,
eds. New York: McGraw-Hill, 1996. Pp. 422– 446.

Miller, L.J. Psychiatric medication during pregnancy: understanding and minimizing risks. *Psychiatr. Ann.* 24:69, 1994.

Calcium Channel Blockers: Diltiazem (Cardizem®), Nicardipine (Nicardipin®), Nifedipine (Procardia®), Verapamil (Calan®, Isoptin®), Nimodipine (Nimotop®), Isradipine (DynaCirc®), Felodipine (Plendil®)

INDICATIONS AND RECOMMENDATIONS

The use of the calcium channel blockers during pregnancy is
indicated for the treatment of specific life-threatening cardiovascular conditions and as adjunctive therapy for the pharmacologic conversion of fetal supraventricular tachyarrhythmias.
They are also reasonable alternatives to standard therapies for
preterm labor and hypertension. Because nifedipine has been
used most commonly and has the most safety information regarding use in pregnancy, it is the calcium channel blocker of
choice for non-arrhythmia indications, pending further research on the newer agents. Because of possible adverse interactions, the combination of calcium channel blockers and magnesium sulfate should be avoided.

The calcium channel blockers are categorized into two
groups. Type 1 agents (diltiazem, verapamil) mainly affect the
cardiac conducting system. Type 2 agents, the dihydropyridine
group (nicardipine, nifedipine, nimodipine, isradipine, and felodipine), mainly relax smooth muscle, particularly vascular
smooth muscle. The type 1 agents are most commonly used as
antiarrhythmic agents, whereas the type 2 agents are most
commonly used to treat hypertension and other vasospastic disorders.

SPECIAL CONSIDERATIONS IN PREGNANCY

Animal studies regarding potential teratogenicity of the calcium channel blockers are reassuring. While many of these
agents have been shown to induce digital defects in rabbit fetuses exposed in utero during the susceptible period, these defects have been documented to be due to maternal hypotension
and decreased uterine blood flow rather than a direct drug effect. These same defects have not been induced in other species.

The use of these agents in human pregnancy was initially
limited due to reports in many animal models (sheep, rhesus
macaques, goats) of reduced uterine blood flow leading to fetal
hypoxia and acidosis. However, experience in human pregnancy

was dissimilar and, more recently, studies of placental blood flow using radioisotopes and by Doppler flow studies indicate that uterine perfusion in human pregnancy is unaffected by these agents.

First-trimester exposure was reported by 78 women in a combined report from six teratogen information services. The proportion of congenital malformations (2/78, or 3%) in the treatment group was not significantly different from that observed in a control group matched for maternal age and smoking (0%). Cumulative experience with the type 2 agents in pregnancy for the treatment of preterm labor or hypertension is large and the data support safety of these agents for use in human pregnancy.

The indication for use of the type 1 agents in pregnancy is maternal or fetal supraventricular tachycardia. Verapamil has been used to successfully treat a supraventricular tachycardia in a digitalized hyperthyroid patient at 36 weeks. A single intravenous dose of 5 mg given over 5 minutes rapidly broke the arrhythmia and the patient remained in sinus rhythm for the remaining 5 weeks of her pregnancy. No adverse maternal or fetal effects were noted, and the neonate had 1- and 5-minute Apgar scores of 8 and 9, respectively. A case has been reported of a fetus at 34 weeks with a tachycardia between 240 and 280 beats/minute and ultrasonic signs of early congestive heart failure that was successfully treated with maternally administered β-acetyldigoxin and verapamil. The mother was maintained on 0.4 mg/day of the digitalis preparation and 80 mg of verapamil 3 times a day. During the 4 days after onset of treatment, the tachyarrhythmia slowed transiently to 180–196 beats/minute. Five days after the onset of therapy, the fetal heart rate was normal at 138–150 beats/minute, and this persisted until delivery 5 weeks later. The infant appeared to be healthy at birth, was in sinus rhythm with a rate of 160–170 beats/minute during the first day of life, had no signs of cardiac hypertrophy or disturbances in repolarization, and had a normal atrioventricular (AV) conduction time.

Type 2 agents have been used successfully for the treatment of the hypertensive disorders of pregnancy. It has recently been hypothesized that the calcium channel blockers may be ideal agents for treating preeclampsia because of their potential for controlling generalized vasospasm, hypertension, and eclamptic seizures. In addition, they have been shown to decrease platelet and erythrocyte aggregation in vitro. Several studies have compared the hemodynamic response to hydralazine to that of nifedipine in the acute management of severe preeclampsia. Although the numbers of patients in the studies are small, nifedipine therapy caused a less precipitous decrease in blood pressure and resulted in fewer episodes of maternal hypotension and resulting fetal distress. In one study, patients were monitored with pulmonary and radial artery catheters. While the decrease in blood pressure was similar in both groups, the decrease in pulmonary capillary wedge pressure was 60% with hydralazine, versus 30% with nifedipine; nifedipine caused less decrease in cardiac preload with the same degree of blood pressure reduction. This is a particularly attractive attribute in the treatment of severe preeclampsia, where the intravascular volume is frequently decreased.

In chronic studies, control of blood pressure was more frequently attained with oral nifedipine (96%) than with oral hydralazine (68%); however, this finding is expected as tachyphylaxis to oral hydralazine is common, limiting its usefulness for chronic therapy. In a randomized trial of oral nifedipine versus bed rest alone in 200 patients with mild preeclampsia remote from term, delivery for severe hypertension occurred less frequently in the nifedipine group. However, the average prolongation of pregnancy and the duration of hospitalization was the same in both groups. There are several anecdotal reports of a significant increase in platelet count after initiation of nifedipine. However, in the chronic trial in patients with mild preeclampsia noted above, the mean platelet count at delivery was the same in both groups, and HELLP syndrome occurred in 5 patients in the nifedipine group versus 2 in the bed-rest-only group. Other complications such as the development of severe proteinuria occurred with similar frequency in both groups. Other authors have suggested that the type 2 calcium channel blockers might be of particular benefit in the treatment of preeclampsia, as they will cause cerebral vasodilatation and therefore might be beneficial in the prevention of eclamptic seizures.

A major concern regarding the use of calcium channel blockers in the treatment of preeclampsia is the potential synergistic action with magnesium sulfate. There have been a small number of case reports of significant complications, including profound hypotension, neuromuscular blockade, and cardiac arrest, with concurrent use of these agents. In all cases, the effect was reversed by administration of calcium gluconate. There are several studies in which concurrent nifedipine and magnesium were used without complications; however, this may be related to the small numbers of patients studied. While there appear to be some significant benefits to the use of nifedipine and related agents in the acute management of severe preeclampsia, in facilities where magnesium sulfate for seizure prophylaxis is the standard of care, the concurrent use of these agents should be limited until more safety information is available.

Type 2 calcium channel blockers have also been used successfully in the treatment of premature labor. There have been a number of randomized trials comparing oral nifedipine to intravenous ritodrine, a single trial comparing nifedipine to subcutaneous terbutaline and another to intravenous magnesium sulfate. Oral nifedipine has appeal due to ease of administration. The trials indicate that efficacy is equivalent to more standard therapies and that side effects limiting therapy are less common. Nifedipine can be recommended as an alternative tocolytic agent. As mentioned above, the concomitant use of calcium channel blockers and magnesium sulfate should be avoided.

All of the type 2 calcium channel blockers have been documented to cross the placental barrier. Cord blood levels are generally lower than maternal levels. Levels in amniotic fluid are lower than cord blood levels. Nifedipine can be measured in breast milk, in levels comparable to maternal blood levels. However, due to protein binding, absorption of drug by the breast-feeding neonate is minimal.

DOSAGE

Nifedipine can be administered sublingually or orally. The usual dose for the treatment of an urgent hypertensive episode is 5–10 mg sublingually. The gelatin capsule should be perforated and the contents extruded under the tongue. Onset of action with a sublingual dose is 3–5 minutes. For chronic control of hypertension, the usual dose is 10–30 mg orally every 8 hours of the short-acting form, or 30–90 mg orally once daily of the long-acting form. Onset of action with oral dosing is 20 minutes, with a peak at 1 hour and a half-life of 2–3 hours. In pregnancy, the half-life of nifedipine is decreased due to more rapid hepatic elimination. Therefore the dosing interval may need to be decreased to achieve adequate therapeutic response. For the treatment of premature labor the most commonly reported protocol is an initial dose of 30 mg orally, followed by 20 mg every 4–8 hours as needed.

ADVERSE EFFECTS

In general, the calcium channel blockers exhibit relatively minor and infrequent side effects. Most studies report the incidence of undesirable side effects to be less than 10%. Fatigue, headache, dizziness, skin rash, and peripheral edema are the adverse sequelae most commonly observed.

These agents are relatively contraindicated in the sick sinus syndrome, second- or third-degree AV block, shock, and congestive heart failure. Both verapamil and nifedipine can increase serum levels of digoxin, and verapamil may also interact with β-adrenergic blockers and the methylxanthines.

MECHANISM OF ACTION

The calcium channel blockers inhibit the inward passage of calcium across myocardial, myometrial, and vascular smooth muscle cells and probably interfere with the intracellular release of calcium. The net effect of these actions is to uncouple the excitation–contraction process, causing smooth muscle relaxation. This results in a reduction in coronary artery and peripheral vascular resistance, as well as myometrial relaxation.

In spite of this common action, these agents constitute a heterogeneous group with different structural, electrophysiologic, and pharmacologic properties. Some of them depress myocardial contractility, whereas others affect the electrical conduction system of the heart.

Verapamil prolongs AV conduction in a dose-dependent fashion. It also decreases sinoatrial (SA) node automaticity, myocardial contractility, and peripheral vascular resistance. Its effect on heart rate and cardiac output is variable. Intravenous verapamil is considered by some authorities to be the drug of choice for treatment of acute paroxysmal supraventricular tachyarrhythmias.

Diltiazem reduces SA node automaticity, AV node conduction, myocardial contractility, and peripheral vascular resistance, but not to the same extent as verapamil. It has a variable effect on heart rate and cardiac output and increases vascular oxygen consumption. The primary use of this drug has been in the treatment of coronary artery spasm associated with variant angina. Because it can improve the balance between myocardial oxygen supply and demand and can reduce cellular injury secondary to ischemia, diltiazem is likely to be of benefit in the treatment of the acutely ischemic myocardium during cardiopulmonary bypass and possibly acute myocardial infarction as well.

Nifedipine, nicardipine, felodipine, and isradipine are potent, long-acting vasodilators. They have mild myocardial depressant effects and no antiarrhythmic properties. These drugs have proven very useful in relieving anginal symptoms caused by coronary vasospasm and have been used successfully in the treatment of essential hypertension and pregnancy-related hypertension.

ABSORPTION AND BIOTRANSFORMATION

The calcium channel blockers are well absorbed after oral administration, but their absolute bioavailability is reduced substantially by a "first-pass" effect in the liver, where they are extensively metabolized. All of these drugs are highly bound to plasma proteins, from 70% to 98%. Verapamil undergoes an 80% to 90% first-pass hepatic elimination after an oral dose. The major metabolite is norverapamil, which maintains 20% of the pharmacologic activity of the parent compound. Seventy-five percent of an oral dose is excreted in the urine. After oral administration, diltiazem undergoes a 60% first-pass metabolism. The major metabolite is desacetyldiltiazem, which maintains 40% to 50% of the pharmacologic activity of the parent compound. Approximately 35% of a dose of diltiazem undergoes renal excretion. Nifedipine is metabolized to inert products, 80% of which are excreted via the kidneys.

RECOMMENDED READING

Belfort, M.A., Saade, G.R., Moise, K.J., Jr., et al. Nimodipine in the management of preeclampsia: maternal and fetal effects. *Am. J. Obstet. Gynecol.* 171:417, 1994.

Ben-Ami, M., Giladi, Y., and Shalev, E. The combination of magnesium sulphate and nifedipine: a cause of neuromuscular blockade. *Br. J. Obstet. Gynaecol.* 101:262, 1994.

Childress, C.H., and Katz, V.L. Nifedipine and its indications in obstetrics and gynecology. *Obstet. Gynecol.* 83:616, 1994.

Danielson, M.K., and Danielsson, B.R. Reproductive toxicity studies of the antihypertensive agent felodipine in the rat. *Arzneimittel Forschung.* 43:106–109, 1993.

Ducsay, C.A., Thompson, J.S., Wu, A.T., and Novy, M.J. Effects of calcium entry blocker (nicardipine) tocolysis in rhesus macaques: fetal plasma concentrations and cardiorespiratory changes. *Am. J. Obstet. Gynecol.* 157:1482, 1987.

Fenakal, K., Fenakal, G., Appelman, Z., Lurie, S., Katz, Z., and Shoham, Z. Nifedipine in the treatment of severe preeclampsia. *Obstet. Gynecol.* 77:331, 1991.

Glock, J.L., and Morales, W.J. Efficacy and safety of nifedipine versus magnesium sulfate in the management of preterm labor: a randomized study. *Am. J. Obstet. Gynecol.* 169:960, 1993.

Harake, B., Gilbert, R.D., Ashwal, S., and Power, G.G. Nifedipine: effects on fetal and maternal hemodynamics in pregnant sheep. *Am. J. Obstet. Gynecol.* 157:1003, 1987.

Holbrook, R.H., Jr., Voss, E.M., and Gibson, R.N. Ovine fetal cardiorespiratory response to nicardipine. *Am. J. Obstet. Gynecol.* 161:718, 1989.

Jegasothy, R., and Paranthaman, S. Sublingual nifedipine compared with intravenous hydralazine in the acute treatment of severe hypertension in pregnancy: potential for use in rural practice. *J. Obstet. Gynaecol. Res.* 22:21, 1996.

Klein, V., and Repke, J.T. Supraventricular tachycardia in pregnancy: cardioversion with verapamil. *Obstet. Gynecol.* 63(S):16s, 1984.

Levin, A.C., Doering, P.L., and Hatton, R.C. Use of nifedipine in the hypertensive diseases of pregnancy. *Ann Pharmacother.* 28:1371, 1994.

Lindow, S.W., Davies, N., Davey, D.A., and Smith, J.A. The effect of sublingual nifedipine on uteroplacental blood flow in hypertensive pregnancy. *Br. J. Obstet. Gynaecol.* 95:1276, 1988.

Lundgren, Y., Thalen, P., and Nordlander, M. Effects of felodipine on utero-placental blood flow in normotensive rabbits. *Pharmacol. Toxicol.* 71:361, 1992.

Lunell, N.O., Bondesson, U., Grunewald, C., Ingemarsson, I., Nisell, H., and Wide-Swensson, D. Transplacental passage of isradipine in the treatment of pregnancy-induced hypertension. *Am. J. Hypertension* 6:110S, 1993.

Magee, L.A., Schick, B., Donnenfeld, A.E., et al. The safety of calcium channel blockers in human pregnancy: a prospective, multicenter cohort study. *Am. J. Obstet. Gynecol.* 174:823, 1996.

Maharaj, B., Khedun, S.M., Moodley, J., Madhanpall, N., and van der Byl, K. Intravenous isradipine in the management of severe hypertension in pregnant and nonpregnant patients. A pilot study. *Am. J. Hypertension* 7:61S–63S, 1994.

Manninen, A.K., and Juhakoski, A. Nifedipine concentrations in maternal and umbilical serum, amniotic fluid, breast milk and urine of mothers and offspring. *Int. J. Clin. Pharm. Res.* 11:231, 1991.

Mari, G., Kirshon, B., Moise, K.J., Jr., Lee, W., and Cotton, D.B. Doppler assessment of the fetal and uteroplacental circulation during nifedipine therapy for preterm labor. *Am. J. Obstet. Gynecol.* 161:1514, 1989.

Rubin, P.C., Butters, L., and McCabe, R. Nifedipine and platelets in preeclampsia. *Am. J. Hypertension* 1:175, 1988.

Scardo, J.A., Vermillion, S.T., Hogg, B.B., and Newman R.B. Hemodynamic effects of oral nifedipine in preeclamptic hypertensive emergencies. *Am. J. Obstet. Gynecol.* 175:336; discussion 338, 1996.

Sibai, B.M., Barton, J.R., Akl, S., Sarinoglu, C., and Mercer, B.M. A randomized prospective comparison of nifedipine and bed rest versus bed rest alone in the management of preeclampsia remote from term. *Am. J. Obstet. Gynecol.* 167:879, 1992.

Snyder, S.W., and Cardwell, M.S. Neuromuscular blockade with magnesium sulfate and nifedipine. *Am. J. Obstet. Gynecol.* 161:35, 1989.

Tranquilli, A.L., Garzetti, G.G., De Tommaso, G., et al. Nifedipine treatment in preeclampsia reverts the increased erythrocyte aggregation to normal. *Am. J. Obstet. Gynecol.* 167:942, 1992.

Visser, W., and Wallenburg, H.C. A comparison between the haemo-dynamic effects of oral nifedipine and intravenous dihydralazine in patients with severe pre-eclampsia. *J. Hypertension* 13:791, 1995.

Waisman, G.D., Mayorga, L.M., Camera, M.I., Vignolo, C.A., and Martinotti, A. Magnesium plus nifedipine: potentiation of hypotensive effect in preeclampsia? *Am. J. Obstet. Gynecol.* 159:308, 1988.

Wide-Swensson, D., Ingemarsson, I., Arulkumaran, S., and Andersson, K.E. Effects of isradipine, a new calcium antagonist, on maternal cardiovascular system and uterine activity in labour. *Br. J. Obstet. Gynaecol.* 97:945, 1990.

Wolff, F., et al. Prenatal diagnosis and therapy of fetal heart rate anomalies: with a contribution on the placental transfer of verapamil. *J. Perinat. Med.* 8:203, 1980.

Camphor (Over-the-Counter)

INDICATIONS AND RECOMMENDATIONS

Camphor is safe to use during pregnancy. This drug is applied topically and produces local anesthetic and antipruritic effects. It is taken orally as an ingredient in paregoric and is used to relieve or prevent flatulence.

SPECIAL CONSIDERATIONS IN PREGNANCY

There are no maternal effects unique to pregnancy. It is theoretically possible for fetal convulsions to occur if large dosages are taken systemically, and at least one fetal death has been reported.

ADVERSE EFFECTS

Camphor is a rubefacient when rubbed on the skin. If not vigorously applied, however, it may cause a feeling of coolness.

When taken systemically, camphor may stimulate the central nervous system. It does not selectively stimulate respiration and has very little effect on the circulation. If children ingest large amounts of solid camphor, convulsions can occur. In small oral dosages, this drug produces a sensation of warmth and comfort in the stomach. It may, however, cause nausea and vomiting in larger dosages.

RECOMMENDED READING

Nelson, M.M., and Forfar, J.O. Associations between drugs administered during pregnancy and congenital abnormalities of the fetus. *Br. Med. J.* 1:523, 1971.

Schenkel, B., and Vorherr, H. Non-prescription drugs during pregnancy: potential teratogenic and toxic effects upon embryo and fetus. *J. Reprod. Med.* 12:27, 1974.

Weiss, J., and Catalano, P. Camphorated oil intoxication during pregnancy. *Pediatrics* 52:713, 1973.

Carbamazepine (Tegretol®)

INDICATIONS AND RECOMMENDATIONS

The use of carbamazepine during pregnancy should be limited to the treatment of trigeminal neuralgia and seizures refractory to therapy with more established agents. As have almost all antiepileptic medications, carbamazepine use during pregnancy has been implicated as a teratogen. In the nonpregnant individual, it is used alone or in combination with other agents in the treatment of simple and complex partial seizures and generalized tonic-clonic seizures. It also has been used for the treatment of bipolar affective disorders, psychosis, and alcohol withdrawal.

SPECIAL CONSIDERATIONS IN PREGNANCY

Carbamazepine crosses the placenta and is present in fetal serum at levels equal to those in maternal serum. At one time carbamazepine was thought to present a lower risk of malformation than phenytoin and was used in women who required anticonvulsant treatment who may have become pregnant. However, more recent reports have indicated that carbamazepine is also a teratogen and that its use should be avoided during pregnancy if possible.

One study, involving both retrospective and prospective phases, found a pattern of malformations including minor craniofacial defects, fingernail hypoplasia, and developmental delay in children born to women who had taken carbamazepine during pregnancy. The authors noted the similarity of these malformations to those of the fetal hydantoin syndrome and speculated that common metabolic pathways could play a part in the teratogenicities.

Maternal use of carbamazepine has also been associated with an increased incidence of spina bifida. One cohort study of women who had taken antiepileptic drugs during pregnancy identified four cases of spina bifida in infants born to 1490 women who had taken anticonvulsant drugs. Among 107 of those women who had taken carbamazepine, 3 gave birth to infants with spina bifida. One of those mothers was also taking valproic acid (also suspected to cause spina bifida) as well, whereas the other two mothers were taking phenytoin, phenobarbital, and/or primidone (none of which were found to have an association with spina bifida). The authors also compiled data from the available cohort studies of prenatal carbamazepine exposure. They concluded from the data that exposure to carbamazepine in utero carries a 1% risk of spina bifida.

The risk of malformation may be increased with multidrug anticonvulsant therapy. One author found a 58% incidence of congenital anomalies in infants born to mothers who took carbamazepine in combination with valproic acid and phenobarbital during pregnancy. The authors hypothesize that this high rate of malformation may be due to metabolic interactions among the drugs.

Studies vary in their conclusions about the effect of pregnancy on carbamazepine clearance and total drug levels. However, free drug plasma concentrations tend to remain stable and should be the parameter to monitor during pregnancy.

Carbamazepine is excreted in breast milk, with milk/plasma ratios of 0.4–0.6. No clinically significant effects have been described in breast-fed infants.

DOSAGE

The initial dose for epilepsy is 200 mg PO bid; dosage may be gradually increased to as high as 1200 mg/day to achieve seizure control. The therapeutic plasma level is approximately 6–8 µg/ml, although considerable variation occurs. Free drug plasma levels are approximately 20% to 25% of total levels.

ADVERSE EFFECTS

The most common side effects include diplopia, ataxia, drowsiness, blurred vision, paresthesias, gastrointestinal disturbances, and headache. Often these occur at the beginning of therapy and are transient, but they may necessitate an adjustment of dosage. A number of cases of bone marrow suppression occasionally resulting in death have been reported, but these cases were confounded by multiple drug therapies and underlying disease and no definite causal connection can be proven. Nevertheless, hematologic parameters should be followed during therapy. Transient mild leukopenia that usually resolves within the first four months of therapy has also been reported. A transient rise in hepatic enzymes may occur and at least one case of fatal hepatitis has been reported. Rarely, a variety of different dermatologic reactions may develop. Drug interactions with coumarin (increased metabolism) and phenytoin (decreased serum levels) have been described.

MECHANISM OF ACTION

Carbamazepine blocks posttetanic potentiation and appears to act selectively on areas of the brain frequently involved in epileptogenesis. Its therapeutic effect in trigeminal neuralgia is particularly related to the blockade of afferent synaptic transmission in the trigeminal nerve.

ABSORPTION AND BIOTRANSFORMATION

Carbamazepine has a variable oral absorption, is highly protein- bound, and is metabolized in the liver. The initial plasma half-life is 25–65 hours, but this decreases to 10–20 hours with repeated doses due to the drug's ability to stimulate its own metabolism. Its major active metabolite, the 10,11-epoxide, has a shorter half-life and is metabolized further to inactive compounds that are excreted in the urine.

RECOMMENDED READING

Bernus, I., et al. Metabolism of carbamazepine and co-administered anticonvulsants during pregnancy. *Epilepsy Res.* 21:65, 1995.

Jones, K.L., et al. Pattern of malformations in the children of women treated with carbamazepine during pregnancy. *N. Engl. J. Med.* 320:1661, 1989.

Kallen, A.J. Maternal carbamazepine and infant spina bifida. *Reprod. Toxicol.* 8:203, 1994.

Lindhout, D., Hoppener, R.J.E.A., and Meinardi, H. Teratogenicity of antiepileptic drug combinations with special emphasis on epoxidation (of carbamazepine). *Epilepsia* 25:77, 1984.

McNamara, J.O. Drugs effective in the therapy of epilepsies. Chapter 20 in *Goodman and Gilman's The Pharmacological Basis of Therapeutics* (9th ed.), J.G. Hardman and L.E. Limbird, eds. New York: McGraw-Hill, 1996. Pp. 473–475.

Pynnonen, S., et al. Carbamazepine: placental transport, tissue concentrations in foetus and newborn, and levels in milk. *Acta Pharmacol. Toxicol.* 41:244, 1977.

Rosa, F.W. Spina bifida in infants of women treated with carbamazepine during pregnancy. *N. Engl. J. Med.* 324:674, 1991.

Tomson, T., et al. Epilepsy and pregnancy: a prospective study of seizure control in relation to free and total plasma concentrations of carbamazepine and phenytoin. *Epilepsia* 35:122, 1994.

Tomson, T., et al. Disposition of carbamazepine and phenytoin in pregnancy. *Epilepsia* 35:131, 1994.

Wilder, B.J., and Bruni, J. *Seizure Disorder: A Pharmacological Approach to Treatment.* New York: Raven Press, 1981.

Woodbury, D.M., Penry, J.K., and Peppenger, C.E. *Antiepileptic Drugs.* New York: Raven Press, 1982.

Cathartics, Contact (Over-the-Counter)

ANTHRACENE CATHARTICS: ALOE, CASCARA, SENNA

Indications and Recommendations

With the exception of aloe, anthraquinone cathartics are safe to use during pregnancy. Despite their safety, however, attention to proper diet and exercise is preferable to dependence on these agents. The anthraquinone cathartics include senna, cascara sagrada, and danthron. Aloe is contraindicated in pregnancy because it can cross the placenta and stimulate the fetal intestine, leading to the passage of meconium. Danthron-containing laxatives were removed from the market in 1987 by the FDA because of carcinogenicity in rats and mice. When an anthraquinone cathartic is indicated, senna is the agent of choice.

Special Considerations in Pregnancy

Aloe should not be used in pregnancy because of the possible increased likelihood of meconium passage. In addition, there has been unsubstantiated speculation that aloe may stimulate uterine contractions. Although data from the Collaborative Perinatal Project suggest an increase in the relative risk for birth defects among infants exposed to cascara derivatives in the first 16 weeks of pregnancy, this was not statistically significant and no confirmatory reports have appeared. Senna is the most widely studied of these drugs. Neither animal studies nor published case series of humans taking senna have found evidence of adverse effects on pregnancy.

The presence of anthraquinone derivatives in breast milk and the incidence of diarrhea among nursing infants whose mothers ingest these substances are controversial. In his book *Drugs in Breast Milk,* Wilson notes that the standard recommendation is for nursing mothers to avoid these medications but that documentation of risk is lacking. The American Academy of Pediatrics considers cascara, danthron, and senna to be compatible with breast-feeding.

Dosage

Senna is taken in a 2 g dose with results in 6 hours. Fluid extract of cascara sagrada, 2.5 ml, will give results in 8 hours. Danthron causes stool softening 6–8 hours after a 25 to 150 mg dose.

Adverse Effects

Side effects include intestinal melanosis with prolonged use. This is reversible when the drug is discontinued.

Mechanism of Action

The anthracene cathartics act directly on the bowel wall to stimulate intestinal motility, which is primarily a large bowel effect. They are hydrolyzed by colonic bacteria with release of the active agent.

CASTOR OIL

Indications and Recommendations

Because of a possible but unproven stimulant effect on uterine motility, castor oil should not be used during pregnancy. It is used as a cathartic agent, most commonly when patients are to have x-rays of the kidney or colon, or both.

DIPHENYLMETHANES: BISACODYL, PHENOLPHTHALEIN

Indications and Recommendations

Diphenylmethanes are safe to use during pregnancy. Despite their safety, however, attention to proper diet and exercise is preferable to dependence on these agents. The diphenylmethanes include phenolphthalein and bisacodyl and are widely used in over-the-counter (OTC) cathartic preparations.

Special Considerations in Pregnancy

There are no special considerations in pregnancy.

Dosage

Phenolphthalein is taken in a dose of 60–200 mg and acts in 6–8 hours. Bisacodyl is taken in a dose of 10–15 mg orally, acting in 6–8 hours, or as a 10 mg rectal suppository acting within 15–60 minutes.

Adverse Effects

Side effects include cramps, mucous stools, and excessive fluid loss in the stools. Allergic skin reactions have been reported with phenolphthalein. Proctitis has been reported with bisacodyl.

Mechanism of Action

Diphenylmethanes act mainly on the large intestine, stimulating peristalsis.

Absorption and Biotransformation

Although phenolphthalein is mainly excreted in the feces, up to 15% may be absorbed, conjugated, and excreted in the urine.

Some is excreted in bowel. The urine or stools, or both, will be pink to red if the pH is alkaline.

Up to 5% of bisacodyl is absorbed and conjugated as a glucuronide appearing in the urine.

RECOMMENDED READING

American Academy of Pediatrics Committee on Drugs. The transfer of drugs and other chemicals into human milk. *Pediatrics* 93:137, 1994.

Anonymous. Risk assessment for senna during pregnancy. *Pharmacology* 44:20, 1992.

Brunton, L.L. Agents affecting gastrointestinal water flux and motility. Chapter 38 in *Goodman and Gilman's The Pharmacological Basis of Therapeutics* (9th ed.), J.G. Hardman and L.E. Limbird, eds. New York: McGraw-Hill, 1996. Pp. 922–924.

Heinonen, O.P., Slone, D., and Shapiro, S. *Birth Defects and Drugs in Pregnancy.* Boston: Wright-PSG, 1977. Pp. 385, 442.

Nelson, M.M., and Forfar, J.O. Associations between drugs administered during pregnancy and congenital abnormalities of the fetus. *Br. Med. J.* 1:523, 1971.

Schenkel, B., and Vorherr, H. Non-prescription drugs during pregnancy: potential teratogenic and toxic effects upon embryo and fetus. *J. Reprod. Med.* 12:27, 1974.

Wilson, J.T. *Drugs in Breast Milk.* Lancaster, UK: MTP, 1981. Pp. 67–68.

Cathartics, Saline (Over-the-Counter): Magnesium Salts, Including Milk of Magnesia and Epsom Salt; Sodium and Potassium Salts

INDICATIONS AND RECOMMENDATIONS

Saline cathartics, which include magnesium, sodium, and potassium salts, are safe to use during pregnancy. Their use, however, should be avoided in patients with significant cardiovascular disease or impairment of renal function. They are used for cathartic cleaning of the bowel before surgery and radiologic or proctologic examination, in patients with functional constipation, and in those with constipation due to inadequate fluid intake or exercise.

SPECIAL CONSIDERATIONS IN PREGNANCY

There are no special considerations in pregnancy.

DOSAGE

Of the magnesium salts, magnesium sulfate (Epsom salt) is given in doses of 10–15 g. It should be dissolved in fruit juice to overcome the objectionable taste. Magnesium citrate is available in a 10-oz bottle of effervescent solution. The usual dose is 5–10 oz. Some patients are nauseated by this preparation, and its action may be quite violent. Magnesium hydroxide is available in an aqueous suspension (milk of magnesia), and the usual dose is 15–40 ml. It also acts as an antacid.

The usual cathartic dose of the phosphate salts of sodium and potassium is from 4 to 20 g. The onset of action for these preparations is 3–6 hours or less.

ADVERSE EFFECTS

There is little systemic effect except for the possibility of dehydration resulting from fluid loss in the feces; this occurs because the preparations are so slowly absorbed that they cause retention of water in the gastrointestinal tract and may even draw fluid into it. Congestive heart failure because of the salt load could occur in patients predisposed to this condition. Magnesium intoxication may occur in patients with impaired renal function.

RECOMMENDED READING

Brunton, L.L. Agents affecting gastrointestinal water flux and motility; emesis and antiemetics; bile acids and pancreatic enzymes. Chapter 38 in *Goodman and Gilman's The Pharmacological Basis of Therapeutics* (9th ed.), J.G. Hardman and L.E. Limbird, eds. New York: McGraw-Hill, 1996. Pp. 921–922.

Nelson, M.M., and Forfar, J.O. Associations between drugs administered during pregnancy and congenital abnormalities of the fetus. *Br. Med. J.* 1:523, 1971.

Schenkel, B., and Vorherr, H. Non-prescription drugs during pregnancy: potential teratogenic and toxic effects upon embryo and fetus. *J. Reprod. Med.* 12:27, 1974.

Cephalosporins: Cefaclor (Ceclor®), Cefadroxil (Duricef®, Ultracef®), Cefamandole (Mandol®), Cefazolin (Ancef®, Kefzol®), Cefonicid (Monocid®), Cefoperazone (Cefobid®), Ceforanide (Precef®), Cefotaxime (Claforan®), Cefoxitin (Mefoxin®), Ceftizoxime (Cefizox®), Ceftriaxone (Rocephin®), Cefuroxime (Zinacef®), Cephalexin (Keflex®), Cephalothin (Keflin®), Cephapirin (Cefadyl®), Cephradine (Anspor®, Velosef®)

INDICATIONS AND RECOMMENDATIONS

The cephalosporins are generally safe to use during pregnancy. However, there are relatively few data regarding the use of the third- generation agents and, until more experience is accumulated in pregnant patients, these newer agents should be reserved for use when no other safer antibiotics are available.

Cephalosporins are categorized as first-, second-, and third-generation agents. In general, higher generation agents have broader gram-negative spectra, are less efficacious against gram-positive organisms, are more efficacious against resistant organisms, and cost more. However, this classification scheme is becoming blurred as newer agents enter the market.

All cephalosporins provide effective coverage against group A and B streptococci and none are effective against group D streptococci (enterococci). Cefoxitin has the best activity against *Bacteroides fragilis.* Ceftriaxone is active against *N. gonorrhoeae,* including strains that produce penicillinase. Ceftazidime and cefoperazone both provide coverage against *Pseudomonas aeruginosa.* Because of the widely differing spectra of these agents, the choice of agent should be based on its individual bactericidal spectrum, route of administration, side effect profile, and indications.

SPECIAL CONSIDERATIONS IN PREGNANCY

The cephalosporins cross the placenta and are found in fetal serum and urine as well as in amniotic fluid. No teratogenic effects have been associated with their use. Pharmacokinetic studies of several cephalosporins have demonstrated that, as with penicillins, mean serum levels are lower in pregnant than in nonpregnant patients receiving equivalent dosages. The half-lives tend to be shorter and the volumes of distribution and clearances larger.

All cephalosporins that have been studied have been shown to be excreted into breast milk in low concentrations. Therefore, the possibility exists that the drug could interfere with neonatal bowel flora. The American Academy of Pediatrics considers cephadroxil, cefazolin, cefotaxime, cefoxitin, cefaprozil, ceftazidime, and ceftriaxone to be compatible with breast-feeding.

DOSAGE

Dosages of Representative Agents

Drug	Route	Dose	Interval
First-Generation Cephalosporins			
Cephalexin	PO	250 mg–1 g	q6°
Cephradine	PO	250 mg–500mg	q6°
	IV/IM	500 mg–1 g	q6°
Cephalothin	IV/IM	500 mg–1 g	q4–6°
Cefazolin	IV/IM	250 mg–1 g	q6–8°
Second-Generation Cephalosporins			
Cefuroxime	PO	250 mg–500 mg	bid
	IV/IM	750 mg–1.5 g	q8°
Cefaclor	PO	250 mg	q8°
Cefoxitin	IV/IM	1–2 g	q6–8°
Cefotetan	IV/IM	1–2 g	q12°
Third-Generation Cephalosporins			
Cefotaxime	IV/IM	1–2 g	q8–12°
Ceftriaxone	IV/IM	1–2 g	qd
Ceftazidime	IV/IM	1 g	q8–12°
Cefoperazone	IV/IM	1–2 g	q12°

ADVERSE EFFECTS

Allergic reactions and gastrointestinal disturbances may occur. The incidence of hypersensitivity reactions to the cephalosporins is higher in patients who have shown an allergic reaction to penicillin. This is apparently related to sensitization to the β-lactam ring common to both drugs. Controversy exists as to the incidence of cross- sensitivity to this drug. With the exception of patients who have had anaphylactic reactions to penicillin, however, cephalosporins are not contraindicated in patients with penicillin allergy. Side effects include thrombophlebitis with intravenous use and a serum sickness–like reaction with prolonged parenteral administration.

Rarely, hemolytic anemia, hepatic dysfunction, blood dyscrasias, and renal damage may occur. Toxic renal damage may be potentiated by the concurrent use of aminoglycosides, probenecid, or potent diuretics such as furosemide or ethacrynic acid.

Cefamandole, cefoperazone, and cefotetan possess a chemical side chain that prevents the activation of prothrombin and cause hypoprothrombinemia with or without bleeding. The hypoprothrombinemia is reversible with administration of vitamin K.

MECHANISM OF ACTION

These drugs inhibit bacterial cell wall synthesis in a manner similar to the penicillins.

RECOMMENDED READING

Bernard, B., et al. Maternal-fetal transfer of cefazolin in the first twenty weeks of pregnancy. *J. Infect. Dis.* 136:377, 1977.

Bourget, P., Quinguis-Desmaris, V., and Fernandez, H. Ceftriaxone distribution and protein binding between maternal blood and milk postpartum. *Ann. Pharmacother.* 27:294, 1993.

Eriksen, N.L., and Blanco, J.D. Extended-spectrum (second- and third-generation) cephalosporins. *Obstet. Gynecol. Clin. North Am.* 19:461, 1992.

Giamarellou, H., et al. A study of cefoxitin, moxalactam, and ceftazidime kinetics in pregnancy. *Am. J. Obstet. Gynecol.* 147:914, 1983.

Gordman, M., et al. A randomized, prospective study of adjunctive ceftizoxime in preterm labor. *Am. J. Obstet. Gynecol.* 172:1546, 1995.

Graham, J.M., Oshiro, B.T., and Blanco, J.D. Limited-spectrum (first-generation) cephalosporins. *Obstet. Gynecol. Clin. North Am.* 19:449, 1992.

Mandell, G.L., and Petri, Jr., W.A. Antimicrobial agents: penicillins, cephalosporins, and other β-lactam antibiotics. Chapter 45 in *Goodman and Gilman's The Pharmacological Basis of Therapeutics* (9th ed.), J.G. Hardman and L.E. Limbird, eds. New York: McGraw-Hill, 1996. Pp. 1089–1096.

Nathorst-Boos, J., et al. Renal elimination of ceftazidime during pregnancy. *Am. J. Obstet. Gynecol.* 172:163, 1995.

Sanchez-Ramos, L., et al. Pyelonephritis in pregnancy: once-a-day ceftriaxone versus multiple doses of cefazolin. *Am. J. Obstet. Gynecol.* 172:129, 1995.

Chloral Hydrate (Noctec™)

INDICATIONS AND RECOMMENDATIONS

The use of chloral hydrate during pregnancy is relatively contraindicated because other therapeutic agents are preferable. It has sedative and hypnotic actions similar to those of paraldehyde, alcohol, and the barbiturates, and it is used primarily as a hypnotic in the treatment of simple insomnia. Chloral hydrate is mutagenic in bacteria and affects mitotic spindle formation in vitro. It and its active metabolite, trichloroethanol, are known to cross the placental barrier rapidly after maternal administration. The effects of its use during pregnancy have not been adequately studied. A British study of the pharmacokinetics of a single antepartum dose of chloral hydrate in 52 pregnant women and their offspring has been published. The authors report that no deleterious effects were noted in either mothers or neonates.

No sedative has been found to be absolutely safe during pregnancy, as most cross the placenta and produce sedation and withdrawal symptoms in the newborn. Should such therapy be required during pregnancy, phenobarbital may be used in the lowest dosage and frequency possible.

Chloral hydrate appears in breast milk, with a milk/plasma ratio of less than 0.5. and has been reported to cause sleepiness in the breast-fed infant.

RECOMMENDED READING

Berstine, J.B., Meyer, A.E., and Berstine, R.L. Maternal blood and breast milk estimation following the administration of chloral hydrate during the puerperium. *J. Obstet. Gynaecol. Br. Emp.* 63:228, 1956.

Berstine, J.B., Meyer, A.E., and Hayman, H.B. Maternal and foetal blood estimation following the administration of chloral hydrate during labor. *J. Obstet. Gynaecol. Br. Emp.* 61:683, 1954.

Committee on Drugs. Transfer of drugs and other chemicals into human milk. *Pediatrics* 93:137, 1994.

Crebelli, R. and Carere, A. Genetic toxicology of 1,1,2-trichloroethylene. *Mutat. Res.* 221:11, 1989.

Hobbs, W.R., Rall, T.W., and Verdoorn, T.A. Hypnotics and sedatives; ethanol. Chapter 17 in *Goodman and Gilman's The Pharmacological Basis of Therapeutics* (9th ed.). New York: McGraw-Hill, 1996. P. 381.

Wilson, J.T. *Drugs in Breast Milk.* Lancaster, UK: MTP, 1981. P. 79.

Chloramphenicol (Chloromycetin®)

INDICATIONS AND RECOMMENDATIONS

Chloramphenicol should be avoided in late pregnancy and during labor because of the potential for the "gray syndrome" in the newborn infant. It should be used during pregnancy only for serious infections with organisms known to be sensitive to the drug. Because of the potential for life-threatening toxicity and hypersensitivity reactions, chloramphenicol should be used only when other antibiotics cannot be substituted. It may be necessary to use chloramphenicol to treat serious anaerobic infections, *Salmonella* infections, and rickettsial diseases. Because of its ability to attain relatively high concentrations in the central nervous system, it is also used against *Haemophilus influenzae* meningitis and brain abscesses.

SPECIAL CONSIDERATIONS IN PREGNANCY

The gray syndrome may be seen in chloramphenicol-treated newborns, especially those born prematurely who are unable to conjugate and excrete the drug fully. It is related to toxic blood levels. The syndrome usually begins 2–9 days after therapy has begun. It consists of vomiting, refusal to suck, rapid irregular respiration, and abdominal distention, followed in 24–48 hours by flaccidity, ashen gray color, and hypothermia. About 40% of these neonates die from circulatory collapse, usually on about the fifth day. Although toxic effects have not been observed in newborns whose mothers received as much as 1 g of chloramphenicol every 2 hours during labor, it is probably best to avoid this drug just prior to delivery. Chloramphenicol readily crosses the placenta.

Chloramphenicol appears in breast milk at levels that are 50% to 60% of maternal plasma levels. Although these levels are too low to precipitate gray syndrome, the theoretical risk of bone marrow depression still exists. Therefore, it is best that nursing mothers not use this drug.

DOSAGE

Chloramphenicol may be given orally or intravenously. The usual oral dose is 50 mg/kg/day given in divided doses every 6 hours. Infections of the central nervous system caused by moderately resistant organisms may require dosage up to 100 mg/kg/day. Therapeutic peak concentrations are 10–20 μg/ml; therapeutic trough concentrations are 5–10 μg/ml.

Patients with renal disease should receive the usual dosage of chloramphenicol, although anemia is more likely to occur. Patients with hepatic disease should receive a reduced dosage and have serum levels monitored.

ADVERSE EFFECTS

Chloramphenicol is the most common drug cause of aplastic anemia and pancytopenia. This effect is not dosage-related but is usually associated with prolonged oral therapy, especially with multiple exposures. The incidence is 1 in 30,000 courses of therapy. The longer the interval between the last dosage of drug and the appearance of the first sign of blood dyscrasia, the greater the likelihood of fatality. When total aplasia of the bone marrow occurs, the fatality rate is almost 100%. Other hypersensitivity reactions include a macular or vesicular skin rash, hemorrhage from skin and mucous membranes, fever, and atrophic glossitis.

A second type of anemia occurs in patients having plasma concentrations of chloramphenicol above 25 μg/ml. It is seen most often with parenteral therapy, is dose-related, and usually disappears completely about 12 days after discontinuance of therapy. The drug inhibits the uptake and incorporation of iron into heme, resulting in anemia, reticulocytopenia, and elevated plasma iron levels.

Chloramphenicol can also cause nausea, vomiting, diarrhea, and perineal irritation. Optic neuritis has also been reported. Large oral dosages may prolong the prothrombin time, presumably by altering the bacterial flora of the gastrointestinal tract.

MECHANISM OF ACTION

Chloramphenicol inhibits protein synthesis in bacteria and rickettsiae, primarily by preventing peptide bond synthesis in ribosomes.

ABSORPTION AND BIOTRANSFORMATION

Chloramphenicol is rapidly absorbed after oral ingestion, with significant plasma concentrations present at 30 minutes and peak levels attained in 2–3 hours. It is well distributed in body fluids and achieves therapeutic concentrations in the cerebrospinal fluid regardless of the presence of meningitis. Its half-life is 3–4 hours.

The drug is inactivated in the liver by conjugation in a step mediated by glucuronyltransferase. The inactive metabolite is rapidly excreted in the urine. More than 80% of an oral dosage can be recovered from the urine.

RECOMMENDED READING

Ambrose, P.J. Clinical pharmacokinetics of chloramphenicol and chloramphenicol succinate. *Clin. Pharmacokinet.* 9:222, 1984.

Kapusnic-Uner, J.E., Sande, M.A., and Chambers, H.F. Antimicrobial agents: tetracyclines, chloramphenicol, erythromycin and miscellaneous antibacterial agents. Chapter 47 in *Goodman and Gilman's The Pharmacological Basis of Therapeutics* (9th ed.), J.G. Hardman and L.E. Limbird, eds. New York: McGraw-Hill, 1996. Pp. 1130–1135.

Kucers, A., and Bennett, N. McK. *The Use of Antibiotics* (2nd ed.). London: Heinemann, 1975. Pp. 244–270.

Schwarz, R.H. Considerations of antibiotic therapy during pregnancy. *Obstet. Gynecol.* 58:95S–99S, 1981.

Chloroquine (Aralen®) and Hydroxychloroquine (Plaquenil®)

INDICATIONS AND RECOMMENDATIONS

The use of chloroquine and hydroxychloroquine during pregnancy should be limited to suppressive therapy in women entering areas with endemic malaria and to treatment of acute attacks of malaria. Although a number of case series have not shown evidence of teratogenicity in human pregnancies, these drugs should be considered only when other regimens are ineffective in the treatment of inflammatory disease states in pregnancy. They are teratogenic in animals at high doses, and higher doses are required to treat inflammatory conditions.

SPECIAL CONSIDERATIONS IN PREGNANCY

Because malaria poses a distinct threat to the pregnant woman and her unborn child, prophylaxis is desirable. No studies have demonstrated untoward fetal effects when chloroquine is given in antimalarial dosages. In a randomized trial involving more than 1400 pregnant women in West Africa, 300 mg of chloroquine weekly decreased the placental infection rate from 19% to 4% but had no significant effect on birth weight.

DOSAGE

When necessary for suppressive therapy of malaria, chloroquine phosphate, one 500 mg tablet (300 mg base), should be given weekly beginning 2 weeks before arrival, throughout the stay, and for 8 weeks after the patient has left the malarious area. The corresponding dose of hydroxychloroquine sulfate is 400 mg (310 mg base) given as two 200 mg tablets. If pretreatment is not possible, then a double loading dose of either drug may be taken in two divided doses 6 hours apart.

An initial loading dose of 1 g of chloroquine phosphate is administered for the treatment of an acute attack of vivax or falciparum malaria. This dose is followed by an additional 500 mg after 6–8 hours and 500 mg again on each of the next 2 consecutive days. A total dose of 2.5 g is given over the 3-day treatment period. The corresponding dose of hydroxychloroquine sulfate is 800 mg, followed by doses of 400 mg for a total of 2 g over 3 days.

Hydroxychloroquine is approved for use in conditions such as lupus erythematosus, and chloroquine is also commonly prescribed in this situation. Antiinflammatory doses of hydroxychloroquine are generally 200 mg twice daily, and of chloroquine 250 mg daily for prolonged periods.

ADVERSE EFFECTS

When used in antimalarial dosages, side effects of chloroquine are mild and include transient headache, visual disturbances, gastrointestinal upset, and pruritus. Long-term therapy with antiinflammatory dosages may be associated with development of retinopathy, and irreversible vision loss may be sustained. Other side effects include dose-dependent myelosuppression, skin rashes, neuromyopathy, tinnitus and deafness, and electrocardiographic changes.

MECHANISM OF ACTION

The exact mechanism of chloroquine's activity is uncertain. Its antimalarial activity is thought to result from its concentration within the food vacuoles of the parasites and its effect on malarial pigment in the host erythrocytes. Chloroquine exerts no significant activity against exoerythrocytic stages of plasmodia.

Chloroquine rapidly controls the parasitemia and clinical symptoms of acute malarial attacks. Fever is controlled within 24–48 hours after administration of therapeutic dosages. With the exception of certain strains, chloroquine completely cures falciparum malaria. Relapses of vivax malaria, however, are not prevented, although the intervals between relapses are substantially increased.

ABSORPTION AND BIOTRANSFORMATION

Chloroquine is rapidly and almost completely absorbed from the gastrointestinal tract. Peak plasma levels are reached within 3–5 hours of oral administration. Much of the drug is bound to plasma proteins and to tissues; approximately 30% is metabolized. Chloroquine is cleared by the kidneys at a very slow rate, which may be increased by acidification of the urine. With single or weekly doses, the plasma half-life is approximately 3 days.

RECOMMENDED READING

Anonymous. Malaria prophylaxis. *Br. Med. J.* 286:787, 1983.

Buchanan, N.M.M., Khamashta, M.A., Morton, K.E., Kerslake, S., Baguley, E.A., and Hughes, G.R.V. A study of 100 high risk lupus pregnancies. *Am. J. Reprod. Immunol.* 28:192, 1992.

Cot, M., Roisin, A., Barro, D., Yada, A., Verhave, J.P., Carnevale, P., and Breart, G. Effect of chloroquine chemoprophylaxis during pregnancy on birth weight: results of a randomized trial. *Am. J. Trop. Med. Hyg.* 46:21, 1992.

Guzzo, C.A., Lazarus, G.S., and Werth, V.P. Dermatological pharmacology. Chapter 64 in *Goodman and Gilman's The Pharmacological Basis of Therapeutics* (9th ed.), J.G. Hardman and L.E. Limbird, eds. New York: McGraw-Hill, 1996. P. 1064.

Heinonen, O.P., Slone, D., and Shapiro, S. *Birth Defects and Drugs in Pregnancy.* Littleton, MA: Wright-PSG, 1977. P. 229.

Levy, M., Buskila, D., Gladman, D.D., Urowitz, M.B., and Koren, G. Pregnancy outcome following first trimester exposure to chloroquine. *Am. J. Perinatol.* 8:174, 1991.

Main, E.K., Main, D.M., and Krogstad, D.J. Treatment of chloroquine-resistant malaria during pregnancy. *J.A.M.A.* 249:3207, 1983.

Tracy, J.W., and Webster, L.T., Jr. Drugs used in the chemotherapy of protozoal infections: malaria. Chapter 40 in *Goodman and Gilman's The Pharmacological Basis of Therapeutics* (9th ed.), J.G. Hardman and L.E. Limbird, eds. New York: McGraw-Hill, 1996. Pp. 970–972.

Chlorpheniramine (Chlor-Trimeton®)

INDICATIONS AND RECOMMENDATIONS

The use of chlorpheniramine during pregnancy should be limited to the provision of symptomatic relief of allergic symptoms caused by histamine release. These include urticaria, rhinitis, and pruritus. Because chlorpheniramine is an antihistamine that merely provides palliative therapy, the avoidance of allergens should be the primary treatment for these symptoms whenever possible. Chlorpheniramine does not appear to have teratogenic effects at recommended dosages; however, no prospective studies are available. This drug is not recommended for use by lactating women.

SPECIAL CONSIDERATIONS IN PREGNANCY

No prospective studies that evaluate the safety of chlorpheniramine use during pregnancy have been conducted. One large retrospective study, however, found no evidence to incriminate this drug as a teratogenic agent.

Due to its anticholinergic properties, chlorpheniramine may inhibit lactation. In addition, small amounts may be secreted into breast milk. This drug and all antihistamines, therefore, should be avoided by the lactating mother.

DOSAGE

The usual oral dose of chlorpheniramine is 4 mg 3–4 times a day. It is available in an extended release formulation, 8–12 mg, that may be given 2–3 times a day.

ADVERSE EFFECTS

Anticholinergic side effects are most common. These include dry mouth and eyes and, rarely, blurred vision. Although it is less likely than other first-generation H_1 antagonists to produce drowsiness, a significant proportion of patients experience sedation. Anorexia, nausea, epigastric distress, and dizziness may also occur.

MECHANISM OF ACTION

Chlorpheniramine is a competitive antagonist of the H_1 receptor and blocks histamine-produced sneezing, pruritis, mucus production, vascular sensitivity, and smooth muscle contraction. It has anticholinergic activity, produces drowsiness, and possesses local anesthetic activity when applied topically.

ABSORPTION AND BIOTRANSFORMATION

The drug is primarily metabolized in the liver, probably by hydroxylation followed by glucuronidation. Excretion is via the kidney.

RECOMMENDED READING

American Pharmaceutical Association. *Handbook of Non- Prescription Drugs.* Washington, DC, 1996. Pp. 140–142.

American Pharmaceutical Association. *Non-Prescription Products: Formulations and Features 96–97.* Washington, DC, 1996. Pp. 62–113.

Babe, Jr., K.S., and Serafin, W.E. Histamine, bradykinin, and their antagonists. Chapter 25 in *Goodman and Gilman's The Pharmacological Basis of Therapeutics* (9th ed.), J.G. Hardman and L.E. Limbird, eds. New York: McGraw-Hill, 1996. Pp. 586–592.

Heinonen O.P., Slone, D., and Shapiro, S. *Birth Defects and Drugs in Pregnancy.* Littleton, MA: Wright-PSG, 1977. Pp. 322–334.

Nishimura, H., and Tanimura, T. *Aspects of the Teratogenicity of Drugs.* Amsterdam: Excerpta Medica, 1976.

Clarithromycin (Biaxin®)

Clarithromycin is contraindicated in pregnancy. It is a macrolide antibiotic that is highly potent against erythromycin-sensitive strains of streptococci and staphylococci, but has only modest activity against *Haemophilus influenzae* and *Neisseria gonorrhoeae.* It also has good activity against *M. catarrhalis, Chlamydia* spp., *L. pneumophila, B. burgdorferi, Mycoplasma pneumoniae,* and *Mycobacterium avium* complex (MAC). Clarithromycin has been associated with adverse outcomes and fetal malformations when given to pregnant monkeys, rats, mice, and rabbits. No data regarding its use in humans are available. Because alternative antibiotics are generally available, there is generally no need to use clarithromycin for treating infections in a pregnant woman.

REFERENCES

Amsden, G.W. Erythromycin, clarithromycin, and azithromycin: are the differences real? *Clin. Ther.* 18:56, 1996.

Clarithromycin and azithromycin. *Med. Lett. Drugs Ther.* 34:45, 1992.

Kapusnic-Uner, J.E., Sande, M.A., and Chambers, H.F. Antimicrobial agents: tetracyclines, chloramphenicol, erythromycin, and miscellaneous antibacterial agents. Chapter 47 in *Goodman and Gilman's The Pharmacological Basis of Therapeutics* (9th ed.), J.G. Hardman and L.E. Limbird, eds. New York: McGraw-Hill, 1996. Pp. 1135–1140.

Class Ic Antiarrhythmic Agents: Flecainide (Tambocor®), Propafenone (Rhythmol®), Moricizine (Ethmozine®)

INDICATIONS AND RECOMMENDATIONS

Class Ic antiarrhythmic agents are Na^+ channel blockers whose common property is a slow rate of block recovery ($\tau_{recovery}$ >10 seconds). Flecainide is effective in maintaining sinus rhythm in adult, pediatric, and fetal patients with supraventricular arrhythmias without structural heart disease. It has been shown to increase mortality, however, in patients recovering from myocardial infarction. Flecainide is used to treat fetal supraventricular tachycardia resistant to digoxin therapy. Its use may be associated with reduced fetal heart rate variability. Human and animal data suggest that flecainide is probably free of teratogenic effects but there are no reports of moricizine safety in human embryos. Propafenone slows conduction in fast-response tissues and is used primarily to maintain sinus rhythm in patients with atrial fibrillation. It has been shown to be effective in treating arrhythmias associated with Wolff-Parkinson-White syndrome and in treating ventricular premature complexes and nonsustained ventricular tachycardias. This agent should be avoided in patients with coronary artery disease or ventricular dysfunction. Moricizine is a phenothiazine analog used in the chronic treatment of ventricular arrhythmias. However, moricizine has been shown to increase mortality in patients with recent myocardial infarction and did not improve long-term survival in a double-blind randomized trial. The lack of reports concerning moricizine safety in the human gravida and fetus suggests that alternative class Ic antiarrhythmic agents be used when indicated. Propafenone may be embryotoxic and should be avoided in the first trimester.

SPECIAL CONSIDERATIONS IN PREGNANCY

Several reports describe successful treatment of fetal supraventricular tachycardia with maternal flecainide in cases with and without congestive failure, most following unsuccessful treatment with digoxin. Most writers regard flecainide as one option among several second-line drugs to be employed after digoxin failure, except in fetuses with atrial flutter. Maternal treatment at usual adult doses is reported to result in flecainide fetal plasma concentrations in the therapeutic range. Transplacental passage of flecainide in the context of fetal and placental hydrops is uncertain. A fetal–maternal plasma concentration ratio of 0.97 has been reported after successful treatment and fetal hemodynamic resolution at term. In cases treated in the second and third trimester for fetal indications, perinatal outcome was good among those in whom normal heart rhythm was restored. Postflecainide reductions of short- and long-term fetal heart rate variability and lack of fetal heart rate accelerations despite continued normal fetal activity have been reported. Writers have speculated that this phenomenon may reflect flecainide-mediated reduced sinoatrial (SA) node sensitivity to autonomic stimulation.

The manufacturer reports sternal defects, ventricular septal abnormalities, and limb clubbing in rabbits treated with 4 times the human dose of flecainide. High doses in rats are fetotoxic and associated with skeletal defects. Adverse effects of prenatal exposure have not been observed in the small number of reported human cases. Moricizine has not been found to be teratogenic in rodents, according to the manufacturer. Doses at 6.7 times that in humans have been associated with fetal growth restriction in rats.

Propafenone and its metabolite have been reported to be present in fetal serum at one-half to two-thirds of maternal values. One series reported no drug-related adverse effects in nine fetuses treated for tachyarrhythmias, though five with hydrops died. Propafenone is reported by its manufacturer as not mutagenic but embryotoxic at 10–40 times human dose in rabbits and rats.

The neonatal dose effect received in breast milk in humans is unlikely to approach therapeutic levels. Milk inhibits gastrointestinal flecainide absorption. No adverse effects in breast-fed neonates of mothers treated with flecainide have been noted; it is considered safe in this context by the American Academy of Pediatrics.

DOSAGE

Flecainide is prescribed twice daily in doses of 50–200 mg in cases of adult tachyarrhythmias. Plasma levels of 0.2–1.0 µg/ml are regarded as therapeutic. Propafenone and moricizine are prescribed 3 times daily in doses of 150–300 mg and 100–300 mg, respectively. A plasma level less than 1.0 µg/ml of propafenone should be maintained to avoid toxicity.

Monitoring of maternal flecainide plasma levels is necessary to confirm adequate maternal dosing and may be sufficient to establish satisfactory fetal exposure in pregnancies undergoing treatment of fetal supraventricular tachycardia.

ADVERSE EFFECTS

Flecainide and propafenone can exacerbate congestive heart failure in patients with myocardial dysfunction. They can also provoke other potentially lethal arrhythmias such as reentrant ventricular tachycardia. In patients with abnormal conduction, flecainide can cause heart block. Flecainide may not be safe for individuals with structurally abnormal hearts with atrial flutter or ventricular arrhythmias. Propafenone can create β-adrenergic blockade with secondary bradycardia and bronchospasm.

MECHANISM OF ACTION

Class Ic agents are Na^+ channel blockers with a slow rate of block recovery ($\tau_{recovery}$ >10 seconds) that block Na^+ current and prolong action potentials in atrial tissue disproportionately at rapid heart rates. Flecainide prolongs the duration of the PR, QRS, and QT intervals, even at normal heart rates. Propafenone prolongs the PR and QRS duration. Moricizine increases QRS duration and shortens the QT interval.

ABSORPTION AND BIOTRANSFORMATION

Flecainide is readily absorbed with a half-life of 10–18 hours, which increases with urinary alkalinization. Propafenone has a half-life of 2–23 hours; its effects may persist due to active metabolites. Flecainide and propafenone are excreted unchanged in urine and metabolized in liver by cytochrome P450 2D6. Activity of this enzyme is functionally absent in 7% of Caucasians and African-Americans, and in others can be inhibited by drugs such as fluoxetine and quinidine.

RECOMMENDED READING

Brunozzi, L.T., Meniconi, L., Chiocchi, P,. Liberati, R., Zuanette, G., and Latini, R. Propafenone in the treatment of chronic ventricular arrhythmias in a pregnant patient. *Br. J. Clin. Pharmacol.* 26:489, 1988.

Committee on Drugs of the American Academy of Pediatrics. The transfer of drugs and other chemicals into human milk. *Pediatrics* 93:137, 1994.

Gembruch, U., Hansmann, M., and Bald, R. Direct intrauterine fetal treatment of fetal tachyarrhythmia withy severe hydrops fetalis by antiarrhythmic drugs. *Fetal Ther.,* 3:210, 1988.

Kofinas, A.D., Simon, N.V., Sagel, H., Lyttle, E., Smith, N., and King, K. Treatment of fetal supraventricular tachycardia with flecainide acetate after digoxin failure. *Am. J. Obstet. Gynecol.* 165:630, 1991.

Libardoni, M., Piovan, D., Busato, E., and Padrini, R. Transfer of propafenone and 5-OH-propafenone to foetal plasma and maternal milk. *Br. J. Clin. Pharmacol.* 32:527, 1991.

McQuinn, R.L., Pisani, A., Wafa, S., et al. Flecainide excretion in human breast milk. *Clin. Pharmacol. Therap.* 48:262, 1990.

Nishimura, O., Okada, F., Ohsumi, I., et al. Reproduction study of flecainide: teratological study in rats with oral administration. *Kiso to Ronsho* 23:17, 1989.

Perry, J.C., and Garson, A., Jr. Flecainide acetate for treatment of tachyarrhythmias in children: review of world literature on efficacy, safety, and dosing. *Am. Heart J.* 124:1614, 1992.

Roden, D.M.: Antiarrhythmic drugs. Chapter 35 in *Goodman and Gilman's The Pharmacological Basis of Therapeutics* (9th ed.), J.G. Hardman and L.E. Limbird, eds. New York: McGraw-Hill, 1996. Pp. 851–874.

The Cardiac Arrhythmia Suppression Trial II Investigators. Effect of the antiarrhythmic agent moricizine on survival after myocardial infarction. *N. Engl. J. Med.* 327:227, 1992.

van Gelder-Hasker, M.R., de Jong, C.L.D., de Vries, J.I.P., and van Geijn, H.P. The effect of flecainide acetate on fetal heart rate variability: a case report. *Obstet. Gynecol.* 86:667, 1995.

Wagner, X., Jouglard, J., Moulin, M., et al. Coadministration of flecainide acetate and sotalol during pregnancy: lack of teratogenic effects, passage across the placenta, and excretion in human breast milk. *Am. Heart J.* 119:700, 1990.

Class III Antiarrhythmic Agents: Amiodarone (Cordarone®), Bretylium (Bretylol®),

INDICATIONS AND RECOMMENDATIONS

Class III antiarrhythmic agents have the primary pharmacologic effect of K^+ channel blockade. Amiodarone is used for oral therapy in patients with recurrent ventricular tachycardia or fibrillation resistant to other drugs and is effective in maintaining sinus rhythm in patients with atrial fibrillation. Bretylium, a quaternary ammonium compound, is used intravenously to treat and prevent recurrence of ventricular fibrillation. Amiodarone may have fetal thyroid effects, possibly because of its structural similarity to thyroid hormone, and so its use should be limited to situations where no safer alternatives are available. Little information exists in the literature regarding bretylium use during pregnancy. However, because ventricular fibrillation is an unusual and life-threatening event, its intravenous use during pregnancy is likely to be justified.

SPECIAL CONSIDERATIONS IN PREGNANCY

Amiodarone appears to be free of teratogenic effects based on a limited number of published observations. Because it is a structural analog of thyroid hormone, binds to nuclear thyroid hormone receptors, and contains 75 mg iodine per 200 mg tablet, amiodarone is a candidate for direct fetal effects. Indeed, neonatal hyper- and hypothyroidism, goiter, and bradycardia have been observed. A cohort study of 12 infants exposed in utero to amiodarone noted one with congenital nystagmus in six exposed in the first trimester, one case each of congenital hypo- and hyperthyroidism, one with developmental delay, and four born small for gestational age. The latter four were also exposed to β-adrenergic blockers. Congenital hypothyroidism has been reported following third-trimester treatment of fetal supraventricular tachycardia. A cohort study of nine gravidas with maternal tachycardia documented lack of neonatal goiter or corneal changes and normal neonatal T_4 and TSH values in eight. The one infant with biochemical evidence of hyperthyroidism showed no clinical signs of the disorder and 12 month follow-up of all infants demonstrated no clinical abnormalities. Another cohort study of five infants of mothers treated with amiodarone noted biochemical evidence of hypothyroidism in one, no evidence of neonatal corneal or liver abnormalities (findings noted in chronic adult exposure), and normal 8-month to 5-year follow-up. Because exposure to a combination of amiodarone and beta blockers has been associated with fetal growth restriction, the combination of these drugs should be avoided in the few months before and during pregnancy. Maternal and cord plasma studies have demonstrated a high maternal-to-fetal concentration gradient in several reports. Intravenous fetal therapy has been observed to correct refractory supraventricular tachycardia not responsive to maternal oral therapy with the same drug. Placental tissue and breast milk had high concentrations of amiodarone and its metabolite, desethylamiodarone. Because adult adverse drug effects are associated with cumulative dose, tissue accumulation may be responsible for drug effects.

Since long-term follow-up after chronic fetal or neonatal exposure is not available, breast-feeding should be viewed as relatively contraindicated in women taking amiodarone.

Bretylium use during pregnancy has not been reported to be associated with neonatal effects, but little information is available.

DOSAGE

Amiodarone is prescribed as a 2- to 4-week loading dose of 800–1600 mg/day followed by a maintenance dose of 100–400 mg/day. Doses used to treat non-life-threatening arrhythmias should be kept at or below 200 mg/day to avoid toxicity. Bretylium is infused intravenously at a loading dose of 150–300 mg and a maintenance dose of 1–4 mg/min.

ADVERSE EFFECTS

Amiodarone may produce hypotension due to vasodilatation and decreased myocardial function when given intravenously. The intravenous formulation of amiodarone is not available in the United States. Adverse effects are uncommon during oral loading. Long-term therapy has been associated with pulmonary fibrosis but generally at doses exceeding 200 mg/day. Other long-term side effects include hypo- or hyperthyroidism (amiodarone is an analog of thyroid hormone), corneal opacities, hepatic dysfunction, peripheral neuropathy, and proximal muscle weakness. Amiodarone has a very long half-life of months duration and plasma levels are of little help in predicting toxicity.

MECHANISM OF ACTION

Amiodarone's many pharmacologic effects (blockade of K^+ channels and inactivated Na^+ channels, decreased Ca^{2+} current and noncompetitive β-adrenergic blockade) may result from alterations of the lipid milieu in which K+ and other channels are located. Amiodarone inhibits abnormal automaticity and results in prolongation of PR, QRS, and QT intervals and may produce sinus bradycardia. Bretylium prolongs cardiac action potentials and interferes with reuptake of norepinephrine, both of which may contribute to its antiarrhythmic properties.

ABSORPTION AND BIOTRANSFORMATION

Amiodarone is insoluble in aqueous phase and is dissolved in dimethylsulfoxide for administration. It has a bioavailability of approximately 30%. Amiodarone is excreted primarily by the liver and bretylium by renal mechanisms. The elimination half-life of bretylium is 7–15 hours. The half-life of amiodarone is of months' duration. Amiodarone can inhibit the metabolism and increase the bioavailability of warfarin, flecainide, procainamide, quinidine, and digoxin.

RECOMMENDED READING

Feit, R.L., and Carr, S.R. Fetal cardiac arrhythmias: diagnosis and management. *Curr. Obstet. Med.* 4:305, 1996.

Gembruch, U., Manz, M., Bald, R., Rüddel, H., Redel, D.A., Schlebusch, H., Nitsch, J., and Hansmann, M. Repeated intravascular treatment with amiodarone in a fetus with refractory supraventricular tachycardia and hydrops fetalis. *Am. Heart J.* 118(6):1335, 1989.

Gutgesell, M., Oberhold, E., and Boyle, R. Oral bretylium tosylate use during pregnancy and subsequent breastfeeding: a case report. *Am. J. Perinatol.* 7:144, 1990.

Magee, L.A., Downar, E., Sermer, M., Boulton, B.C., Allen, L.C., and Koren, G. Pregnancy outcome after gestational exposure to amiodarone in Canada. *Am. J. Obstet. Gynecol.* 172:1307, 1995.

Matsumura, L.K., Born, D., Kunii, I.S., Branco, D.B., and Maciel, R.M. Outcome of thyroid function in newborns from mothers treated with amiodarone. *Thyroid* 2:279, 1992.

Plomp, T.A., Bulsma, T., and de Vijlder, J.J. Use of amiodarone during pregnancy. *Eur. J. Obstet. Gynecol. Reprod. Biol.* 43:201, 1992.

Roden, D.M. Antiarrhythmic drugs. Chapter 35 in *Goodman and Gilman's The Pharmacological Basis of Therapeutics* (9th ed.), J.G. Hardman and L.E. Limbird, eds. New York: McGraw-Hill, 1996. Pp. 851–874.

The WHO Working Group, Bennet, P.N., ed. *Drugs and Human Lactation. New York:* Elsevier Science, 1988. Pp. 112–113.

Widerhorn, J., Bhandari, A.K., Bughi, S., Rahimtoola, S.H., and Elkayam, U. Fetal and neonatal adverse effects profile of amiodarone treatment during pregnancy. *Am. Heart J.* 122:112, 1991.

Clindamycin (Cleocin®)

INDICATIONS AND RECOMMENDATIONS

The use of clindamycin during pregnancy includes the treatment of anaerobic infections, particularly *Bacteroides fragilis*, and gram-positive infections, with the exception of *Streptococcus faecalis*. In patients who cannot tolerate erythromycin, it has been used for the treatment of *Chlamydia trachomatis*. Due to its efficacy against *Mobiluncus* and other anaerobes, it has been used to treat bacterial vaginosis. In the penicillin-allergic patient, it has also been employed for the treatment of chorioamnionitis and the treatment of group B streptococcus.

Clindamycin has an antibacterial spectrum similar to that of lincomycin and erythromycin, although it is slightly more effective against anaerobic bacteria, especially *B. fragilis*. If diarrhea develops during the administration of this drug, stool cultures for *Clostridium difficile* should be obtained. The diarrhea usually resolves within 10–14 days after discontinuation of the drug.

SPECIAL CONSIDERATIONS IN PREGNANCY

There are no unusual maternal effects during pregnancy. The drug rapidly crosses the placenta and is 90% bound to serum protein. It appears to concentrate within the chorion and amnion. Cord concentrations of the drug are approximately 50% of those found in the maternal circulation. There are no reports of adverse fetal reactions to clindamycin administration; however, there are no controlled studies in pregnancy.

Clindamycin is excreted in small amounts in breast milk. It is not known if these doses may induce pseudomembranous colitis in the infant. Prescribing the drug to nursing mothers is therefore best avoided when possible, although the drug is considered compatible with breast-feeding by the American Academy of Pediatrics.

DOSAGE

The oral dose of clindamycin is 150–450 mg every 6 hours. The intramuscular or intravenous dose is 300–600 mg every 6 hours. A topical preparation used in the treatment of acne is applied twice daily. The peak serum level is obtained within 45–60 minutes of intravenous administration, with a half-life of 2–3 hours.

ADVERSE EFFECTS

Common side effects include diarrhea (20% of patients), nausea, vomiting, and allergic reactions. Pseudomembranous colitis, sometimes fatal, has been reported in 2% to 10% of patients receiving clindamycin. This condition can occur both during treatment and up to 3–4 weeks after completion of therapy. It occurs with both oral and parenteral therapy. Therapy should be discontinued if pseudomembranous colitis is suspected; once confirmed, this side effect can be treated with metronidazole.

MECHANISM OF ACTION

Clindamycin is bacteriostatic and inhibits bacterial protein synthesis by binding to the 50S ribosomal subunit. It also stimulates leukocyte host–defense mechanisms.

ABSORPTION AND BIOTRANSFORMATION

Clindamycin is nearly completely absorbed after oral administration. Approximately 4% to 5% of a topical dose is systemically absorbed, but this amount may be increased in certain individuals. The drug is widely distributed throughout the body but does not gain access to the cerebrospinal fluid. Most of the drug is metabolized in the liver to products excreted in the urine and bile. Only 10% of the drug is excreted unchanged in the urine. Little adjustment of dosage is required for patients with renal failure, but the dosage may need adjustment in patients with hepatic decompensation.

RECOMMENDED READING

American Academy of Pediatrics, Committee on Drugs. The Transfer of Drugs and Other Chemicals into Human Milk. *Pediatrics* 93: 137, 1994.

Dhawan, V.K., and Haragopal, T. Clindamycin: a review of fifty years of experience. *Rev. Infect. Dis.* 4:1133, 1982.

Kapusnik-Uner, J.E., Sande, M., and Chamber, H.F. Antimicrobial agents: tetracyclines, chloramphenicol, erythromycin, and miscellaneous antibacterial agents. Chapter 47 in *Goodman and Gilman's The Pharmacological Basis of Therapeutics* (9th ed.), J.G. Hardman and L.E. Limbird, eds. New York: McGraw-Hill, 1996. Pp. 1141–1143.

Soper, D.E. Clindamycin. *Obstet. Gynecol. Clin. North Am.* 19:483, 1992.

Steen, B., and Rane, A. Clindamycin passage into human milk. *Br. J. Clin. Pharmacol.* 13:661, 1982.

Weinstein, A.J., Gibbs, R.S., and Gallagher, M. Placental transfer of clindamycin and gentamicin in term pregnancy. *Am. J. Obstet. Gynecol.* 124:688, 1976.

Zambrano, D. Clindamycin in the treatment of obstetric and gynecologic infections: a review. *Clin. Ther.* 13:58, 1991.

Clomiphene Citrate (Clomid®)

INDICATIONS AND RECOMMENDATIONS

Clomiphene is contraindicated during pregnancy. There is no indication for its use during pregnancy because it is utilized to induce ovulation. However, some women not knowing of their pregnancy might inadvertently continue to take clomiphene citrate during the first trimester.

Clomiphene works on the central nervous system at the hypothalamic level to block estrogen uptake. This results in increased follicle-stimulating hormone (FSH) production by the pituitary with a consequent increase in follicular estradiol production. The elevated estradiol level stimulates a luteinizing hormone (LH) surge during midcycle, which in turn causes ovulation to occur. Clomiphene is taken approximately 7–12 days before ovulation, and studies have shown most of it to be cleared at the time of conception. Maternal side effects when this drug is taken during the first trimester include scotomas, nausea, and abdominal pain. Epidemiologic studies have raised the possibility that clomiphene, or other ovulation-inducing agents, may be associated with an increased risk for the later development of ovarian cancer in women treated for infertility.

Although such a relationship has not been firmly established, the Association for the Study of Reproductive Medicine has recommended that clomiphene be administered for no more than six cycles to a single individual.

Effects on the fetus are unknown. Exposure of pregnant rats to a single dose of clomiphene was associated with abnormalities in the reproductive tract reminiscent of diethylstilbestrol (DES) exposure. Two cases of babies born with anomalies after inadvertent exposure in early pregnancy have been published, but of course denominator figures are unavailable. Human data are so scanty that no conclusions can be drawn.

In addition to the usual questions about fetal effects of the drug taken after conception, it is also legitimate to inquire as to whether pregnancies resulting from clomiphene induction of ovulation are at any particular risk. There have been case reports in humans of neural tube defects (NTDs), cleft lip and palate, Down syndrome, congenital heart defects, and other anomalies. However, when large series were reviewed there did not appear to be a significant difference from the general population with regard to malformation rates. In one large retrospective series from Sweden, the incidence of malformations when ovulation was induced with clomiphene was similar to that observed in a series of pregnancies induced with gonadotropin therapy and, at 5.4%, was slightly higher than the 3.2% observed in the general population. It may be that this represents an expression of the subfertility that made ovulation induction necessary. A number of more recent case reports and case series have raised the possibility that neural tube defects are more common in clomiphene-induced pregnancies than in the general population. A case-control, population-based series from California detected no excess of NTDs among clomiphene-induced pregnancies. The various published series are limited by small sample size and potentially by reporting and ascertainment bias. To date, no convincing evidence supporting a role for clomiphene in the genesis of NTDs has emerged.

RECOMMENDED READING

Ahlgren, M., Kallen, B., and Rannevik, G. Outcome of pregnancy after clomiphene therapy. *Acta Obstet. Gynecol. Scand.* 55:371, 1976.

Asch, R.H., and Greenblatt, R.B. Update on the safety and efficacy of clomiphene citrate as a therapeutic agent. *J. Reprod. Med.* 17:175, 1976.

Goldfarb, A.F., et al. Critical review of 160 clomiphene-related pregnancies. *Obstet. Gynecol.* 31:342, 1968.

Huppert, L.C., and Wallach, E.C. Induction of ovulation with clomiphene citrate. *J. Reprod. Med.* 18:201, 1977.

McCormack, S., and Clark, J.H. Clomid administration to pregnant rats causes abnormalities of the reproductive tract in offspring and mothers. *Science* 204:629, 1979.

Mills J.L., Simpson, J.L., Rhoads, G.G., et al. Risk of neural tube defects in relation to maternal fertility and fertility drug use. *Lancet* 336:103, 1990.

Rossing, M.A., Daling, J.R., Weiss, N.S., Moore, D.E., and Self, S.G. Ovarian tumors in a cohort of infertile women. *N. Engl. J. Med.* 331:771, 1994.

Shaw, G.M., Lammer, E.J., and Velie, E.M. Ovulation induction by clomiphene and neural tube defects. *Reprod. Toxicol.* 9:399, 1995.

Singhi M., and Singhi, S. Possible relationship between clomiphene and neural tube defects. *J. Pediatrics* 93:152, 1978.

Spirtas, R., Kaufman, S.C., and Alexander, N.J. Fertility drugs and ovarian cancer: red alert or red herring? *Fertil. Steril.* 59:291, 1993.

Van Loon, K., Besseghir, K., and Eshkol, A. Neural tube defects after infertility treatment: a review. *Fertil. Steril.* 58:875, 1992.

Werler, M.M., Louik, C., Shapiro, S., and Mitchell, A.A. Ovulation induction and risk of neural tube defects. *Lancet* 344:445, 1994.

Ylikorkala, O. Congenital anomalies and clomiphene. *Lancet* 2:1262, 1975.

Clotrimazole
(Gyne-Lotrimin®, Lotrimin®)

INDICATIONS AND RECOMMENDATIONS

The use of clotrimazole during pregnancy should be limited to the topical treatment of vaginal and skin infections caused by susceptible yeast and fungi. These include *Candida albicans* and *Trichophyton* species. At this time there are no data implicating clotrimazole as a teratogen. This medication should not be applied vaginally after membranes have ruptured.

SPECIAL CONSIDERATIONS IN PREGNANCY

The use of clotrimazole for the treatment of vaginal candidiasis during pregnancy has been extensively studied. First-trimester vaginal use of clotrimazole was not associated with an increased rate of birth defects in a retrospective hospital discharge study. One report noted the efficacy of clotrimazole in eliminating neonatal thrush and maternal nipple soreness. No studies implicate clotrimazole as a teratogen. No data are available to address the safety of clotrimazole for nursing mothers.

DOSAGE

For the treatment of vaginal candidiasis, one vaginal tablet or one applicator dose of the vaginal cream should be inserted high into the vagina for 7 consecutive nights.

ADVERSE EFFECTS

Untoward effects of clotrimazole therapy are uncommon and may include erythema, burning, stinging, edema, pruritus, urticaria, and general irritation of the skin or vagina. Rarely, patients complain of lower abdominal cramps and slight urinary frequency.

MECHANISM OF ACTION

Clotrimazole is structurally unrelated to the other antifungal agents and appears to act by interfering with the phospholipid layer of the fungal membrane. It has broad-spectrum antifungal activity. Clotrimazole therapy is effective in the treatment of vulvovaginal candidiasis, tinea pedis, tinea cruris, tinea corporis, and tinea versicolor.

ABSORPTION AND BIOTRANSFORMATION

Clotrimazole has been found to be only slightly absorbed from skin and vaginal mucosa. Only 0.15% of the dose was recovered in the urine after it had been applied to inflamed skin. Serum levels of 0.05 µg/ml were achieved after administration of a single intravaginal 100 mg tablet.

RECOMMENDED READING

Bennett, J.E. Antimicrobial agents: antifungal agents. Chapter 49 in *Goodman and Gilman's The Pharmacological Basis of Therapeutics* (9th ed.), J.G. Hardman and L.E. Limbird, eds. New York: McGraw-Hill, 1996. Pp. 1180–1188.

Frerich, W., and Gad, A. The frequency of *Candida* infections in pregnancy and their treatment with clotrimazole. *Curr. Opin. Med. Res.* 4:640, 1977.

Haram, K., and Digranes, A. Vulvovaginal candidiasis in pregnancy treated with clotrimazole. *Acta Obstet. Gynecol. Scand.* 57:453, 1978.

Johnstone, H.A., and Marcinak, J.F. Candidiasis in the breastfeeding mother and infant. *J. Obstet. Gynecol. Neonat. Nurs.* 19: 171, 1990.

Lindeque, B.G., and Niekirk, W.A. Treatment of vaginal candidiasis in pregnancy with a single clotrimazole 500 mg vaginal pessary. *S. Afr. Med. J.* 65:123, 1984.

Rosa, F.W., Baum, C., and Shaw, M. Pregnancy outcomes after first-trimester vaginitis drug therapy. *Obstet. Gynecol.* 69:751, 1987.

Tan, C.G. A comparative trial of six day therapy with clotrimazole and nystatin in pregnant patients with vaginal candidiasis. *Postgrad. Med.* 50 (Suppl. 1):102, 1974.

Clozapine (Clozaril®)

INDICATIONS AND RECOMMENDATIONS

The use of clozapine during pregnancy should be limited to the treatment of the schizophrenic woman who does not respond to other antipsychotics and for whom discontinuation of therapy would pose a danger to herself or the fetus. Because of its significant risk of agranulocytosis, clozapine is indicated only for use in severely ill schizophrenic patients who fail to respond adequately to standard antipsychotic drug treatment.

SPECIAL CONSIDERATIONS IN PREGNANCY

Maternal and newborn clozapine levels have been reported from one maternal–infant pair only. In that patient, on the day of delivery, clozapine concentrations were similar in maternal plasma and in amniotic fluid; however, fetal plasma level was almost double the maternal level. On the day after delivery, the level in breast milk was almost 6 times the level in maternal plasma. One week later, the breast milk concentration was slightly less than 3 times plasma level.

The literature contains two reports of infants exposed to clozapine throughout gestation. In one, the patient became pregnant while on therapy and did not reveal her pregnancy until the sixth month. She continued clozapine throughout her pregnancy and delivered a healthy infant at 38 weeks. The second patient (in whom the blood and breast milk levels above were measured) also became pregnant while on therapy. She took 100 mg/day, which was reduced to 50 mg/day during the last 9 weeks of pregnancy in an attempt to avoid possible sedation of the newborn. She gave birth to a 3600 g infant at 41 weeks. The infant's Apgar scores were 5 at 1 minute and 8 at 5 minutes. The patient did not breast-feed her baby. The infant showed no psychomotor abnormalities at 6 months of age.

Because of the paucity of information regarding clozapine use during pregnancy, in spite of the apparently good outcomes in the above cases, patients on clozapine therapy should be counseled to avoid pregnancy.

DOSAGE

The dose of clozapine is gradually increased from 25 mg qd or qid to a target dose of 300–450 mg/day after 2 weeks. Some patients require doses of up to 900 mg/day.

ADVERSE EFFECTS

The most significant adverse effect is agranulocytosis, which can be fatal if not detected early. White blood cell counts should be performed weekly throughout therapy. Seizures are reported to occur, especially with higher doses. Other side effects include orthostatic hypotension, tachycardia and ECG changes, drowsiness, dizziness, and constipation.

MECHANISM OF ACTION

Clozapine is a tricyclic dibenzodiazepine that differs from the more typical antipsychotic agents in its relative affinities for various neuroreceptors. Its exact mechanism of action is unknown. It is thought to bind preferentially dopaminergic receptors in the limbic system. It also acts as an antagonist at adrenergic, cholinergic, histaminergic, and serotonergic receptors.

ABSORPTION AND BIOTRANSFORMATION

Clozapine is well absorbed from the gastrointestinal tract. It is approximately 95% bound to serum proteins. It is almost completely metabolized with 50% of the dose excreted in the urine and 30% in the feces. Its half-life is 12 hours at steady state.

RECOMMENDED READING

Baldessarini, R.J. Drugs and the treatment of psychiatric disorders: psychosis and anxiety. Chapter 18 in *Goodman and Gilman's The Pharmacological Basis of Therapeutics* (9th ed.), J.G. Hardman and L.E. Limbird, eds. New York: McGraw-Hill, 1996. Pp. 403, 406.

Barnas, C. et al. Clozapine concentrations in maternal and fetal plasma, amniotic fluid, and breast milk. *Am. J. Psychiatry* 151: 945, 1994.

Waldman, M.D., and Safferman, A.Z. Pregnancy and clozapine. *Am. J. Psychiatry* 150:168, 1993.

Cocaine

INDICATIONS AND RECOMMENDATIONS

Cocaine is contraindicated during pregnancy. This drug is a local anesthetic and has no other indications. Other local anesthetic agents have now replaced cocaine. It is most widely used as a social drug, taken intranasally or intravenously (cocaine hydrochloride), smoked (crack cocaine or cocaine base), or taken orally (chewing coca leaves or smoking coca paste), rectally, sublingually, subcutaneously, or intramuscularly because it brings about a feeling of well-being and euphoria. Such uses are illegal. In addition, a withdrawal syndrome has been described for cocaine, which consists of craving for the drug, fatigue, hyperphagia, and depression, as well as suppression of REM sleep. Cocaine acts by binding to the dopamine reuptake transporter at synapses, leading to persistence of high concentrations of dopamine. There appears to be greater propensity for abuse when cocaine is smoked or taken intravenously, presumably because of the more rapid onset of action, greater magnitude of effect, and shorter duration with these routes. Acute intoxication with cocaine may include convulsions and cardiac arrhythmias, as with other local anesthetics, as well as vasoconstriction, hypertension, and respiratory arrest.

Cocaine has not been shown to be teratogenic in animal studies. However, its effects on the pregnant woman and her fetus have not been thoroughly investigated. A meta-analysis of 45 studies of possible teratogenicity found a trend toward increased overall malformation rates (RR = 4; CI = 0.7–23.6), which was not statistically significant. Urogenital tract anomalies have been reported to occur with increased frequency in exposed pregnancies, and this effect was statistically significant in the above meta-analysis.

Although possibly confounded by the concomitant use of other drugs, intrauterine growth restriction, prematurity, premature rupture of the membranes, abruptio placentae, prenatal intracranial hemorrhage, and uterine rupture have all been reported to occur more often with cocaine use in pregnancy. The primary cardiovascular effect of cocaine is vasoconstriction. This phenomenon has been demonstrated in the uterine arteries of gravid primates. Transient myocardial ischemia has been reported in 29% of 35 cocaine-exposed infants compared to 5% of control neonates. A population-based case-control series of 355 cocaine-exposed infants and 199 controls demonstrated an approximate tripling of neonatal hospital costs when cocaine exposure was present. This was extrapolated to a national cost of $500 million annually.

In one study, women who used cocaine at the time of conception and during most of pregnancy had a significantly higher incidence of previous spontaneous abortion, and the offspring of the pregnancies under study had significant depression of interactive behavior and a poor organizational response to environmental stimuli. Early data suggested that exposure to cocaine in utero was associated with mental and motor function impairment in the offspring. These preliminary conclusions were not confirmed in large-scale, long-term prospective studies, and at the present time the long-term effects of cocaine on the offspring are unclear.

Because this drug has no therapeutic value, it is clearly contraindicated in pregnancy.

RECOMMENDED READING

Acker, D., et al. Abruptio placentae associated with cocaine use. *Am. J. Obstet. Gynecol.* 146:220, 1983.

Carr, S.R., Coustan, D.R. Nonprescription drugs and alcohol: use and abuse. In *Medicine of the Fetus and Mother* (2nd ed.), E.A. Reece, J.C. Hobbins, and M.J. Mahoney. In press.

Chasnoff, I.J., Griffith, D.R., MacGregor, S., Dirkes, K., and Burns, W.J. Temporal patterns of cocaine use in pregnancy: perinatal outcome. *J.A.M.A.* 261:1741, 1989.

Coles, C., Platzman, K., and Smith, I. Effects of cocaine and alcohol use in pregnancy on neonatal growth and neurobehavioral status. *Neurotoxicol. Teratol.* 14:23, 1992.

Fantel, A.G., and MacPhail, B.J. The teratogenicity of cocaine. *Teratol.* 26:17, 1982.

Hatsukami, D.K., and Fischman, M.W. Crack cocaine and cocaine hydrochloride: are the differences myth or reality? *J.A.M.A.* 276:1580, 1996.

Leshner, A.I. Molecular mechanisms of cocaine addiction. *N.E.J.M.* 335:128, 1996.

Lutiger, B., Graham, K., Einarson, T.R., and Koren, G. Relationship between gestational cocaine use and pregnancy outcome: a meta-analysis. *Teratol.* 44:405, 1991.

Mehta, S.K., Finkelhor, R.S., Anderson, R.L. et al. Transient myocardial ischemia in infants prenatally exposed to cocaine. *J. Pediatrics* 122:945, 1993.

Morgan, M.A., Silavin, S.L., Randolph, M., Payne, G.G., Jr., et al. Effect of intravenous cocaine on uterine blood flow in the gravid baboon. *Am. J. Obstet. Gynecol.* 164:1021, 1991.

Phibbs, C.S., Bateman, D.A., and Schwartz, R.M. The neonatal costs of maternal cocaine use. *J.A.M.A.* 266:1521, 1991.

Colchicine

INDICATIONS AND RECOMMENDATIONS

Animal studies as well as colchicine's mode of action would suggest teratogenicity, and this drug should probably be avoided where other equally effective treatments are available. However, colchicine has been used safely during pregnancy in the treatment of familial Mediterranean fever (FMF), an inherited disorder of unknown etiology. FMF occurs predominantly in those of Sephardic Jewish, Armenian, and Arabic ancestry but is not restricted to these groups.

Colchicine is a mitotic spindle poison that acts by binding tubulin and blocking its polymerization. This results in metaphase arrest of actively dividing cells. There are also data suggesting that colchicine inhibits protein synthesis and cholesterol metabolism in embryonal and ovarian tissue.

Colchicine's use in the treatment of gout is based on its ability to decrease the inflammatory response to the deposition of urate crystals in joint tissue, in part by inhibiting leukocyte metabolism and chemotaxis. Experience with colchicine treatment of pregnant women is limited, as gout is unusual in women of reproductive age. There is a wider experience in treatment of the pregnant patient with colchicine for FMF. Chronic colchicine prophylaxis is routine. In one report, 91 patients continued colchicine treatment throughout the entire pregnancy and delivered at term, and another 40 patients had conceptional exposure but interrupted treatment for the first trimester. There was no unusual frequency of fetal abnormality noted in either population. Further, in follow-up of the children to 10 years of age, no growth disturbances or other deviations from the norm have been observed.

Colchicine is a major teratogen and embryotoxin in chicks, mice, rats and rabbits, with abnormalities seen in facial and central nervous system structures. In humans, colchicine use has been associated with sperm abnormalities, including azoospermia. A single case report notes a trisomic infant born to a couple in which the man was receiving colchicine. Cause and effect has been debated.

Indications for use of colchicine in the pregnant patient are few. No cases of congenital malformations or untoward outcome directly attributable to maternal colchicine have been reported. However, caution in its use is necessary given the very limited human data and teratogenicity in animals. Paternal use of colchicine prior to conception is unlikely a significant reproductive risk.

RECOMMENDED READING

Ehrenfeld, M., et al. The effects of longterm colchicine therapy on male fertility in patients with familial Mediterranean fever. *Andrologia* 118:420, 1986.

Ferreira, N.R., and Buoniconti, A. Trisomy after colchicine therapy. *Lancet* 2: 1304, 1968.

Hsu, T.C., and Satya-Prakash, K.L. Aneuploidy induction by mitotic arrestants in animal cell systems: possible mechanisms. *Basic Life Sci.* 36:279, 1985.

Insel, P.A. Analgesic-antipyretic and antiinflammatory agents and drugs employed in the treatment of gout. Chapter 27 in *Goodman and Gilman's The Pharmacological Basis of Therapeutics* (9th ed.), J.G. Hardman and L.E. Limbird, eds. New York: McGraw-Hill, 1996. Pp. 647–649.

Kaufman, S.S., et al. Increasing inhibition of hepatic protein secretion by colchicine during development. *Am. J. Physiol.* 247: 6311, 1984.

Merlin, H.E. Azoospermia caused by colchicine: a case report. *Fertil. Steril.* 23:180, 1972.

Rabinovitch, O., et al. Colchicine treatment in conception and pregnancy: two hundred thirty-one pregnancies in patients with familial Mediterranean fever. *Am. J. Reprod. Immunol.* 28:245, 1992.

Szabo, K.T., and Kang, J.Y. Comparative teratogenic studies with various therapeutic agents in mice and rabbits. *Teratology* 2: 270, 1969.

Venable, J.H. The effect of colchicine on the rat embryo. *Anat. Rec.* 94:528, 1946.

Walker, F.A. Trisomy after colchicine therapy (letter). *Lancet* 1: 257, 1969.

Contraceptives, Oral

INDICATIONS AND RECOMMENDATIONS

The use of oral contraceptives is contraindicated during pregnancy because there is no reason for their use. Some patients, however, not knowing that they have conceived, may inadvertently continue to take oral contraceptives early in the first trimester.

Most combination oral contraceptive pills in the United States contain a 19-nortestosterone progestin and a synthetic estrogen. When taken during pregnancy, these drugs may increase maternal nausea and vomiting and cause cholestatic jaundice. Newer progestational agents, such as desogestrel and norgestimate, have recently been introduced. Little information is available concerning their inadvertent use in pregnancy.

The ingestion of large dosages of synthetic estrogens during the first trimester, e.g., diethylstilbestrol (DES), has been associated with vaginal adenosis and adenocarcinoma of the vagina, as well as reproductive problems, in female offspring. Testicular cysts, oligospermia, and hypospadias have been reported in male offspring. Although these disturbances have not been associated with oral contraceptives inadvertently taken during the first trimester, extrapolation from DES data suggests the theoretical possibility of such a risk.

Presumably because of the weak androgenic effect of many of the 19-nortestosterone derivatives used as progestational agents, masculinization of exposed female fetuses has been reported, particularly with older, very high dosage formulations.

There are inconclusive data to link early pregnancy oral contraceptive exposure with neural tube defects, limb defects, cardiac abnormalities, and cleft palate. Large-scale case-control studies (including the report from the Finnish Register of Congenital Malformations containing 3002 mothers of infants with malformations) have failed to confirm any strong association. Interestingly, one large study suggested that the combination of maternal smoking and oral contraceptive use during early pregnancy may be a risk factor for malformations. Two recent meta-analyses found no association between oral contraceptive exposure in early pregnancy and congenital malformations in general, congenital heart defects, limb reduction defects, and external genital malformations. There are two case reports of camptomelic dwarfism and sex reversal in female infants exposed to oral contraceptives in utero. There is a single provocative case report of an infant with transposition of the great vessels born to a mother who attempted to induce abortion by the ingestion of 120–150 oral contraceptive pills early in the first trimester.

Other effects of oral contraceptives taken within 2 months of conception may include a decrease in the spontaneous abortion rate of chromosomally normal fetuses, and a doubling of the dizygous twinning rate, as reported in one study.

The steroid hormones in oral contraceptives pass into the breast milk in measurable amounts. Combined oral contraceptive pill ingestion, but not the use of progestin only pills, during lactation has been associated with a measurable diminution in the milk supply, but not with clinically significant problems in the nursing infant. Oral contraceptives are deemed compatible with breast-feeding according to the American Academy of Pediatrics.

The oral contraceptives are contraindicated in pregnancy because of potential adverse effects on the fetus. It goes without saying that they have no therapeutic value in pregnant women. Although there may be an association between congenital anomalies and oral contraceptives taken during the first trimester, the preponderance of current evidence suggests that the risk, if any, is small when compared to the background risk for birth defects.

RECOMMENDED READING

Borglin, N., and Sandholm, L. Effect of oral contraceptives on lactation. *Fertil. Steril.* 22:39, 1971.

Bracken, M.B. Oral contraception and twinning: an epidemiologic study. *Am. J. Obstet. Gynecol.* 133:432, 1979.

Bracken, M.B., and Srisuphan, W. Oral contraception as a risk factor for preeclampsia. *Am. J. Obstet. Gynecol.* 142:191, 1982.

Bracken, M.B. Oral contraception and congenital malformations in offspring: a review and meta-analysis of the prospective studies. *Obstet. Gynecol.* 76:552, 1990.

Chez, R.A. Proceedings of the symposium: progesterone, progestins, and fetal development. *Fertil. Steril.* 30:16, 1978.

Committee on Drugs of the American Academy of Pediatrics. The transfer of drugs and other chemicals into human milk. *Pediatrics* 93:137, 1994.

Compodonico, I., Guerro, B., and Landa, L. Effect of a low-dose oral contraceptive (150 g of levonorgestrel and 30 g ethinylestradiol) on lactation. *Clin. Ther.* 1:454, 1978.

Croxatto, H.B., Diaz, S., Peralta, O., et al. Fertility regulation in nursing women. IV. Long-term influence of a low-dose combined oral contraceptive initiated at day 30 postpartum upon lactation and infant growth. *Contraception* 27:13, 1983.

Keith, L., and Berger, S.L. The relationship between congenital defects and the use of exogenous progestational (contraceptive) hormones during pregnancy: a 20 year review. *Int. J. Gynecol. Obstet.* 15:115, 1977.

Kim, M.R., Qazi, Q.H., Anderson, V.M., and Valencia, G.B. A genetic male infant with female phenotype in camptomelic syndrome: a possible relationship to exposure to oral contraceptives during pregnancy. *Am. J. Obstet. Gynecol.* 172:1042, 1995.

Linn, S., et al. Lack of association between contraceptive usage and congenital malformations in offspring. *Am. J. Obstet. Gynecol.* 147:923, 1983.

Nilsson, S., Nygren, K., and Johansson, E.D.B. D-Norgestrel concentrations in maternal plasma, milk and child plasma during administration of oral contraceptives to nursing women. *Am. J. Obstet. Gynecol.* 129:178, 1977.

Raman-Wilms, L., Tseng, A.L., Wighardt, S., Einarson, T.R., Koren, G. Fetal genital effects of first-trimester sex hormone exposure: a meta-analysis. *Obstet. Gynecol.* 85:141, 1995.

Redline, R.W., and Abramowsky, C.R. Transposition of the great vessels in an infant exposed to massive doses of oral contraceptives. *Am. J. Obstet. Gynecol.* 141:468, 1981.

Sackoff, J., Kline, J., and Susser, M. Previous use of oral contraeptives and spontaneous abortion. *Epidemiology* 5:422, 1994.

Savolainen, E., Saksela, E., and Saxen, L. Teratogenic hazards of oral contraceptives analyzed in a national malformation register. *Am. J. Obstet. Gynecol.* 140:521, 1981.

Williams, C.L., and Stancel, G.M. Estrogens and progestins. Chapter 57 in *Goodman and Gilman's The Pharmacological Basis of Therapeutics* (9th ed.), J.G. Hardman and L.E. Limbird, eds. New York: McGraw-Hill, 1996. Pp. 1411–1440.

Co-trimoxazole: Trimethoprim-Sulfamethoxazole (Bactrim®, Septra®)

INDICATIONS AND RECOMMENDATIONS

The use of co-trimoxazole during pregnancy is relatively contraindicated because for most of its indications there are more desirable alternatives. Its use should be limited to treatment of life-threatening infections, such as those caused by *Pneumocystis carinii,* which are not amenable to treatment with less hazardous antibiotics. It should not be administered in the third trimester because of the danger of kernicterus to the neonate.

SPECIAL CONSIDERATIONS IN PREGNANCY

Despite favorable outcomes in a few limited studies that used co-trimoxazole to treat bacteriuria during various stages of pregnancy, the use of this agent should be avoided whenever possible.

Both trimethoprim and sulfamethoxazole cross the placenta and appear in measurable amounts in fetal blood. Although no instances have been documented, there is a theoretical possibility that trimethoprim will inhibit the reduction of dihydrofolate to tetrahydrofolate in the fetus, thereby causing congenital anomalies. In addition, the use of sulfonamides in the last 3 months of pregnancy is contraindicated because of the danger of kernicterus in the neonate (see "Sulfonamides").

DOSAGE

The usual adult dose is 800 mg sulfamethoxazole plus 160 mg trimethoprim every 12 hours for 10–14 days. Larger dosages have been used in patients with serious or life-threatening diseases. The dosage must be reduced in patients with renal disease.

ADVERSE EFFECTS

Sulfonamide use is often associated with skin reactions, and the same spectrum of reactions is seen with co-trimoxazole therapy. Nausea and vomiting are common side effects, as are glossitis and stomatitis. While there is no evidence that co-trimoxazole causes folate deficiency in normal people at recommended dosages, megaloblastosis, leukopenia, or thrombocytopenia may be seen in those who are folate- deficient. Additional hematologic reactions include other types of anemia and coagulation disorders.

MECHANISM OF ACTION

The antimicrobial activity of the trimethoprim-sulfamethoxazole combination results from their individual and synergistic actions on the tetrahydrofolate synthesis pathway. Sulfamethoxazole inhibits the incorporation of para-aminobenzoic acid (PABA) into folic acid, and trimethoprim prevents the reduction of dihydrofolate to tetrahydrofolate. The toxicity is selective for microorganisms, as mammalian cells do not utilize PABA and trimethoprim is a highly selective inhibitor of enzyme activity in lower organisms.

Because of this unique mechanism of action, co-trimoxazole has a broad spectrum of action against gram-positive and gram-negative organisms and is effective in the treatment of *P. carinii* infections in impaired hosts.

ABSORPTION AND BIOTRANSFORMATION

The individual ingredients of co-trimoxazole have been selected to achieve optimal blood and tissue concentration ratios of 20:1. While trimethoprim is absorbed more quickly than sulfamethoxazole, their half-lives are well matched at approximately 11 and 10 hours, respectively.

Trimethoprim is rapidly distributed and concentrated in tissues. It enters the cerebrospinal fluid and sputum readily. Up to 60% is excreted in the urine in 24 hours. Metabolites of trimethoprim are also excreted. The rate of excretion is significantly decreased in uremia.

Sulfamethoxazole is approximately 65% bound to plasma proteins. In 24 hours, 25% to 50% is excreted in the urine, approximately one-third as conjugates. The rate of excretion is significantly decreased in uremia.

RECOMMENDED READING

Bailey, R.R., Bishop, V., and Peddie, B.A. Comparison of single dose with a five day course of co-trimoxazole for asymptomatic (covert) bacteriuria of pregnancy. *Aust. N. Z. J. Obstet. Gynecol.* 23:139, 1983.

Connelly, R.T., and Lourwood, D.L. Pneumocystis carinii pneumonia prophylaxis during pregnancy. *Pharmacotherapy* 14:424, 1994.

Czeizel, A. A case-control analysis of the teratogenic effects of co-trimoxazole. *Reprod. Toxicol.* 4:305, 1990.

Hicks, M.L., et al. Acquired immunodeficiency syndrome and *Pneumocystis carinii* infection in a pregnant woman. *Obstet. Gynecol.* 76:480, 1990

Mandell, G.L., and Petri, Jr., W.A. Antimicrobial agents: Sulfonamides, trimethoprim-sulfamethoxazole, quinolones, and agents for urinary tract infections. Chapter 44 in *Goodman and Gilman's The Pharmacological Basis of Therapeutics* (9th ed.), J.G. Hardman and L.E. Limbird, eds. New York: McGraw-Hill, 1996. Pp. 1063–1065.

Pedler, S.J., and Bint, A.J. Management of bacteriuria in pregnancy. *Drugs* 33:413, 1987.

Vercaigne, L.M., and Zhanel, G.G. Recommended treatment for urinary tract infection in pregnancy. *Ann. Pharmacother.* 28:248, 1994.

Ylikorkala, O., et al. Trimethoprim-sulfonamide combination administered orally and intravaginally in the first trimester of pregnancy: Its absorption into serum and transfer to amniotic fluid. *Acta Obstet. Gynecol. Scand.* 52:229, 1973.

Coumarin Anticoagulants: Warfarin (Coumadin®)

INDICATIONS AND RECOMMENDATIONS

The use of oral anticoagulants in the warfarin family is contraindicated during pregnancy. During the first trimester, these compounds have the potential for causing warfarin embryopathy. During the second and third trimesters, their use can result in the development of central nervous system and ocular anomalies. In addition, because these drugs readily cross the placental barrier they anticoagulate the fetus. Deaths from fetal hemorrhage occurring before and during labor have been reported.

Warfarins inhibit vitamin K epoxide reductase and vitamin K reductase, blocking conversion of vitamin K to its active form. Fetal abnormalities associated with maternal ingestion of warfarin anticoagulants include nasal hypoplasia, stippling of bone, hydrocephalus, microcephaly, ophthalmologic abnormalities, intrauterine growth retardation, and developmental delays. In addition, two cases of urinary tract abnormalities have been reported after in utero exposure to warfarin.

Some authors have advocated the use of warfarin anticoagulants during the second trimester and up to 3 weeks before the estimated date of delivery. The rationale for this regimen is that it avoids first-trimester exposure and also reduces the risk of fetal hemorrhage at the time of labor and delivery at term. It has been found, however, that while the warfarin embryopathy syndrome results from exposure in the first trimester, central nervous system abnormalities may develop at any gestational age. In addition, the onset of premature labor cannot be anticipated and, consequently, the infant could be fully anticoagulated at the time of an early delivery. We therefore recommend that heparin be used as the drug of choice in any patient who requires anticoagulation throughout pregnancy.

Postpartum administration of warfarin poses no hazard to the nursing infant since only an inactive form of the drug appears in human milk.

RECOMMENDED READING

Åstedt, B. Antenatal drugs affecting vitamin K status of the fetus and newborn. *Semin. Thromb. Hemost.* 21:364, 1995.

Hall, B.D. Warfarin embryopathy and urinary tract anomalies: possible new association. *Am. J. Med. Genet.* 34:292, 1989.

Hall, J.G., Pauli, R.M., and Wilson, K.M. Maternal and fetal sequelae of anticoagulation during pregnancy. *Am. J. Med.* 68:122, 1980.

Israel D.H., Sharma S.K., and Fuster, V. Antithrombotic therapy in prosthetic heart valve replacement. *Am. Heart J.* 127:400, 1994.

Shaul, W.L., Emery, H., and Hall, J.G. Chondroplasia puncta and maternal warfarin use during pregnancy. *Am. J. Dis. Child.* 129:360, 1975.

Cromolyn Sodium (Aarane®, Gastrocrom®, Intal®, Nasalcrom®)

INDICATIONS AND RECOMMENDATIONS

Cromolyn sodium may be administered via inhalation to pregnant asthmatics before unavoidable exposure to allergens that are known to cause severe bronchospasm and to prevent exercise-induced bronchospasm. It may also be administered nasally to treat and prevent allergic rhinitis and orally for the treatment of mastocytosis. Cromolyn sodium has no role in the treatment of acute asthmatic attacks. This drug seems to be well tolerated in pregnancy, and its systemic absorption is minimal.

SPECIAL CONSIDERATIONS IN PREGNANCY

No unusual maternal effects are reported. No information is available regarding the passage of cromolyn sodium across the placenta.

Teratogenicity has not been reported in humans. In one series of 296 pregnant asthmatics treated with cromolyn sodium, malformations were observed in only four newborns (1.4%), an incidence lower than the usual 2% to 3% seen in the general population. Studies in animals have failed to produce teratogenesis after prolonged intravenous administration of the drug. Decreased fetal weight, however, has been reported in association with dosages close to those that produce maternal toxicity in animals.

DOSAGE

The usual inhaled dose is 20 mg q6h at regular intervals. A clinical response to this drug is often seen within 3–5 days but may take as long as a month. The prophylactic dose is 20 mg inhaled no more than 1 hour prior to exercise or allergen exposure. This drug should not be given during an acute asthmatic attack because it can aggravate the existing bronchial irritation. For allergic rhinitis, the dose is one spray into each nostril 3–6 times daily at regular intervals. The oral dose is 200 mg qid, one-half hour before meals and at bedtime.

ADVERSE EFFECTS

Side effects are uncommon and usually minor. They include mild sore throat, nasal congestion, cough, transient wheezing, urticaria, and maculopapular rash. Occasionally, angioedema, fever, nausea, vomiting, pulmonary infiltrates, muscular weakness, pericarditis, and, very rarely, anaphylaxis may occur.

MECHANISM OF ACTION

Cromolyn sodium inhibits the release of histamine and slow-reacting substance of anaphylaxis by mast cells. These are the chemical mediators of a bronchospastic response after either immunologic or nonimmunologic stimulation. This drug does not have direct bronchodilator, antihistaminic, or antiinflammatory effects. The amount of drug absorbed into the circulation following inhalation of therapeutic dosages does not appear to exert any generalized pharmacologic action.

ABSORPTION AND BIOTRANSFORMATION

For asthma, cromolyn is given via inhalation of either a solution or the powdered drug. The pharmacologic effects are from the topical deposition of the drug in the lung. Only 1–2 mg of a 20 mg dose reaches the alveoli. The remainder is retained in the trachea and oropharynx and is swallowed later. About 1% of an oral dose and 7% to 8% of the inhaled dose is absorbed systemically through the gastrointestinal tract. Eighty percent of the absorbed cromolyn sodium is eliminated in the feces. The absorbed drug is excreted unchanged in the urine. The plasma half-life is 60–90 minutes.

RECOMMENDED READING

Berstein, I.L., et al. A controlled study of cromolyn sodium sponsored by the Drug Committee of the American Academy of Allergy. *J. Allergy Clin. Immunol.* 50:235, 1972.

Falliers, C.J. Cromolyn sodium prophylaxis. *Pediatr. Clin. North Am.* 22:141, 1975.

Gwin, E., Kerby, G., and Ruth, W. Cromolyn sodium in the treatment of asthma associated with aspirin hypersensitivity and nasal polyps. *Chest* 72:148, 1977.

Khurana, S., and Hyde, J.S. Cromolyn sodium, five to six years later. *Ann. Allergy* 39:94, 1977.

Noble, S.L., Forbes, R.C., and Woodbridge, H.B. Allergic rhinitis. *Am. Fam. Physician* 51:837, 1995.

Serafin, W.E. Drugs used in the treatment of asthma. Chapter 28 in *Goodman and Gilman's The Pharmacological Basis of Therapeutics* (9th ed.), J.G. Hardman and L.E. Limbird, eds. New York: McGraw-Hill, 1996. Pp. 667–669.

Silverman, M., and Andrea, T. Time course of effect of disodium cromoglycate on exercise-induced asthma. *Arch. Dis. Child.* 47:419, 1972.

Turner, E.S., Greenberger, P.A., and Patterson, R. Management of the pregnant asthmatic patient. *Ann. Intern. Med.* 93:905, 1980.

Wilson, J. Utilisation du cromoglycate de sodium au cours de la grossesse. *Acta Ther.* 8 (Suppl.):45, 1982.

Cyclizine (Marezine®)

INDICATIONS AND RECOMMENDATIONS

Cyclizine is safe to use during pregnancy for the prevention of nausea, vomiting, and dizziness associated with motion sickness. This drug is probably effective for control of postoperative nausea and vomiting when used parenterally or rectally. Although cyclizine has been shown to be teratogenic in rodents, this effect has not been demonstrated in humans when recommended dosages are used.

SPECIAL CONSIDERATIONS IN PREGNANCY

Cyclizine crosses the placenta and has been shown to be teratogenic in rodents. However, large-scale studies in humans show that the rate of severe congenital anomalies in children of mothers who took cyclizine during pregnancy is not significantly different than in the offspring of mothers who did not receive antinauseants.

DOSAGE

The dose for prevention of motion sickness is 50 mg a half-hour before departure, repeated every 4–6 hours as necessary. Dose should not exceed 200 mg/day.

ADVERSE EFFECTS

The more common side effects of cyclizine include drowsiness, dry mouth, and, rarely, blurred vision.

MECHANISM OF ACTION

Cyclizine is a piperazine antihistamine that depresses labyrinth excitability and vestibular-cerebellar pathway conduction. It inhibits the effects of histamine on capillary permeability and on smooth muscle by competitive inhibition at H_1 receptors. Either stimulation or depression of the central nervous system may occur through an unknown mechanism. It has anticholinergic activity, although no significant effects on the cardiovascular system occur at normal therapeutic dosages.

ABSORPTION AND BIOTRANSFORMATION

Cyclizine is readily absorbed from the gastrointestinal tract and is widely distributed to body tissues. The exact nature of elimination in humans is unknown, but it appears to be extensively metabolized in the liver and excreted in the urine.

RECOMMENDED READING

American Pharmaceutical Association. *Handbook of Non-Prescription Drugs.* Washington, DC, 1996. Pp. 290–291.

American Pharmaceutical Association. *Non-Prescription Products: Formulations and Features 96–97.* Washington, DC, 1996. P. 162.

Babe, Jr., K.S., and Serafin, W.E. Histamine, bradykinin, and their antagonists. Chapter 25 in *Goodman and Gilman's The Pharmacological Basis of Therapeutics* (9th ed.), J.G. Hardman and L.E. Limbird, eds. New York: McGraw-Hill, 1996. P. 591.

Biggs, J.S.G. Vomiting in pregnancy: causes and management. *Drugs* 9:299, 1975.

Heinonen, D., Slone, D., and Shapiro, S. *Birth Defects and Drugs in Pregnancy.* Littleton, MA: Wright-PSG, 1977. Pp. 323–333.

Milkovich, L., and Van den Berg, B.J. An evaluation of the teratogenicity of certain antinauseant drugs. *Am. J. Obstet. Gynecol.* 125:244, 1976.

Nishimura, H., and Tanimura. T. *Clinical Aspects of the Teratogenicity of Drugs.* Amsterdam: Excerpta Medica, 1976.

Cyclobenzaprine (Flexeril®)

INDICATIONS AND RECOMMENDATIONS

Cyclobenzaprine is a tricyclic amine used as a skeletal muscle relaxant to treat muscle spasm associated with acute musculoskeletal conditions. It is considered an adjunct to rest and physical therapy. This agent is structurally related to the tricyclic antidepressants. Animal studies have not demonstrated teratogenicity for this drug. However, because no published reports of use in human pregnancy could be found, and because the conditions for which cyclobenzaprine is prescribed tend to be self-limited, cyclobenzaprine is not recommended for use during pregnancy.

RECOMMENDED READING

Merck and Co. Flexeril tablets (cyclobenzaprine HCl). Entry in *Physicians Desk Reference* (52nd ed.). Montvale, NJ: Medical Economics, 1998. Pp. 1656–1657.

Cyclosporine (Sandimmune®, Neoral®) and Tacrolimus (Prograf®)

INDICATIONS AND RECOMMENDATIONS

The use of cyclosporines in pregnant women should be limited to clinical situations in which immunosuppression is critical to maternal survival. These drugs are most commonly used to prophylax against rejection in allogenic organ transplant recipients but also have therapeutic value in a number of other disorders such as autoimmune diseases when standard therapy is ineffective.

SPECIAL CONSIDERATIONS IN PREGNANCY

In studies on rats and rabbits, embryotoxicity occurred when cyclosporine doses high enough to be toxic to the mother were administered. However, at dosages that were well tolerated by the mother, no embryotoxicity was demonstrated. When organ culture studies were performed using rat embryos, cyclosporine did not induce malformations, whereas azathioprine did so.

Cyclosporine crosses the placenta, with fetal levels between 37% and 64% of maternal plasma levels in various reports. There have been a number of case reports and case series documenting successful pregnancy outcome with maternal cyclosporine therapy. Although congenital malformations were not reported to occur more frequently than in the general population, spontaneous abortion, prematurity, and growth restriction appear to be more common. Whether these problems are related to the cyclosporine, or to the underlying disease states, or to other drugs prescribed concomitantly is impossible to ascertain. As yet, there is no evidence for human teratogenicity with this drug.

Transient neonatal thrombocytopenia, as well as immunosuppression (demonstrated by suppression of third-party lymphocyte culture growth), has occurred in infants of mothers taking this drug. One study (Pilarski et al., 1994) found slight delays in T-cell development in neonates who were exposed in utero to cyclosporine. The authors concluded that "the immune system in humans appears to be remarkably resilient, and successfully adapts to the presence of cyclosporine during its early developmental stages." In addition, breast milk cyclosporine levels were in the same range as maternal serum levels. The Committee on Drugs of the American Academy of Pediatrics considers breast-feeding to be contraindicated while taking cyclosporine.

DOSAGE

Cyclosporine is available as an oral solution (100 mg/ml), as soft gelatin capsules (25, 50, and 100 mg), and as an intravenous preparation (250 mg/5 ml). The initial dose is given 4–12 hours before transplantation. The drug is started at a single oral dose of 15 mg/kg/day; this dosage is continued for 1–2 weeks after surgery, then gradually tapered (5% per week) to a maintenance dose of 5–10 mg/kg/day. Surveys of transplant centers suggest that lower initial doses are commonly used, ranging from 9 ± 3 mg/kg/day for renal transplant patients to 7 ± 3 mg/kg/day for heart transplant patients. The daily dosage is commonly divided into two. Neoral is a microemulsion of cyclosporine, which is more predictably absorbed orally and generally requires approximately 10% lower dosing than Sandimmune. It is supplied as 25 and 100 mg tablets, and an oral solution of 100 mg/ml. Blood concentration monitoring is used to guide therapy, with trough levels being most critical. Because of differences among assays, specific recommendations for target blood or plasma levels are beyond the scope of this book. Tacrolimus (Prograf) is supplied as 1 and 5 mg capsules and as an intravenous preparation in 1 ml ampules containing 5 mg/ml. Its potency is approximately 100 times that of cyclosporine.

Intravenous administration of cyclosporine has been associated with anaphylaxis, so that the use of this route should be limited to patients unable to take the drug orally. When used intravenously, the dosage of cyclosporine is one-third the oral dosage.

Corticosteroid therapy is generally used as an adjunct to cyclosporine, with initial high doses (as much as 200 mg/day prednisone in some series) but slow tapering to maintenance doses, often as low as 10–20 mg prednisone each day. Adjustments in dosage of cyclosporine and corticosteroids should be the responsibility of individuals experienced in the use of these drugs and in the care of transplant recipients.

ADVERSE EFFECTS

Dose-related nephrotoxicity is seen in a high proportion of transplant recipients treated with cyclosporine. In the case of renal transplant recipients, nephrotoxicity may be difficult to distinguish from rejection. If it does not improve with adjustment in dosage, it may be necessary to switch to other forms of immunosuppressive therapy. Hypertension was reported in 26% of 227 renal transplant recipients receiving this drug in a randomized trial, as opposed to 18% of 228 receiving azathioprine. Hepatotoxicity, consisting of elevated liver enzymes and bilirubin, was reported in 4% to 7% of treated patients and usually responded to reduction in dosage. Hirsutism, tremors, paresthesias, gum dysplasia, nausea, and vomiting have all been reported. Anaphylaxis was reported in approximately 1 in 1000 patients receiving cyclosporine intravenously, and for this reason, all such patients should be closely observed for at least 30 minutes after beginning the infusion. Anaphylactic reactions have not been reported with the oral route of administration.

MECHANISM OF ACTION

Cyclosporine (cyclosporin A) is a cyclic polypeptide containing 11 amino acids. It is a product of the fungus *Tolypocladium inflatum Gams*. Tacrolimus (FK506) is a macrolide antibiotic produced by *Streptomyces tsukubaensis*. These drugs inhibit cell-mediated immunity, such as allograft rejection, presumably by suppressing the activation of T lymphocytes. They must be administered before these T lymphocytes have undergone proliferation in response to exposure to a specific antigen. B-cell function is not altered.

ABSORPTION AND BIOTRANSFORMATION

Gastrointestinal absorption of cyclosporine is incomplete and variable. Peak concentrations are achieved at 3–4 hours, and bioavailability is approximately 20% to 50% compared to intravenous dosing. The newer microemulsion formulation appears to be absorbed much more uniformly and predictably, and exhibits increased bioavailability, so that similar plasma levels of cyclosporine can be achieved with 10% lower dosing. Only about 40% of absorbed cyclosporine is distributed in plasma, with the remainder being taken up by erythrocytes, granulocytes, and lymphocytes. Approximately 90% of plasma cyclosporine is protein-bound. Elimination is mainly via the biliary system, with a half-life of approximately 19 hours.

RECOMMENDED READING

Committee on Drugs of the American Academy of Pediatrics. The transfer of drugs and other chemicals into human milk. *Pediatrics* 93:137, 1994.

Diasio, R.B., and LoBuglio, A.F. Immunomodulators: immunosuppresive agents and immunostimulants. Chapter 52 in *Goodman and Gilman's The Pharmacological Basis of Therapeutics* (9th ed.), J.G. Hardman and L.E. Limbird, eds. New York: McGraw-Hill, 1996. Pp. 1296–1300.

Doria, A., Di Lenardo, L., Vario, S., Calligaro, A., Vaccaro, E., and Gambari, P.F. Cyclosporin A in a pregnant patient affected with lupus erythematosus. *Rheumatol. Int.*12:77, 1992.

Flechner, S.M., Katz, A.R., Rogers, A.J., Van Buren, C., and Kahan, B.D. The presence of cyclosporine in body tissues and fluids during pregnancy. *Am. J. Kidney Dis.* 5:60, 1985.

Haugen, G., Fauchald, P., S dal, G., Leivestad, T., and Moe, N. Pregnancy outcome in renal allograft recipients in Norway. *Acta Obstet. Gynecol. Scand.* 73:541, 1994.

Laifer, S.A. Pregnancy after transplantation. Chapter 1 in *Current Obstetric Medicine,* Vol. 2(R.V. Lee, W.M. Barron, D.B. Cotton, and D. Coustan, eds.). St. Louis: Mosby–Yearbook, 1993. Pp. 1–24.

Neoral. *Physicians' Desk Reference* (50th ed.). Montvale, NJ: Medical Economics, 1996. Pp. 2276–2280.

Olshan A.F., Mattison, D.R., Zwanenburg, T.S.B., and the Working Group on the Toxicity of Cyclosporine A. Cyclosporine A: review of genotoxicity and potential for adverse human reproductive and developmental effects. *Mutat. Res.* 317:163, 1994.

Pilarski L.M., Yacyshyn, B.R., and Lazarovits, A.I. Analysis of peripheral blood lymphocyte populations and immune function from children exposed to cyclosporine or to azathioprine in utero. *Transplantation* 57:133, 1994.

Prograf. *Physicians' Desk Reference* (50th ed.). Montvale, NJ: Medical Economics, 1996. Pp. 1042–1045.

Sandimmune. *Physicians' Desk Reference* (50th ed.). Montvale, NJ: Medical Economics, 1996. Pp. 2286–2290.

Takahashi, N., Nishida, H., and Hoshi, J. Severe B cell depletion in newborns from renal transplant mothers taking immunosuppressive agents. *Transplantation* 57:1617, 1994.

Yoshimura, N., Oka, T., Fujiwara, Y., Ohmori, Y., Yasumura, T., and Honjo, H. A case report of pregnancy in renal transplant recipient treated with FK506 (tacrolimus). *Transplantation* 61:1552, 1996.

Cyproheptadine (Periactin®)

INDICATIONS AND RECOMMENDATIONS

Cyproheptadine, an antihistamine and serotonin antagonist, is teratogenic at relatively high dosages in some laboratory animals. It has no clear advantages over other antihistamines when used to treat allergic reactions such as rhinitis, urticaria, and angioedema, but its serotonin antagonism is useful in treating postgastrectomy dumping syndrome and the intestinal hypermotility of carcinoid, although somatostatin analogs are generally preferred. Therefore, its use in pregnancy should be limited to the latter indications.

SPECIAL CONSIDERATIONS IN PREGNANCY

Whereas some studies of cyproheptadine given to rats show no teratogenic or embryotoxic effects at subcutaneous doses up to 5 mg/kg/day (the usual oral dose is approximately 0.2 mg/kg/day), others show teratogenic effects with single intraperitoneal doses of 10–50 mg/kg on day 7, 10, 13, or 15 of a 22-day gestation. Chronic intraperitoneal dosing at 2 mg/kg/day throughout pregnancy resulted in increased perinatal mortality. Finally, rats given cyproheptadine by gastric intubation on days 6–15 of pregnancy manifested increased anomalies among their offspring when doses of 15 mg/kg/day were exceeded. In a recent study, rats were given cyproheptadine orally (11 mg/kg/day) on days 13–20. When the offspring were tested at 50 days of age, they manifested glucose intolerance, higher insulin levels in the pancreas, and an exaggeration of the insulin-lowering effect of cyproheptadine on the pancreas. For these reasons it seems prudent to avoid this drug in pregnancy when other equally effective alternatives exist.

There is a single case report of a patient treated with cyproheptadine throughout pregnancy for Cushing's syndrome (because adrenocorticotropic hormone [ACTH] secretion may be dependent on serotonergic neurons) who delivered a normal baby at term. The baby died of gastroenteritis at 4 months. In another case, the drug was discontinued at the end of the first trimester. The pregnancy outcome was normal.

Sadovsky and colleagues have reported the use of cyproheptadine to prevent recurrent abortion, but appropriate control groups were not described. Interestingly, when 29 women were given 4–16 mg/day during the first and second trimesters, no teratogenic effects were seen in the 23 term and 5 premature infants. Unfortunately, follow-up information on these neonates is not available. Although the rationale for this application was the ability of cyproheptadine to block serotonin-induced abortion in rats, this drug appears to be incapable of prolonging normal pregnancy in laboratory animals.

No data on breast-feeding by women taking cyproheptadine are currently available.

DOSAGE

Cyproheptadine is available as a 4 mg tablet and as a syrup (2 mg/5 ml). The usual dose is 12–16 mg/day. Doses should not exceed 0.5 mg/kg/day.

ADVERSE EFFECTS

Atropine-like effects include drowsiness, dry mouth, blurred vision, palpitations, tachycardia, thickening of bronchial secretions, and urinary retention. Hypotension may occur. Allergic manifestations, including anaphylactic shock, have also been reported.

MECHANISM OF ACTION

Cyproheptadine blocks both H_1 receptors and serotonin (5-hydroxytryptamine) receptors. Of particular value is its ability to block serotonin receptors in vascular smooth muscle and in the gastrointestinal tract. It also has anticholinergic and sedative effects.

ABSORPTION AND BIOTRANSFORMATION

This drug is only administered orally. Much of its elimination is urinary and is diminished in the presence of renal insufficiency.

RECOMMENDED READING

Chow, S.A., and Fischer, L.J. Alterations in rat pancreatic B-cell function induced by prenatal exposure to cyproheptadine. *Diabetes* 33:572, 1984.

De la Fuente, M., and Alia, M. The teratogenicity of cyproheptadine in two generations of Wistar rats. *Arch. Intern. Pharmacodyn. Ther.* 257:168, 1982.

Kasperlik-Zaluska, A., et al. Two pregnancies in a woman with Cushing's syndrome treated with cyproheptadine. *Br. J. Obstet. Gynaecol.* 87:1171, 1980.

Khir, A.S.M., How, J., and Bewsher, P.D. Successful pregnancy after cyproheptadine treatment for Cushing's disease. *Eur. J. Obstet. Gynecol. Reprod. Biol.* 13:343, 1982.

Rodrigues Gonzalez, M.D., Lima Perez, M.T., and Sanabria Negrin, J.G. The effect of cyproheptadine chlorhydrate on rate embryonic development. *Teratogen. Carcinogen. Mutagen* 3:439, 1983.

Sadovsky, E. Attempts to delay labor in rats by a serotonin antagonist, cyproheptadine. *Isr. J. Med. Sci.* 9:1590, 1974.

Sadovsky, E., et al. The use of antiserotonin-cyproheptadine HCl in pregnancy: an experimental and clinical study. *Adv. Exp. Med. Biol.* 27:399, 1972.

Sanders-Bush, E., and Mayer S.E. 5-Hydroxytryptamine (serotonin) receptor agonists and antagonists. Chapter 11 in *Goodman and Gilman's The Pharmacological Basis of Therapeutics* (9th ed.), J.G. Hardman and L.E. Limbird, eds. New York: McGraw-Hill, 1996. P. 261.

Weinstein, D., et al. Teratogenicity of cyproheptadine in pregnant rats. *Arch. Int. Pharmacodyn. Ther.* 215:345, 1975.

Danazol (Danocrine®)

INDICATIONS AND RECOMMENDATIONS

Danazol is contraindicated in pregnancy. This drug is a testosterone derivative and a weak androgen, and there are a number of case reports of masculinization of female fetuses with its use. It was originally developed for the treatment of endometriosis. Ovulation is usually, but not always, suppressed when danazol is taken, and pregnancy has a suppressive effect on endometriosis, so it is unlikely that a woman known to be pregnant would be prescribed danazol. However, danazol is also used in the treatment of hereditary angioneurotic edema, an autosomal dominant disorder that can be life threatening. Its effectiveness in this condition appears to be related to an androgenic side effect on the liver, causing increased production of an inhibitor of the complement cascade. Fortunately, most case series seem to indicate that pregnancy decreases the frequency of attacks of angioneurotic edema. Prophylactic administration of fresh-frozen plasma is often recommended for patients with this disorder who are undergoing cesarean section because fresh-frozen plasma contains C-1 esterase inhibitor, which is lacking in patients with this disorder. Danazol is also occasionally used for the treatment of severe fibrocystic breast disease, hemophilia type A, and as a third-line treatment of immune thrombocytopenic purpura.

As of 1984, 10 in 15 female fetuses exposed to danazol (800 mg/day) in utero and reported to the FDA had virilization of the external genitalia. All had fused labia, and 7 in 10 had clitoral hypertrophy. In each of these cases, it is presumed that the pregnancies were established at the time danazol exposure was commenced. No case of virilization was reported in which danazol had been discontinued before the eighth week of embryogenesis. Another case has been reported in which danazol was started in a dose of 400 mg/day at the time of the last menstrual period prior to conception. The fetus was exposed to danazol until the 18th week of pregnancy (documented by ultrasound), at which time the medication was discontinued. The female neonate had fused, scrotalized labia, clitoromegaly, and a well-defined median raphe. Internal genitalia have been female in all of these cases. Unfortunately, no satisfactory denominator figures are available for danazol exposure during pregnancy. Reports of urogenital sinus formation in danazol-exposed pregnancies have recently appeared, and the possibility exists that this anomaly might be induced by the drug.

RECOMMENDED READING

Ahn, Y.S., et al. Danazol for the treatment of idiopathic thrombocytopenic purpura. *N. Engl. J. Med.* 308:1396, 1983.

Boulos, A.N., Brown, R., Hukin, A., and Williams, R.M. Danazol prophylaxis for delivery in hereditary angioneurotic edema. *Br. J. Obstet. Gynaecol.* 101:1094, 1994.

Brunskill, P.J. The effects of fetal exposure to danazol. *Br. J. Obstet. Gynaecol.* 99:212, 1992.

Gralnick, H.R., et al. Benefits of danazol treatment in patients with hemophilia A (classic hemophilia). *J.A.M.A.* 253:1151, 1985.

Peress, M.R., et al. Female pseudohermaphroditism with somatic chromosomal anomaly in association with in utero exposure to danazol. *Am. J. Obstet. Gynecol.* 142:708, 1982.

Quagliarello, J., and Greco, M.A. Danazol and urogenital sinus formation in pregnancy. *Fertil. Steril.* 43:939, 1985.

Rosa, F.W. Virilization of the female fetus with maternal danazol exposure. *Am. J. Obstet. Gynecol.* 149:99, 1984.

Schiavotto, C., Castaman, G., and Rodeghiero, F. Treatment of idiopathic thrombocytopenic purpura (ITP) in patients with refractoriness to or with contraindication for corticosteroids and/or splenectomy with immunosuppressive therapy and danazol. *Hematologica* 78 (Suppl 2):29, 1993.

Shaw, R.W. Female pseudohermaphroditism associated with danazol exposure in utero. Case report. *Br. J. Obstet. Gynaecol.* 91:386, 1984.

Stiller, R.J., Kaplan, B.M., and Andreoli, J.W., Jr. Hereditary angioedema and pregnancy. *Obstet. Gynecol.* 64:133, 1984.

Wilson, J.D. Androgens. Chapter 58 in *Goodman and Gilman's The Pharmacological Basis of Therapeutics* (9th ed.), J.G. Hardman and L.E. Limbird, eds. New York: McGraw-Hill, 1996. Pp. 1441–1457.

Dextran: Dextran 40 (Rheomacrodex®), Dextran 70 (Macrodex ®)

INDICATIONS AND RECOMMENDATIONS

Dextrans are relatively contraindicated during pregnancy because other, more physiologic plasma expanders are preferable. Dextran is used as a plasma expander and for prophylaxis of thromboembolism. If dextran therapy is unavoidable, use of low molecular weight dextran is preferable because its use is associated with fewer anaphylactoid reactions.

Although dextrans have been used with success to produce volume expansion in patients with preeclampsia, the risk of anaphylactoid reactions is so great that they should not be used in pregnancy unless no other plasma volume expander is available. In one prospective study of 5745 gynecologic and obstetric patients who received dextran-70 during surgery, the incidence of severe reactions was 1:821 and the overall incidence of reactions was 1:383. One neonatal death occurred following dextran-induced cardiac arrest in a woman about to undergo cesarean section. While the above patients were not treated with dextran 1 (a hapten used to decrease the incidence and severity of anaphylactoid reactions to dextran), another author reports three obstetric patients who experienced anaphylactoid reactions due to dextran 70 despite treatment with hapten. One of the mothers experienced a mild reaction but gave birth to a child with serious brain damage; one mother died from myocardial infarction; the third mother recovered without sequelae.

RECOMMENDED READING

Berg, E.M., Fasting, S., and Sellevold, O.F. Serious complications with dextran-70 despite hapten prophylaxis. Is it best avoided prior to delivery? *Anaesthesia* 46:1033, 1991.

Paull, J. A prospective study of dextran-induced anaphylactoid reactions in 5745 patients. *Anaesthesia Intensive Care* 15:163, 1987.

Sehgal, N.N., and Hitt, J.R. Plasma volume expansion in the treatment of pre-eclampsia. *Am. J. Obstet. Gynecol.* 138:165, 1980.

Dextromethorphan (Over-the-Counter)

INDICATIONS AND RECOMMENDATIONS

Dextromethorphan is safe to use during pregnancy. It is indicated for the suppression of dry, hacking, nonproductive coughs.

SPECIAL CONSIDERATIONS IN PREGNANCY

A recent report has identified dextromethorphan as a teratogen in the chick embryo, causing an increased incidence of embryonic death and congenital defects of the neural crest and neural tube.

Studies in humans, however, have shown no link between dextromethorphan and birth defects. The Collaborative Perinatal Project reported a standardized relative risk of 1.18 among the offspring of 300 women who used dextromethorphan during the first 4 lunar months of pregnancy. The only specific anomaly associated with dextromethorphan's use during this time period was inguinal hernia, with a standardized risk of 1.3. A smaller cohort study that included 59 women who used dextromethorphan during the first trimester of pregnancy similarly showed no increased incidence of fetal malformations.

The only report possibly associating dextromethorphan use with congenital anomalies in humans discusses 5 infants with agenesis of the cloacal membrane, a distinctive pattern of malformations of the genitourinary structures and hindgut resulting in complete bladder and bowel obstruction and deformation of the hollow viscera. Of these infants, the mothers of 4 may have possibly taken cough syrup containing dextromethorphan. Given the frequency of such symptoms and treatment in normal pregnancies and the unusual and severe nature of the defect, it seems unlikely that dextromethorphan played a causal role. Indeed, the authors of the report implicated doxylamine as the likely cause of these defects. No similar reports of substantiating evidence for an association between dextromethorphan and this set of anomalies has come to light in the 14 year interim.

DOSAGE

The usual dose is 10–20 mg 3 or 4 times a day. It is generally administered in syrup form, with 5 ml containing 5–15 mg dextromethorphan. It is also available in lozenge form. An effect is usually observed within 30 minutes.

ADVERSE EFFECTS

Unlike codeine, dextromethorphan only occasionally produces drowsiness or gastrointestinal disturbances. Its toxicity is low, but in very high dosages, it may produce central nervous system depression or intoxication with bizarre behavior.

MECHANISM OF ACTION

Dextromethorphan acts centrally to decrease the sensitivity of respiratory system cough receptors or to interrupt the transmission of cough impulses. It is the d-isomer of the codeine analog of levorphanol, but it has no significant analgesic or addictive properties.

ABSORPTION AND BIOTRANSFORMATION

Metabolism is believed to occur in the liver with excretion in the kidney.

RECOMMENDED READING

American Pharmaceutical Association. *Handbook of Non-Prescription Drugs.* Washington, DC, 1996. Pp. 150–151.

American Pharmaceutical Association. *Non-Prescription Products: Formulations and Features 96–97.* Washington, DC, 1996. Pp. 62–113.

Andaloro, V.J., Monaghan, D.T., and Rosenquist, T.H. Dextromethorphan and other N-methyl D-aspartate receptor antagonists are teratogenic in the avian embryo model. *Pediatric Research* 43:1, 1998.

Aselton, P., et al. First-trimester drug use and congenital disorders. *Obstet. Gynecol.* 65:451, 1985.

Heinonen, O.P., Slone, D., and Shapiro, S. *Birth Defects and Drugs in Pregnancy.* Littleton, MA: Wright-PSG, 1977. Pp. 378, 496.

Reisine, T., and Pasternak, G. Opioid analgesics and antagonists. Chapter 23 in *Goodman and Gilman's The Pharmacological Basis of Therapeutics* (9th ed.), J.G. Hardman and L.E. Limbird, eds. New York: McGraw-Hill, 1996. P. 551.

Robinson, H.B., Tross, K. Agenesis of the cloacal membrane. A possible teratogenic anomaly. *Persp. Pediatr. Pathol.* 8:79, 1984.

Schenkel, B., and Vorherr, H. Non-prescription drugs during pregnancy: potential teratogenic and toxic effects upon embryo and fetus. *J. Reprod. Med.* 12:27, 1974.

Diazoxide (Hyperstat®)

INDICATIONS AND RECOMMENDATIONS

The use of diazoxide during pregnancy is controversial and, if used at all, should be reserved for patients with severe acute hypertensive episodes. This drug is a potent and rapidly acting antihypertensive agent and is marketed for the intravenous therapy of hypertensive emergencies. An oral preparation is available for the treatment of hypoglycemia, but this should not be used during pregnancy.

Diazoxide is rarely the drug of choice for the treatment of hypertension during pregnancy. If this drug is used, the fetal heart rate should be monitored continuously during therapy. Maternal blood sugars should be monitored regularly and a cord blood glucose obtained from the neonate immediately after delivery. Studies suggest that during pregnancy minibolus therapy is as effective as standard administration schedules and is far less likely to cause significant side effects. Whenever possible, this drug should not be used in combination with either hydralazine or methyldopa.

Hypotensive episodes following diazoxide administration should be treated with the rapid infusion of 1 or more liters of 5% dextrose in normal saline. The use of sympathomimetic agents such as norepinephrine to restore the blood pressure should be avoided unless there is no response to the infusion of fluid. This should almost never be necessary.

SPECIAL CONSIDERATIONS IN PREGNANCY

The most serious potential side effect after the intravenous administration of a 150 or 300 mg bolus of diazoxide to a preeclamptic patient is significant hypotension. Several series have shown some diastolic pressure drops to 50–60 mm Hg in patients with initial readings of 100 mm Hg or higher. In a number of these patients, there was also concomitant fetal bradycardia. Severe hypotensive responses have been specifically related to the potentiating effects of other vasodilators (e.g., hydralazine) or catecholamine-depleting drugs (e.g., methyldopa or reserpine) given either before or subsequent to the administration of diazoxide.

Because sodium and water are retained when diazoxide is used, the concomitant use of furosemide has been advised for the medical patient. The use of potent diuretics, however, is ill advised in preeclamptic patients, who may be significantly hypovolemic.

Diazoxide slows uterine contractions. As delivery is an integral part of the management of severely hypertensive, preeclamptic patients, intravenous oxytocin may be needed to induce labor in women receiving diazoxide. Glucose levels should be monitored in both mother and neonate.

Diazoxide crosses the placenta, but when it is given intravenously, it seems to have little effect on the fetus if there is no concomitant maternal hypotension. Fetal hyperglycemia may be produced. Several cases of prolonged neonatal hyperglycemia have been reported in premature infants of women treated with standard bolus doses. The term fetus seems to rapidly clear the drug. The authors of one animal study in which diazoxide was given intravenously for 4 days described necrosis of the fetal pancreatic islet cells.

When diazoxide is given orally to pregnant women for several weeks, persistent alopecia, lanuginous hypertrichosis, and decreased bone age have been reported in the neonate.

DOSAGE

The standard recommendation is to rapidly inject a bolus of 300 mg or 5 mg/kg body weight of diazoxide within a period of 10–30 seconds. The dependence of the hypotensive effect on the injection rate is related to the rapidity with which the drug is bound by serum albumin. The hypotensive effect will be noted within 5 minutes; thereafter, blood pressure increases gradually and returns to pretreatment levels within 3–15 hours. If the initial response is unsatisfactory, the dose may be repeated in 30 minutes.

Studies have indicated that low-bolus or minibolus diazoxide therapy in severely hypertensive pregnant women can be as efficacious as standard bolus treatment while significantly reducing maternal and fetal morbidity. In one study, 11 gravid hypertensive patients with diastolic blood pressures of 110 mm Hg or greater were given 60 mg boluses of diazoxide and compared with 10 matched patients who were given 150 mg boluses at similar intervals. Only one patient in the first group, but three in the second, became hypotensive and had associated fetal heart rate decelerations. Another investigation utilized 30 mg boluses given over 30–60 seconds in 34 gravid women with blood pressures in excess of 160/115 mm Hg. These boluses were administered every 1–2 minutes until the diastolic blood pressure fell below 90 mm Hg. The average dose required to achieve this goal was 120 mg, and all 34 patients responded within 5–10 minutes. Each of these women was delivered within 6 hours of initiating therapy. No hypotensive episodes were noted, and no neonatal hyperglycemia was observed. Maternal hyperglycemia and sodium and water retention were also minimal with this regimen.

It is possible that the decrease in maternal protein concentration that occurs during pregnancy results in higher levels of free drug and proportionally lower amounts of the protein-bound fraction when small boluses of diazoxide are injected. This could explain why smaller dosages can be given more slowly to pregnant patients, yet lower their blood pressure effectively while minimizing significant side effects.

ADVERSE EFFECTS

Because cardiovascular reflexes and the sympathetic nervous system function normally, diazoxide rarely causes postural hypotension. Sodium and water retention usually occur because of the drug's direct tubular antinatriuretic effect. Hyperglycemia may occur because of reduced insulin secretion by the pancreatic beta cells as well as a direct effect on the liver to increase its rate of glucose release. Mild hyperuricemia may be noted. A direct relaxation of uterine musculature can cause labor to stop. Finally, symptoms associated with the sympathetic reflex response to vasodilatation may occur.

MECHANISM OF ACTION

Diazoxide primarily relaxes arteriolar smooth muscle in all circulatory beds, which results in a reduction of vascular resistance. In association with this reduction in arterial pressure, there is a reflex increase in heart rate, stroke volume, and cardiac output, which may partially counteract the hypotensive effect of the vascular dilatation. Blood flow through all circulatory beds is generally well maintained, and renal blood flow and glomerular filtration rate are usually unchanged or increased.

ABSORPTION AND BIOTRANSFORMATION

The drug is primarily eliminated from the body by glomerular filtration. The serum half-life is normally 20–30 hours, but 90% of the drug is rapidly bound to albumin after intravenous administration. Because only the free drug is active, diazoxide must be administered every 4–12 hours, despite the long half-life in serum.

RECOMMENDED READING

Boulous, M.M., et al. Placental transfer of diazoxide and its hazardous effect on the newborn. *J. Clin. Pharmacol.* 11:206, 1971.

Davey, M., Moodley, J., and Soutter, P. Adverse effects of a combination of diazoxide and hydralazine therapy. *S. Afr. Med. J.* 59:496, 1981.

Dudley, D.K.L. Minibolus diazoxide in the management of severe hypertension in pregnancy. *Am. J. Obstet. Gynecol.* 151:196, 1985.

Kelly, J.V. Drugs used in the management of toxemia of pregnancy. *Clin. Obstet. Gynecol.* 20:395, 1977.

Koch-Weser, J. Diazoxide. *N. Engl. J. Med.* 294:1271, 1976.

Michael, C.A. Intravenous diazoxide in the treatment of severe preeclamptic toxaemia and eclampsia. *Aust. N. Z. J. Obstet. Gynaecol.* 13:143, 1973.

Milner, R.D.G., and Chouksey, S.K. Effects of fetal exposure to diazoxide in man. *Arch. Dis. Child.* 47:537–543, 1972.

Milsap, R.L., and Auld, P.A. Neonatal hyperglycemia following maternal diazoxide administration. *J.A.M.A.* 243:144, 1980.

Morris, J.A., et al. The management of severe pre-eclampsia and eclampsia with intravenous diazoxide. *Obstet. Gynecol.* 49:675, 1977.

Neuman, J., et al. Diazoxide for the acute control of severe hypertension complicating pregnancy: a pilot study. *Obstet. Gynecol.* 53(Suppl.):50S, 1979.

Redman, C.W.G. The use of antihypertensive drugs in hypertension in pregnancy. *Clin. Obstet. Gynecol.* 4:685, 1977.

Smith, M.J., Aynsley-Green, A., and Redman, C.W. Neonatal hyperglycemia after prolonged maternal treatment with diazoxide. *Br. Med. J. Clin. Res.* 284:1234, 1982.

Digoxin (Lanoxin®)

INDICATIONS AND RECOMMENDATIONS

Digoxin is safe for use in pregnancy if the mother's blood level is monitored frequently to avoid toxicity and to ensure adequate digitalization. Digoxin is the most frequently prescribed of the digitalis glycosides, a group of drugs used in the treatment of congestive heart failure and atrial fibrillation and in the prevention of paroxysmal atrial tachycardia. Digoxin has been used successfully for the transplacental treatment of fetal arrhythmias and unexplained fetal hydrops.

SPECIAL CONSIDERATIONS IN PREGNANCY

Serum levels should be monitored in pregnant women near term to ensure maintenance of therapeutic levels. Digoxin levels in the mother at term are usually significantly lower than levels taken several weeks postpartum on the same maintenance dosage.

The digitalis glycosides readily cross the placenta. They seem to be preferentially concentrated in the fetal heart during the second half of pregnancy. Amniotic fluid levels of digoxin have been used to monitor fetal levels. Levels of the drug in the amniotic fluid slightly exceed those in fetal serum. In a study of 11 mothers who received digoxin throughout pregnancy for rheumatic heart disease, paired cord and maternal blood samples obtained at parturition showed lower digoxin levels in cord blood than that of the mother. The total tissue-bound digoxin level in the placenta, however, correlated closely with maternal digoxin levels. Neonates and, presumably, the fetus seem to tolerate high serum levels of digoxin (2–4 ng/ml) much better than adults do. The only reported adverse fetal outcome followed a maternal overdose with 8.9 mg of digoxin in the third trimester. Autopsy findings suggested intrauterine anoxia from prolonged fetal bradycardia as the cause of death. There was no increase in fetal anomalies associated with first trimester use of digoxin in 142 women.

Digoxin has been used to treat a variety of fetal arrhythmias. When the drug is used for this indication, the mother should be fully digitalized and then followed with determination of serum digoxin and potassium levels. When digoxin is used for the treatment of fetal arrhythmias, toxicity should be defined both by maternal serum concentrations and by the presence of maternal symptoms and/or ECG changes. The therapeutic effect on the fetus can be followed with serial fetal echocardiograms.

Compromised fetuses may require direct injection of rapidly active agents to achieve desired results.

Digoxin is excreted in maternal milk, but far below the usual therapeutic dosage for a newborn. Digoxin milk/plasma ratios vary from 0.6 to 0.9 in several pharmacokinetic studies. The total daily amount excreted, however, is far below the usual therapeutic dosage for a newborn. The American Academy of Pediatrics and the WHO Working Group on Drugs and Human Lactation have stated that digoxin use is compatible with breast-feeding.

DOSAGE

The usual initial digitalizing dose of approximately 1.0 mg for maternal indications may be given orally or parenterally in several divided doses. Digoxin given for fetal indications may require larger initial doses. The usual maintenance dose is between 0.25 and 0.5 mg/day. The therapeutic plasma levels are 0.5–2.0 ng/ml in adults. In some patients with atrial fibrillation, levels of 2.5–4.0 ng/ml may be required to slow the maternal ventricular rate. Fetal response to maternal digitalization is usually observed within 6–12 hours of achieving adequate maternal levels.

ADVERSE EFFECTS

Side effects of digoxin, which are rare when the drug is given in therapeutic dosages, include skin rashes, eosinophilia, and gynecomastia (in males). Toxic effects of the digitalis derivatives include gastrointestinal symptoms of anorexia, nausea, and vomiting; visual changes; and alterations of cardiac rate and rhythm, especially extrasystoles and heart block. These toxic effects may be seen in patients with digoxin levels greater than 3 ng/ml. Digitalis toxicity can be potentiated by hypokalemia.

MECHANISM OF ACTION

The exact mechanism of action of digoxin is not known. The main pharmacologic action of all digitalis glycosides is to increase the force and velocity of the myocardial contraction. They have a direct action on both the failing and nonfailing heart. When given to patients in congestive heart failure, cardiac output is increased, systolic emptying is more complete, and end-diastolic volumes and pressures are reduced. Sympathetic tone is reduced, and in edematous patients diuresis results. Digitalis glycosides also decrease conduction velocity through the atrioventricular node. This effect is most apparent in patients with supraventricular tachyarrhythmias.

ABSORPTION AND BIOTRANSFORMATION

Approximately 65% to 80% of an oral digoxin dose is absorbed. Only about 25% is bound to plasma proteins, and it is primarily excreted unchanged in the urine. The half-life of digoxin is approximately 36 hours and increases as renal function diminishes.

RECOMMENDED READING

Allonen, H., Kanto, J., and Iisalo, E. The foeto-maternal distribution of digoxin in early human pregnancy. *Acta Pharmacol. Toxicol.* 39:477, 1976.

Aselton, P.A., et al. First trimseter drug use and congenital disorders. *Obstet. Gynecol.* 65:451, 1985.

Committee on Drugs, American Academy of Pediatrics. The transfer of drugs and other chemicals into human breast milk. *Pediatrics* 93:137, 1994.

Feit, L.R., and Carr, S.R. Fetal cardiac arrhythmias: diagnosis and treatment. *Curr. Obstet. Med.* 4:305, 1996.

Finley, J.P., et al. Digoxin excretion in human milk (letter). *J. Pediatrics* 94:339, 1979.

Kohl, T., Tercanli, S., Kececioglu, D., and Holzgreve, W. Direct fetal administration of adenosine for the termination of incessant supraventricular tachycardia. *Obstet. Gynecol.* 85(2):873, 1995.

Levy, M., Granit, L., and Laufer, N. Excretion of drugs in human milk. *N. Engl. J. Med.* 297:789, 1977.

Loughnan, P.M. Digoxin excretion in human breast milk. *J. Pediatrics* 92:1019, 1978.

Rasmussen, R., Nawaz, M., and Steiness. E. Mammary excretion of digoxin goats. *Acta Pharmacol. Toxicol.* 36:377, 1975.

Rogers, M.C., et al. Serum digoxin concentrations in the human fetus, neonate and infant. *N. Engl. J. Med.* 287:1010, 1972.

Saarikoski, S. Placental transfer and fetal uptake of 3H digoxin in humans. *Br. J. Obstet. Gynaecol.* 83:879, 884, 1976.

Seyka, L.F. Digoxin: placental transfer, effects on the fetus, and therapeutic use in the newborn. *Clin. Perinatol.* 2:23, 1975.

Sherma, J.L., Jr., and Locke, R.V. Transplacental neonatal digitalis intoxication. *Am. J. Cardiol.* 6:834, 1960.

WHO Working Group, and Bennet, P.N., eds. *Drugs and Human Lactation.* New York: Elsevier Science, 1988. Pp. 104–105.

Dimenhydrinate (Dramamine®)

INDICATIONS AND RECOMMENDATIONS

Dimenhydrinate is contraindicated during pregnancy because other agents are preferred. It is an antihistamine used in the prevention and treatment of nausea and vomiting associated with motion sickness. There is no evidence that dimenhydrinate is teratogenic. A number of reports have described an oxytocic effect with intravenous dimenhydrinate. In one placebo-controlled study, the intravenous injection of dimenhydrinate was associated with uterine hyperstimulation and fetal distress. Meclizine is therefore preferable for the treatment of motion sickness during pregnancy.

The short-term use of dimenhydrinate by a breast-feeding mother appears to have little effect on the infant.

RECOMMENDED READING

Babe, Jr., K.S., and Serafin, W.E. Histamine, bradykinin, and their antagonists. Chapter 25 in *Goodman and Gilman's The Pharmacological Basis of Therapeutics* (9th ed.), J.G. Hardman and L.E. Limbird, eds. New York: McGraw-Hill, 1996. P. 592.

Ito, S., et al. Prospective follow-up of adverse reactions in breast-fed infants exposed to maternal medication. *Am. J. Obstet. Gynecol.* 168:1393–1399, 1993.

Leathem, A.M. Safety and efficacy of antiemetics used to treat nausea and vomiting in pregnancy. *Clin. Pharm.* 5:60, 1986.

Shephard, B., Cruz, A., and Spellacy, W. The acute effects of Dramamine on uterine contractility during labor. *J. Reprod. Med.* 16:27, 1976.

Dinoprostone (Prostaglandin E_2, Cervidil®, Prepidil®, Prostin E_2®)

INDICATIONS AND RECOMMENDATIONS

Dinoprostone is indicated during pregnancy as an abortifacient from the 12th to the 20th week of pregnancy (up to 28 weeks in the management of missed abortion or intrauterine fetal death) and for cervical ripening for induction of labor. Except for these uses, it is contraindicated during pregnancy.

SPECIAL CONSIDERATIONS DURING PREGNANCY

Dinoprostone is the naturally occurring form of prostaglandin E_2. In pregnancy, prostaglandin plays an important role in the final events leading to the initiation of labor. Prostaglandins stimulate the myometrium of the gravid uterus to contract in a manner similar to that seen in the term uterus during labor. The contractions are strong enough to induce delivery of the fetus if treatment is given during the first two trimesters of pregnancy. While prostaglandins of both the E and F series produce uterotonic activity, dinoprostone is more specific for uterine action than prostaglandin $F_{2\alpha}$, the most commonly studied alternative.

At term, dinoprostone plays an important role in the complex changes involved in cervical ripening. Dinoprostone has been shown to be superior to placebo or no therapy in producing cervical softening. It is also more likely than either placebo or no therapy to initiate labor. It has also been reported to increase the chance of successful induction, decrease the incidence of prolonged labor, and reduce the total dose of oxytocin required for labor induction.

DOSAGE

For the termination of pregnancy, one 20 mg suppository is inserted high into the vagina at 3 to 5 hour intervals until abortion occurs. Continuous administration for more than 2 days is not advised.

For cervical ripening, 0.5 mg of vaginal gel is administered into the cervical canal via syringe and catheter. A repeat dose may be given after 6 hours if there is no cervical or uterine response to the initial dose. Alternatively, a 10 mg vaginal insert, designed to release 0.3 mg/hour over 12 hours, may be placed in the posterior fornix of the vagina. The insert should be removed upon onset of labor or 12 hours after insertion.

ADVERSE EFFECTS

The principal side effects of the prostaglandins are nausea, vomiting, and diarrhea due to stimulation of the gastrointestinal tract. Pretreatment with antiemetic and antidiarrheal drugs decreases the incidence of these effects. In addition, many patients experience transient pyrexia, probably due to actions on the thermoregulatory centers in the hypothalamus. In addition, when used for cervical ripening, uterine hyperstimulation with and without fetal distress has been reported.

MECHANISM OF ACTION

The exact mechanism of action of the prostaglandins is unclear. They are naturally occurring substances that bind to fairly specific receptors on the cell membrane or intracellular organelles to produce their physiologic or pharmacologic effect.

ABSORPTION AND BIOTRANSFORMATION

Dinoprostone applied topically to the cervix is probably absorbed to some extent in the bloodstream. It is then completely metabolized, primarily in the lung but with further metabolism in the liver and kidney. Metabolites are then excreted in the urine. The half-life is estimated to be 2.5–5 minutes.

REFERENCES

Campbell, W.B., and Halushka, P.V. Lipid-derived autacoids, eicosanoids, and platelet-activating factor. Chapter 26 in *Goodman and Gilman's The Pharmacological Basis of Therapeutics* (9th ed.), J.G. Hardman and L.E. Limbird, eds. New York: McGraw-Hill, 1996. P. 601.

Graves, C.R. Agents that cause contraction or relaxation of the uterus. Chapter 39 in *Goodman and Gilman's The Pharmacological Basis of Therapeutics* (9th ed.), J.G. Hardman and L.E. Limbird, eds. New York: McGraw-Hill, 1996. Pp. 942–943.

O'Brien, W.F. The role of prostaglandins in labor and delivery. *Clin. Perinatol.* 22:973, 1995.

Xenakis, E. M.-J., and Piper, J.M. Chemotherapeutic induction of labour. A rational approach. *Drugs* 54:61, 1997.

Diphenhydramine (Benadryl®, AllerMax®)

INDICATIONS AND RECOMMENDATIONS

Diphenhydramine may be administered during pregnancy for the treatment of allergic disorders characterized by urticaria, pruritus, and rhinitis. It is also used to reverse the extrapyramidal side effects caused by phenothiazines and to control drug and blood transfusion reactions. Because of its possible association with an increased incidence of oral clefts, some authors recommend that diphenhydramine not be used in the first trimester for reducing self-limited symptoms or the discomfort of allergies.

SPECIAL CONSIDERATIONS IN PREGNANCY

No prospective studies have been conducted that evaluate the safety of diphenhydramine's use during pregnancy. One study comparing 599 children with oral clefts to controls found that the intake of diphenhydramine was significantly more common among the mothers of children with clefts. This was not true for mothers who had taken cyclizine. However, the association between the use of diphenhydramine and cleft palate has never been confirmed, and several large analyses have found no association between its use and any congenital anomaly.

A presumed withdrawal syndrome has been reported in a single newborn exposed to large doses (150 mg/day, duration of therapy not stated) in utero. In another case report, a woman took diphenhydramine 50 mg and temazepam 30 mg and 3 hours later delivered a stillborn term infant. No mechanism of action for this effect was suggested.

Diphenhydramine is not recommended for use by nursing mothers because it may inhibit lactation and cause drowsiness in the infant.

DOSAGE

The usual oral dose is 50 mg taken 3 or 4 times a day. If parenteral administration is required, 10–50 mg may be given intravenously or by deep intramuscular injection. The maximum daily dose is 400 mg.

ADVERSE EFFECTS

Anticholinergic side effects are most common; these include drowsiness, dry mouth and eyes, and, rarely, blurred vision. Anorexia, nausea, epigastric distress, and dizziness can also occur.

MECHANISM OF ACTION

Diphenhydramine is a competitive antagonist of histamine at the H_1 receptor. It decreases edema formation by diminishing capillary dilatation and permeability. It has anticholinergic activity and therefore reduces the tremor and rigidity of Parkinsonism. It produces drowsiness and possesses local anesthetic ability when used topically.

ABSORPTION AND BIOTRANSFORMATION

Diphenhydramine is rapidly absorbed from the gastrointestinal tract. When taken orally, the maximum effects are noted within 1 hour, and the duration of action is 4–6 hours; that is, it reaches peak tissue concentrations in about 1 hour, and the tissues are almost depleted of the drug in about 6 hours. Diphenhydramine is metabolized in the liver and metabolites are excreted in the urine.

RECOMMENDED READING

American Pharmaceutical Association. *Handbook of Non-Prescription Drugs.* Washington, DC, 1996. P. 64.

Babe, Jr., K.S., and Serafin, W.E. Histamine, bradykinin and their antagonists. Chapter 25 in *Goodman and Gilman's The Pharmacological Basis of Therapeutics* (9th ed.), J.G. Hardman and L.E. Limbird, eds. New York: McGraw-Hill, 1996. Pp. 586–592.

Greenberger, P., and Patterson, R. Safety of therapy for allergic symptoms during pregnancy. *Ann. Intern. Med.* 89:234, 1978.

Heinonen, O.P., Slone, D., and Shapiro, S. *Birth Defects and Drugs in Pregnancy.* Littleton, MA: Wright-PSG, 1977. Pp. 323–334.

Kargas, G.A., et al. Perinatal mortality due to interaction of diphenhydramine and temazepam. *N. Engl. J. Med.* 313:1417, 1985.

Leatham, A.M. Safety and efficacy of antiemetics used to treat nausea and vomiting in pregnancy. *Clin. Pharm.* 5:660, 1986.

Nashimura, H., and Tanimura, T. *Aspects of the Teratogenicity of Drugs.* Amsterdam: Excerpta Medica, 1976.

Parkin, D.E. Probable Benadryl withdrawal manifestations in a newborn infant. *J. Pediatrics* 85:580, 1974.

Saxen, I. Cleft palate and maternal diphenhydramine intake. *Lancet* 1:407, 1974.

Diphenoxylate (Lomotil®, When Combined with Atropine)

INDICATIONS AND RECOMMENDATIONS

Diphenoxylate is safe to use during pregnancy based on the limited data available. It is combined with atropine (to prevent abuse) and used as an antidiarrheal agent. Because it provides symptomatic relief only, primary treatment should be directed to the underlying condition, together with correction of fluid and electrolyte depletion. It should not be used for diarrhea associated with organisms that penetrate the intestinal mucosa or in pseudomembranous colitis associated with broad-spectrum antibiotics.

SPECIAL CONSIDERATIONS IN PREGNANCY

Only two case reports of congenital malformations in infants exposed to diphenoxylate in utero were found. Neither implicates the drug as a teratogen. One infant was exposed to the drug on days 104–110 of gestation, long after the cleft palate, cardiac defect, absent tibiae, and polydactyly had developed. In addition, the infant was exposed to at least five other drugs (excluding vitamins) in utero. The second infant, exposed to diphenoxylate and atropine during the 10th week of gestation, had developed Ebstein's anomaly, an isolated cardiac defect presumed to develop around day 48 of gestation.

In the Collaborative Perinatal Project, seven infants were exposed to diphenoxylate in utero during the first 4 months and no congenital malformations were found. Despite this paucity of data, the similarity of diphenoxylate to meperidine suggests that the drug is probably safe for pregnant women.

This drug is excreted in breast milk. Because diphenoxylate is considered to be contraindicated in children up to 2 years of age (severe toxic reactions may occur at presumably therapeutic dosages), breast-feeding mothers should not take the drug.

DOSAGE

Diphenoxylate is available as a tablet containing 2.5 mg combined with 0.025 mg atropine, and as a liquid containing the same dose in 5 ml. The usual adult dose is two tablets or 10 ml of liquid 4 times a day until diarrhea is controlled, usually within 48 hours.

ADVERSE EFFECTS

Allergic reactions have been reported. In addition, some patients have reported abdominal discomfort, drowsiness, dizziness, depression, restlessness, nausea, headache, and blurred vision. Intestinal obstruction and toxic megacolon have occurred in patients with inflammatory bowel disease or parasitic colitis. Overdosage can lead to morphine-like symptoms.

The atropine added to this compound can give rise to typical atropinic side effects, especially when overdosage occurs.

MECHANISM OF ACTION

Diphenoxylate, a congener of meperidine, exerts a direct effect on the muscles of the small and large intestines to inhibit propulsive movements. Hyperperistalsis is diminished, allowing reabsorption of water and electrolytes. This effect occurs at dosages considerably lower than those necessary to cause euphoria or physical dependence. However, acute or chronic use increases the risk of physical dependence.

ABSORPTION AND BIOTRANSFORMATION

Diphenoxylate is rapidly absorbed after oral dosing, reaching peak plasma levels at approximately 2 hours. The half-life is approximately 12 hours. The drug is rapidly hydrolyzed to its active metabolite, diphenoxylic acid. Approximately 15% of diphenoxylate is excreted in the urine, and 50% is excreted in the stool.

RECOMMENDED READING

Brunton, L.L. Agents affecting gastrointestinal water flux and motility; emesis and antiemetics; bile acids and pancreatic enzymes. Chapter 38 in *Goodman and Gilman's The Pharmacological Basis of Therapeutics* (9th ed.), J.G. Hardman and L.E. Limbird, eds. New York: McGraw-Hill, 1996, P. 926.

Gattuso, J.M., and Kamm, M.A., Adverse effects of drugs used in the management of constipation and diarrhea. *Drug Safety* 10:47, 1994.

Heinonen, O.P., Slone, D., and Shapiro, S. *Birth Defects and Drugs in Pregnancy.* Boston: Wright-PSG, 1977. P. 287.

Ho, C.K., Kaufman, R.L., and McAllister, W.H. Congenital malformations: cleft palate, congenital heart disease, absent tibiae, and polydactyly. *Am. J. Dis. Child.* 129:714, 1975.

Siebert, J.R., et al. Ebstein's anomaly and extracardiac defects. *Am. J. Dis. Child.* 143:570, 1989.

Dipyridamole (Persantine®)

INDICATIONS AND RECOMMENDATIONS

Dipyridamole is indicated during pregnancy for the prevention of arterial thrombosis in patients with prosthetic heart valves and for the prevention and treatment of thrombotic thrombocytopenic purpura (TTP). It is not indicated for the prophylaxis or treatment of venous thromboembolic disease.

SPECIAL CONSIDERATIONS IN PREGNANCY

TTP is a severe hemorrhagic disorder that also affects neurologic, cardiovascular, and renal function. It is usually fatal to mother and/or fetus if untreated in pregnancy. The most effective treatment for a fulminant episode of TTP during pregnancy appears to be plasmapheresis. Dipyridamole is used as an adjunct to plasmapheresis. Patients undergoing plasmapheresis who are maintained on anticoagulant treatment of aspirin plus dipyridamole have a 70% to 80% survival rate with minimal or no sequelae. In addition, aspirin and dipyridamole prophylaxis for prevention of a pregnancy-associated relapse of TTP significantly reduces the severity of any relapse, allowing delivery of healthy babies at term.

Because warfarin is contraindicated in the pregnant patient, alternative anticoagulants must be used for prevention of thrombosis in artificial heart valves during pregnancy. Several studies have reported the successful and safe use of aspirin plus dipyridamole or dipyridamole alone in these patients.

Dipyridamole has been used in combination with aspirin to decrease the risk of preeclampsia-toxemia in women at risk for that condition and to prevent fetal growth retardation. For these uses, the addition of dipyridamole to aspirin did not significantly increase the effect of aspirin alone. Dipyridamole should not be used routinely for these indications.

There are no data available on the ability of dipyridamole to cross the placenta. In the cases reported to date, no adverse fetal effects have been noted.

Dipyridamole is excreted in breast milk.

DOSAGE

The usual oral dose for prophylaxis of thromboembolism is 75–100 mg qid as an adjunct to warfarin treatment. For the treatment and prevention of TTP, the usual dose of dipyridamole has been 75 mg tid along with aspirin.

ADVERSE EFFECTS

In standard dosages, dipyridamole's side effects are usually minimal and transient, and include nausea, vomiting, and diarrhea as well as headache and vertigo. Rarely, liver dysfunction may occur.

MECHANISM OF ACTION

Dipyridamole's action is not understood. It acts to selectively dilate coronary arteries and also interferes with platelet function. When combined with warfarin, it inhibits embolization from prosthetic heart valves and when combined with aspirin, it reduces thrombosis in patients with thrombotic diseases. It interferes with platelet function by increasing the intracellular concentration of cyclic AMP.

ABSORPTION AND BIOTRANSFORMATION

After an oral dose, peak concentrations are reached in about 75 minutes. Its initial half-life is approximately 40 minutes and its terminal half-life about 10 hours. The drug is metabolized in the liver and is excreted unchanged or as its glucuronide conjugate in feces.

RECOMMENDED READING

Beaufils, M., et al. Prevention of pre-eclampsia by early antiplatelet therapy. *Lancet* 1:840, 1985.

Biale, Y., et al. The course of pregnancy in patients with artificial heart valves treated with dipyridamole. *Int. J. Gynaecol. Obstet.* 18:128, 1980.

Ezra, Y., Rose, M., and Eldor, A. therapy and prevention of thrombotic thrombocytopenic purpura during pregnancy: a clinical study of 16 pregnancies. *Am. J. Hematol.* 51:1, 1996

Fitzgibbons, J.F., et al. Survival following thrombotic thrombocytopenic purpura in pregnancy. *Obstet. Gynecol.* 50 (Suppl):66s, 1977.

Lauchkner, W., Schwarz, R., and Retzke, U. Cardiovascular action of dipyridamole in advanced pregnancy. *Zentralbl. Gynakol.* 103: 220, 1981.

Lubbe, W.F., et al. Lupus anticoagulant in pregnancy. *Br. J. Obstet. Gynaecol.* 91:357, 1984.

Majerus, P.W., et al. Anticoagulant, thrombolytic, and antiplatelet drugs. Chapter 54 in *Goodman and Gilman's The Pharmacological Basis of Therapeutics* (9th ed.), J.G. Hardman and L.E. Limbird, eds. New York: McGraw-Hill, 1996. Pp. 1353–1354.

Moncada, S., and Korbut, R. Dipyridamole and other phosphodiesterase inhibitors act as antithrombotic agent by potentiating endogenous prostacyclin. *Lancet* 1:1286, 1978.

Rozdzinski, E., et al. Thrombotic thrombocytopenic purpura in early pregnancy with maternal and fetal survival. *Ann. Hematol.* 64: 245, 1992.

Disulfiram (Antabuse®)

INDICATIONS AND RECOMMENDATIONS

The use of disulfiram (tetraethylthiuram disulfide) is contraindicated in pregnancy. This substance, if taken in combination with alcohol, causes extremely high acetaldehyde concentrations, which lead to generalized vasodilatation, feelings of warmth, throbbing headache, nausea, vomiting, respiratory difficulties, chest pain, hypotension, thirst, and other adverse signs and symptoms. Collectively, these are called the acetaldehyde syndrome. As a consequence, the drug is useful in helping to motivate alcoholic individuals to avoid alcohol.

Disulfiram has not been shown to be teratogenic in laboratory animals. Among nine exposed human infants uncovered by a literature search, two had clubfoot anomalies, one had phocomelia, one had a constellation of anomalies of the extremities and vertebral column, one had microcephaly and mental retardation, one had Pierre Robin syndrome, and three were normal. The true number of exposures in the population is not known. Although alcohol is known to be a teratogen, the mothers of these infants were reported to be alcohol-free during their pregnancies. It is currently not known if alcohol intake before conception may be teratogenic.

Since alternative psychosocial interventions may be successful in treating alcoholism, the use of disulfiram appears to be unjustified during pregnancy. When a pregnant individual who has been taking disulfiram is counseled, she should be made aware of the available data and supported in whatever decision she makes regarding continuation of the pregnancy.

RECOMMENDED READING

Dehaene, P., Titran, M., and DuBois, D. Syndrome de Pierre Robin et malformations cardiaques chez un nouveau-ne-role du disulfirame pendant la grossesse? *Presse Med.* 13:1394, 1984.

Favre-Tissot, M., and DeLatour, P. Psychopharmacologie et teratogenese a propos du disulfirame: essai experimental. *Ann. Med. Psychol.* 1:735, 1965.

Gardner, R.J.M., and Clarkson, J.E. A malformed child whose previously alcoholic mother had taken disulfiram. *N. Z. Med. J.* 93:184, 1981.

Hobbs, W.R., Rall, T.W., and Verdoorn, T.A. Hypnotics and sedatives; ethanol. Chapter 17 in *Goodman and Gilman's The Pharmacological Basis of Therapeutics* (9th ed.), J.G. Hardman and L.E. Limbird, eds. New York: McGraw-Hill, 1996. Pp. 391–393.

Jones, K.L., et al. The effect of disulfiram on the unborn baby. *Teratology* 43:438, 1991.

Nora, A.H., Nora, J.J., and Blu, J. Limb-reduction anomalies in infants born to disulfiram-treated alcoholic mothers. *Lancet* 2:664, 1977.

Robens, J.F. Teratologic studies of carbaryl, diazinon, norea, disulfiram, and thiram in small laboratory animals. *Toxicol. Appl. Pharmacol.* 15:152, 1969.

Loop diuretics: Furosemide (Lasix®), Bumetanide (Bumex ®)

INDICATIONS AND RECOMMENDATIONS

Furosemide may be administered to pregnant women for the treatment of pulmonary edema, congestive heart failure, and some cases of chronic renal disease. It is a powerful loop diuretic that may rapidly decrease maternal intravascular volume and, consequently, diminish uteroplacental perfusion. For this reason it must be used with extreme care in the obstetric patient. It is not indicated for the routine treatment of hypertension or peripheral edema during pregnancy.

Furosemide has also been used, in combination with digoxin, to treat the fetus with hydrops secondary to congenital heart block. It has been administered orally to the mother or directly to the fetus.

There is little information in the literature regarding the use of bumetanide during pregnancy.

SPECIAL CONSIDERATIONS IN PREGNANCY

Furosemide must be administered with great caution in the pregnant patient. As indicated above, hypovolemia may lead to decreased uterine blood flow, which can affect the fetus adversely. If the drug is used, the fetus should be carefully monitored for evidence of intrauterine compromise.

Animal studies have shown that furosemide causes unexplained maternal deaths and abortions in rabbits as well as an increased incidence of fetal hydronephrosis in rats. Administration of furosemide to late gestation pregnant rats results in abnormal ossification of the ribs.

Using ultrasonic measurements of human fetal bladder volume, Wladimiroff reported that the maternal administration of furosemide resulted in an increase of 80% to 150% in the hourly fetal urine production rate. As a result of this observation, the "furosemide challenge test" was advocated as a diagnostic tool for evaluating renal function in utero. However, both animal studies and case series have demonstrated that failure to visualize the fetal bladder after maternal intravenous furosemide injection does not prove that the fetal kidneys are absent.

In a placental transfer study, furosemide was administered orally to 18 pregnant women on the day of delivery. The ratio between drug concentrations in maternal plasma and umbilical cord plasma decreased with time and was equal 8–10 hours after administration. The plasma half-life appeared to be longer in the mothers than in healthy nonpregnant volunteers.

The pharmacokinetics of furosemide have been studied in 12 newborns who had been exposed to the drug transplacentally and 21 neonates who received it therapeutically after birth. In the transplacental group, plasma half-lives ranged from 6.8–96.0 hours, and there was a significant inverse relationship between the gestational age and elimination rate. In neonates who received intravenous furosemide postnatally for therapeutic indications, premature neonates had prolonged plasma half-lives (26.8 ± 12.2 hours) as compared to the full-term group (13.4 ± 8.6 hours). Furosemide administered intraamniotically to ovine pregnancies causes a rapid and prolonged increase in fetal urine flow. Because this was true despite surgical ligation of the fetal esophagus, the investigators suggest that the furosemide was absorbed through the amniotic membranes.

It has been reported that furosemide may increase the incidence of patent ductus arteriosus in premature infants with the respiratory distress syndrome (RDS). This presumably is due to stimulation of the renal synthesis of prostaglandin E_2. Furosemide readily crosses the placenta, and amniotic fluid may act as a reservoir for this drug. Its half-life in neonates is eightfold longer than that in adults and, as mentioned previously, this is increased further in premature infants. Because in normal infants the ductus arteriosus may not close until several days after birth, exposure to furosemide in utero may be detrimental, especially in the case of premature neonates who go on to develop RDS.

DOSAGE

Furosemide may be given intravenously in dosages ranging from 10 to 40 mg, injected over 1–2 minutes. The usual oral dosage ranges from 20 mg to 80 mg up to 4 times daily. The maximum dose is generally considered to be 600 mg daily.

SIDE EFFECTS

The most serious side effect of furosemide is severe hypovolemia. Hyponatremia, hypokalemia, hypochloremia, hyperuricemia, and metabolic alkalosis may also occur. Glucose intolerance, hearing loss, and interstitial nephritis have been reported.

Occasionally, skin rash, photosensitivity, paresthesias, gastrointestinal disturbances, thrombocytopenia, and neutropenia are seen.

MECHANISM OF ACTION

Furosemide acts directly on the ascending limb of the loop of Henle. It works primarily by blocking the function of the Na^+-K^+-$2Cl^-$ symporter. In the normally functioning kidney, furosemide causes excretion of 25% of the filtered sodium load and produces a prompt diuresis where maximal sodium and water reabsorption has not already taken place in the proximal tubule. The drug's effectiveness decreases as the glomerular filtration rate approaches 20 ml/minute.

ABSORPTION AND BIOTRANSFORMATION

Furosemide is readily absorbed from the gastrointestinal tract and is strongly bound to plasma proteins. Half-life is 30 minutes to 3 hours. Two-thirds of an oral dose is excreted in the urine, with the remainder being metabolized. Urinary excretion is accomplished by both glomerular filtration and proximal tubular secretion.

RECOMMENDED READING

Anandakumar, C., Biswas, A., Chew, S.S.L., Chia, D., Wong, Y.C., and Ratnam, S.S. Direct fetal therapy for hydrops secondary to congenital atrio-ventricular heart block. *Obstet. Gynecol.* 87:835, 1996.

Aranda, J.V., et al. Pharmacokinetic disposition and protein-binding of furosemide in newborn infants. *J. Pediatrics* 93:507, 1978.

Beerman, B., et al. Placental transfer of furosemide. *Clin. Pharmacol. Ther.* 24:560, 1978.

Chamberlain, P.F., et al. Ovine fetal urine production following maternal intravenous furosemide administration. *Am. J. Obstet. Gynecol.* 151:815, 1985.

Cohen, J.I. Promotion of patent ductus arteriosus by furosemide (letter). *N. Engl. J. Med.* 309:432, 1983.

Gant, N.F. The metabolic clearance rate of dehydroisoandrosterone sulfate: III. The effect of thiazide diuretics in normal and future preeclamptic pregnancies. *Am. J. Obstet. Gynecol.* 123: 159, 1975.

Gifford, R.W., Jr. A guide to the practical use of diuretics. *J.A.M.A.* 235:1890, 1976.

Gilbert, W.M., Newman, P.S., Brace, R.A.: Potential route for fetal therapy: intramembranous absorption of intraamniotically injected furosemide. *Am. J. Obstet. Gynecol.* 172:1471, 1995.

Green, T.P., et al. Furosemide promotes patent ductus arteriosus in premature infants with the respiratory distress syndrome. *N. Engl. J. Med.* 308:743, 1983.

Harris, J.P., Alexson, C.G., Manning, J.A., and Thompson, H.O. Medical therapy for the hydropic fetus with congenital complete atrioventricular block. *Am. J. Perinatol.* 10:217, 1993.

Jackson, E.K. Diuretics. Chapter 29 in *Goodman and Gilman's The Pharmacological Basis of Therapeutics* (9th ed.), J.G. Hardman and L.E. Limbird, eds. New York: McGraw-Hill, 1996. Pp. 697–701.

Krunlovsky, F.A., and del Grew, C. Diuretic agents: mechanism of action and clinical uses. *Postgrad. Med.* 59:105, 1976.

Nakatsuka, T., Fujikake, N., Hasebe, M., and Ikeda, H. Effects of sodium bicarbonate and ammonium chloride on the incidence of furosemide-induced fetal skeletal anomaly, wavy rib, in rats. *Teratology* 48:139, 1993.

Raghavendra, B.N., Young, B.K., Greco, M.A., Lustig-Gillman, I., Horrii, S.C., Hirsch, M.A., and Yee, J. Use of furosemide in pregnancies complicated by oligohydramnios. *Radiology* 165:455, 1987.

Riva, E., et al. Pharmacokinetics of furosemide in gestosis of pregnancy. *Eur. J. Clin. Pharmacol.* 14:361, 1978.

Vert, P., et al. Pharmacokinetics of furosemide in neonates. *Eur. J. Clin. Pharmacol.* 22:39, 1982.

Wladimiroff, J.W. Effect of furosemide on fetal urine production. *Br. J. Obstet. Gynaecol.* 82:221, 1975.

Potassium-Sparing Diuretics: Triamterene (Dyrenium®, Maxzide®), Amiloride (Midamor®)

INDICATIONS AND RECOMMENDATIONS

Triamterene and amiloride, as diuretics, are relatively contraindicated in pregnancy. Both are potassium-sparing diuretics and act on the luminal sodium channels of the distal tubules and collecting ducts; neither antagonizes aldosterone. Diuretics in general have a limited indication in the pregnant patient with cardiovascular disorders, such as pulmonary edema, congestive heart failure, and severe hypertension. The effects of triamterene on uterine blood flow have not been studied. Triamterene diffuses across the human placenta rapidly; the rate of transfer between maternal and fetal compartments, however, has not been studied. A retrospective review of 271 exposures (5 of which were first trimester) did not detect an increased adverse outcome rate attributable to triamterene. Reported use of amiloride in pregnant patients exists; however, there is inadequate experience to conclude safety.

The effects of other diuretics in pregnancy, such as a thiazide or furosemide, have been more thoroughly investigated. With their use, potassium levels are followed closely. If hypokalemia develops, potassium supplementation is indicated and effective. Therefore, triamterene or amiloride has no advantage over these better known drugs.

RECOMMENDED READING

Ching, M., et al. Mechanism of triamterene transfer across human placenta. *J. Pharm. Exp. Ther.* 246:1093, 1988.

Christianson, R., and Page E.W. Diuretic drugs and pregnancy. *Obstet. Gynecol.* 48:647, 1976.

Heinonen, O.P., et al. *Birth Defects and Drugs in Pregnancy.* Littleton, MA: Wright-PSG, 1977. Pp. 372, 441.

Jackson, E.W. Diuretics. Chapter 29 in *Goodman and Gilman's The Pharmacological Basis of Therapeutics* (9th ed.), J.G. Hardman and L.E. Limbird, eds. New York: McGraw-Hill, 1996. Pp. 704–706.

Lindheimer, M.D., and Katz, A.L. Sodium and diuretics in pregnancy. *N. Engl. J. Med.* 288:891, 1973.

Pruitt, A.W., et al. Transfer characteristics of triamterene and its analogs. Central nervous system, placenta and kidney. *Drug Metab. Dispos.* 3:30, 1995.

Robson, D.J., et al. Use of amiodarone during pregnancy. *Postgrad. Med. J.* 61:75, 1985.

Stokes, G.S., et al. Bartter's syndrome presenting during pregnancy: results of amiloride therapy. *Med. J. Aust.* 2:360, 1974.

Diuretics, Thiazide: Chlorothiazide (Diuril®), Hydrochlorothiazide (Esidrix®, HydroDiuril®, Oretic®), Hydroflumethiazide (Diucardin®), Methylclothiazide (Enduron®),

INDICATIONS AND RECOMMENDATIONS

The use of the thiazides during pregnancy is controversial. If used at all, they should be restricted to very specific situations. These drugs are diuretics and have antihypertensive activity in some patients with essential hypertension. The administration of thiazides does not prevent the development of preeclampsia, and these drugs have no role in the therapy of that condition. They also should not be used for the treatment of peripheral edema in the pregnant woman.

Since thiazides may decrease placental perfusion, controversy exists over the use of these drugs during pregnancy in patients with chronic hypertension. If started before conception, there is no strong evidence to suggest that continued therapy will compromise fetal growth. Some authors therefore recommend leaving a patient on this medication if it has been successfully used to control documented hypertension prior to the pregnancy. If, on the other hand, it becomes necessary to initiate treatment after the patient has become pregnant, the combination of a thiazide and methyldopa may reduce the potential for decreased placental perfusion. Some authors have recommended that the initiation of therapy with the thiazides be limited to the first half of pregnancy. There is a case report describing the use of thiazides, along with a low-sodium diet, to limit renal calcium excretion in a pregnant patient with hypoparathyroidism unresponsive to dietary phosphate restriction and calcium and vitamin D supplementation.

Frequent determinations of serum electrolytes should be made in pregnant women taking thiazide diuretics. Such women will frequently need oral potassium supplementation.

Fetal growth should also be monitored closely throughout the period of therapy.

SPECIAL CONSIDERATIONS IN PREGNANCY

It is known that in preeclampsia many patients have a decreased intravascular volume. The administration of thiazides will reduce this further. Gant and colleagues demonstrated a reduced metabolic clearance rate of dehydroepiandrosterone sulfate (MCRDS) in 9 of 10 pregnant women studied on the seventh day of thiazide therapy, which may represent decreased placental perfusion. These facts suggest that the administration of thiazides may compromise optimal fetal oxygenation and nutrition, especially in fetuses of patients with preeclampsia.

Sibai, Grossman, and colleagues performed a randomized prospective investigation on 20 women with mild chronic hypertension who were receiving diuretics when seen in the first trimester. Half of these women were allowed to continue their diuretic medication throughout the pregnancy, whereas the other 10 patients had this medication discontinued at the time of their first visit. The initial plasma volumes were similar in both groups, but serial studies showed a marked reduction of plasma volume in the diuretic group as compared to the control group. Whereas those who stopped taking the diuretics had a mean increase of 52% in plasma volume, as pregnancy progressed the diuretic group had a mean increase of only 18%. The difference was most pronounced at 26–32 weeks. Two patients in the diuretic group and one of the control subjects required the addition of methyldopa for blood pressure control. Despite the relative reduction in plasma volume in the treated group, there was no significant difference in gestational age at birth, birth weight, placental weight, or superimposed preeclampsia when compared to the control group. Although the number of patients studied was small, this well-designed study suggests that in chronic hypertensive pregnancies, diuretics may prevent normal plasma expansion without influencing perinatal outcome.

An additional problem that may occur when thiazides are given to pregnant women is maternal hyperuricemia. This rarely requires therapy but may mask the increase in serum uric acid that is often seen in association with developing preeclampsia. The thiazides cross the placenta and may cause symptomatic neonatal hyponatremia, hypokalemia, and thrombocytopenia.

Placental transfer of hydrochlorothiazide was studied in 10 term pregnancies in which mothers being treated for edema or hypertension were given 50 mg/day at least 2 weeks before delivery. Maternal and umbilical venous blood and amniotic fluid were collected at delivery in each of these cases. Analysis of the samples revealed that hydrochlorothiazide concentrations in umbilical cord plasma approached those in maternal plasma, whereas amniotic fluid levels were higher than those in either maternal or fetal blood.

The drugs are excreted in breast milk, but the amount of chlorothiazide that appears in the milk is probably too small to cause an adverse effect in the nursing infant. The American Academy of Pediatrics considers thiazides to be compatible with breast-feeding.

DOSAGE

These drugs are usually given orally, with the diuretic effect occurring within 1–2 hours of absorption. The peak effect occurs in 4 hours and lasts about 6–12 hours. Chlorothiazide is usually administered in doses of 500–750 mg bid while hydrochlorothiazide doses are generally 50–75 mg bid.

ADVERSE EFFECTS

Side effects include hyponatremia, hypokalemia, and metabolic alkalosis. Hyperglycemia and allergic dermatitis with photosensitivity may occur. Occasionally pancreatitis, leukopenia, thrombocytopenia, and vasculitis may occur. Hydrochlorothiazide has been demonstrated to increase cholesterol and lipoprotein levels in nonpregnant individuals.

MECHANISM OF ACTION

The primary mode of action of thiazide diuretics is inhibition of electrolyte reabsorption in the distal tubules of the nephron. This results in an increase in sodium, chloride, and potassium excretion along with accompanying water. Uric acid excretion is also inhibited.

The thiazides cause an initial reduction in extracellular and plasma volume and a concurrent decrease in cardiac output. In nonpregnant patients, the effect is transient, and in 1–2 weeks the plasma volume and cardiac output return to normal levels, although a reduction in peripheral resistance is maintained. The persistent hypotensive effect may be secondary to either a direct action on the arteriolar smooth muscle or to changes of electrolyte concentration in the vessel wall. The latter could influence tone or pressor responsiveness. The autonomic reflexes essential for cardiovascular homeostasis are unimpaired. Plasma renin increases in response to sodium depletion and may remain increased throughout the time the drug is administered.

ABSORPTION AND BIOTRANSFORMATION

The thiazides are not metabolized in the body. They are rapidly absorbed from the gastrointestinal tract, distributed throughout the extracellular space, and then excreted unchanged in the urine.

RECOMMENDED READING

Beermann, B., et al. Placental transfer of hydrochlorothiazide. *Gynecol. Obstet. Invest.* 11:45, 1980.

Committee on Drugs of the American Academy of Pediatrics. The transfer of drugs and other chemicals into human milk. *Pediatrics* 93:137, 1994.

Gant, N.F., et al. The metabolic clearance rate of dehydroisoandrosterone sulfate: III. The effect of thiazide diuretics in normal and future pre-eclamptic pregnancy. *Am. J. Obstet. Gynecol.* 123:159, 1975.

Jackson, E.K. Diuretics. Chapter 29 in *Goodman and Gilman's The Pharmacological Basis of Therapeutics* (9th ed.), J.G. Hardman and L.E. Limbird, eds. New York: McGraw-Hill, 1996. Pp. 701– 704.

Kurzel, R.B., Hagen, G.A.: Use of thiazide diuretics to reduce the hypercalciuria of hypoparathyroidism during pregnancy. *Am. J. Perinatol.* 7:333, 1990.

Pollare, T., Lithell, H., and Berne, C. A comparison of the effects of hydrochlorothiazide and captopril on glucose and lipid metabolism in patients with hypertension. *N. Engl. J. Med.* 321:868, 1989.

Pritchard, J.A. Standardized treatment of 154 consecutive cases of eclampsia. *Am. J. Obstet. Gynecol.* 123:543, 1975.

Sibai, B.M., Grossman, R.A., and Grossman, H.G. Effects of diuretics on plasma volume in pregnancies with long-term hypertension. *Am. J. Obstet. Gynecol.* 150:831, 1984.

Sibai, B.M., et al. Plasma volume findings in pregnant women with mild hypotension: therapeutic considerations. *Am. J. Obstet. Gynecol.* 145:539, 1983.

Werthmann, M.W., Jr., and Krees, S.V. Excretion of chlorothiazide in human breast milk. *J. Pediatrics* 81:781, 1972.

Docusates (Over-the-Counter)
Docusate Sodium (Colace®, Doxinate®), Docusate Calcium (Surfak®), Docusate Potassium (Kasof®)

INDICATIONS AND RECOMMENDATIONS

Docusates are safe to use during pregnancy. These drugs are used as stool softeners in people with hemorrhoids, anorectal disorders, hernias, and cardiovascular disease. They are widely used for women recovering from third- and fourth-degree perineal lacerations after delivery of their infants.

SPECIAL CONSIDERATIONS IN PREGNANCY

There are no special considerations to be kept in mind during pregnancy.

DOSAGE

Docusates vary in dosage from 50 to 500 mg/day taken by mouth in fruit juice or milk. An effect is seen within 24–48 hours. Rectal preparations of 50–100 mg are also available.

ADVERSE EFFECTS

Docusates may produce cramping. They also may increase gastrointestinal absorption of concomitantly administered drugs. An overdose may cause anorexia, diarrhea, and vomiting.

MECHANISM OF ACTION

Docusates are anionic surfactants and act to soften the fecal mass by lowering surface tension, thus facilitating penetration of water and fats.

ABSORPTION AND BIOTRANSFORMATION

Docusates manifest no systemic effects because of their limited absorption, although a small portion is absorbed from the gastrointestinal tract and excreted in the bile.

RECOMMENDED READING

Brunton, L.L. Agents affecting gastrointestinal water flux and motility; emesis and antiemetics; bile acids and pancreatic enzymes. Chapter 38 in *Goodman and Gilman's The Pharmacological Basis of Therapeutics* (9th ed.), J.G. Hardman and L.E. Limbird, eds. New York: McGraw-Hill, 1996. P. 924.

Nelson, M.M., and Forfar, J.O. Associations between drugs administered during pregnancy and congenital abnormalities of the fetus. *Br. Med. J.* 1:523, 1971.

Schenkel, B., and Vorherr, H. Non-prescription drugs during pregnancy: potential teratogenic and toxic effects upon embryo and fetus. *J. Reprod. Med.* 12:27, 1974.

Dopamine (Intropin®)

INDICATIONS AND RECOMMENDATIONS

The use of dopamine in pregnancy should be limited to the treatment of cardiogenic, traumatic, or hypovolemic shock. It is a potent sympathomimetic drug that has been used safely during pregnancy.

SPECIAL CONSIDERATIONS IN PREGNANCY

When dopamine was administered in doses of 2–4 μg/kg/min to chronically instrumented pregnant sheep near term, a statistically significant increase in uterine blood flow was noted. When doses of 8–16 μg/kg/min were given the responses were variable. In another study, instrumented near-term pregnant sheep were subjected to autonomic blockade with spinal anesthesia. These animals demonstrated decreased systemic arterial pressure, heart rate, and uterine blood flow as well as increased uterine vascular resistance. Dopamine administered intravenously during the spinal hypotension corrected these disturbed circulatory parameters. Dopamine use in pregnant baboons has resulted in decreased uterine artery blood flow. As a result, other pressors, such as milrinone, have been suggested for use in pregnancy.

Published experience with the use of this drug during human pregnancy is limited. In one study, dopamine was given to 26 patients and found to be as effective as ephedrine in correcting postspinal hypotension before repeat cesarean section. No differences in Apgar scores or neonatal blood gases were observed in the two groups.

A Viennese series describes the use of dopamine to prevent renal failure in nine eclamptic patients. The drug was administered by continuous infusion at a dose of 3 μg/kg/min in conjunction with a diuretic to improve renal perfusion and promote diuresis. All of the patients showed initial improvement in renal function with this regimen, and seven went on to complete recovery, but the other two died. Obviously, more data are needed before dopamine can be recommended for this indication.

Dopamine is a major suppressor of prolactin, and its use may result in failure of successful lactation. No information is available at present on dopamine's disposition in breast milk.

DOSAGE

Dopamine is administered parenterally at an initial rate of 2–5 µg/kg/min, and this may be gradually increased to 20–50 µg/kg/min as the clinical situation demands. All patients require monitoring of blood volume, myocardial function, and urine production during therapy. Reduced urinary output, tachycardia, or the development of an arrhythmia may be an indication for slowing or terminating the infusion. Since the duration of action of dopamine is brief, the rate of administration can be used to control the intensity of effect.

ADVERSE EFFECTS

Nausea, vomiting, tachycardia, anginal pain, arrhythmias, headache, hypertension, and vasoconstriction may be encountered during infusion of dopamine. Before dopamine is administered to patients in shock, hypovolemia should be corrected by transfusion of whole blood, plasma, or appropriate fluids. No adverse fetal or neonatal effects attributed to the drug have been described.

MECHANISM OF ACTION

Dopamine exerts a positive inotropic effect on the myocardium, acting as an agonist at β_1-adrenergic receptors. In low dosages, it causes renal and splanchnic vasodilatation through activation of dopaminergic receptors. Slightly higher dosages cause beta stimulation of the heart to increase cardiac output. Further increases in dosage elicit an increase in heart rate, although tachycardia is less prominent during infusions of dopamine than of isoproterenol. Still higher dosages cause alpha stimulation and vasoconstriction, which may impair generalized peripheral as well as renal and mesenteric perfusion.

ABSORPTION AND BIOTRANSFORMATION

Dopamine is ineffective when given orally. When administered parenterally, absorbed drug is rapidly biotransformed, primarily to 3,4-dihydroxyphenylacetic acid (DOPAC) and 3-methoxy-4-hydroxyphenylacetic acid (HVA); small amounts are also converted to norepinephrine and other compounds. About 80% of the metabolites are excreted in the urine within 24 hours. Very little, if any, dopamine crosses the blood–brain barrier.

RECOMMENDED READING

Cabalum, T., et al. Effect of dopamine on hypotension induced by spinal anesthesia. *Am. J. Obstet. Gynecol.* 133:630, 1979.

Clark, R.B., and Brunner, J.A. Dopamine for the treatment of spinal hypotension during cesarean section. *Anesthesiology* 35:514, 1980.

Escalada, J., Cacicedo, L., Ortego, J., Melian, E., Sanchez-Franco, F. Prolactin gene expression and secretion during pregnancy and lactation in the rat: role of dopamine and vasoactive intestinal peptide. *Endocrinology* 137:631–637, 1996.

Fishburne, J.I., Jr., et al. Effects of amrinone and dopamine on uterine blood flow and vascular responses in the gravid baboon. *Am. J. Obstet. Gynecol.* 158:829–837, 1988.

Gerstner, G., and Grunberger, W. Dopamine treatment for prevention of renal failure in patients with severe eclampsia. *Clin. Exp. Obstet. Gynecol.* 7:219, 1980.

Hoffman, B.B., and Lefkowitz, R.J. Catecholamines, sympathomimetic drugs, and adrenergic receptor antagonists. Chapter 10 in *Goodman and Gilman's The Pharmacological Basis of Therapeutics* (9th ed.), J.G. Hardman and L.E. Limbird, eds. New York: McGraw-Hill, 1996. Pp. 211–212.

Grunberger, W., and Szalay, S. Uterine and systemic vascular responses to dopamine in pregnant ewes. *Arch. Gynecol.* 233:259, 1983.

Katz, V.L., et al. Low dose dopamine in the treatment of persistent oliguria in pre-eclampsia. *Int. J. Gynecol. Obstet.* 31:57, 1990.

Santos, A.C., Baumann, A.L., Wlody, D., Pedersen, H., Morishima, H.O., and Finster, M. The maternal and fetal effects of milrinone and dopamine in normotensive pregnant ewes. *Am. J. Obstet. Gynecol.* 166:257, 1992.

Doxylamine (Bendectin®, When Combined with Pyridoxine)

INDICATIONS AND RECOMMENDATIONS

The combination of doxylamine and pyridoxine (Bendectin) was removed from the market in 1983 in the United States—not by the FDA, but by the manufacturer. This drug had been used widely and studied intensively in the pregnant woman. The manufacturer estimates that it was used in 29 million pregnancies between 1956 and 1979. Large epidemiologic studies failed to demonstrate an association between use of the drug and the occurrence of birth defects in the offspring. Although a few of the studies have shown an association between some subcategories of birth defects and Bendectin, the specific defects implicated were generally not the same from one study to another. It should be noted that when one is evaluating statistical significance, the test that is usually applied is the 0.05 level of probability. When this standard is met, it means that the likelihood of an association being due to chance is 5% (i.e., the odds are 20:1 that the finding is not artifactual). On the other hand, this also means that if no real association exists, it is likely that every 20 times such an association is looked for, one will by chance appear to be found. Thus, it is not surprising that when a myriad of individual birth defects are investigated, some will appear to be significantly associated with the drug under investigation. If the associations were real, one would expect that the same type of birth defects would recur from study to study; this has not been the case with Bendectin to date. Two studies reported a positive association between maternal Bendectin use and the occurrence of pyloric stenosis in the offspring. However, other studies and meta-analyses have failed to confirm such an association.

The manufacturer removed this product from the market for economic reasons. Beginning in 1981, an increasing number of lawsuits were filed against the manufacturer. They alleged that Bendectin was responsible for a multitude of birth defects in children whose mothers had taken it during pregnancy. It should be noted that approximately 3% of all children have an identifiable birth defect and that estimates of the percentage of pregnant women taking Bendectin when it was available range from 5% to 25%. Thus, even if the drug reduced the occurrence of birth defects by half (no one has suggested that it does), there would be, among the 3–4 million babies born in the United States each year, between 2250 and 15,000 babies with birth defects who were exposed to Bendectin in utero. If we make the more reasonable assumption that this drug has no effect on birth defects, the numbers of such babies would be between 4500 and 30,000 each year. By the time the manufacturer removed Bendectin from the market in 1983, there had been well over 300 suits instituted, with no end in sight. Only two cases had been decided, one in favor of the manufacturer and the other in favor of the plaintiff (although this case was under appeal). In view of these events, the manufacturer made the projection that, even if it won all of the suits filed, the cost of defending them would make the continued marketing of this drug financially prohibitive, and so the production of Bendectin was discontinued. In addition, the manufacturer set up a fund to settle all outstanding and potential claims.

We have undertaken such a long discussion of an unavailable drug to explain why it is no longer being made and to point out that its discontinuance left a therapeutic gap in the care of pregnant women. Most cases of nausea in pregnancy can be dealt with by simple measures. However, shortly after the withdrawal of Bendectin from the market, national statistics in both the United States and Canada demonstrated a measurable increase in hospitalizations for nausea and vomiting in pregnancy per thousand births, with an estimated cost in the United States of $73 million over 5 years. Persistent nausea in the first trimester continues to be a real clinical problem, and the physician is now faced with the prospect of prescribing medications about which much less is known when the usual nonpharmacologic forms of therapy fail. It is by no means clear that the removal of this drug from the market represents a "victory" for the pregnant consumer, as some have claimed.

RECOMMENDED READING

Aselton, P.A., et al. Pyloric stenosis and maternal Bendectin exposure. *Am. J. Epidemiol.* 120:251, 1984.

Brent, R.L. Bendectin: review of the medical literature of a comprehensively studied human nonteratogen and the most prevalent tortogen-litigen. *Reprod. Toxicol.* 9:337, 1995.

Eskenazi, B., and Bracken, M.B. Bendectin (Debendox) as a risk factor for pyloric stenosis. *Am. J. Obstet. Gynecol.* 144:919, 1982.

Jick, H., et al. First trimester drug use and congenital disorders. *J.A.M.A.* 5246:343, 1981.

McKeigue, P.M., Lamm, S.H., Linn, S., Kutcher, J.S. Bendectin and birth defects: I. A meta-analysis of the epidemiologic studies. *Teratology* 50:27, 1994.

Michaelis, J., et al. Prospective study of suspected associations between certain drugs administered during early pregnancy and congenital malformations. *Teratology* 27:57, 1983.

Milkovich, L., and Van den Berg, B.J. An evaluation of the terato-genicity of certain antinauseant drugs. *Am. J. Obstet. Gynecol.* 125:244, 1976.

Neutel C.I., and Johansen, H.L. Measuring drug effectiveness by default: the case of Bendectin. *Can. J. Public Health* 86:66, 1995.

Ornstein, M., Einarson, A., and Koren, G. Editorial: Bendectin/di-clectin for morning sickness: a Canadian follow-up of an Ameri-can tragedy. *Reprod. Toxicol.* 9:1, 1995.

Shiono, P.H., and Klebanoff, M.A. Bendectin and human congenital malformations. *Teratology* 40:151, 1989.

Dronabinol (Marinol®)

Dronabinol, or Δ-9-tetrahydrocannabinol, is an orally active cannabinoid used in the treatment of nausea and vomiting as-sociated with cancer chemotherapy, and also in treating the anorexia and weight loss that is often present in AIDS patients. Its use in pregnancy should be limited to the above situations, and patients should be informed of the lack of credible human data regarding reproductive toxicity.

SPECIAL CONSIDERATIONS IN PREGNANCY

There are no credible data to describe the impact of dronabi-nol use on pregnancy outcomes. Presumably the same concerns as arise with marijuana use (see marijuana) exist with regard to this drug. However, because dronabinol is pure Δ-9-tetrahy-drocannabinol, need not be smoked, and does not contain the myriad of other substances found in marijuana, some of the potential risks should be ameliorated. Furthermore, because dronabinol's use is confined to specific very serious medical sit-uations and it may have a beneficial impact on appetite, nutri-tion, and well-being for such patients, it seems reasonable to counsel AIDS patients and cancer chemotherapy recipients about the availability of this drug, with appropriate warnings about the lack of data regarding fetal effects.

DOSAGE

Dronabinol is available as capsules containing 2.5, 5, and 10 mg of Δ-9-tetrahydrocannabinol. In AIDS patients being treated for anorexia and weight loss, the usual starting dose is 2.5 mg twice daily. The dose may be gradually increased to a maximum of 20 mg/day. When the drug is used as an antiemetic in chemotherapy patients, it is usually given in a dose of 5 mg/m^2 of body surface area, 1–3 hours before the administra-tion of chemotherapy and every 2–4 hours afterward, for a total of 4–6 doses per day. The dose can be gradually increased as necessary in 2.5 mg/m^2 increments to a maximum of 15 mg/m^2 per dose. Dose escalation should be done cautiously as most of the side effects of dronabinol are dose-related.

ADVERSE EFFECTS

Dronabinol is considered by the government as a drug of abuse and is classified as a schedule II drug. It is not clear as to whether the changes reported in marijuana users (decreased motivation, cognition, judgment, and perception) are drug-induced or related to other factors. They have not been reported in AIDS patients treated with dronabinol. However, an abstinence syndrome has been reported in patients who discontinued dronabinol after taking 210 mg/day for approximately 2 weeks. This included insomnia, irritability, and restlessness, progressing to "hot flashes," sweating, rhinorrhea, loose stools, hiccups, and anorexia over 24 hours, and then abating over another 48 hours.

A relatively large proportion of patients (8% to 24%, depending on dosage) reported experiencing a cannabinoid "high." A third of patients reported central nervous system effects. These included amnesia, anxiety, ataxia, confusion, depersonalization, dizziness, hallucination, paranoid reaction, somnolence, and abnormal thinking. Cardiovascular effects included palpitations, tachycardia, vasodilatation and flushing, hypertension and hypotension. Gastrointestinal disturbances included pain, nausea, and vomiting. Dronabinol also has the potential for significant drug interactions when taken with alcohol or central nervous system depressants. The manufacturer's package insert contains an extensive list of other reported drug interactions, and this should be consulted before the drug is prescribed.

MECHANISM OF ACTION

The mechanism of action of cannabinoids is not completely understood. However, a cannabinoid receptor has been identified in the central nervous system, and an endogenous ligand has been discovered.

ABSORPTION AND BIOTRANSFORMATION

Dronabinol is almost completely absorbed after oral dosing. Because of high lipid solubility and extensive first-pass hepatic metabolism, between 10% and 20% of the oral dose appears in the circulation. The drug is highly protein-bound. Peak concentrations are reached approximately 2–4 hours after oral dosing. The initial half- life is approximately 4 hours, but there is a much slower second half- life lasting 25–36 hours. The drug is primarily eliminated through biliary excretion into the stools. Because of its high fat solubility, dronabinol has a long elimination time, and small amounts may be recovered from the stool for as long as 5 weeks after a single oral dose.

RECOMMENDED READING

Doyle, E., and Spence, A.A. Cannabis as a medicine? *Br. J. Anaesth.* 74:359, 1995.

O'Brien, C.P. Drug addiction and drug abuse. Chapter 24 in *Goodman and Gilman's The Pharmacological Basis of Therapeutics* (9th ed.), J.G. Hardman and L.E. Limbird, eds. New York: McGraw-Hill, 1996. Pp. 572–573.

Roxane Laboratories. Marinol (dronabinol). Manufacturer's package insert in *Physicians Desk Reference* (52nd ed.). Montvale, NJ: Medical Economics, 1998. Pp. 2544–2546.

Ephedrine

INDICATIONS AND RECOMMENDATIONS

Ephedrine is the vasopressor agent of choice for use in pregnancy as it preserves uterine blood flow in contrast to the more commonly used pressors such as norepinephrine. However, use of pressors should be limited to correction of maternal hypotension unresponsive to appropriate fluid infusion, left lateral uterine displacement, and other appropriate resuscitative measures. This drug should not be used to treat asthma in pregnant women as other agents for that purpose are preferable.

SPECIAL CONSIDERATIONS IN PREGNANCY

Ephedrine crosses the placenta and appears in umbilical cord blood at a concentration 70% of maternal blood level. When given to normal gravidas receiving epidural anesthesia for elective cesarean section, ephedrine did not decrease uterine blood flow and appeared to preserve uterine perfusion in the face of systemic maternal hypotension. With prophylactic use of ephedrine prior to regional anesthesia for cesarean delivery, there is an increase in neonatal catecholamine levels but no alteration in neonatal acid–base status. Neurologic examinations of newborns exposed in utero to prophylactic ephedrine were identical to those in a control group of neonates. However, subtle electroencephalographic findings consistent with central nervous system stimulation were present for the first 2 hours of life. In one study, the administration of ephedrine to women who had been given epidural anesthesia was associated with significant increases in fetal heart rate and beat-to-beat variability. These changes were dose-related but did not have an observed effect on scalp blood pH or Apgar scores when compared with those of control subjects. When ephedrine is used in combination with oxytocics, severe hypertension may develop. It must be used with extreme caution in patients with hypertension.

Prophylactic administration of intramuscular ephedrine in doses of 25 or 50 mg given 15–30 minutes before epidural anesthesia to women undergoing cesarean section was no more successful than intramuscular placebo in preventing hypotension. Furthermore, persistent hypertension developed in 8 of 12 women given the 50 mg dose. In another study, ephedrine was administered to 44 healthy women undergoing elective, repeat cesarean section under spinal anesthesia. Twenty of these patients were given an infusion, starting at a dose of 5 mg/min, immediately after induction of the anesthesia to maintain the maternal systolic blood pressure between 90% and 100% of the baseline value. The mean dose administered was 31.6 mg. The remaining 24 patients received a 20 mg intravenous bolus and additional 10 mg boluses if needed when the systolic blood pressure fell to 80% of baseline levels. The mean dose administered to this group was 26.8 mg. The infusion group had significantly less deviation of the systolic blood pressure from the baseline, and reactive hypertension did not occur. Furthermore, the group receiving ephedrine by infusion had significantly less nausea and vomiting. No appreciable difference was noted in Apgar scores, fetal blood gas tensions, or time for onset of neonatal respirations.

DOSAGE

For the treatment of hypotension, ephedrine is usually administered intravenously in 5 to 20 mg doses every 60 seconds as needed to keep the systolic blood pressure above 100 mm Hg or within 80% of baseline blood pressure. It is rarely necessary to use more than 60 mg for this purpose. Ephedrine's duration of action is several hours.

ADVERSE EFFECTS

Side effects associated with the use of ephedrine include hypertension, cardiac arrhythmias, palpitations, insomnia, tremor, and anxiety.

MECHANISM OF ACTION

Ephedrine has both α- and β-adrenergic actions. It acts by stimulating the release of stored norepinephrine and by direct stimulation of adrenergic receptors. The predominant cardiovascular effect is beta stimulation. Therefore, in comparison to other vasopressor agents, vasoconstriction has a minor role in its action.

The effects of ephedrine in the body are widespread. Because it produces mild bronchodilatation, it has been used as an adjunct to theophylline therapy in asthma. It increases both systolic and diastolic blood pressures and decreases pulse pressure; heart rate is generally unchanged; cardiac output is increased; renal and splanchnic blood flow are decreased; and coronary, cerebral, and muscle blood flow are increased. Ephedrine decreases uterine activity (β_2 effect). It also produces mydriasis when applied topically.

ABSORPTION AND BIOTRANSFORMATION

Ephedrine is well absorbed when given orally. Most of the drug is metabolized by deamination and conjugation. Both metabolites and unchanged drug are excreted in the urine.

RECOMMENDED READING

Chen, K.K., and Schmidt, C.F. Ephedrine and related substances. *Medicine* 9:1, 1930.

Eng, M., Berges, P.V., and Ueland, K. The effects of methoxamine and ephedrine in normotensive pregnant primates. *Anesthesia* 35:354, 1970.

Hollmen, A.I., Jouppila, R., Albright, G.A., Jouppila, P., Vierola, H., and Koivula, A. Intervillous blood flow during caesarean section with prophylactic ephedrine and epidural anesthesia. *Acta Anaesthiol. Scand.* 28:396, 1984.

Hughes, S.C., Ward, M.G., Levinson, G., Shnider, S.M., Wright, R.G., Gruenke, L.D., and Craig, J.C. Placental transfer of ephedrine does not affect neonatal outcome. *Anesthesiology* 63:217, 1985.

Kang, Y.G., Abouleish, E., and Caritis, S. Prophylactic intravenous ephedrine infusion during spinal anesthesia for cesarean section. *Anesth. Analg.* 61:839, 1982.

Kangas-Saarela, T., Hollmen, A.I., Tolonen, U., Eskelinen, P., Alahuhta, S., Jouppila, R., Kivela, A., and Huttunen, P. Does ephedrine influence newborn neurobehavioral responses and spectral EEG when used to prevent maternal hypotension during cesarean section? *Acta Anaesthesiol. Scand.* 34:8, 1990.

Ralstow, D.H., Schnider, S.M., and deLorimier, A.A. Effect of equipotent doses of ephedrine, metaraminol, mephentermine, and methoxamine on uterine blood flow in the pregnant ewe. *Anesthesia* 40:354, 1974.

Rolbin, S.H., et al. Prophylactic intramuscular ephedrine before epidural anaesthesia for cesarean section: Efficacy and actions on the fetus and newborn. *Can. Anaesth. Soc. J.* 29:148, 1982.

Schnider, S.M., deLorimier, A.A., and Holl, J.W. Vasopressor in obstetrics: I. Correction of fetal acidosis with ephedrine during spinal hypotension. *Am. J. Obstet. Gynecol.* 102:911, 1968.

Weinberger, M. Use of ephedrine in bronchodilator therapy. *Pediatr. Clin. North Am.* 22:121, 1975.

Wright, R.G., et al. The effect of maternal administration of ephedrine on fetal heart rate and variability. *Obstet. Gynecol.* 57:734, 1981.

Ergonovine Maleate (Ergotrate®), Methylergonovine Maleate (Methergine®)

INDICATIONS AND RECOMMENDATIONS

Ergot alkaloids such as ergonovine maleate and methylergonovine maleate are contraindicated during pregnancy prior to delivery of the infant. Their use is indicated for the prevention and treatment of postpartum and postabortal hemorrhage due to uterine atony. They may also be used during the puerperium to promote involution of the uterus. They are direct stimulants of gravid and nongravid uterine muscle, although the gravid uterus is much more sensitive to their effects. Due to the high degree of uterine stimulation produced, ergot preparations are not recommended for antepartum use, nor should they be administered prior to delivery of the placenta. They should not be used for the induction or augmentation of labor because of their tendency to produce tetanic contractions.

The ergot alkaloids can induce coronary spasm, and there have been case reports of acute myocardial infarction following both intramuscular injection and oral administration of methylergonovine.

Several studies have shown ergonovine to interfere with normal secretion of prolactin in the immediate puerperium. Lactation thus may be delayed or inhibited in nursing mothers when it has been administered. One randomized trial found that women treated with ergometrine (methylergonovine) during the third stage of labor were more likely to discontinue breast-feeding within 4 weeks than were those not given this drug.

RECOMMENDED READING

Asgaonkar, D.S., Jagose, J., Jaykar, V.V., et al. Ergot poisoning: a report of two cases. *J. Assoc. Physicians India* 35:603, 1987.

Begley, C.M. The effect of ergometrine on breast feeding. *Midwifery* 6:60, 1990.

Canales, R., et al. Effect of ergonovine on prolactin secretion and milk letdown. *Obstet. Gynecol.* 48:228, 1976.

Floss, H., Cassidy, J., and Robbers, J. Influence of ergot alkaloids on pituitary prolactin and prolactin-dependent processes. *J. Pharm. Sci.* 62:699, 1973.

Fujiwara, Y., Yamanaka, O., Nakamura, T., et al. Acute myocardial infarction induced by ergonovine administration for artificially induced abortion. *Jpn. Heart J.* 34:803, 1993.

Graves, C.R. Agents that cause contraction or relaxation of the uterus. Chapter 39 in *Goodman and Gilman's The Pharmacological Basis of Therapeutics* (9th ed.), J.G. Hardman and L.E. Limbird, eds. New York: McGraw-Hill, 1996. Pp. 943–945.

Liao, J.K., Cockrill, B.A., and Yurchak, P.M. Acute myocardial infarction after ergonovine administration for uterine bleeding. *Am. J. Cardiol.* 68:823, 1991.

Ergotamine Tartrate (Cafergot®, with Caffeine; Ergomar®; Ergostat®; Gynergen®)

INDICATIONS AND RECOMMENDATIONS

Ergotamine tartrate is contraindicated during pregnancy. This drug, which is used to abort migraine and cluster headaches, produces α-adrenergic blockade and, more importantly, acts on the central nervous system and directly stimulates smooth muscle. It should not be used during pregnancy because it can create tetanic uterine contractions. Cases of uterine tachysystole, fetal distress, and stillbirth following Cafergot ingestion have been published. It may also cause a significant increase in blood pressure at therapeutic dosages. Administration of this drug during organogenesis has produced an increased incidence of fetal wastage in rats and fetal growth retardation in rats, mice, and rabbits. A case has been reported of a woman who ingested ergotamine tartrate daily during six pregnancies. Four ended in spontaneous abortion, one in the premature delivery of a small-for-date infant and one in the premature delivery of an infant with multiple areas of jejunal atresia. The authors speculate that the atresia may have been due to the vascular effects of the drug. There have been other case reports of apparent fetal vascular injury after ergotamine was ingested during pregnancy.

RECOMMENDED READING

deGroot, A.N.J.A., van Dongen, P.W.J., van Roosmalen, J., and Eskes, T.K.A.B. Ergotamine-induced fetal stress: review of side effects of ergot alkaloids during pregnancy. *Eur. J. Obstet. Gynecol. Reprod. Biol.* 51:73, 1993.

Floss, H., Cassidy, J., and Robbers, J. Influence of ergot alkaloids on pituitary prolactin and prolactin-dependent processes. *J. Pharm. Sci.* 62:699, 1973.

Graham, J.M., Jr., Marin-Padilla, M., and Hoefnagel, D. Jejunal atresia associated with Cafergot ingestion during pregnancy. *Clin. Pediatrics* 22:226, 1983.

Grauwiler, J., and Schön, H. Teratological experiments with ergotamine in mice, rats and rabbits. *Teratology* 7:227, 1973.

Hosking, S.P. Ergotamine use in pregnancy. *Aust. N. Z. J. Obstet. Gynaecol.* 36:159, 1996.

Peroutka, S.J. Drugs effective in the therapy of migraine. Chapter 21 in *Goodman and Gilman's The Pharmacological Basis of Therapeutics* (9th ed.), J.G. Hardman and L.E. Limbird, eds. New York: McGraw-Hill, 1996. Pp. 491–496.

Raymond, G.V. Teratogen update: ergot and ergotamine. *Teratology* 51:344, 1995.

Silberstein, S.D. Headaches and women: treatment of the pregnant and lactating migraineur. *Headache* 33:533, 1993.

Verloes, A., Emonts, P., Dubois, M., et al. Paraplegia and arthrogryposis multiplex of the lower extremities after intrauterine exposure to ergotamine. *J. Med. Genet.* 27:213, 1990.

Erythromycin (E-Mycin®, Erythrocin®)

INDICATIONS AND RECOMMENDATIONS

Erythromycin is safe to use during pregnancy; however, preparations of the estolate ester should be avoided. It is an antibiotic primarily used to treat gram-positive bacterial infections in penicillin-allergic patients. It is also effective against gonococci, *Haemophilus* sp., *Legionella pneumophila*, *Mycoplasma pneumoniae*, and *Chlamydia trachomatis*. Although it is effective in the treatment of syphilis, its use for this indication is not recommended in pregnancy.

SPECIAL CONSIDERATIONS IN PREGNANCY

Fetal plasma concentrations are 5% to 20% of those found in maternal plasma. This drug is safe for the fetus, but because it reaches inadequate fetal levels, erythromycin is not recommended for treatment of syphilis during pregnancy. Penicillin desensitization should be considered for the penicillin-allergic patient.

While erythromycin is the approved first-line drug for the treatment of *Chlamydia* infections during pregnancy, its side effects (primarily nausea and vomiting) often prevent patients from completing a full course of therapy. If erythromycin cannot be tolerated, amoxicillin is the recommended alternative based on cure rate, patient compliance, and cost.

Concentrations of erythromycin in breast milk are approximately 50% of those in maternal serum. The American Academy of Pediatrics considers its use compatible with breastfeeding.

In one study, a significant proportion of pregnant women (10% to 15%) who received erythromycin estolate for 3 weeks developed subclinical, reversible hepatic toxicity. It is therefore recommended that erythromycin estolate be avoided during pregnancy.

Use of oral erythromycin has been associated with declining maternal urinary estriol levels, with an almost immediate rise after cessation of therapy. The decline has been attributed to an alteration in the normal intestinal flora, which results in interference with estriol hydrolysis and reabsorption.

DOSAGE

The usual oral dose is 250–500 mg q6h. The usual intravenous dose is 1–4 g/day. Parenteral administration is rarely indicated because of the severe pain and frequent phlebitis associated with its use.

ADVERSE EFFECTS

Gastrointestinal disturbances are the most frequent side effect encountered with oral erythromycin use. Severe pain at the injection site is common with parenteral administration. Allergic reactions and transient deafness are rare side effects. Cholestatic hepatitis has been associated with erythromycin estolate use in adults.

MECHANISM OF ACTION

Erythromycin is an orally effective macrolide antibiotic that inhibits protein synthesis by reversibly binding to the 50S ribosomal subunits of sensitive microorganisms.

ABSORPTION AND BIOTRANSFORMATION

Erythromycin is well absorbed orally, but absorption varies with the salt and dosage form administered. It is concentrated in the liver and excreted in the bile. Only 2% to 5% of the oral dose is excreted by the kidneys, whereas 12% to 15% appears in the urine after parenteral administration.

RECOMMENDED READING

Centers for Disease Control and Prevention. Guidelines for the prevention and control of congenital syphilis. *M.M.W.R.* 37(S-1):9, 1988.

Centers for Disease Control and Prevention. 1989 Sexually transmitted diseases treatment guidelines. *M.M.W.R.* 38(S-8):6, 1989.

Committee on Drugs. The transfer of drugs and chemicals into human milk. *Pediatrics* 93:137, 1994.

Gallagher, J.C., Ismail, M.A., and Aladjem, S. Reduced urinary estriol levels with erythromycin therapy. *Obstet. Gynecol.* 56:381, 1980.

Graham, E.M. Erythromycin. *Obstet. Gynecol. Clin. North Am.* 19:539, 1992.

Kapusnic-Uner, J.E., Sande, M.A., and Chambers, H.F. Antimicrobial agents: tetracyclines, chloramphenicol, erythromycin and miscellaneous antibacterial agents. Chapter 47 in *Goodman and Gilman's The Pharmacological Basis of Therapeutics* (9th ed.), J.G. Hardman and L.E. Limbird, eds. New York: McGraw-Hill, 1996. Pp. 1135–1140.

McCormack, W.M., et al. Hepatotoxicity of erythromycin estolate during pregnancy. *Antimicrob. Agents Chemother.* 12:630, 1977.

Philipson, A., Sabath, L.D., and Charles, D. Transplacental passage of erythromycin and clindamycin. *N. Engl. J. Med.* 288:1219, 1973.

Turrentine, M.A., and Newton, E.R. Amoxicillin or erythromycin for the treatment of antenatal chlamydial infection: a meta-analysis. *Obstet. Gynecol.* 86:1021, 1995.

Wendel, G.D., et al. Penicillin allergy and desensitization in serious infections during pregnancy. *N. Engl. J. Med.* 312:1229, 1985.

Erythropoietin (Epoetin Alfa, Epogen®, Procrit®)

Recombinant erythropoietin, a glycoprotein that stimulates red blood cell production, may be used during pregnancy. Erythropoietin is used to increase endogenous red blood cell production in those with conditions of chronic anemia such as chronic renal failure, zidovudine-treated AIDS patients, cancer patients on chemotherapy, and persons with any of a few primary hematopoietic disorders. It is not effective in patients with aplastic anemia or myelodysplasia. Erythropoietin is sometimes used preoperatively to increase hematopoiesis in preparation for autologous transfusion or to decrease the requirement for transfusions. Routine use for this indication is not justified in pregnancy, although specific circumstances may warrant the treatment.

SPECIAL CONSIDERATIONS IN PREGNANCY

The available evidence suggests that erythropoietin does not cross the human placenta to any appreciable extent. There have been numerous case reports and case series in which pregnant women were treated with erythropoietin, without apparent adverse effects. In a pilot study series, erythropoietin plus parenteral iron immediately stimulated red cell production in 8 of 11 cases of severe iron deficiency anemia in pregnancy. The investigators suggested erythropoietin as a possible alternative for anemic gravidas who refuse blood transfusions or don't respond to iron therapy alone.

DOSAGE

Erythropoietin may be given intravenously or subcutaneously. The usual initial dose is 50–100 U/kg, given intravenously 3 times a week to patients in renal failure. The dose is subsequently titrated against the patient's hematocrit. Because patients with adequate endogenous erythropoietin production are unlikely to respond to exogenous erythropoietin, the manufacturer recommends that patients with AIDS being treated with zidovudine have their serum erythropoietin levels measured prior to therapy. If the level is more than 500 mU/ml, a response is unlikely. For patients with serum erythropoietin levels below 500 mU/ml, the usual starting dose is 100 U/kg given either intravenously or subcutaneously, 3 times a week. The dosage is then titrated against the hematocrit. The usual dose for cancer patients receiving chemotherapy is 150 U/kg, given subcutaneously 3 times per week. In preoperative patients, the recommended dose is 300 U/kg/day for 10 days, on the day of surgery, and for 4 days following surgery.

In order for erythropoietin to be effective, the patient must have adequate iron stores. Thus concomitant administration of oral or parenteral iron may be necessary if iron deficiency is present. The response to erythropoietin therapy in patients with chronic renal disease may take 2–6 weeks in some patients.

ADVERSE EFFECTS

Adverse effects directly attributable to erythropoietin administration have been rare, and have included local skin reactions and arthralgia. However, complications secondary to increased hematocrit, including thrombotic events and hypertension, have been reported, particularly in patients with chronic renal failure. Caution should be exercised to avoid too rapid a rise in hematocrit during the initial weeks of therapy.

MECHANISM OF ACTION

Produced primarily in the renal cortex, erythropoietin is the most significant enhancer of proliferation of committed red cell progenitors. It binds to a receptor on erythroid precursor cells.

ABSORPTION AND BIOTRANSFORMATION

Following subcutaneous injection, peak plasma levels occur within 5–24 hours. The half-life is approximately 10 hours.

RECOMMENDED READING

Amgen Company. Epogen (Epoietin Alfa Recombinant). Entry in *Physicians Desk Reference* (52nd ed.). Montvale, NJ: Medical Economics, 1998. Pp. 505–512.

Braga, J., Marques, R., Branco, A., et al: Maternal and perinatal implications of the use of human recombinant erythropoietin. *Acta Obstet. Gynecol. Scand.* 75:449, 1996.

Breymann, C., Major, A., Richter, C., et al: Recombinant human erythropoietin and parenteral iron in the treatment of pregnancy anemia: a pilot study. *J. Perinat. Med.* 23:89, 1995.

Harris, S.A., Payne, G.Jr., and Putnam, J.M. Erythropoietin treatment of erythropoietin-deficient anemia without renal disease during pregnancy. *Obstet. Gynecol.* 87:812, 1996.

Hillman, R.S. Hematopoietic agents.Chapter 53 in *Goodman and Gilman's The Pharmacological Basis of Therapeutics* (9th ed.), J.G.Hardman and L.E. Limbird, eds. New York: McGraw-Hill, 1996. Pp. 1312–1315.

Koenig, H.M., Levine, E.A., Resnick, D.J., et al. Use of recombinant human erythropoietin in a Jehovah's Witness. *J. Clin. Anesth.* 5:244, 1993.

Malek, A., Sager, R., Eckhardt, K.U., et al: Lack of transport of erythropoietin across the human placenta studies by an in vitro perfusion system. *Pflugers Arch. Eur. J. Physiol.*427:157, 1994.

Reisenberger, K., Egarter, C., Kapiotis, S., et al. Transfer of erythropoietin across the placenta perfused in vitro. *Obstet. Gynecol.* 89:738, 1997.

Schneider, H., and Malek, A. Lack of permeability of the human placenta for erythropoietin. *J. Perinat. Med.*23:71, 1995.

Scott, L.L., Ramin, S.M., Richey, M., et al. Erythropoietin use in pregnancy: two cases and a review of the literature. *Am. J. Perinatol.* 12:22, 1995.

Widness, J.A., Schmidt, R.L., and Sawyer, S.T. Erythropoietin transplacental passage- review of animal studies. *J. Perinat. Med.* 23:61, 1995.

Zanjani, E.D., Pixley, J.S., Slotnick, N., et al. Erythropoietin does not cross the placenta into the fetus. *Pathobiology* 61:211, 1993.

Estrogens (Synthetic and Natural, Including Diethylstilbestrol and Tamoxifen)

INDICATIONS AND RECOMMENDATIONS

Both steroidal and nonsteroidal estrogens are contraindicated in pregnancy. In the past, nonsteroidal estrogens were often prescribed for maintenance of diabetic pregnancies and the prevention of spontaneous abortions. However, it is now known that they are not effective for these therapeutic objectives.

Maternal side effects may include nausea, vomiting, skin changes, thrombophlebitis, pulmonary embolism, and cholestatic jaundice. Important fetal effects have been noted when nonsteroidal estrogen [specifically diethylstilbestrol (DES)] was administered during the first trimester. These include an increased incidence of adenocarcinoma and adenosis of the vagina, as well as cervical, uterine, and tubal deformities in females. Clear cell adenocarcinoma of the vagina and cervix has been reported to occur in 1 of 1000 DES- exposed women, with median age of diagnosis at 19 years. A well-controlled prospective study found that the incidence of cervical and vaginal dysplasia among DES daughters was approximately twice that seen in a matched control group of unexposed women. There are a number of reports of increased reproductive loss among DES daughters who become pregnant, with the strong possibility that incompetent cervix syndrome may be common among such patients. However, most of these studies were based on selected groups of DES daughters, generally those presenting for care at a DES program. One nonrandomized study of pregnancy outcome among DES daughters found that placement of a cervical cerclage in subjects with hypoplastic cervices or prior reproductive loss resulted in better pregnancy outcomes than did expectant management of patients with normal-appearing cervices. Infertility was assessed among surviving female offspring in a follow-up study of a randomized prospective trial of DES. Primary infertility was significantly more common in exposed than unexposed subjects. Duration and amount of menstrual bleeding were also diminished in DES-exposed daughters. Testicular cysts and oligospermia have been noted when developing male gonadal tissue has been exposed to these compounds in utero. In a second follow-up study of the aforementioned randomized prospective trial, it was determined that surviving male offspring exposed to DES prior to 11 weeks gestation were 3 times as likely as placebo-exposed controls to have congenital malformations of the genital tract but were no less fertile. The estrogens are secreted in breast milk.

Tamoxifen, a nonsteroidal estrogen/antiestrogen compound, is often used for treatment of malignancy, including breast cancer. There has been one case report of a woman who used the drug throughout pregnancy and delivered a baby with Goldenhar's syndrome (a heterotopic field defect of facial and vertebral anomalies).

It is recommended that estrogens, both steroidal and nonsteroidal, natural and synthetic, not be utilized during pregnancy. There is no proof that they are beneficial, and there is good evidence that the nonsteroidal estrogens may produce fetal genital tract anomalies and disease.

RECOMMENDED READING

Bibbo, N., et al. Followup study of male and female offspring of DES exposed mothers. *Obstet. Gynecol.* 49:1, 1977.

Cullins, S.L., Pridjian, G., Sutherland, C.M. Goldenhar's syndrome associated with tamoxifen given to the mother during gestation. *J.A.M.A.* 271:1905, 1994.

Herbst, A.L., and Bern, H.A., eds. *Developmental Effects of Diethylstilbestrol (DES) in Pregnancy.* New York: Thieme-Stratton, 1981.

Hornsby, P.P., Wilcox, A.J., Weinberg, C.R., and Herbst, A.L. Effects on the menstrual cycle of in utero exposure to diethylstilbestrol. *Am. J. Obstet. Gynecol.* 170:709, 1994.

Jefferies, J.A., et al. Structural anomalies of the cervix and vagina in women enrolled in the Diethylstilbestrol Adenosis (DESAD) Project. *Am. J. Obstet. Gynecol.* 148:59, 1984.

Kaufman, R.H., et al. Upper genital tract abnormalities and pregnancy outcome in diethylstilbestrol-exposed progeny. *Am. J. Obstet. Gynecol.* 148:973, 1984.

Ludmir, J., Landon, M.B., Gabbe, S.G., Samuels, P., and Mennuti, M.T. Management of the diethylstilbestrol-exposed pregnant patient: a prospective study. *Am. J. Obstet. Gynecol.* 157:665, 1987.

Melnick, S., Cole, P., Anderson, D., and Herbst, A. Rates and risks of diethylstilbestrol-related clear-cell adenocarcinoma of the vagina and cervix. *N. Engl. J. Med.* 316:514, 1987.

Robboy, S.J., et al. Increased incidence of cervical and vaginal dysplasia in 3,980 diethylstilbestrol-exposed young women. *J.A.M.A.* 252:2979, 1984.

Sandberg, E.C., et al. Pregnancy outcome in women exposed to diethylstilbestrol in utero. *Am. J. Obstet. Gynecol.* 140:194, 1981.

Senekjian, E.K., Potkul, R.K., Frey, K., Herbst, A.L. Infertility among daughters either exposed or not exposed to diethylstilbestrol. *Am. J. Obstet. Gynecol.* 158:493, 1988.

Stillman, R.J. In utero exposure to diethylstilbestrol: Adverse effects on the reproductive tract and reproductive performance in male and female offspring. *Am. J. Obstet. Gynecol.* 142:905, 1982.

Wilcox, A.J., Baird, D.D., Weinberg, C.R., Hornsby, P.P., and Herbst, A.L. Fertility in men exposed prenatally to diethylstilbestrol. *N. Engl. J. Med.* 332:1411, 1995.

Wilson, J.G., and Brent, R.L. Are female sex hormones teratogenic? *Am. J. Obstet. Gynecol.* 141:567, 1981.

Ethacrynic Acid (Edecrin®)

INDICATIONS AND RECOMMENDATIONS

The use of ethacrynic acid is relatively contraindicated during pregnancy because other therapeutic agents are preferable. It is a loop diuretic with activity similar to that of furosemide. The major complications associated with the use of ethacrynic acid in pregnancy are ototoxicity and hypokalemic alkalosis. These sequelae have been observed in both pregnant women and their offspring.

Maternal use of ethacrynic acid has been implicated as the cause of fetal polyhydramnios, neonatal polyuria, and nephrolithiasis. The cause of the nephrolithiasis was hypothesized to be drug-induced hypercalciuria, similar to that seen in premature infants exposed chronically to furosemide. In this case, the fetus had also been exposed to nifedipine, also known to increase urinary calcium during the last 3 weeks of gestation, after the polyhydramnios was documented.

It should be noted that reports describing the uneventful use of this drug during pregnancy have been published. If a loop diuretic is indicated for an obstetric patient, furosemide is the drug of choice.

RECOMMENDED READING

Finnerty, F.A. Hypertension in pregnancy. *Clin. Obstet. Gynecol.* 18:145, 1975.

Fischer, A.F., Parker, B.R., and Stevenson, D.K. Nephrolithiasis following in utero diuretic exposure: an unusual case. *Pediatrics* 81:712, 1988.

Fort, A.T., Morrison, J.C., and Fish, S.A. Iatrogenic hypokalemia of pregnancy by furosemide and ethacrynic acid. *J. Reprod. Med.* 6:207, 1971.

Harrison, K.A. Ethacrynic acid in blood transfusion—its effects on plasma volume and urine flow in severe anaemia in pregnancy. *Br. Med. J.* 4:84, 1986.

Jackson, E.K. Diuretics. Chapter 29 in *Goodman and Gilman's The Pharmacological Basis of Therapeutics* (9th ed.), J.G. Hardman and L.E. Limbird, eds. New York: McGraw-Hill, 1996. Pp. 697–701.

Jones, H.C. Intrauterine ototoxicity—a case report and review of the literature. *J. Natl. Med. Assoc.* 65:201, 1973.

Young, B.K., and Haft, J.I. Treatment of pulmonary edema with ethacrynic acid during labor. *Am. J. Obstet. Gynecol.* 107:330, 1970.

Ethambutol (Myambutol®)

INDICATIONS AND RECOMMENDATIONS

Ethambutol is recommended as an adjunct to isoniazid in the treatment of active tuberculosis in pregnancy. It is a synthetic tuberculostatic agent that is used in conjunction with other antitubercular drugs because of the rapid development of resistance when it is used alone.

SPECIAL CONSIDERATIONS IN PREGNANCY

Ethambutol appears to have no maternal effects unique to pregnancy. Large-scale studies of women who received combination isoniazid-ethambutol therapy during pregnancy indicate that in the usual antitubercular dosages the treatment is not associated with an increase in fetal anomalies when compared to untreated mothers.

In a review of 650 women who received ethambutol during 655 pregnancies, 14 infants or fetuses with congenital anomalies were found, for an incidence of approximately 2%. This rate is similar to that observed in the general population. No pattern to the anomalies was noted, and the rates of stillbirth and prematurity were not increased.

DOSAGE

The usual adult dose is 15 mg/kg/day in a single dose, given in combination with isoniazid, for a total of 18–24 months.

ADVERSE EFFECTS

Ethambutol use is relatively free of side effects. The most important adverse reaction is optic neuritis, which occurs primarily in patients who receive more than 25 mg/kg/day or in those with renal impairment. It appears gradually, usually as blurred vision, color blindness, and restriction of visual fields, and is generally reversible with prompt discontinuation of therapy. Hyperuricemia due to impaired urinary excretion of uric acid may occur. Other side effects include diminished visual acuity, rash, and drug fever.

MECHANISM OF ACTION

The precise mechanism of action of ethambutol is unknown, but it appears to be related to inhibition of incorporation of mycolic acid into the mycobacterial cell wall. It has no effect on bacteria other than mycobacteria. Primary resistance among mycobacteria is rare, but resistance develops rapidly in vivo when the drug is used alone.

ABSORPTION AND BIOTRANSFORMATION

About 80% of an oral dose is absorbed. The drug is concentrated in erythrocytes, which may serve as a depot from which ethambutol slowly enters the plasma. Of the absorbed dose, nearly 100% is recovered in the urine within 24 hours, 80% as unchanged ethambutol. The half-life is 3–4 hours and increases significantly with renal failure.

RECOMMENDED READING

Bobrowitz, I.D. Ethambutol in pregnancy. *Chest* 66:20, 1974.

Good, J.T., Jr., et al. Tuberculosis in association with pregnancy. *Am. J. Obstet. Gynecol.* 140:492, 1981.

Lewat, M.D., et al. Ethambutol in pregnancy: observations on embryogenesis. *Chest* 6:25, 1974.

Mandell, G.L., and Petri, Jr., W.A. Antimicrobial agents: drugs used in the chemotherapy of tuberculosis and leprosy. Chapter 44 in *Goodman and Gilman's The Pharmacological Basis of Therapeutics* (9th ed.), J.G. Hardman and L.E. Limbird, eds. New York: McGraw-Hill, 1996. Pp. 1161–1162.

Scheinhorn, D.J., and Angelillo, V.A. Antituberculosis therapy in pregnancy: risks to the fetus. *West. J. Med.* 127:195, 1977.

Snider, D.E., et al. Treatment of tuberculosis during pregnancy. *Am. Rev. Resp. Dis.* 122:65, 1980.

Snider, D. Pregnancy and tuberculosis. *Chest* 86:10S, 1984.

Ethchlorvynol (Placidyl®)

INDICATIONS AND RECOMMENDATIONS

The use of ethchlorvynol is relatively contraindicated during pregnancy because other therapeutic agents are preferable. It is used primarily as a hypnotic agent in the treatment of insomnia. This drug offers no therapeutic advantage over barbiturate or nonbarbiturate sedatives. Little is known about its effects on the pregnant woman or fetus. In dogs, it has been shown to achieve significant fetal blood levels within 90 minutes of maternal ingestion. Symptoms resembling congenital narcotic withdrawal have been described in the human newborn after the mother has ingested ethchlorvynol.

No sedative has been found to be absolutely safe during pregnancy as most cross the placenta and produce sedation and withdrawal symptoms in the newborn. Should such therapy be required during pregnancy, phenobarbital may be used (see "Phenobarbital").

RECOMMENDED READING

Hobbs, W.R., Rall, T.W., and Verdoorn, T.A. Hypnotics and sedatives; ethanol. Chapter 17 in *Goodman and Gilman's The Pharmacological Basis of Therapeutics* (9th ed.), J.G. Hardman and L.E. Limbird, eds. New York: McGraw-Hill, 1996. Pp. 381–382.

Hume, A.S., Williams, J.M., and Douglas, B.H. Disposition of ethchlorvynol in maternal blood, fetal blood, amniotic fluid and chorionic fluid. *J. Reprod. Med.* 6:229, 1971.

Rumack, B.H., and Walravens, P.A. Neonatal withdrawal following maternal ingestion of ethchlorvynol. *Pediatrics* 52:714, 1973.

Ethosuximide (Zarontin®)

INDICATIONS AND RECOMMENDATIONS

Ethosuximide may be administered to pregnant women who require treatment for absence seizures. This condition is rare in women of childbearing age, so the drug's effects on the fetus have not been studied in depth. If absence seizures persist during childbearing years and require treatment, therapy with ethosuximide may be continued through pregnancy. Use of ethosuximide is preferred over the use of trimethadione during pregnancy.

SPECIAL CONSIDERATIONS IN PREGNANCY

In a study of 10 pregnant women taking ethosuximide for the treatment of seizures during pregnancy, the fetal/maternal serum concentration ratio was 0.97, indicating that the fetus is exposed to similar drug concentrations as the mother. Of the 13 infants born to these mothers, two had major malformations (hare lip and bilateral clefting). The number of minor malformations was higher in the treated group than in the controls. The significance of these data is difficult to determine because all but two of the women were on multi-drug therapy including phenobarbital, primidone, phenytoin, and carbamazepine.

Breast milk concentrations of ethosuximide are similar to those in maternal serum (milk/serum ratio = 0.86). Nursed infants have been reported to maintain serum levels of 15–40 µg/ml.

DOSAGE

The initial dose should be 500 mg/day, which may be slowly increased by 250 mg increments until seizures are controlled or up to 20 mg/kg/day. Dosage should be adjusted to maintain a therapeutic plasma level of 40–100 µg/ml.

ADVERSE EFFECTS

Side effects include drowsiness, headache, hiccup, euphoria, and disequilibrium. Ethosuximide may cause local irritation of the stomach, with anorexia, gastric discomfort, nausea, and vomiting. These problems often occur at the onset of therapy, are usually transient, and are not clearly dose-related. Other reported associations include urticarial rash, Stevens-Johnson syndrome, a lupus-like syndrome, and, rarely, leukopenia, pancytopenia, and aplastic anemia.

MECHANISM OF ACTION

Ethosuximide reduces low threshold calcium ion currents (T currents) in thalamic neurons, the neurons that play an important role in the generation of the characteristic electroencephalographic patterns of absence seizures.

ABSORPTION AND BIOTRANSFORMATION

Absorption is fairly rapid and complete from the alimentary tract, with peak plasma levels occurring within 3 hours after a single oral dose. It has been demonstrated that ethosuximide is absorbed faster from a syrup preparation than from capsules. It is fairly uniformly distributed throughout the body, except in adipose tissue, where levels are lower than elsewhere. The drug is minimally bound to plasma and spinal fluid proteins. Twenty-five percent of ethosuximide is excreted unchanged in the urine. The remaining drug is metabolized in the liver. The adult plasma half-life is between 40 and 50 hours.

RECOMMENDED READING

Kuhnz, W., et al. Ethosuximide in epileptic women during pregnancy and lactation period. Placental transfer, serum concentrations in nursed infants and clinical status. *Br. J. Clin. Pharmacol.* 18:671, 1984.

McNamara, J.O. Drugs effective in the therapy of epilepsies. Chapter 20 in *Goodman and Gilman's The Pharmacological Basis of Therapeutics* (9th ed.), J.G. Hardman and L.E. Limbird, eds. New York: McGraw-Hill, 1996. Pp. 475–476.

Sullivan, F.M., and McElhatton, P.R. A comparison of the teratogenic activity of the antiepileptic drugs carbamazepine, clonazepam, ethosuximide, phenobarbital, phenytoin, and primidone
in mice. *Toxicol. Appl. Pharmacol.* 40:365, 1977.

Wilder, B.J., and Bruni, J. *Seizure Disorders: A Pharmacological Approach to Treatment.* New York: Raven Press, 1981.

Woodbury, D.M., Penry, J.K., and Pippenger, C.E. *Antiepileptic
Drugs* (2nd ed.). New York: Raven Press, 1982.

Evans Blue Dye (T1824)

INDICATIONS AND RECOMMENDATIONS

Evans blue dye, an azo dye used in the determination of maternal plasma volume, may be used during pregnancy. Although
one series of studies has suggested teratogenicity in rats, another found that intravenously injected Evans blue dye did not
appear in the amniotic fluid or cord blood at term. Although
Evans blue dye has also been injected intraamniotically to diagnose rupture of membranes and as a marker when perform-
ing amniocentesis in multiple gestations, indigo carmine is
more commonly used for this purpose.

SPECIAL CONSIDERATIONS IN PREGNANCY

In a series of experiments in which 1 ml of a 1% solution of
various azo dyes was injected subcutaneously into female rats
on days 1, 8, and 9 of gestation, Evans blue dye was associated
with a 10% maternal death rate, a 25% fetal reabsorption rate,
and a 14% malformation rate among surviving fetuses. These
rates were higher than those observed with any of the 14 other
dyes utilized, with the exception of trypan blue. The malformations seen were primarily in the central nervous system. No information is available as to the mechanism of these problems,
nor are dose–response curves described. Nevertheless, it would
appear prudent to avoid the use of this agent during the time of
organogenesis.

In a single case report, bluish, followed by greenish, discoloration of the neonatal skin followed an apparent subcutaneous
fetal injection of Evans blue dye at the time of amniocentesis.
No adverse effects were noted.

An association between reduced intravascular volume and
both hypertensive disorders of pregnancy and intrauterine
growth disorders has led to the use of plasma volume determination as an investigative tool in patients at risk for these complications. Evans blue dye is the standard agent used in such
measurements. There is evidence that this dye may disappear
more rapidly from the circulation of women with preeclampsia
than from that of normal pregnant women. Adverse pregnancy
effects of the intravenous use of Evans blue dye have not been
reported.

DOSAGE

With the patient lying on her side, Evans blue dye is injected
intravenously in a known quantity (usually 2 ml of 0.5% solu-

tion). Preinjection and timed postinjection blood samples are obtained. These are then centrifuged and the optical density of the plasma is measured, optimally at two different wavelengths. Optical density values are compared with those obtained when samples of the same lot of dye are diluted with pooled plasma, so that the concentration of the dye can be calculated from the following formula:

Plasma volume (ml) = dye injected (mg)
÷ concentration obtained (mg/ml)

Investigators have generally either extrapolated back to time zero or used the dye concentration at 10 minutes after injection to calculate plasma volume.

ADVERSE EFFECTS

No information is available.

MECHANISM OF ACTION

See "Dosage."

ABSORPTION AND BIOTRANSFORMATION

Little information is available concerning the half-life of Evans blue dye in the circulation. It is known to be strongly protein-bound. In one study, 5% of the dye had disappeared from the circulation by 1 hour after injection and 41% by 24 hours. Another study demonstrated a linear decline in plasma concentrations from 10 to 60 minutes after intravenous injection.

RECOMMENDED READING

Atlay, R.D., and Sutherst, J.R. Premature rupture of the fetal membranes confirmed by intraamniotic injection of dye (Evans blue T1824). *Am. J. Obstet. Gynecol.* 108:993, 1970.

Brans Y.W., Dutton, E.B., Schwartz, C.A., Carey, K.D. Dilution kinetics of chemicals used for estimation of water content of body compartments in perinatal medicine. *Pediatr. Res.* 25:377, 1989.

Brown, M.A., Mitar, D.A., and Whitworth, J.A. Measurement of plasma volume in pregnancy. *Clin. Sci.* 83:29, 1992.

Campbell, D.M., and Campbell, A.J. Evans blue disappearance rate in normal and pre-eclamptic pregnancy. *Clin. Exp. Hypertension* B2:163, 1983.

Chesley, L.C., and Duffus, G.M. Posture and apparent plasma volume in late pregnancy. *J. Obstet. Gynaecol. Br. Commw.* 78:406, 1971.

Durocher, J., and Moutquin, J. Standardisation de la méthode de mesure du volume serique par le bleu Evans, chez la femme enceinte. *Clin. Biochem.* 16:234, 1983.

Giacoia, G.P. Green baby: a consequence of intrauterine exposure to Evan's blue dye. *Am. J. Perinatol.* 5:234, 1988.

Goodlin, R.C., et al. Clinical signs of normal plasma volume expansion during pregnancy. *Am. J. Obstet. Gynecol.* 145:1001, 1983.

Hays, P.M., Cruikshank, D.P., and Dunn, L.J. Plasma volume determination in normal and preeclamptic pregnancies. *Am. J. Obstet. Gynecol.* 151:958, 1985.

Sibai, B.M., et al. Plasma volume determination in pregnancies complicated by chronic hypertension and intrauterine fetal demise. *Obstet. Gynecol.* 60:174, 1982.

Soffronoff, E.C., Kauffmann, B.M., and Connaughton, J.F. Intravascular volume determinations in hypertensive diseases of pregnancy. *Am. J. Obstet. Gynecol.* 127:4, 1977.

Thompson, K.J., Hirsheimer, A., Gibson, J.G., II, Evans, W.A., Jr. Studies on the circulation in pregnancy: III. Blood volume changes in normal pregnant women. *Am. J. Obstet. Gynecol.* 36:48, 1938.

Wilson, J.G. Teratogenic activity of several azo dyes chemically related to trypan blue. *Anat. Rec.* 123:313, 1955.

Famciclovir (Famvir®)

INDICATIONS AND RECOMMENDATIONS

Famciclovir is contraindicated in pregnancy because other therapeutic agents are preferable. Famciclovir is an antiviral agent indicated for the treatment of acute herpes zoster (shingles) and recurrent episodes of genital herpes. Shingles poses no threat to maternal or fetal health and need not be treated during pregnancy. Should treatment be necessary for a recurrent episode of genital herpes during pregnancy, acyclovir, for which there are more clinical data, would be the drug of choice.

RECOMMENDED READING

Hayden, F.G. Antimicrobial agents: antiviral agents. Chapter 50 in *Goodman and Gilman's The Pharmacological Basis of Therapeutics* (9th ed.), J.G. Hardman and L.E. Limbird, eds. New York: McGraw-Hill, 1996. Pp. 1193–1204.

Nelson, C.T., and Demmler, G.J. Cytomegalovirus infection in the pregnant mother, fetus, and newborn infant. *Clin. Perinatol.* 24:151, 1997

Whitley, R.J., and Kimberlin, D.W. Treatment of viral infections during pregnancy and the neonatal period. *Clin. Perinatol.* 24: 267, 1997.

Felbamate (Felbatol®)

Felbamate is an anticonvulsant used as a second-line drug in the treatment of partial seizures. There is little or no information available regarding felbamate's effects in pregnancy other than one study demonstrating that it crosses the rat placenta. However, because of the known risk of aplastic anemia and liver failure in patients taking this drug, it is rarely used except when other treatments fail and its use should be avoided in pregnancy if at all possible.

RECOMMENDED READING

Adusumalli, V.E., Yang, J.T., Wong, K.K., et al. Felbamate pharmacokinetics in the rat, rabbit and dog. *Drug Metab. Dispos.* 19:1116, 1991.

McNamara, J.O. Drugs effective in the therapy of the epilepsies. Chapter 20 in *Goodman and Gilman's The Pharmacological Basis of Therapeutics* (9th ed.), J.G. Hardman and L.E. Limbird, eds. New York: McGraw-Hill, 1996. P. 481.

Wallace Laboratories. Felbatol (felbamate): Entry in *Physicians Desk Reference* (52nd ed.). Montvale, NJ: Medical Economics, 1998. Pp. 2960–2964.

Fluconazole (Diflucan®)

INDICATIONS AND RECOMMENDATIONS

Fluconazole is contraindicated during the first trimester of pregnancy if given in high dose for treatment of systemic fungal infections.

Animal studies have shown that fluconazole can be teratogenic in high doses. Pregnant rats given doses equivalent to 20–40 times a usual human dose produced pups with structural abnormalities, including supernumerary or wavy ribs, dilatation of the renal pelvis, delays in ossification, cleft palate, and abnormal craniofacial ossification. Pregnant rabbits given similar doses had an increased incidence of abortion but no fetal anomalies.

Human data include one report describing three infants (two siblings) with craniofacial, skeletal, and cardiac defects born to two women who received high doses (800 mg/day) of fluconazole throughout the first trimester of pregnancy for treatment of disseminated *Coccidioides immitis*. Their anomalies were similar to those observed in animal studies, including thin, wavy ribs and ossification defects. High-dose fluconazole has been given to a pregnant woman from the 16th week of gestation, for a total of 50 days, for the treatment of *Candida albicans* sepsis without apparent deleterious effects to the fetus.

Studies of its use at low doses and in short durations for the treatment of vaginal candidiasis appear to indicate that such use is not associated with an increased incidence of congenital anomaly, spontaneous abortion, or other adverse outcome of pregnancy. One published prospective study in humans reported no fetal anomalies among the 44 births of 43 women exposed to fluconazole, with all but one exposed to a single 150 mg dose. Unfortunately, no information regarding the gestational week of exposure was obtained. A second prospective study examined first-trimester exposure to low-dose, short-term fluconazole treatment in 226 women. The results showed no significantly increased risk of congenital anomaly or other major adverse pregnancy outcome.

In spite of the promising data regarding use of low-dose fluconazole in the first trimester of pregnancy, the case reports documenting congenital anomalies similar to those seen in animal studies during pregnancy would indicate that fluconazole use should be avoided in the first trimester. However, the data do indicate that low-dose, short-duration exposure during the first trimester is not necessarily an indication for termination of pregnancy.

RECOMMENDED READING

Bennett, J.E. Antimicrobial agents: antifungal agents. Chapter 49 in *Goodman and Gilman's The Pharmacological Basis of Therapeutics* (9th ed.), J.G. Hardman and L.E. Limbird, eds. New York: McGraw-Hill, 1996. Pp. 1183–1184.

Inman, W., et al. Safety of fluconazole in the treatment of vaginal candidiasis. A prescription-event monitoring study, with special reference to the outcome of pregnancy. *Eur. J. Clin. Pharmacol.* 46:115, 1994.

Lee, B.E., et al. Congenital malformations in an infant born to a woman treated with fluconazole. *Pediatr. Infect. Dis. J.* 11:1062, 1992.

Mastroiacovo, P., et al. Prospective assessment of pregnancy outcomes after first-trimester exposure to fluconazole. *Am. J. Obstet. Gynecol.* 175:1645, 1996.

Pursley, T.J., et al. Fluconazole-induced congenital anomalies in three infants. *Clin. Infect. Dis.* 22:336, 1996.

Wiesinger, E.C., et al. Fluconazole in *Candida albicans* sepsis during pregnancy: case report and review of literature. *Infection* 24:263, 1996.

Fluoroquinolone Antibiotics: Ciprofloxacin (Cipro®), Enoxacin (Penetrex®), Lomefloxacin (Maxaquin®), Norfloxacin (Noroxin®), Ofloxacin (Floxin®)

INDICATIONS AND RECOMMENDATIONS

The fluoroquinolone antibiotics are antimicrobial agents frequently prescribed for the treatment of a wide range of infections. The older quinolones, such as nalidixic acid, had limited utility due to narrow spectra and rapid development of bacterial resistance. The new fluorinated 4-quinolones have rapidly gained acceptance in the general population due to broad-spectrum antimicrobial activity, excellent bioavailability and tissue penetration, and relative lack of side effects. The agents are effective in the treatment of many respiratory, genitourinary, gastrointestinal, skin, soft tissue, and bone infections. However, reported use in pregnancy to date has been limited and theoretical concerns of mutagenesis and carcinogenesis have been expressed. Although available information is reassuring, if antibiotic agents with better documentation of safe use in pregnancy are an option, then use of the quinolones should be avoided.

SPECIAL CONSIDERATIONS IN PREGNANCY

Concern regarding malformations, particularly of the musculoskeletal system, has been raised by pediatric reports of arthralgia, joint swelling, and gait abnormalities in children exposed to fluoroquinolones. In addition, at high doses the quinolones will inhibit type II topoisomerase, an enzyme involved in DNA replication. Human reports are limited to a study of 38 pregnant women self-reporting to a registry for advice following treatment with ciprofloxacin or norfloxacin. Thirty-five of the women were exposed during the first trimester. Follow-up was performed by interview following birth and at a mean age of 27 months, and there were no congenital or developmental abnormalities reported by the mothers or pediatricians.

The fluoroquinolones have been documented to cross the placenta in human and animal studies. In humans, amniotic fluid concentrations of ciprofloxacin were 57% to 1000% and of ofloxacin were 35% to 257% of maternal serum concentrations. In macaque monkeys embryonic tissue levels are similar to maternal plasma levels.

Ciprofloxacin is found in breast milk in rabbits following an intravenous dose, at mean levels 3 times greater than serum levels. In developing animals, exposure to fluoroquinolones has been shown to induce cartilage damage. Therefore, until further information is available, breast-feeding is not recommended during therapy with these agents.

DOSAGE

Usual oral doses are 200–400 mg every 12 hours for ofloxacin and enoxacin, 400 mg every 12 hours for norfloxacin, 400 mg every 24 hours for lomefloxacin, and 250–750 mg every 12 hours for ciprofloxacin. The intravenous dose of ciprofloxacin or ofloxacin is 200–400 mg every 12 hours, administered over a minimum of 60 minutes. Monitoring of serum levels is recommended for patients with renal impairment.

ADVERSE EFFECTS

The fluoroquinolones are usually very well tolerated. The most common side effects are nausea, diarrhea, abdominal discomfort, headache, dizziness, skin rash, and photosensitivity. Serious complications are rare. Arthralgia, joint swelling, and gait abnormalities have been observed in young children and juvenile animals exposed to the new quinolones. Therefore pediatric use has been discouraged.

MECHANISM OF ACTION

The quinolones inhibit the action of the bacterial enzyme DNA gyrase. This enzyme is involved in the proper unwinding of DNA during replication. This enzyme is not found in mammalian cells, although a structurally related eukaryotic enzyme, type II topoisomerase, is inhibited at much higher concentrations. The fluoroquinolones are bactericidal to most gram-negative organisms. Ciprofloxacin and ofloxacin have good activity against many gram-positive organisms and many intracellular organisms such as *Legionella, Mycoplasma,* and *Chlamydia.* They have limited efficacy against anaerobic organisms.

ABSORPTION AND BIOTRANSFORMATION

With the exception of norfloxacin, good serum levels are achieved with oral administration, with peak levels at 1–3 hours. Food may delay the time to peak concentration but will not impair absorption. The serum half-life is 3–5 hours for norfloxacin and ciprofloxacin, 10–11 hours for perfloxacin and fleroxacin.

Bioavailability ranges from 50% to 95% and tissue penetration is excellent. Drug elimination is renal and hepatic. Intravenous formulations are available for ciprofloxacin and ofloxacin.

RECOMMENDED READING

Andriole, V.T. *Infectious Diseases.* Philadelphia: W.B. Saunders, 1992. Pp. 244–253.

Aramayona J.J., Mora J., Fraile L.J., Garcia M.A., Abadia A.R., et al. Penetration of enrofloxacin and ciprofloxacin into breast milk, and pharmacokinetics of the drugs in lactating rabbits and neonatal offspring. *Am. J. Vet. Res.* 57:547, 1996.

Berkovitch, M., Pastuszak, A., Gazarian, M., Lewis, M., and Koren, G. Safety of the new quinolones in pregnancy. *Obstet. Gynecol.* 84:535, 1994.

Giamarellou, H., Kolokythas, E., Petrikkos, G., Gazis, J., Aravatinos, D., and Skikakis, P. Pharmacokinetics of three newer quinolones in pregnant and lactating women. *Am. J. Med.* 87 (Suppl 5A):49S, 1989.

Hummler, H., Richter, W.F., and Hendrick, A.G. Developmental toxicity of fleroxacin and comparative pharmacokinetics of four fluoroquinolones in the cynomolgus macaque. *Toxicol. Appl. Pharmacol.* 122:34, 1993.

Mantel, G.L., and Petri, W.A. Antimicrobial agents: sulfonamides, trimethoprim-sulfamethoxazole, quinolones, and agents for urinary tract infections. Chapter 44 in *Goodman and Gilman's The Pharmacological Basis of Therapeutics* (9th ed.), J.G. Hardman and L.E. Limbird, eds. New York: McGraw-Hill, 1996. Pp. 1065–1068.

Gabapentin (Neurontin®)

INDICATIONS AND RECOMMENDATIONS

Gabapentin is an anticonvulsant medication used as adjunctive therapy in the treatment of partial seizures with and without secondary generalization. Based on the lack of data regarding use in pregnancy, gabapentin should be avoided during pregnancy unless the clinical situation is severe and alternatives are ineffective or unavailable.

SPECIAL CONSIDERATIONS IN PREGNANCY

Little information is available regarding gabapentin's use in human pregnancy. The manufacturer reported fetotoxicity and teratogenicity in rats and increased fetal losses in rabbits. A published study of various animal species did not report teratogenicity or toxicity. There is a published description of two cases of cranial abnormalities (holoprosencephaly, absence of an auditory canal) in offspring exposed to gabapentin in utero.

DOSAGE

Gabapentin is added to other agents when partial seizures are not adequately controlled. The drug is available in 100, 300, and 400 mg capsules. The starting dose is generally 100 mg 3 times daily, which can then be titrated rapidly to the usual effective dose range of 900–1800 mg total daily dose in three divided doses.

ADVERSE EFFECTS

Side effects include somnolence, dizziness, ataxia, and fatigue, all of which usually resolve within 2 weeks of starting therapy.

ABSORPTION AND BIOTRANSFORMATION

Gabapentin is well absorbed after oral administration and food has no effect on its absorption. The drug is not appreciably metabolized and is eliminated by the kidneys, with a half-life of 5–9 hours. There is no appreciable interaction with absorption and biotransformation of other anticonvulsants.

RECOMMENDED READING

McNamara, J.O. Drugs effective in the therapy of the epilepsies. Chapter 20 in *Goodman and Gilman's The Pharmacological Basis of Therapeutics* (9th ed.), J.G. Hardman and L.E. Limbird, eds. New York: McGraw-Hill, 1996. P. 480.

Parke-Davis Pharmaceutical Company. Neurontin (Gabapentin capsules): Entry in *Physicians Desk Reference* (52nd ed.). Montvale, NJ: Medical Economics, 1998. Pp. 2110–2113.

Petrere, J.A., and Anderson, J.A. Developmental toxicity studies in mice, rats, and rabbits with the anticonvulsant gabapentin. *Fund. Appl. Toxicol.* 23:585, 1994.

Rosa, F. Holoprosencephaly and antiepileptic exposures (letter). *Teratology* 51:230, 1995.

Gamma Benzene Hexachloride, Lindane (Kwell®)

INDICATIONS AND RECOMMENDATIONS

Gamma benzene hexachloride may be administered to pregnant women for the treatment of scabies and lice. Head lice *(Pediculus humanus capitis)* and crab lice *(Phthirus pubis)* are treated with the cream, lotion, or shampoo form of the drug. Scabies *(Sarcoptes scabiei)* is treated with the cream or lotion form. Treatment should be such that only a minimal amount of drug is absorbed percutaneously.

SPECIAL CONSIDERATIONS IN PREGNANCY

There is a single case report of fetal deaths in a twin pregnancy at 16 weeks, in which the mother drank a large amount of lindane in an apparent suicide attempt. Although some studies have demonstrated embryotoxicity in mice and rats, there have thus far been no reports of adverse fetal effects associated with the topical use of gamma benzene hexachloride during pregnancy. Because it can be absorbed through the skin and is known to cause severe neurologic reactions in cases of overdosage, attempts should be made to minimize the amount of drug absorbed. For the treatment of scabies, the lotion or cream should be applied to dry, cool skin and washed off after 8 hours. Pediculosis should be treated with the shampoo, which must be rinsed thoroughly after application. Simultaneous application of lotions, ointments, or oils may enhance percutaneous absorption and should be avoided. Reapplication and retreatment should not be undertaken routinely.

DOSAGE

In the treatment of scabies a thin layer of the cream or lotion should be applied to the entire skin surface. It should be allowed to remain on the skin for 8 hours and then the skin should be washed thoroughly. A second or third application may be made at weekly intervals if necessary.

In the treatment of pediculosis, the affected and surrounding hairy areas should be wet with 30 ml shampoo. Water should then be added and the shampoo worked into a lather for at least 4 minutes. The area should then be rinsed thoroughly and dried with a towel. A fine-tooth comb should be used to remove any remaining nit shells. If necessary, the treatment may be repeated in 24 hours but not more than twice in a week.

ADVERSE EFFECTS

Side effects are rare but may be dangerous when they occur. Fatal cases of aplastic anemia have resulted from prolonged exposure to the vaporized drug. In addition, very high doses applied percutaneously or taken orally have produced convulsions in humans.

MECHANISM OF ACTION

The mechanism of action of gamma benzene hexachloride is similar to that of DDT. It is absorbed through the exoskeletons of many arthropods and acts directly on their nervous tissue to produce convulsions and death. It is an excellent miticide and pediculicide that produces relief of symptoms usually within 24 hours of application.

ABSORPTION AND BIOTRANSFORMATION

The exact pharmacokinetics of gamma benzene hexachloride are unknown. The drug is absorbed through the skin. After local application of a 0.3% lotion, it reaches levels of 2–6 ng/ml in patients with intact skin and 30–200 ng/ml in patients with excoriated skin. The preparations available in the United States are 1% concentrations and would be expected to produce correspondingly higher levels. The toxic level measured in a child who had ingested the drug and had severe neurologic sequelae was 86 g/ml.

RECOMMENDED READING

Konje, J.C., Otolorin, E.O., Sotunmbi, P.T., and Ladipo, O.A. Insecticide poisoning in pregnancy. A case report. *J. Reprod. Med.* 37: 992, 1992.

Lange, M., Nitzsche, K., and Zesch, A. Percutaneous absorption of lindane in healthy volunteers and scabies patients. *Arch. Dermatol. Res.* 271:387, 1981.

Lee, B., and Groth, P. Scabies: transcutaneous poisoning during treatment. *Pediatrics* 59:643, 1977.

McNutt, T.L., and Harris, C. Lindane embryotoxicity and differential alteration of cysteine and glutathione levels in rat embryos and visceral yolk sacs. *Reprod. Toxicol.* 8:351, 1994.

Rasmussen, J.E. Lindane: a prudent approach. *Arch. Dermatol.* 123:1008, 1987.

Schacter, B. Treatment of scabies and pediculosis with lindane preparations: an evaluation. *J. Am. Acad. Dermatol.* 5:517, 1981.

Sircar, S., and Lahiri, P. Lindane (τ-HCH) causes reproductive failure and fetotoxicity in mice. *Toxicology* 59:171, 1989.

Zesch, A., Nitzsche, K., and Lange, M. Demonstration of the percutaneous resorption of a lipophilic pesticide and its possible storage in the human body. *Arch. Dermatol. Res.* 273:43, 1982.

Gancyclovir (Cytovene®)

INDICATIONS AND RECOMMENDATIONS

Gancyclovir is contraindicated in pregnancy. It is used for the treatment of cytomegalovirus (CMV) retinitis in patients who are immunocompromised. It has a narrow therapeutic index with significant hematologic toxicity. It is known to cross the placenta, probably by simple diffusion. Because of its toxicity, there are no studies investigating its use during pregnancy. One attempt to prevent CMV infection in a fetus by maternal treatment was ineffective in preventing the fetal infection; the infant was stillborn.

RECOMMENDED READING

Gilstrap, L.C., et al. The transfer of the nucleoside analog ganciclovir across the perfused human placenta. *Am. J. Obstet. Gynecol.* 170:967, 1994.

Nicolini, U., et al. Prenatal diagnosis of congenital human cytomegalovirus infection. *Prenatal Diagn.* 14:906, 1994.

Gemfibrozil (Lopid®)

INDICATIONS AND RECOMMENDATIONS

Gemfibrozil is contraindicated in pregnancy because other therapeutic modalities are preferable. This drug is a fibric acid derivative that decreases serum triglycerides and very-low-density lipoprotein cholesterol and increases high-density lipoprotein cholesterol. It is used in the treatment of hypertriglyceridemia (types IV and V hyperlipidemias) in those who represent a risk of pancreatitis and who do not respond to diet therapy.

Gemfibrozil is known to cross the placenta, but there are no data regarding its effects on the human fetus. One case report documents a patient with severe hypertriglyceridemia who received gemfibrozil from 35 to 36 weeks gestation at which time she delivered a 2670-g infant whose 1-minute Apgar score was 9. No other information about the infant was given.

It is generally recommended that severe hypertriglyeridemia during pregnancy be treated with a careful restriction of calories and fat. For prevention of acute pancreatitis, hospitalization for intravenous fluid therapy and plasma exchange may be required.

RECOMMENDED READING

Perrone, G., and Critelli, C. Severe hypertriglyceridemia in pregnancy. A clinical case report. *Minerva Ginecologica* 48:573, 1996.

Saravanan, P., et al. Plasma exchange for dramatic gestational hyperlipidemic pancreatitis. *J. Clin. Gastroenterol.* 22:295, 1996.

Watts, G.F., et al. Management of patients with severe hypertriglyceridaemia during pregnancy: report of two cases with familial lipoprotein lipase deficiency. *Br. J. Obstet. Gynecol.* 99:163, 1992.

Witzham, J.L. Drugs used in the treatment of hyperlipoproteinemias. Chapter 36 in *Goodman and Gilman's The Pharmacological Basis of Therapeutics* (9th ed.), J.G. Hardman and L.E. Limbird, eds. New York: McGraw-Hill, 1996. Pp. 893–895.

Gentian Violet

INDICATIONS AND RECOMMENDATIONS

Gentian violet is relatively contraindicated in pregnancy because other therapeutic agents are preferable. When applied topically, this triphenylmethane (rosaniline) dye is bacteriostatic and bactericidal to gram-positive bacteria and many fungi. Gram-negative and acid-fast bacteria are very resistant. It is used for the treatment of vaginal candidiasis and has largely been replaced by other antifungal agents because of its propensity to stain skin and clothing. One study has demonstrated mouse embryotoxicity in vitro, but this has not been confirmed with in vivo studies. Gentian violet has not demonstrated teratogenicity in either rabbits or rats. The Collaborative Perinatal Project documented 40 pregnancies with exposure to gentian violet, four of which had malformations. One or two percent solutions of gentian violet to treat nipple thrush may cause irritation and oral mucous tissue ulceration in the breast-feeding infant. A 0.25% or 0.5% solution is nearly as efficacious and less irritating. Should treatment for *Candida* vaginitis become necessary during pregnancy, nystatin is the drug of choice.

RECOMMENDED READING

Buttar, H.S., Moffat J.H., Bura, C., and St-Vil, J. The in vitro embryotoxicity of gentian violet in pre-implantation mouse embryos. *Teratology* 41:541, 1990.

Heinonen, O.P., et al. *Birth Defects and Drugs in Pregnancy.* Littleton, MA: Wright-PSG, 1977. P. 302.

Uttar, A.R. Gentian violet treatment for thrush: can its use cause breastfeeding problems? *J. Hum. Lact.* 6:178, 1990.

Glucocorticosteroids: Betamethasone (Celestone®), Cortisone (Cortone® Hydrocortisone (Cortef®, Hydrocortone®, Solu-Cortef®), Methylprednisolone (Medrol®, Solu-Medrol®), Prednisolone, Prednisone (Deltasone®), Triamcinolone (Aristocort®, Kenalog®)

INDICATIONS AND RECOMMENDATIONS

Glucocorticosteroid therapy may be administered during pregnancy and lactation if it is medically indicated. These agents are used as replacement therapy for acute or chronic adrenal insufficiency, as suppressive therapy for congenital adrenal hyperplasia, and in the treatment of a large number of pathologic states as antiinflammatory agents. They are also commonly used in obstetrics for the prevention of respiratory distress syndrome (RDS) and intraventricular hemorrhage (IVH) in the neonate in situations in which premature delivery of the infant is likely.

SPECIAL CONSIDERATIONS IN PREGNANCY

Animal studies have shown a consistent link between maternal ingestion of corticosteroids and fetal malformations, especially cleft palate. Substantial data in humans do not indicate that corticosteroid use results in a significant increase in fetal malformations. However, there have been scattered reports of cleft palate, growth retardation, neonatal cataracts, and adrenal suppression in infants born to women exposed to steroids during pregnancy.

Maternal glucocorticoid therapy has been shown to decrease the incidence of mortality, RDS and IVH in the offspring of women who deliver their infants before 34 weeks. Dexamethasone and betamethasone are the preferred corticosteroids for this use because they readily cross the placenta in their biologically active forms. In addition, they have no mineralocorticoid activity, weak immunosuppressive activity, and a relatively long duration of action. The benefits of steroid use can be seen starting at 24 hours and lasting up to 7 days after treatment. In addition, the evidence suggests that the fetuses benefit even if treatment is begun less than 24 hours before delivery. All fetuses between 24 and 30 weeks gestation threatened with premature delivery are candidates for prenatal corticosteroid therapy. This treatment is not recommended for mothers expected to deliver after 34 weeks gestation because the risk of RDS and IVH is low. In preterm premature rupture of membranes at less than 30–32 weeks gestation in the absence of clinical chorioamnionitis, antenatal corticosteroid use is appropriate because of the high risk of IVH.

A fetal deficiency of 21-hydroxylase, an enzyme required for normal adrenal hormone secretion, predisposes a female fetus to congenital adrenal hyperplasia with prenatal development of ambiguous genitalia. Treatment with dexamethasone 20–25 mg/kg/day in 2–3 divided doses, begun before the 10th week of gestation and continued through term, is effective in reducing masculinization of the genitalia. Careful maternal monitoring should be performed. This fetal therapy spares the daughter and family the consequences of genital ambiguity including surgery, sex misassignment, and gender confusion.

Corticosteroid therapy may be necessary for the treatment of maternal diseases including rheumatoid arthritis, systemic lupus erythematosus, and asthma during pregnancy. Because fetal levels of prednisone are 8–10 times lower than maternal levels, prednisone is the glucocorticoid of choice to be given for women who take corticosteroids during pregnancy. If a pregnant woman has received chronic glucocorticoid therapy during pregnancy, she should receive stress doses for labor and delivery.

When administered for the treatment of maternal asthma, inhaled agents are preferable to oral corticosteroids because of their minimal systemic absorption. In one study of 824 pregnant women with asthma, maternal use of oral corticosteroids was independently associated with the occurrence of preeclampsia. Steroid dependent asthmatics, as well as gravidas treated with prednisone for phospholipid antibody syndrome, have been reported to have a greater likelihood of preterm PROM. Still, because of the significant morbidity of maternal asthma, risk–benefit considerations favor the use of oral steroids when indicated for severe asthma during pregnancy.

Studies have shown that small amounts of prednisone and prednisolone are detectable in breast milk. Following a 10 mg dose of prednisone, milk concentrations of prednisone and prednisolone after 2 hours were 0.03 and 0.002 mg/ml, respectively. Use of low-dose prednisone (less than 20 mg) is considered safe when breast-feeding.

DOSAGE

The dosage of glucocorticoids varies depending on the condition treated and the relative potency of the agent used. For acute adrenal insufficiency, after an initial intravenous bolus of 100 mg, hydrocortisone is given by continuous infusion at a rate of 100 mg q8h to approximate the maximum daily rate of cortisol secretion in response to stress. After stabilization, 25 mg IM may be given q6–8h. The usual dose of hydrocortisone for the treatment of chronic adrenal insufficiency is 20 mg every am and 10 mg every pm, which may be adjusted according to the patient's blood pressure and sense of well-being. Depending on the form of steroid given and the patient's electrolyte status, mineralocorticoids may need to be added.

Higher than physiologic doses are employed in the treatment of rheumatic disorders, renal diseases, allergic disease, autoimmune hemolytic anemia, renal transplantation, and other conditions that respond to therapeutic doses of corticosteroids.

The antenatal regimens for the prevention of RDS and IVH are betamethasone 12 mg IM q24h × 2 or dexamethasone 6 mg IM q12h × 4. These doses have been shown to deliver concentrations of steroid to the fetus that are comparable to physiologic stress levels of cortisol occurring after birth in untreated premature infants who develop RDS. Higher doses do not increase benefits.

ADVERSE EFFECTS

Side effects of corticosteroid use at supraphysiologic doses are often severe and may be life threatening. They include fluid and electrolyte imbalance, hyperglycemia, peptic ulcers (that may bleed or perforate), increased susceptibility to infections (including reactivation of latent tuberculosis), osteoporosis, psychosis, myopathy, striae, ecchymoses, acne, cataracts, and fat deposition characteristic of Cushing's syndrome. In addition, rapid withdrawal of corticosteroids after prolonged treatment can result in acute adrenal insufficiency. A less severe glucocorticoid withdrawal syndrome consists of fever, myalgia, arthralgia, and malaise. Inhaled corticosteroids have minimal systemic effects but have been reported to cause adrenal suppression and other metabolic changes, although significantly less than with oral therapy.

MECHANISM OF ACTION

Corticosteroids are a family of 21-carbon compounds. They appear to interact with specific receptor proteins in target tissues to regulate the effect of corticosteroid responsive genes and influence protein synthesis. Their physiologic effects are widespread. They stabilize lysosomal membranes, inhibiting the production and release of inflammatory mediators and decreasing chemotaxis. They also decrease mast cell activity and lymphocyte lysis, which consequently disturbs cell-mediated immunity.

Hematologic effects include granulocytosis (due to demargination of white blood cells), increased platelets, and decreased eosinophils.

Metabolic effects include increased peripheral gluconeogenesis, hepatic glycogenolysis, and hepatic gluconeogenesis. In the presence of growth hormone, corticosteroids promote lipolysis. Electrolyte changes include sodium and water retention, along with potassium loss in the urine.

ABSORPTION AND BIOTRANSFORMATION

Most corticosteroid compounds are well absorbed orally. Others are given parenterally to order to achieve high concentrations rapidly in bodily fluids. As a general rule, the glucocorticoids are metabolized by the sequential addition of oxygen or hydrogen atoms followed by conjugation to form water-soluble compounds that are excreted in the urine.

Approximately 10% to 20% of a dose of inhaled corticosteroids reaches the lung. Approximately 50% is deposited in the oral pharynx.

RECOMMENDED READING

Andersen, G.E., and Friis-Hansen, B. Hypercholesterolemia in the newborn: occurrence after antepartum treatment with betamethasone-phenobarbital-ritodrine for the prevention of the respiratory distress syndrome. *Pediatrics* 62:8, 1978.

Challis, J.R., Kendall, J.Z., and Robinson, J.S. The regulation of corticosteroids during late pregnancy and their role in parturition. *Biol. Reprod.* 16:57, 1977.

Collaborative Group on Antenatal Steroid Therapy. Effect of antenatal dexamethasone administration on the prevention of respiratory distress syndrome. *Am. J. Obstet. Gynecol.* 141:276, 1981.

Cowchock, F.S., Reece, E.A., Balabon, D., et al. Repeated fetal losses associated with antiphospholipid antibodies. *Am. J. Obstet. Gynecol.* 166:1318, 1992.

David, M., and Forest, M.G. Prenatal treatment of congenital adrenal hyperplasia resulting from 21-hydroxylase deficiency. *J. Pediatrics* 105:799, 1984.

Dombrowski, M.P. Pharmacologic therapy of asthma during pregnancy. *Obstet. Gynecol. Clin. North Am.* 24:559, 1997.

Effect of corticosteroids for fetal maturation on perinatal outcomes. NIH Consensus Development Panel on the Effect of Corticosteroids for Fetal Maturation on Perinatal Outcomes. *J.A.M.A.* 273:413, 1995.

Fraser, F.C., and Sajoo, A. Teratogenic potential of corticosteroids in humans. *Teratology* 51:45, 1995.

Katz, F.H., and Duncan, B.R. Entry of prednisone into human milk. *N. Engl. J. Med.* 293:1154, 1975.

Kauppila, A., et al. Cell-mediated immunocompetence of children exposed in utero to short- or long-term action of glucocorticoids. *Gynecol. Obstet. Invest.* 15:41, 1983.

Levine, L.S., and Pang, S. Prenatal diagnosis and treatment of congenital adrenal hyperplasia. *J. Pediatr. Endocrinol.* 7:193, 1994.

MacArthur, B.A., et al. School progress and cognitive development of 6-year-old children whose mothers were treated antenatally with betamethasone. *Pediatrics* 70:99, 1982.

Mercado, A.B., et al. Prenatal treatment and diagnosis of congenital adrenal hyperplasia owing to steroid 21-hydroxylase deficiency. *J. Clin. Endocrinol. Metab.* 80:2014, 1995.

Murphy, B.E.P., Patrick, J., and Denton, R.L. Cortisol in amniotic fluid during human gestation. *J. Clin. Endocrinol. Metab.* 40:164, 1975.

Nelson, J.L., and Ostensen, M. Pregnancy and rheumatoid arthritis. *Rheum. Dis. Clin. North Am.* 23:195, 1997.

Otero, L., et al. Neonatal leukocytosis associated with prenatal administration of dexamethasone. *Pediatrics* 68:778, 1981.

Perlow, J.H., Montgomery, D., Morgan, M.A., et al. Severity of asthma and perinatal outcome. *Am. J. Obstet. Gynecol.* 167:963, 1992.

Ramsey-Goldman, R., and Schilling, E. Immunosuppressive drug use during pregnancy. *Rheum. Dis. Clin. North Am.* 23:149–167.

Ricke, P.S., Elliott, J.P., and Freeman, R.K. Use of corticosteroids in pregnancy-induced hypertension. *Obstet. Gynecol.* 55:206, 1980.

Schapiro, S. Some physiologic biochemical and behavioral consequences of neonatal hormone administration: cortisol and thyroxin. *Gen. Comp. Endocrinol.* 10:214, 1968.

Schatz, M., et al. The safety of asthma and allergy medications during pregnancy. *J. Allergy Clin. Immunol.* 100:301, 1997.

Schimmer, B.P., and Parker, K.L. Adrenocorticotropic hormone; adrenocortical steroids and their synthetic analogs: inhibitors of the synthesis and actions of adrenocortical hormones. Chapter 59 in *Goodman and Gilman's The Pharmacological Basis of Therapeutics* (9th ed.), J.G. Hardman and L.E. Limbird, eds. New York: McGraw-Hill, 1996. Pp. 1465–1483.

Speiser, P.W. and New, M.I. Prenatal diagnosis and treatment of congenital adrenal hyperplasia. *J. Pediatr. Endocrinol.* 7:183, 1994.

Update: Drugs in breast milk. *Med. Lett. Drugs Ther.* 21:21, 1979.
Yackel, D.B., Kempers, R.D., and McConahey, W.M. Adrenocortico-
steroid therapy in pregnancy. *Am. J. Obstet. Gynecol.* 96:985, 1966.

Glycopyrrolate (Robinul®)

INDICATIONS AND RECOMMENDATIONS

Glycopyrrolate appears to be safe when used as indicated
during pregnancy. Glycopyrrolate is a synthetic, anticholinergic, quaternary ammonium compound used parenterally to decrease gastrointestinal secretions before elective surgery. This
drug appears to be as effective as atropine as a preanesthetic
agent and, on a theoretical basis, offers greater safety to the fetus because its transfer across the placenta is minimal.

SPECIAL CONSIDERATIONS IN PREGNANCY

The effectiveness of glycopyrrolate in reducing the volume
and acidity of gastric secretions, especially when combined with
magnesium trisilicate, has been demonstrated in obstetric patients treated before elective cesarean sections. Several studies
have shown that this drug causes an increase in maternal heart
rate and decrease in beat-to-beat variability as a result of vagal
inhibitory effects on the sinoatrial pacemaker. Unlike atropine,
however, glycopyrrolate crosses the placenta poorly and concentrations in arterial and venous umbilical blood, and in amniotic
fluid, remain low and clinically insignificant. No adverse effects
on neonates born to women who were premedicated with this
drug have thus far been reported. One case has documented the
development of supraventricular tachycardia in a parturient
treated simultaneously with ritodrine and glycopyrrolate. Such
coadministration should probably be avoided. Glycopyrrolate
use during organogenesis was not associated with an increased
incidence of birth defects in either mice or rats.

DOSAGE

The drug is given parenterally in a single dose of 1–2 mg.
Glycopyrrolate may be given orally in doses of 1–2 mg q4–6h.

ADVERSE EFFECTS

As with other anticholinergic drugs, side effects include dryness of mucous membranes, thirst, and constipation. Larger
dosages may produce slurred speech, blurred vision, occasional
disorientation, hallucinations, delirium, loss of taste, urinary
retention, headache, tachycardia, and palpitations. Glycopyrrolate is contraindicated for use in patients with glaucoma, bladder neck or gastrointestinal obstruction, paralytic ileus, and severe ulcerative colitis.

MECHANISM OF ACTION

Glycopyrrolate acts as a competitive antagonist of acetylcholine at postganglionic muscarinic sites. Because it is a
quaternary ammonium compound, physicochemical laws of
membrane transport suggest that glycopyrrolate should be

transferred poorly across the blood–brain and placental barriers. This is probably why the drug causes fewer maternal central nervous system and fetal side effects than do other anticholinergic agents.

ABSORPTION AND BIOTRANSFORMATION

Glycopyrrolate undergoes biotransformation in the liver and renal excretion.

RECOMMENDED READING

Abboud, T.K., et al. Use of glycopyrrolate in the parturient: effect on the maternal and fetal heart and uterine activity. *Obstet. Gynecol.* 57:224, 1981.

Ali-Melkkila, T., Kaila, T., Kanto, J., and Iisalo, E. Pharmacokinetics of glycopyrronium in perturients. *Anaesthesia* 45:634, 1990.

Agiwada, K., et al. [Effects of glycopyrrolate on pre- and post-natal developement of the offspring in pregnant mice and rats.] *Oyo Yakuri* 7:617, 1973.

Diaz, D.M., Diaz, S.F., and Mary, G.F. Cardiovascular effects of glycopyrrolate and belladonna derivatives in obstetric patients. *Bull. N.Y. Acad. Med.* 56:245, 1980.

Kennedy, S.K., and Longnecker, D.E. History and principles of anesthesiology. Chapter 13 in *Goodman and Gilman's The Pharmacological Basis of Therapeutics* (9th ed.), J.G. Hardman and L.E. Limbird, eds. New York: McGraw-Hill, 1996. P. 304.

Roper, R.E., and Salem, M.G. Effects of glycopyrrolate and atropine combined with antacid on gastric acidity. *Br. J. Anaesthesiol.* 53:1277, 1981.

Simpson, J.I., and Griffin, J.P. A glycopyrrolate-ritodrine drug–drug interaction. *Can. J. Anaesth.* 35:187, 1988.

Gonadotropin-Releasing Hormone Agonists: Leuprolide acetate (Lupron®, Lupron Depot®), Histrelin acetate (Supprelin®), Nafarelin acetate (Synarel®), Goserelin acetate (Zoladex®)

INDICATIONS AND RECOMMENDATIONS

Gonadotropin-releasing hormone agonists (GnRH agonists) are contraindicated during pregnancy. They are synthetic analogs of the endogenous decapeptide GnRH. Pulsatile GnRH stimulates the release of gonadotropins from the pituitary, whereas continuous GnRH suppresses gonadotropin release. The GnRH agonists are used to suppress pre-ovulatory gonadotropin surges in patients undergoing assisted reproduction, and also for the suppression of endometriomas, uterine leiomyomas, hirsutism, and polycystic ovarian syndrome. They are also used in the management of estrogen-dependent breast cancers. Because of their suppressive effect on gonadotropin release it would be unlikely for a woman to ovulate and conceive while receiving GnRH agonists, other than in the special setting of assisted reproduction where the drugs are given only before, and not after, ovulation. On the other hand, on theoretical grounds, the use of GnRH analogs during early pregnancy might be expected to suppress gonadotropins and lead to spontaneous abortion. There is no indication for the use of GnRH agonists during pregnancy. In premarketing animal studies, GnRH agonists were teratogenic in rabbits but not in rats. One of the manufacturers maintains a registry of patients unintentionally exposed to leuprolide during pregnancy, and thus far no excess of congenital malformations has been observed in over 300 such patients whose follow-up results are available. A number of case reports and case series have also failed to demonstrate an increased malformation rate. Patients who inadvertently take these drugs during pregnancy should be counseled regarding the available animal and human data.

RECOMMENDED READING

Ascoli, M., and Segaloff, D.L. Adenohypophyseal hormones and their hypothalamic releasing factors. Chapter 55 in *Goodman and Gilman's The Pharmacological Basis of Therapeutics* (9th ed.), J.G. Hardman and L.E. Limbird, eds. New York: McGraw-Hill, 1996. Pp. 1378–1380.

Chang, S.Y., and Soong, Y.-K. Unexpected pregnancies exposed to leuprolide acetate administered after the mid-luteal phase for ovarian stimulation. *Hum Reprod* 10:204, 1995.

Tap Holdings, Inc. Unpublished data from Jones, K.L. Leuprolide acetate and pregnancy. March 1994.

Tap Pharmaceuticals, Inc. Lupron (Leuprolide acetate). Entry in *Physicians Desk Reference* (52nd ed.). Montvale, NJ: Medical Economics, 1998. Pp. 2904–2918.

Wilshire, G.B., Emmi, A.M., Gagliardi, A.C., et al: Gonadotropin-releasing hormone agonist administration in early human pregnancy is associated with normal outcomes. *Fertil. Steril.* 60:980, 1993.

Young, D.C., Snabes, M.C., and Poindexter, A.N. III. GnRH agonist exposure during the first trimester of pregnancy. *Obstet. Gynecol.* 81:587, 1993.

Gold Salts: Auranofin (Ridaura®), Aurothioglucose (Solganal®), Gold Sodium Thiomalate (Aurolate®, Myochrysine®)

INDICATIONS AND RECOMMENDATIONS

The administration of gold salts during pregnancy for the treatment of rheumatoid arthritis is controversial. Animal data suggest teratogenicity when high dosages are used. However, approximately 75 uneventful human pregnancies have been reported. Because gold salts are extremely toxic, their use should be reserved for patients with rheumatoid arthritis refractory to other forms of treatment, such as NSAIDs and physiotherapy, and they should be discontinued before conception if possible. Patients who conceive while receiving gold therapy or within months of discontinuing therapy should be informed of the theoretic risks to the fetus and of the generally favorable pregnancy outcomes reported in humans.

SPECIAL CONSIDERATIONS IN PREGNANCY

Gold salts have been shown to be teratogenic in rats and rabbits, with ventral wall defects being the predominant anomaly in the rabbits. Dosages were considerably higher than those generally used in humans.

Gold was detected in the liver, kidney, and placenta of a human fetus whose gold-treated mother chose termination when pregnancy was discovered at 20 weeks' gestation. When another woman, treated with gold throughout gestation, delivered a healthy baby at term, umbilical cord serum gold concentration was 225 μg/dl, while simultaneous maternal venous plasma gold concentration was 392 μg/dl. These cases demonstrate that gold salts cross the placenta. Anecdotal reports of human fetal exposure to gold salts in the first trimester include 79 cases. One baby died of severe malformations; two had congenital hip dislocation; a fourth was stillborn due to a true knot in the umbilical cord but was normally formed. Thus, the incidence of major anomalies was 1 in 79 (1.3%). These anecdotal data do not support the recommendation that pregnancies conceived inadvertently during the administration of gold salts be terminated.

DOSAGE

Aurothioglucose is given by intramuscular injection and is available as a 50 mg/ml solution in oil. Gold sodium thiomalate is also given intramuscularly and is marketed in concentrations of 10, 25, 50, and 100 mg/ml. Various dosing regimens have been proposed. Most commonly, 10 mg is given in the first week as a test dose, followed by 25 mg in the second and third weeks, and 50 mg/week thereafter, up to a total dose of 1 gm. If no favorable response is seen at this point or if toxicity occurs, treatment should be discontinued. If remission occurs, dosage is reduced or the dosage interval increased. If a relapse occurs during the year of low-dose therapy, the dosage is increased. If a relapse occurs after the course of treatment has ended, it is reinstituted.

Auranofin, an oral form of gold, is manufactured in capsules containing 3 mg. The usual dose is 3–6 mg/day, with an increase to 9 mg/day if the response is inadequate after 6 months.

ADVERSE EFFECTS

Gold salts are exceedingly toxic, with an estimated incidence of adverse effects between 25 and 50% of treated individuals. Serious toxicity occurs in about 10% of patients. The mortality related to this drug is estimated to be approximately 0.4%.

Toxicity most commonly involves the skin and oral mucous membranes. These reactions may range from erythema to severe exfoliative dermatitis. Stomatitis, pharyngitis, tracheitis, gastritis, colitis, glossitis, and vaginitis may occur. A characteristic gray-blue pigmentation (chrysiasis) may appear in skin and mucous membranes, especially with exposure to light.

Severe blood dyscrasias may also result. Thrombocytopenia may be fatal and may not develop until many months after the initiation of therapy. It is believed to be related to an immunologic mechanism causing accelerated platelet destruction. Leukopenia, agranulocytosis, and aplastic anemia have been reported. Eosinophilia is common and may be an indication for temporary discontinuance of therapy.

Renal damage, localized in the proximal tubules, results in heavy proteinuria and hematuria. The predominant lesion is membranous glomerulonephritis when nephrosis occurs.

Encephalitis, peripheral neuritis, hepatitis, pulmonary infiltrates, and nitritoid crisis (resembling anaphylaxis) have all been reported.

Oral gold appears to be better tolerated than the injectable compounds and the incidence and severity of mucocutaneous and hematological side effects is less. However, it produces a high incidence of gastrointestinal disturbances requiring discontinuation of therapy in approximately 5% of patients.

Chelating agents have been used in cases of severe toxicity or overdosage.

MECHANISM OF ACTION

The mechanism of action of gold salts in rheumatoid arthritis is poorly understood. These compounds can suppress or prevent the development of symptoms but do not cure the disease. They can decrease concentrations of rheumatoid factor and immunoglobulins and impair mitogen-induced proliferation of lymphocytes. Their activity is most likely related to their ability to inhibit the maturation and function of mononuclear phagocytes and of T-cells, thereby suppressing immune responsiveness.

ABSORPTION AND BIOTRANSFORMATION

Aurothioglucose and gold sodium thiomalate are more water soluble and are given by intramuscular injection. They are rapidly absorbed from the injection site, reaching peak plasma concentrations in 2–6 hours unless the salt is suspended in oil, in which case the absorption is more gradual. Approximately 25% of the gold in an oral dose of auranofin is absorbed.

In the blood, gold is first bound to albumin (about 95%). Early in the course of treatment, much of the gold is transferred to erythrocytes. Synovial fluid concentrations are approximately half the plasma levels. As therapy continues, gold is preferentially deposited in the joints affected by rheumatoid arthritis, as opposed to skeletal muscle, bone, and fat. Gold deposits are also found in macrophages, in renal tubular epithelium, and in many other tissues.

The plasma half-life is approximately 7 days for a single 50 mg dose, but lengthens with chronic therapy, and may be as long as weeks to months after prolonged therapy. Gold remains in tissues for many years after therapy is discontinued.

Excretion is approximately 75% renal and 25% fecal (via biliary secretion). After a cumulative dose of 1,000 mg, blood concentrations fall to normal in 40–80 days, but urinary excretion can be detected for at least 1 year. Sulfhydryl chelating agents increase the excretion of gold.

RECOMMENDED READING

Chaffman, M., et al. Auranofin: A preliminary review of its pharmacological properties and therapeutic use in rheumatoid arthritis. *Drugs* 27:378, 1984.

Cohen, D.L., and Orzel, J. Infants of mothers receiving gold therapy. *Arthritis Rheum.* 24:104, 1981.

Hollander, J.L. Gold therapy for rheumatoid arthritis. In J. L. Hollander (ed.), *Arthritis and Allied Conditions*. Philadelphia: Lea & Febiger, 1972.

Kidston, M.E., Beck, F., and Lloyd, J.B. The teratogenic effect of Myochrysine injection in rats. *J. Anat.* 108:590, 1971.

Miyamoto, T., et al. Gold therapy in bronchial asthma-special emphasis upon blood levels in gold and its teratogenicity. *Nippon Naika Gakkai Zasshi* 63:1190, 1974.

Moller-Madsen, B., and Danscher, G. Transplacental transport of gold in rats exposed to sodium aurothiomalate. *Exp. Mol. Pathol.* 39:327, 1983.

Rocker, I., and Henderson, W.J. Transfer of gold from mother to fetus. *Lancet* 2:1246, 1976.

Rogers, J.G., et al. Possible teratogenic effects of gold. *Aust. Paediatr. J.* 16:194, 1980.

Szabo, K.T., DiFebbo, M.E., and Phelan, D.G. The effects of gold-containing compounds on pregnant rabbits and their fetuses. *Vet. Pathol.* 15(Suppl. 5):97, 1978.

Szabo, K.T., Guerriero, F.J., and Kang, Y.J. The effects of gold-containing compounds on pregnant rats and their fetuses. *Vet. Pathol.* 15(Suppl. 5):89, 1978.

Tarp, U., and Graudal, H. A followup study of children exposed to gold compounds in utero. *Arthritis Rheum.* 28:235, 1985.

Griseofulvin (Fulvicin®, Grifulvin V®, Grisactin®)

INDICATIONS AND RECOMMENDATIONS

Griseofulvin use is contraindicated during pregnancy. It is a systemic agent used to treat fungal infections of the skin, hair, and nails. Griseofulvin is a known teratogen in rats, dogs, cats, and mice and has been shown to cross the human placenta. Its use during early pregnancy has been anecdotally associated with the birth of two sets of conjoined twins. This association has not been substantiated by reviews of other congenital anomaly registries. Because griseofulvin is used to treat non-life-threatening infections, its use should be postponed until after delivery.

RECOMMENDED READING

Bennett, J.E. Antimicrobial agents: antifungal agents. Chapter 49 in *Goodman and Gilman's The Pharmacological Basis of Therapeutics* (9th ed.), J.G. Hardman and L.E. Limbird, eds. New York: McGraw-Hill, 1996. Pp. 1184.

Klein, M.F., and Beall, J.R. Griseofulvin: a teratogenic study. *Science* 175:1483, 1972.

Knudsen, L.B. No association between griseofulvin and conjoined twinning (letter). *Lancet* 2:1097, 1987.

Metneki, J., and Czeizel, A. Griseofulvin teratology (letter). *Lancet* 1:1042, 1987.

Rosa, F.W., Hernandez, C., and Carlo, W.A. Griseofulvin teratology, including two thoracopagus conjoined twins (letter). *Lancet* 1:171, 1987.

Rubin, A., and Dvornik, D. Placental transfer of griseofulvin. *Am. J. Obstet. Gynecol.* 92:882, 1965.

Guanethidine (Ismelin®)

INDICATIONS AND RECOMMENDATIONS

Guanethidine is contraindicated during pregnancy because other agents are better characterized, more effective, and have fewer side effects. This drug is a powerful postganglionic sympatholytic compound and is no longer widely used as an antihypertensive agent, except in patients whose hypertension is uncontrolled by, or who cannot tolerate, other more effective drugs. It acts by blocking norepinephrine release from nerve endings, which exposes more of the neurotransmitter to metabolic inactivation in the neuron and results in a depletion of the storage site.

Many of the observed side effects of guanethidine are due to the combination of adrenergic inhibition and unopposed parasympathetic function. Adverse effects include significant orthostatic and exercise hypotension, bradycardia, increased gastric secretion, and frequent bowel movements or diarrhea. The drug must be present within neuronal endings in order to have an effect. Any agents that inhibit the storage of guanethidine or its transport across the neuronal membrane will therefore block its action. These agents include the tricyclic antidepressants, phenothiazines, amphetamines, methylphenidate, and reserpine.

Experience with guanethidine in the pregnant woman is limited, and its effects on the fetus are unknown. Pronounced postural hypotension and other annoying sequelae of this drug make it a poor choice for the therapy of hypertension in pregnancy. Guanethidine appears in breast milk in very small quantities and can probably be given to nursing mothers.

RECOMMENDED READING

Oates, J.A. Antihypertensive agents and the drug therapy of hypertension. Chapter 33 in *Goodman and Gilman's The Pharmacological*

Basis of Therapeutics (9th ed.), J.G. Hardman and L.E. Limbird, eds. New York: McGraw-Hill, 1996. Pp. 790–791.

H₂ Receptor Antagonists: Cimetidine (Tagamet®), Famotidine (Pepcid®), Nizatidine (Axid®), Ranitidine (Zantac®)

INDICATIONS AND RECOMMENDATIONS

Cimetidine and ranitidine are safe to use at term to prevent Mendelson's syndrome. At other times during pregnancy, they should be used when antacid therapy is inadequate. Famotidine and nizatidine, newer agents for which there is less clinical experience, should not be used during pregnancy until they have been further studied. These agents are used clinically to treat duodenal ulcer disease as well as gastric hypersecretory states. They are also used for preanesthetic prophylaxis against gastric acid aspiration pneumonitis prior to surgeries including cesarean section.

SPECIAL CONSIDERATIONS IN PREGNANCY

Nizatidine use during pregnancy has been associated with congenital malformations in rabbits. Except for the cimetidine effects on rats discussed below, administration of cimetidine and ranitidine during organogenesis to rats, rabbits, and mice, in dosages far exceeding the usual recommendations for humans, was associated with no adverse fetal effects.

Both cimetidine and ranitidine cross the human placenta resulting in fetal/maternal ratios of up to 0.84 and 0.9, respectively. The safety of the H₂ receptor antagonists during the first trimester was examined in a prospective cohort study involving 178 mothers with known exposures to ranitidine (71%) and cimetidine (16%) as well as famotidine (8%) and nizatidine (5%). There was no increase in major malformations or relationship between drug exposure and birth weight, gestational age, or preterm delivery. Although these data support the safety of H₂ blockers, the authors could not rule out a small teratogenic risk.

Cimetidine alone of the H₂ receptor antagonists is known to have weak antiandrogenic effects. These are primarily seen in men receiving large doses (more than 3 g/day) for hypersecretory conditions. Early studies indicated that male rats exposed to cimetidine in utero showed measurable effects on testicular, prostatic, and seminal vesicular weight and testosterone levels. However, later investigators have found no or insignificant effect on these and other parameters of androgenic effects, leading them to conclude that cimetidine given during gestation does not significantly affect the rat fetus. Unfortunately, there are no human data available regarding this effect.

In one report of three cases of cimetidine use for various lengths of time beginning at 16 weeks, 12 weeks, and 31 weeks gestation, all three patients delivered healthy newborns without congenital defects or metabolic disturbances. Another woman, who took 1000 mg daily from the 16th to the 20th week of gestation, gave birth to an apparently normal 2500-g child. There is a single case report of transient impaired hepatic excretory function in a neonate whose mother took 1200 mg daily for treatment of an ulcer during the month prior to delivery.

Ranitidine has been used to treat gastroesophageal reflux disease (GERD) after 20 weeks gestation with favorable results. Patients responded well to a dose of 150 mg bid, reporting less severe heartburn and the need for fewer antacids; once daily therapy did not provide adequate relief. No adverse fetal effects were reported. Ranitidine in doses of 150 mg bid and 150 mg tid was used throughout pregnancy in two patients with Zollinger-Ellison syndrome. Both pregnancies resulted in healthy infants, although one had reduced fetal heart rate prior to delivery.

Both ranitidine and cimetidine are effective in the prophylaxis of aspiration pneumonitis (Mendelson's syndrome). This syndrome is more frequently seen in pregnancy because the gravid uterus can compress the stomach and increase intragastric pressure while progestin relaxes the gastroesophageal sphincter. It is most likely to develop if the aspirated material has a pH less than 2.5. Cimetidine and ranitidine effectively increase the gastric fluid pH and can also decrease fluid volume. However, they must be given at least 90 minutes before induction of anesthesia for maximum effectiveness. These drugs have been given in this situation at term without adverse neonatal effect.

Some investigators have reported that cimetidine and ranitidine can change the pharmacokinetics of local anesthetics by inhibiting hepatic enzymes and reducing liver blood flow. Because treatment with H₂ receptor antagonists is associated with the use of local anesthetics for anesthesia for cesarean section, several studies have examined this issue in the obstetric patient. The available studies generally conclude that single doses of cimetidine and ranitidine do not significantly affect the dispositions of lidocaine or bupivacaine in this setting.

Both cimetidine and ranitidine appear in breast milk in greater concentration than in maternal serum, but as yet no adverse effects in the nursing infant have been reported. They have been classified by the American Academy of Pediatrics as being compatible with breast-feeding.

DOSAGE

The usual oral dose of cimetidine for duodenal ulcer is 800 mg at bedtime for 4–6 weeks. The dose may also be divided, 400 mg bid. Gastric ulcers may take longer to heal and GERD and hypersecretory states require higher doses. Hospitalized patients unable to take the medication orally may be given 300 mg IV every 6 hours. Dosage should be reduced with renal impairment.

The usual oral dose of ranitidine for duodenal ulcer is 300 mg at bedtime for 4–6 weeks. The dose may be divided, 150 mg bid. As with cimetidine, dosage adjustment is required for gastric ulcer, GERD, and hypersecretory states. The usual IV dose is 50 mg q8h. Dosage should be reduced with renal impairment.

ADVERSE EFFECTS

Side effects of the H$_2$ receptors antagonists are uncommon and usually minor. Headache, dizziness, fatigue, muscle pains, constipation, diarrhea, and skin rashes have been reported. Increases in serum creatinine and in liver enzymes have occurred. In elderly patients and those with impaired renal function, neurologic effects including confusion, slurred speech, delirium, hallucinations, and coma have occurred. Fever has occasionally been reported. Cimetidine has been associated with gynecomastia in men and galactorrhea in women, especially when given in high dosages for long periods. These effects are presumed to be due to cimetidine's ability to enhance the secretion of prolactin and to competitively bind to androgen receptors.

MECHANISM OF ACTION

These agents act as reversible competitive antagonists at H$_2$ (histamine) receptors. They are highly selective and have little or no effect on H$_1$ receptors. Although H$_2$ receptors are present in numerous tissues, these agents almost exclusively inhibit receptors responsible for gastric acid secretion, which is diminished in a dose-dependent manner. Gastrin- and pentagastrin-invoked acid secretion are also effectively blocked, whereas the acid–secretion stimulating effects of acetylcholine and muscarinic drugs are only partially blocked. All phases of gastric secretion (basal, food induced, gastric distention induced, and hormonally induced) are inhibited. The volume and hydrogen ion concentration of gastric juice are both diminished.

ABSORPTION AND BIOTRANSFORMATION

H$_2$ receptor antagonists are rapidly and well absorbed after oral administration. There is, however, significant first-pass hepatic metabolism of cimetidine, famotidine, and ranitidine, which limits their bioavailability to 50%. The half-lives of those three agents are 2–3 hours whereas that of nitazidine is shorter. Most of an oral dose of any of these agents is excreted unchanged in the urine within 24 hours, and renal impairment requires dosage reduction. Ranitidine is sufficiently metabolized that its half-life is significantly prolonged with hepatic dysfunction.

RECOMMENDED READING

Brunton, L.L. Agents for control of astric acidity and treatment of peptic ulcers. Chapter 27 in *Goodman and Gilman's The Pharmacological Basis of Therapeutics* (9th ed.), J.G. Hardman and L.E. Limbird, eds. New York: McGraw-Hill, 1996. Pp. 904–907.

Flynn, R.J., et al. Does pretreatment with cimetidine and ranitidine affect the disposition of bupivacaine? *Br. J. Anaesth.* 62:87, 1989.

Glade, G., Saccar, C.L., and Pereira, G.R. Cimetidine in pregnancy: apparent transient liver impairment in the newborn. *Am. J. Dis. Child.* 134:87, 1980.

Hodgkinson, P., et al. Comparison of cimetidine with antacid for safety and effectiveness in reducing gastric acidity before elective cesarean section. *Anesthesiology* 59:86, 1983.

Hoie, E.B., et al. Development of secondary sex characteristics in male rats after fetal and perinatal cimetidine exposure. *J. Pharm. Sci.* 83:107, 1994.

Johnston, J.R., et al. Use of cimetidine as an oral antacid in obstetric anesthesia. *Anesth. Analg.* 62:720, 1983.

Lagace, E. Safety of first trimester exposure to H$_2$ blockers. *J. Fam. Pract.* 43:342, 1996.

Larson, J.D., et al. Double-blind, placebo-controlled study of ranitidine for gastroesphageal reflux symptoms during pregnancy. *Obstet. Gynecol.* 90:83, 1997.

Magee, L.A., et al. Safety of first trimester exposure to histamine H$_2$ blockers. A prospective cohort study. *Dig. Dis. Sci.* 41:1145, 1996.

McGowan, W.A.W. Safety of cimetidine in obstetric patients. *J. R. Soc. Med.* 72:902, 1979.

Schenker, S., et al. Human placental transport of cimetidine. *J. Clin. Invest.* 80:1428, 1987.

Shapiro, B.H., and Bitar, M.S. Developmental levels and androgen responsiveness of hepatic mono-oxygenases of male rats perinatally exposed to maternally administered cimetidine. *Toxicol. Lett.* 55:85, 1991.

Somogyi, A., and Gugler, R. Cimetidine excretion into breast milk. *Br. J. Clin. Pharmacol.* 7:627, 1979.

Stewart, C.A., et al. Management of the Zollinger-Ellison syndrome in pregnancy. *Am. J. Obstet. Gynecol.* 176:224, 1997.

Haloperidol (Haldol®)

INDICATIONS AND RECOMMENDATIONS

Haloperidol may be administered to pregnant women for the treatment of psychosis and for the treatment of Gilles de la Tourette disease. Haloperidol is similar to the phenothiazine antipsychotics and is used to treat delusions, hallucinations, disordered thought processes, paranoid symptoms, and withdrawal psychoses. It has also been used successfully to treat chorea gravidarum during the second and third trimesters of pregnancy. Because of isolated case reports of teratogenicity, haloperidol use in pregnancy should be avoided in the first trimester if possible.

SPECIAL CONSIDERATIONS IN PREGNANCY

Congenital anomalies, including phocomelia, have been noted in infants whose mothers have taken haloperidol during pregnancy. However, only isolated cases have been reported. In one series of 38 infants with severe limb reduction defects, none of the mothers could recall having taken haloperidol during the index pregnancies. In a study of 100 patients treated with haloperidol for hyperemesis gravidarum in the first trimester, no malformations were found and no effect was seen on birth weight, duration of pregnancy or fetal or neonatal mortality. As there have been no prospective studies to date, the available data are insufficient to implicate haloperidol as the cause of malformations.

Haloperidol is excreted in breast milk, with a calculated daily dose to the suckling infant in the range of 10–25 µg/day. This is equivalent to 6 µg/kg/day and should be compared with a daily dose of 14 µg/kg in an average 70 kg individual taking 1.0 mg haloperidol each day. To date there are no reports of adverse effects in human infants nursed by mothers taking this drug.

DOSAGE

Haloperidol is available in tablets of 0.5, 1.0, 2.0, 5.0, 10.0, and 20.0 mg; as an oral concentrate of 2 mg/ml; and as a 5 mg/ml solution for intramuscular injection. The usual dosage is between 0.5 and 2.0 mg 2–3 times a day. Some patients given long-term treatment become drug-resistant and may require 3–5 mg 2–3 times a day. In rare cases, haloperidol has been used in doses in excess of 100 mg daily. The reported cases of chorea gravidarum were treated initially with 1 mg 4 times a day, then reduced to 0.5 mg 4 times daily. It is also available in a long-acting form for intramuscular injection. This preparation has a 4-week duration and is used only in chronic psychotic patients who require prolonged parenteral antipsychotic therapy.

ADVERSE EFFECTS

The most important side effects are those on the central nervous system (acute dystonia, akasthisia, Parkinsonism, neuroleptic malignant syndrome, and tardive dyskinesia). More common and less severe side effects include faintness, palpitation, and anticholinergic effects. Occasionally, haloperidol will cause blood dyscrasias, rashes, menstrual irregularities, and galactorrhea.

MECHANISM OF ACTION

The mechanism of action of haloperidol is only partly known and is thought to be similar to that of the piperazine phenothiazines. Its effects may be due to blockage of dopamine receptors in the basal ganglia, hypothalamus, limbic system, brainstem, and medulla.

ABSORPTION AND BIOTRANSFORMATION

Haloperidol is readily absorbed from the gastrointestinal tract, with peak effect being achieved approximately 3 hours after oral dosing. The drug is extensively degraded in the liver, so that less than 1% is excreted unchanged in the urine.

RECOMMENDED READING

Ayd, F.J., Jr. Excretion of psychotropic drugs in human breast milk. *Int. Drug Ther. Newslett.* 8:33, 1973.

Baldessarini, R.J. Drugs and the treatment of psychiatric disorders: psychosis and anxiety. Chapter 18 in *Goodman and Gilman's The Pharmacological Basis of Therapeutics* (9th ed.), J.G. Hardman and L.E. Limbird, eds. New York: McGraw-Hill, 1996. Pp. 404–417.

Donaldson, J.O. Control of chorea gravidarum with haloperidol. *Obstet. Gynecol.* 59:381, 1982.

Hanson, J.W., and Oakley, G.P., Jr. Haloperidol and limb deformity (letter). *J.A.M.A.* 231:26, 1975.

McCullar, F.G.W., and Heggeness, L. Limb malformations following maternal use of haloperidol. *J.A.M.A.* 231:62, 1975.

Patterson, J.F. Treatment of chorea gravidarum with haloperidol. *South. Med. J.* 72:1220, 1979.

Schatzberg, A.F., and Memeroff, C.B. *Textbook of Psychopharmacology.* Washington, DC: American Psychiatric Press, 1995. Pp. 823–837.

Stewart, R.B., Karas, B., and Springer, P.K. Haloperidol excretion in breast milk. *Am. J. Psychiatry* 137:849, 1980.

Van Waes, A., and Van De Velde, E. Safety evaluation of haloperidol in the treatment of hyperemesis gravidarum. *J. Clin. Pharmacol.* 9:224, 1969.

Whalley, L.J., Blain, P.G., and Prime, J.K. Haloperidol secreted in breast milk. *Br. Med. J.* 282:1746, 1981.

Hemorrhoidal Preparations (Anusol® Suppository or Ointment, Anusol-HC®)

INDICATIONS AND RECOMMENDATIONS

Hemorrhoidal suppositories and ointments are safe for use in pregnancy. These preparations are used for the symptomatic relief of pain or discomfort related to external or internal hemorrhoids, proctitis, cryptitis, fissures, and incomplete fistulas, and for relief of local pain following anorectal surgery. The use of hydrocortisone-containing agents is controversial and if used at all should be restricted to very specific situations.

SPECIAL CONSIDERATIONS IN PREGNANCY

Anusol-HC-25 contains 25 mg hydrocortisone acetate and is often used for severe acute discomfort. Because steroids are absorbed systemically from the rectum, especially from inflamed tissues, this drug should be used during pregnancy with the same precautions as other steroid preparations.

DOSAGE

One hemorrhoidal suppository may be inserted rectally in the morning, another at bedtime, and one after each bowel movement. Ointments can be applied externally or inserted rectally with a plastic applicator. The ointment should be applied every 3–4 hours.

MECHANISM OF ACTION AND ADVERSE EFFECTS

Hemorrhoidal suppositories and ointments contain various combinations of local anesthetics, vasoconstrictors, protectants, and astringents. These combinations provide a soothing, lubricating action on the mucous membranes, which relieves discomfort secondary to the passage of stool. The primary side effects of these agents are skin sensitivity reactions caused primarily by the local anesthetics. Therefore, agents containing local anesthetics should be used with caution.

RECOMMENDED READING

American Pharmaceutical Association. *Handbook of Nonprescription Drugs.* Washington, DC, 1996. Pp. 261–271.

American Pharmaceutical Association. *Nonprescription Products: Formulations and Features 96–97.* Washington, DC, 1996. Pp. 261–271.

Heparin; Low Molecular Weight Heparin: Enoxaparin (Lovenox®), Dalteparin (Fragmin®), Ardeparin (Normiflo®); Heparinoids: Danaparoid (Orgaran®)

INDICATIONS AND RECOMMENDATIONS

Heparin is the anticoagulant of choice during pregnancy. Some researchers have recommended the use of oral anticoagulants during the second trimester, but as these compounds may induce fetal abnormalities throughout pregnancy, it is preferable to administer heparin whenever anticoagulation is necessary in an undelivered patient.

Anticoagulants are indicated in the treatment and prophylaxis of pulmonary embolism, venous thromboembolic disease, and atrial fibrillation with embolization; prevention of clotting in arterial and cardiac surgery; and the prevention of clotting with implanted prosthetic devices such as heart valves. Controversy exists regarding the latter indication. Some case series suggest that serious prosthetic valve thrombosis during pregnancy is more likely with heparin than with warfarin anticoagulation, particularly with the use of older prostheses. However, controlled studies are lacking and advocates of heparin point out the risk of warfarin embryopathy and fetal hemorrhage at any trimester of pregnancy. In addition, it is not clear as to whether cases of valve thrombosis despite heparin therapy represent inadequate dosage. Heparin is also commonly recommended for the treatment of patients with phospholipid antibodies or lupus anticoagulant who are at risk for fetal compromise on this basis.

When initiated before elective surgery, a course of heparin given subcutaneously and in subtherapeutic dosages has been reported to be effective in preventing postoperative deep vein phlebitis. Minidose therapy has also been given as prophylaxis against phlebitis in obese patients confined to bed for prolonged periods and in women with a history of deep vein problems in prior pregnancies.

Patients who are being fully anticoagulated with heparin may require continuous hospitalization throughout the course of the therapy, although selected individuals can be instructed to give their own intravenous or subcutaneous injections with outpatient monitoring. Minidose heparin prophylaxis can be given entirely on an outpatient basis with periodic monitoring. Heparin can be administered to breast-feeding mothers.

Low molecular weight heparin is now available for prophylaxis. Although these preparations are quite expensive compared to standard heparin, there are some potential theoretic advantages to their use in pregnancy. They have greater bioavailability and are longer acting, and so can be used once or twice daily. They have little effect on the activated partial thromboplastin time (APTT), and so monitoring with this test is not useful nor is it necessary, since their plasma concentrations are more predictable than that of standard heparin. The likelihood of thrombocytopenia, osteoporosis, and bleeding complications appears to be less than with standard heparin. Some studies of the treatment of venous thrombosis have shown low molecular weight heparins to be at least equally effective to unfractionated heparin. In December of 1997 the Food and Drug Administration issued an advisory to health care providers, noting that there have been more than 30 cases reported to the agency of epidural or spinal hematomas developing in patients concurrently receiving low molecular weight heparin and epidural/spinal anesthesia. Most were elderly women undergoing orthopedic surgery. The risk was apparently increased with the use of indwelling epidural catheters or with the concomitant use of drugs affecting hemostasis.

SPECIAL CONSIDERATIONS IN PREGNANCY

Because heparin does not cross the placenta, it has no direct effect on the fetus. An increased risk of spontaneous abortion and premature labor has been reported by some authors. Prospective studies, however, have not confirmed these findings. Heparin given to breast-feeding women does not have any demonstrable ill effect on the nursing infant.

Low molecular weight heparin was demonstrated to prevent fetal resorption better than standard heparin in a mouse model of antiphospholipid syndrome. A number of case series have described the use of low molecular weight heparins during pregnancy for prophylaxis of thromboembolism and treatment of antithrombin deficiency with apparent success. In all likelihood low molecular weight heparins do not cross the placenta, as their presence in umbilical cord blood could not be demonstrated 2 hours after maternal injection.

DOSAGE

The anticoagulant potency of a given weight of heparin may vary from one preparation to another. It should always be ordered in USP units as opposed to milliliters of solution. The effect is variable among patients, and the dosage therefore must be monitored with APTT. With subcutaneous heparin, the mid-interval APTT should be 1.5–2.5 times control values, although with very sensitive APTT assays the therapeutic range may be higher. Requirements for heparin may dramatically decrease as the thrombophlebitic process is brought under control. When prophylactic low-dose heparin is utilized the APTT is not generally raised. Studies in which heparin levels were monitored suggest that heparin requirements to achieve a given level may be higher in pregnancy than in the nonpregnant individual and are quite variable. Doses as high as 7500–10,000 units every 12 hours may be needed to replicate levels seen at 5000 unit doses outside of pregnancy.

Intravenous heparin administered by a dosing nomogram (starting dose 80 units/kg body weight bolus followed by 18 units/kg/h infusion) was demonstrated to be more effective at rapidly reaching the therapeutic goal than standard (5000 units bolus followed by 1000 units/h) dosage in a randomized controlled trial in nonpregnant patients requiring heparin. To date, no such trials in pregnancy have been published.

In the case of overdose, heparin is immediately discontinued. If it is necessary to reverse the anticoagulant effect, protamine sulfate is administered as a 1% solution in a dose of 1 mg for each 100 units of heparin thought to be present at the time of neutralization. (Consider 30 minutes to be the half-life of intravenous heparin and 60 minutes the half-life of subcutaneous heparin.) If protamine is given in excess, it may itself act as an anticoagulant by interfering with the action of thrombin on fibrinogen. Some clinicians therefore will give half of the projected dose and observe the effect on the APTT.

Low molecular weight heparins are given subcutaneously. The dosage is fixed and not adjusted. When these compounds are used for prophylaxis, the dose is generally administered once or twice daily. The usual dose of delteparin is 2500 units once daily. When enoxaparin is used for prophylaxis in hip surgery the dose recommended to be given every 12 hours in a dose of 30 mg subcutaneously. One study suggested that, with enoxaparin, 40 mg injected once daily provided more appropriate blood levels of heparin than 20 mg. These standard doses have not yet been validated by clinical studies in pregnancy, and some clinicians suggest measuring anti-factor Xa levels as an assay for heparin. Again, critical values for pregnancy have not been determined. Based on studies of hip replacement patients and other clinical situations, goals for prophylactic anticoagulation with low molecular weight heparin are generally in the range of 0.1 to 0.2 unit/ml, whereas for therapeutic anticoagulation they may be as high as 0.4 to 0.8 unit/ml. Generally speaking, each laboratory offers its own critical values.

ADVERSE EFFECTS

The most important side effect associated with heparin administration is hemorrhage in the mother. The anticoagulant action of this substance can be rapidly reversed with protamine sulfate. The following conditions have been considered by some authors to be contraindications to the use of heparin:

1. Any condition in which an increased bleeding tendency exists
2. Subacute bacterial endocarditis
3. Acute pericarditis
4. Threatened abortion
5. Suspected intracranial bleeding

Prolonged use of heparin has been associated with maternal osteoporosis. The exact mechanism is unknown, although interference with the metabolism of vitamin D has been observed. The development of osteoporosis seems to be related to the dose of heparin administered and the duration of treatment. Spinal fractures are unusual and have not been reported in patients receiving less than 10,000 units/day regardless of the duration of therapy. Conversely, the shortest reported time from initiation of therapy to radiologic demonstration of spinal fractures is approximately 4 months.

A retrospective analysis of 20 women treated during and after pregnancy has been performed within 2 years of terminating therapy. These patients had received subcutaneous heparin at doses ranging from 16,000 to 20,000 units/day for 6–32 weeks, and none showed evidence of thoracolumbar spine osteoporosis. However, significant phalangeal demineralization was found in patients after long-term therapy (more than 25 weeks) as compared to short-term therapy (less than 7 weeks). Whether these changes are reversible remains to be determined because prospective long-term follow-up studies are lacking. A prospective cohort study of 14 gravidas on heparin and 14 controls found significant decreases in proximal femoral bone density in 5 of 14 cases but none of the controls. The difference continued to be statistically significant at 6 months post partum.

Hypersensitivity reactions are usually manifested by chills, fever, and urticaria, but true anaphylactoid reactions have also occurred. Unusual side effects include transient alopecia, reversible thrombocytopenia, and rebound hyperlipemia when the drug is discontinued.

When given simultaneously with heparin, the following drugs may cause excessive bleeding: aspirin and aspirin derivatives, phenylbutazone, indomethacin, clofibrate, glyceryl guaiacolate (guaifenesin), and dipyridamole. Drugs that may decrease the anticoagulant effect when given with heparin include d-tubocurarine and the quinine derivatives.

MECHANISM OF ACTION

Heparin is a complex anionic mucopolysaccharide with a molecular weight of approximately 12,000. It is stored, and probably formed in, the mast cells of animal tissues. Heparin inhibits factors involved in the conversion of prothrombin to thrombin. Its anticoagulant effect requires the presence of an α-globulin known as antithrombin III, the heparin cofactor. Heparin combines with antithrombin III and in doing so alters the configuration of that molecule. Antithrombin III is then able to combine with many coagulation proteins and inhibit their activity. Heparin also directly interferes with platelet aggregation.

ABSORPTION AND BIOTRANSFORMATION

Heparin is not well absorbed after oral administration. Subcutaneous, intravenous, and intramuscular routes of administration are effective. Peak plasma heparin concentration after a given dose of heparin has been reported to be lower in pregnancy than in the nonpregnant state, and the time from injection to peak plasma concentration shorter (113 versus 222 minutes). Intramuscular injections may cause local or dissecting retroperitoneal hematomas. The drug is metabolized in the liver. A partially degraded form of heparin, called *uroheparin*, is excreted in the urine. Heparin does not cross the placenta or pass into the mother's milk.

RECOMMENDED READING

Barbour, L.A., Kick, S.D., Steiner, J.F., et al. A prospective study of heparin-induced osteoporosis in pregnancy using bone densitometry. *Am. J. Obstet. Gynecol.* 170:862, 1994.

Barbour, L.A., Smith, J.M., and Marlar, R.A. Heparin levels to guide thromboembolism prophylaxis during pregnancy. *Am. J. Obstet. Gynecol.* 173:1869, 1995.

Brancazio, L.R., Roperti, K.A., Stierer, R., and Laifer, S.A. Pharmacokinetics and pharmacodynamics of subcutaneous heparin during the early third trimester of pregnancy. *Am. J. Obstet. Gynecol.* 173:1240, 1995.

Buckley, M.M., and Sorkin, E.M. Enoxaparin: a review of its pharmacology and clinical applications in the prevention and treatment of thromboembolic disorders. *Drugs* 44:465, 1992.

de-Swiet, M., et al. Prolonged heparin therapy in pregnancy causes bone demineralization. *Br. J. Obstet. Gynaecol.* 90:1129, 1983.

Dulitzki, M., Pauzner, R., Langevitz, P. et al. Low-molecular weight heparin during pregnancy and delivery: preliminary experience with 41 pregnancies. *Obstet. Gynecol.* 87:380–383, 1996.

Elkayam, U. Anticoagulation in pregnant women with prosthetic heart valves: a double jeopardy. *J. Am. Coll. Cardiol.* 27:1704, 1996.

Hall, J.G., Pauli, R.M., and Wilson, K.M. Maternal and fetal sequelae of anticoagulation during pregnancy. *Am. J. Med.* 68:122, 1980.

Harenberg, J., Schneider, D., Heilmann, L., and Wolf, H. Lack of anti-factor Xa activity in umbilical cord samples after subcutaneous administration of heparin or low molecular mass heparin in pregnant women. *Hemostasis* 23:314, 1993.

Hirsh, J., and Fuster, V. Guide to anticoagulant therapy. Part 1: Heparin. *Circulation* 89:1449, 1994.

Howell, R., et al. The risks of antenatal subcutaneous heparin prophylaxis: a controlled trial. *Br. J. Gynaecol.* 90:1124, 1983.

Hull, R.D., Raskob, G.E., Pineo, G.F., et al. Subcutaneous low-molecular-weight heparin compared with continuous intravenous heparin in the treatment of proximal-vein thrombosis. *N. Engl. J. Med.* 326:975, 1992.

Inbar, O., Blank, M., Faden, D., et al. Prevention of fetal loss in experimental antiphospholipid syndrome by low-molecular-weight heparin. *Am. J. Obstet. Gynecol.* 169:423, 1993.

Levine, M., Gent, M., Hirsh, J., et al. A comparison of low-molecular-weight heparin administered primarily at home with unfractionated heparin administered in the hospital for proximal deep-vein thrombosis. *N. Engl. J. Med.* 334:677, 1996.

Macklon, N.S., Greer, I.A., Reid, A.W., and Walker, I.D. Thrombocytopenia, antithrombin deficiency and extensive thromboembolism in pregnancy: treatment with low-molecular-weight heparin. *Blood Coag. Fibrinol.* 6:672, 1995.

Magnani, H.N. Heparin-induced thrombocytopenia: an overview of 230 patients treated with Orgaran. *Thromb. Hemost.* 70:554, 1993.

Majerus, P.W., Broze, G.J., Jr., Miletich, J.P., and Tollefsen, D.M. Anticoagulant, thrombolytic and antiplatelet drugs. Chapter 54 in *Goodman and Gilman's The Pharmacological Basis of Therapeutics* (9th ed.), J.G. Hardman and L.E. Limbird, eds. New York: McGraw-Hill, 1996. Pp. 1341–1359.

Medical Letter: Ardeparin and danaparoid for prevention of deep vein thrombosis. *Med. Lett.* 39:94, 1997.

Rai, R., Cohen, H., Dave, M., and Regan, L. Randomized controlled trial of aspirin and aspirin plus heparin in pregnant women with recurrent miscarriage associated with phospholipid antibodies. *Br. Med. J.* 314:253, 1997.

Raschke, R.A., Reilly, B.M., and Guidry, J.R. The weight-based heparin dosing nomogram compared with a "standard care" nomogram. *Arch. Intern. Med.* 119:874, 1993.

Salazar, E., Izagurine, R., Verdejo, J., and Mutchinick, O. Failure of adjusted doses of subcutaneous heparin to prevent thromboembolic phenomena in pregnant patients with mechanical cardiac valve prostheses. *J. Am. Coll. Cardiol.* 27:1698, 1996.

Sturridge, F., de Swiet, M., and Letsky, E. The use of low molecular weight heparin for thrombo prophylaxis in pregnancy. *Br. J. Obstet. Gynaecol.* 101:69, 1994.

Food and Drug Administration. FDA Public Health Advisory. Subject: Reports of epidural or spinal hematomas with the concurrent use of low molecular weight heparin and spinal/epidural anesthesia or spinal puncture. US Dept of Health and Human Services, Public Health Service, FDA. 15 Dec 97.

Heroin

INDICATIONS AND RECOMMENDATIONS

Heroin, or diacetylmorphine, is contraindicated during pregnancy. It is a class I drug, meaning that there are no valid indications for its use in the United States. It is highly addictive and the pregnant woman addicted to heroin represents a significant economic, social, and medical problem to our society.

Heroin easily crosses the placenta, and fetal withdrawal may occur if the mother undergoes rapid withdrawal. Fetal death in utero has been reported under these circumstances. Infants of heroin-addicted mothers tend to be of low birth weight, and other obstetric complications occur with increased frequency. Fetal movements may be diminished transiently after heroin injection. On the other hand, it appears that fetal hepatic and pulmonary maturation are accelerated. It is not clear as to whether congenital anomalies are more common among infants of heroin-addicted mothers, although some evidence suggests this to be the case. Overall perinatal mortality is increased. Neonatal withdrawal symptoms are common.

It is not clear whether the effects of maternal heroin use on the offspring persist into later childhood. Sudden infant death syndrome has been reported to occur with increased frequency. Some studies have found measurable effects in preschool youngsters, but possible confounding by environmental and other factors makes interpretation difficult. Many treatment programs have been aimed at this group of individuals, and some success at improving outcome has been reported. See "Methadone" and "Narcotic Analgesics" for discussion of fetal and maternal effects.

RECOMMENDED READING

Carr, S.R., and Coustan, D.R. Nonprescription drugs and alcohol: abuse and effects in pregnancy. Chapter 22 in *Medicine of the Fetus and Mother* (2nd ed.), E.A. Reece, J.C. Hobbins, M.J. Mahoney, and R.H. Petrie, eds. Philadelphia: Lippincott-Raven, in press.

Farrell, T., Owen, P., and Harrold, A. Fetal movements following intrapartum maternal opiate administration. *Clin. Exp. Obstet. Gynecol.* 23:144, 1996.

Glass, L., Rajegowda, B.K., and Evans, H.E. Absence of respiratory distress syndrome in premature infants of heroin-addicted mothers. *Lancet* 2:685, 1971.

Kandall, S.R., Gaines, J., Habel, L., et al. Relationship of maternal substance abuse to subsequent sudden infant death syndrome in offspring. *J. Pediatrics* 123:120, 1993.

Nathenson, G., et al. The effect of maternal heroin addiction on neonatal jaundice. *J. Pediatrics* 81:899, 1972.

Reisine, T., and Pasternak, G. Opioid analgesics and antagonists. Chapter 23 in *Goodman and Gilman's The Pharmacological Basis of Therapeutics* (9th ed.), J.G. Hardman and L.E. Limbird, eds. New York: McGraw-Hill, 1996. Pp. 536–540.

Rementeria, J.L., and Nunag, N.N. Narcotic withdrawal in pregnancy: stillbirth incidence with a case report. *Am. J. Obstet. Gynecol.* 116:1152, 1973.

Van Baar, A., and dew Graaff, B.M.T. Cognitive development at preschool age of infants of drug-dependent mothers. *Dev. Med. Child. Neurol.* 36:1063, 1994.

Wilson, G.S., et al. The development of preschool children of heroin-addicted mothers: a controlled study. *Pediatrics* 63:135, 1979.

Heterocyclic Antipsychotics: Loxapine (Loxitane®), Molindone (Moban®), Pimozide (Orap®), Risperidone (Risperdal®); see also Clozapine

INDICATIONS AND RECOMMENDATIONS

The heterocyclic antipsychotics are relatively contraindicated during pregnancy because other therapeutic agents are preferable. Loxapine, molindone, and risperidone are indicated for management of the manifestations of psychotic disorders. Pimozide is indicated for the suppression of severely compromising motor and phonic tics in patients with Tourette's disorder who have failed to respond satisfactorily to standard treatment.

None of these agents have been studied in pregnant women. In laboratory animals, risperidone is known to cross the placenta and its use is associated with an increased stillborn rate and an increased number of pup deaths on days 1–4 during lactation. The manufacturer's literature reports that pimozide causes a decreased number of pregnancies and retarded fetal development in rats. In rabbits its use during pregnancy is associated with maternal toxicity and mortality, decreased weight gain, and embryotoxicity.

A woman who is taking these drugs should be counseled to avoid pregnancy. If she desires to become pregnant, she should be switched to one of the phenothiazines, which have been better studied during pregnancy, if such a switch would not harm the patient.

RECOMMENDED READING

Baldessarini, R.J. Drugs and the treatment of psychiatric disorders: psychosis and anxiety. Chapter 18 in *Goodman and Gilman's The Pharmacological Basis of Therapeutics* (9th ed.), J.G. Hardman and L.E. Limbird, eds. New York: McGraw-Hill, 1996. Pp. 402–419.

Goldberg, H.L. Psychotropic drugs in pregnancy and lactation. *Int. J. Psychiatr. Med.* 24:129–147, 1994.

Schatzberg, A.F., and Nemeroff, C.B. *Textbook of Psychopharmacology.* New York: American Psychiatric Press, 1995. Pp. 247–280, 828—829.

HMG-CoA Reductase Inhibitors Atorvastatin (Lipitor®), Fluvastatin (Lescol®), Lovastatin (Mevacor®), Pravastatin (Pravachol®), Simvastatin (Zocor®)

INDICATIONS AND RECOMMENDATIONS

HMG-CoA reductase inhibitors are contraindicated in pregnancy. These drugs block the synthesis of cholesterol in the liver by competitively inhibiting HMG-CoA reductase, a key enzyme in early cholesterol biosynthesis.

Early studies in laboratory animals have shown lovastatin to cause fetal skeletal malformations. Because of these early reports, all of these agents have been labeled as drugs that may cause fetal harm when given to pregnant women. No studies of the use of these drugs during pregnancy has been performed.

In a single case report, the use of lovastatin during the first trimester of pregnancy was associated with the birth of a child with multiple congenital anomalies including vertebrae anomalies, anal atresia, tracheoesophageal fistula, and renal and radial dysplasia (VATER syndrome). The mother had concurrently taken dextroamphetamine.

Simvastatin has been found to suppress human testicular testosterone synthesis in vitro when used in concentrations probably exceeding those achieved with therapeutic use.

RECOMMENDED READING

Dostal, L.A., Schardein, J.L., and Anderson, J.A. Developmental toxicity of the HMG-CoA reductase inhibitor, atorvastatin, in rats and rabbits. *Teratology* 50:387, 1994.

Ghidini, A., Sicherer, S. and Willner, J. Congenital abnormalities (VATER) in baby born to mother using lovastatin. *Lancet* 339: 1416, 1992.

Masters, B.A., et al. In vitro myotoxicity of the 3-hydroxy-3-methyl-glutaryl coenzyme A reductase inhibitors, pravastatin, lovastatin, and simvastatin, using neonatal rat skeletal myocytes. *Toxicol. Appl. Pharmacol.* 131:163–74, 1995.

Smals, A.G., et al. The HMG-CoA reductase inhibitor simvastatin suppresses human testicular testosterone synthesis in vitro by a selective inhibitory effect on 17-ketosteroid-oxidoreductase enzyme activity. *J. Steroid Biochem. Mol. Biol.* 38:465, 1991.

Tse, F.L., and Labbadia, D. Absorption and disposition of fluvastatin, an inhibitor of HMG-CoA reductase, in the rabbit. *Biopharm. Drug Disp.* 13:285, 1992.

Witzham, J.L. Drugs used in the treatment of hyperlipoproteinemias. Chapter 36 in *Goodman and Gilman's The Pharmacological Basis of Therapeutics* (9th ed.), J.G. Hardman and L.E. Limbird, eds. New York: McGraw-Hill, 1996. Pp. 884–885.

Hydantoins; Phenytoin (Dilantin®) and Phenacemide (Phenurone®)

INDICATIONS AND RECOMMENDATIONS

Hydantoins may be prescribed during pregnancy for individuals with clear indications for their use that outweigh the risk of fetal hydantoin syndrome. Counseling such patients is crucial. The epileptic gravida can be reassured that most pregnant women with epilepsy have a successful pregnancy, although there is an increased risk of congenital malformations (two to three times that seen in the normal population). Whenever possible, a single medication for control of seizures is preferable to multiple drug regimens.

Phenytoin is most commonly used as an anticonvulsant in the treatment of generalized tonic-clonic, simple complex, and partial seizures. It is ineffective against absence seizures and may even exacerbate them. It is also, more rarely, used as an intravenous antiarrhythmic agent in the treatment of ventricular arrhythmias, but alternative agents are preferred during pregnancy. Phenacemide is a congener of the hydantoins that is useful in the treatment of severe seizure disorders poorly responsive to other drugs. It is useful in the treatment of complex partial seizures. It should not be used unless other agents have proven ineffective in seizure control.

SPECIAL CONSIDERATIONS IN PREGNANCY

Dosage requirements for phenytoin have been reported to increase during pregnancy and fall in the puerperium, although this remains controversial. Phenytoin readily crosses the placenta, and identical maternal and fetal plasma levels have been reported at delivery. Elimination of the drug by the full-term neonate has been shown to be similar to that of adults.

The risk of congenital abnormalities in infants exposed to hydantoins is 6% to 8%, or 2–3 times the rate of malformations in the general population. This increase in congenital abnormalities may be due to elevated levels of epoxides, the oxidative metabolites of the hydantoins. Genetic defects in either epoxide hydrolase activity or free radical scavengers have been postulated as explanations of why some exposed infants display teratogenic effects and some do not. A combination of defects termed the fetal hydantoin syndrome has been described. This consists of craniofacial abnormalities, growth retardation, mental retardation, and nail and digital hypoplasia. The syndrome's degree of expression is variable. Its more serious consequences can be found in 10% of exposed neonates, whereas manifestations of its mildest form may be present in 30% of cases. Numerous case reports have also suggested a correlation between maternal phenytoin administration and fetal neuroblastoma, gastrointestinal and genitourinary defects, and melanotic neuroectodermal tumors. Phenacemide has been found to cause birth defects in mice at the lowest dose tested. The manufacturer has stated that Phenurone can cause fetal harm when administered to pregnant women.

As with phenobarbital, the hydantoins have been associated with a vitamin K–deficient coagulopathy in the neonate. This tendency can be reversed by administration of vitamin K_1 (10 mg/day) to the mother during the last month of the pregnancy. It is also almost universal that vitamin K is administered at birth, so a vitamin K–dependent coagulopathy appears unlikely. If an institution does not routinely administer vitamin K at birth, measurement of cord blood prothrombin time followed by vitamin K administration as necessary is indicated. Neonatal glucose levels should be checked shortly after birth. Breastfeeding is not contraindicated. All anticonvulsants interfere with folic acid metabolism. Periconceptional and first-trimester folic acid supplementation (0.4 mg/day) is recommended. Serial complete blood count and liver function tests should be performed if phenacemide is used, as leukopenia and liver toxicity have been described.

DOSAGE

The usual adult maintenance dose of phenytoin in anticonvulsant therapy is about 300 mg/day. This dosage should produce serum levels in the therapeutic range of 10–20 µg/ml. As the half-life of phenytoin is relatively long, steady-state serum levels are reached in 6–10 days when no loading dose is given. These can be reached more quickly if a load of 1000 mg in divided doses over 1–2 days is given before institution of maintenance therapy. Dosage alterations should await achievement of a plateau level and should be attempted in small stepwise increments. Since phenytoin exhibits dose-dependent kinetics, dosage increases may lead to larger than expected increases in serum levels. Phenacemide is usually started at 1.5 g/day, given in divided doses of 500 mg each. This may be increased by 500 mg/day weekly when seizure control is still poor. The total adult daily dose is usually 2–3 g.

Intravenous therapy is sometimes indicated when a patient is not able to take oral medications and in the treatment of status epilepticus. This drug must be given slowly at a rate of less than 50 mg/min, preferably with concurrent maternal cardiac monitoring. Phenytoin should not be given intramuscularly because the drug is erratically absorbed from the site of administration.

Changes in the serum hydantoin levels secondary to drug interactions may adversely affect the therapeutic response. Carbamazepine, folic acid, and alcohol may decrease steady-state hydantoin levels, whereas isoniazid, chloramphenicol, primidone, and warfarin (Coumadin) may increase such levels. When phenobarbital is given concurrently, it may either increase or decrease hydantoin plasma concentrations by either increasing or competitively inhibiting their metabolism.

ADVERSE EFFECTS

A variety of adverse effects have been reported, including nystagmus, ataxia, vertigo, diplopia, peripheral neuropathy, deterioration in intellect, hyperactivity, drowsiness, and hallucinations. Gastrointestinal symptoms, gingival hyperplasia, osteomalacia, megaloblastic anemia, hirsutism, and decreased insulin secretion with hyperglycemia can also occur. Some of these effects are dose related, but they may be seen with serum levels in the upper portion of the therapeutic range.

Idiosyncratic reactions include skin rash, Stevens-Johnson syndrome, systemic lupus erythematosus, aplastic anemia, hepatic necrosis, and nonspecific lymphadenopathy. With rapid intravenous administration, cardiovascular collapse and central nervous system depression can occur.

MECHANISM OF ACTION

The hydantoins block the spread of electrical activity from a seizure focus by stabilizing the neuronal membrane and preventing posttetanic potentiation. They are effective in the treatment of generalized tonic-clonic seizures, as well as simple complex and partial seizures. They are ineffective against absence seizures and may even exacerbate them.

ABSORPTION AND BIOTRANSFORMATION

Phenytoin is absorbed through the duodenum and is readily bound to albumin and α-globulins. The plasma protein binding is not significantly altered in pregnancy. Phenytoin and phenacemide are metabolized by the liver and the metabolite is excreted via the kidneys. The rate of metabolism of phenytoin is variable, with a half-life usually ranging from 17 to 56 hours. The pharmacokinetics of phenacemide in humans have not been well determined.

RECOMMENDED READING

Brown, N.A., Shull, G., Kao, J., Goulding, E.H., and Fabro, S. Teratogenicity and lethality of hydantoin derivatives in the mouse: structure-toxicity relationships. *Toxicol. Appl. Toxicol.* 64:271, 1982.

Kaneko, S.K. Antiepileptic drug therapy and reproductive consequences: functional and morphologic effects. *Reprod. Toxicol.* 5:179, 1991.

Kelly, T.E. Teratogenicity of anticonvulsant drugs. I. Review of the literature. *Am. J. Med. Genet.* 19:413, 1984.

Kochenour, N.K., Emery, M.G., and Sawchuk, R.J. Phenytoin metabolism in pregnancy. *Obstet. Gynecol.* 56:577, 1980.

McNamara, J.O. Drugs effective in the therapy of the epilepsies. Chapter 20 in *Goodman and Gilman's The Pharmacological Basis of Therapeutics* (9th ed.), J.G. Hardman and L.E. Limbird, eds. New York: McGraw-Hill, 1996. Pp. 468–471.

Monson, R.R., et al. Dilantin and selected congenital malformations. *N. Engl. J. Med.* 289:1049, 1973.

Seizure Disorders in Pregnancy. American College of Obstetricians and Gynecologists Educational Bulletin No. 231, December 1996.

Wilder, B.J., and Bruni, J. *Seizure Disorders: A Pharmacological Approach to Treatment.* New York: Raven Press, 1981.

Woodbury, D.M., Penry, J.K., and Pippenger, C.E. *Antiepileptic Drugs* (2nd ed.). New York: Raven Press, 1982.

Yerby, M.S. Pregnancy, teratogenesis and epilepsy. *Neurol. Clin.* 12:749, 1994.

Hydralazine (Apresoline®)

INDICATIONS AND RECOMMENDATIONS

Hydralazine is safe to use during pregnancy. It traditionally has been the drug of choice for the acute control of moderate to severe hypertension in patients with preeclampsia. This drug may also be used in combination with other agents to control chronic hypertension in obstetric patients.

Significant iatrogenic hypotension can develop when hydralazine is used to treat an acute hypertensive episode in an intravascularly depleted patient with preeclampsia. In order to minimize the chances of this occurring, the drug should be administered in 5 mg boluses intravenously not more frequently than every 15–20 minutes. Administration of hydralazine by intravenous bolus is preferable to continuous intravenous infusion in preeclampsia as several studies have demonstrated an increased risk for hypotension and fetal distress with the latter mode of therapy. This is related to a cumulative effect of the administered hydralazine, as the plasma elimination half-life is approximately 2–4 hours, and the antihypertensive effect is even more prolonged.

Tachyphylaxis is common when hydralazine is used as a single agent, making it a poor choice for the management of patients with chronic hypertension. In order to maximize its long-term effectiveness, it may be necessary to add diuretics and possibly propranolol to the regimen. Since there are objections to the use of these agents during pregnancy, we do not recommend hydralazine as primary therapy for the obstetric patient with chronic hypertension.

SPECIAL CONSIDERATIONS IN PREGNANCY

Acute hypotensive episodes can occur in response to an intravenous bolus of hydralazine given to a preeclamptic patient who is intravascularly volume depleted. The effect on the fetus of lowering maternal blood pressure with intravenous hydralazine has been studied in 33 women with diastolic pressures of 110 mm Hg or greater. All of these pregnancies were beyond 30 weeks gestation. Thirty of the women responded to a dose of 12.5 mg hydralazine with a decrease in diastolic pressure to values between 70 and 90 mm Hg. Nineteen fetuses demonstrated evidence of heart rate decelerations with or without bradycardia, whereas the other 14 fetuses did not show any evidence of fetal heart rate abnormalities. In the first group, there were 3 stillborns and 13 neonates born with weights below the 10th percentile for gestational age. In the second group, there was only one neonate below the 10th percentile and no perinatal deaths. Despite the fact that this older study utilized an initial dose that is more than twice the currently recommended dose, the majority of patients did not have a fall in diastolic values below 70 mm Hg. However, even with drops in pressure into the range of 70–90 mm Hg, it appears that growth-retarded fetuses are far more likely to demonstrate heart rate changes than those who are appropriately grown.

Tachycardia and increased cardiac work and oxygen consumption accompany the intravenous use of hydralazine. This may precipitate angina or myocardial ischemia in a patient with occlusive coronary artery disease. The treatment for symptoms related to increased cardiac work is intravenous propranolol.

Specific fetal side effects related to hydralazine therapy for the mother have only rarely been described in humans. An isolated case of neonatal thrombocytopenia has been reported, but there is very little supportive evidence to implicate hydralazine as the cause of this problem. In animals, however, skeletal defects can be produced that resemble those observed in experimentally induced manganese deficiency states.

Older studies that could not distinguish uterine from placental blood flow indicated that hydralazine increased uteroplacental blood flow in sheep with hypertension. Newer techniques demonstrated that whereas treatment of hypertensive pregnant rats with hydralazine results in a 57% increase in flow to the uterus, placental blood flow was decreased by 44%. In sheep, blood flow to the uterus increased, but blood flow to the placenta was unchanged. In human hypertensive pregnancy, administration of intravenous hydralazine caused a decrease in intervillous blood flow in 6 of 10 patients as measured by the [133]xenon perfusion method. In contrast, in this study and others, umbilical flow was increased by hydralazine, suggesting a possible direct effect on umbilical vessels. In vitro studies have failed to demonstrate a direct vasodilatory effect of hydralazine on umbilical arteries or veins. Adverse effects on placental perfusion leading to fetal distress can best be avoided by proper dosing of the drug to avoid systemic hypotension. An appropriate therapeutic goal would be a diastolic blood pressure between 90 and 100 mm Hg.

DOSAGE

Intravenous hydralazine should be given in 5 mg boluses not more frequently than every 20 minutes. The onset of action is 10–20 minutes, with maximum effect at 20–40 minutes. Therefore, caution should be used with repeat dosing at 20 minutes if the blood pressure is continuing to decline. In a study of 70 pre-eclamptic patients requiring acute blood pressure control, 43% required a second dose of 5 mg, and only 13% required a third 5 mg bolus to achieve the therapeutic goal of a mean arterial pressure less than 125 mm Hg. If good blood pressure control is not achieved after a total of 20 mg, then an alternate antihypertensive agent should be considered. The duration of antihypertensive action of an intravenous dose ranges from 4 to 8 hours. The usual starting oral dose is 20 mg twice daily for 2–3 days, then 50 mg twice daily for the remainder of the first week of therapy. Subsequent increases can be by 100 mg/week as needed to reach therapeutic goals. Doses beyond 400 mg/day are unlikely to achieve further benefit.

ADVERSE EFFECTS

Side effects include palpitations, flushing, nasal congestion, headache, dizziness, anginal attacks, and electrocardiographic changes of myocardial ischemia. Side effects related to chronic use in doses greater than 200 mg/day include drug fever, skin eruptions, peripheral neuropathy, blood dyscrasias, mild gastrointestinal symptoms, and an acute rheumatoid state that can progress to the hydralazine-lupus syndrome. Up to 10% to 20% of patients who receive more than 400 mg/day will develop this last problem. Occasionally, central nervous system toxicity may be manifested as an acute psychotic episode.

MECHANISM OF ACTION

Hydralazine reduces vascular resistance by directly relaxing arteriolar smooth muscle. Postcapillary capacitance vessels are much less affected than precapillary resistance vessels. It has been postulated that hydralazine may be able to chelate certain trace metals required for smooth muscle contraction.

Peripheral arterial vasodilatation is not uniform. Vascular resistance in the coronary, cerebral, splanchnic, and uterine circulations decreases more than in skin and muscle. Renovascular resistance decreases more than that in other vascular beds. Blood flow in the more dilated circulatory beds usually increases unless the hypotensive effect of the drug is profound. Both supine and standing blood pressures are decreased.

Hydralazine has no direct action on the heart; homeostatic circulatory reflexes mediated by the autonomic nervous system remain fully functional. Decreased arterial pressure activates baroreceptors to mediate a sympathetic discharge. This results in increased heart rate, stroke volume, and cardiac output. Because this increase in cardiac output partially offsets the effect of arteriolar dilatation and limits the hypotensive effectiveness of the drug, hydralazine is usually combined with a drug that limits the increase in cardiac output when prescribed for long-term use.

Renal blood flow and glomerular filtration rates are either unaffected or increased. Hydralazine causes sodium and water retention, with expansion of plasma and extracellular volumes. This is a result of a direct renal mechanism as well as an increase in peripheral plasma renin activity. Increases in renin activity during hydralazine therapy are effectively minimized in the nonpregnant woman by the coadministration of propranolol.

ABSORPTION AND BIOTRANSFORMATION

Hydralazine is fairly completely absorbed after oral administration. Peak serum concentrations are reached 1–2 hours after administration of an oral dose. Intravenous administration of a given dose results in higher serum levels than the same dose given orally. About 85% of the circulating drug is bound to albumin.

Acetylation in the liver is the major pathway of biotransformation. The rate of acetylation is dependent on the genetically determined activity of hepatic N-acetyltransferase. Therefore, when treated with the same dose of hydralazine, slow acetylators have higher serum concentrations than rapid acetylators. In addition, slow acetylators seem to be more prone to develop the hydralazine-lupus syndrome.

Very high serum levels may be found in patients with renal insufficiency. Renal excretion of the active drug is not usually an important route of elimination, so that uremia probably interferes with biotransformation.

RECOMMENDED READING

Belfort, M.A., Saade, G.R., Suresh M., Johnson, D., and Vedernikov, Y.P. Human umbilical vessels: responses to agents frequently used in obstetric patients. *Am. J. Obstet. Gynecol.* 172:1395, 1995.

Gudmundsson, S., Gennser, G., and Marsal K. Effects of hydralazine on placental and renal circulation in preeclampsia. *Acta Obstet. Gynecol. Scand.* 74:415, 1995.

Harper A., and Murnaghan, G.A. Maternal and fetal hemodynamics in hypertensive pregnancies during maternal treatment with intravenous hydralazine or labetalol. *Br. J. Obstet. Gynaecol.* 98: 453, 1991.

Jouppila, P., Kirkinen, P., Koivula, A., and Ylikorkala, O. Effects of dihydralazine infusion on the fetoplacental blood flow and maternal prostanoids. *Obstet. Gynecol.* 65:115, 1985.

Koch-Weser, J. Hydralazine. *N. Engl. J. Med.* 295:320, 1976.

Lipshitz, J., Ahokas R.A., and Reynolds, S.L. The effect of hydralazine on placental perfusion in the spontaneously hypertensive rat. *Am. J. Obstet. Gynecol.* 156:356,1987.

Lodeiro, J.G., Feinstein, S.J., and Lodeiro, S.B. Fetal premature atrial contractions associated with hydralazine. *Am. J. Obstet. Gynecol.* 160:105, 1989.

Paterson-Brown, S., Robson, S.C., Redfern, N., Walkinshaw, S.A., and DeSwiet, M. Hydralazine boluses for the treatment of severe hypertension in pregnancy. *Br. J. Obstet. Gynaecol.* 101:409, 1994.

Pedron, S.L., Reid, D.L., Barnard, J.M., Henry, J.B., Phernetton, T.M., and Rankin, J.H.G. Differential effects of intravenous hydralazine on myoendometrial and placental blood flow in hypertensive pregnant ewes. *Am. J. Obstet. Gynecol.* 167:1672, 1992.

Pryde, P.G., Abel, E.L., Hannigan, J., Evans, M.I., and Cotton, D.B. Effects of hydralazine on pregnant rats and their fetuses. *Am. J. Obstet. Gynecol.* 169:1027, 1993.

Spinnato, J.A., Sibai, B.M., and Anderson, G.D. Fetal distress after hydralazine therapy for severe pregnancy-induced hypertension. *South. Med. J.* 79:559, 1986.

Vink, G.J., Moodley, J., and Philpott, R.H. Effect of dihydralazine on the fetus in the treatment of maternal hypertension. *Obstet. Gynecol.* 55:519, 1980.

Widerlov, E., Karlman, I., and Storsater, J. Hydralazine-inducted neonatal thrombocytopenia (letter). *N. Engl. J. Med.* 303:1235, 1980.

Yemini, M., Shoham, Z., Dgani, R., Lancet, M., Mogilner, B.M., Nissim, F., and Bar-Khayim, Y. Lupus-like syndrome in a mother and newborn following administration of hydralizine; a case report. *Eur. J. Obstet. Gynecol. Reprod. Biol.* 30:193, 1989.

Hydroxyzine (Atarax®, Vistaril®)

INDICATIONS AND RECOMMENDATIONS

Hydroxyzine, a piperazine H_1 receptor antihistamine, is safe to use after the first trimester of pregnancy and is commonly administered, alone or in combination with analgesic agents, for the relief of pain and anxiety during labor. In addition, it is often used as an antipruritic and antianxiety agent. Although human data are lacking, there is evidence that hydroxyzine in large dosages is teratogenic in laboratory animals, and therefore use of the drug is best avoided during the first trimester of pregnancy. Antihistamines are not recommended for lactating women.

SPECIAL CONSIDERATIONS IN PREGNANCY

In the Collaborative Perinatal Project, there were 3248 infants with malformations among the more than 50,000 mother–infant pairs studied. Five in 50 mother–infant pairs exposed to hydroxyzine during the first four lunar months of pregnancy had congenital abnormalities, whereas three anomalies would have been expected. Thus, there appeared to be a relative risk of 1.55 for birth defects in neonates exposed to this drug during the first 4 months in utero. In a study of 100 mother–infant pairs exposed in the first trimester, there was no significant difference in anomalies compared to untreated controls. Animal studies have demonstrated an increased incidence of facial clefts when hydroxyzine was administered in excessive dosages (200 mg/kg) during organogenesis and this association has also been questioned in one human study.

Although one study has demonstrated a statistically significant decrease in fetal heart rate beat-to-beat variability when hydroxyzine was administered to laboring mothers, this effect was said to be clinically insignificant.

There is a single case report of an apparent neonatal withdrawal syndrome in a newborn whose mother required 600 mg/day of hydroxyzine for pruritus throughout the pregnancy. The cord blood hydroxyzine level was 180 μg/dl (usual adult therapeutic level is 50 μg/dl). This infant was also exposed to phenobarbital in the last 3 weeks in utero.

Due to its anticholinergic properties, hydroxyzine might be expected to inhibit lactation. Such an effect has not yet been demonstrated.

DOSAGE

Hydroxyzine is available in capsules containing 25, 50, and 100 mg, and in 25, 50, 75, and 100 mg vials for intramuscular injection. When used as an antipruritic, the usual dose is 25 mg tid or qid. When used orally as an antianxiety drug, the starting dose is usually 50–100 mg qid. When used intramuscularly as an antianxiety agent or in combination with an analgesic, doses of 25–100 mg are employed and may be repeated at 4- to 6-hour intervals.

ADVERSE EFFECTS

Although hydroxyzine is often used intentionally to potentiate the effects of narcotic analgesics, it should be remembered that this drug also potentiates other central nervous system depressants, such as barbiturates and alcohol. Other adverse effects include drowsiness and dry mouth. Rarely, excessively high doses have been associated with involuntary motor activity, tremor, and convulsions. Tissue damage has been reported with inadvertent subcutaneous injection.

MECHANISM OF ACTION

Hydroxyzine is a piperazine antihistamine that is a competitive blocker of the H_1 receptor in effector cells. It inhibits the smooth muscle response to histamine in the gastrointestinal and respiratory tracts, antagonizes the increased capillary permeability induced by histamine (the wheal and flare), and suppresses the stimulant effect of histamine on the autonomic nervous system. It does not inhibit histamine release. The central nervous system and antimotion sickness effects are poorly understood, as is the potentiation of narcotics, depressants, and alcohol. Anticholinergic side effects appear to be due to blockage of muscarinic receptors.

ABSORPTION AND BIOTRANSFORMATION

Hydroxyzine is rapidly absorbed after oral dosing, and clinical effects are noted within 15–30 minutes after ingestion. Effects are maximal within 1–2 hours and last for 3–6 hours. The drug is metabolized in the liver, with degradation products excreted in the urine within 24 hours.

RECOMMENDED READING

Babe, K.S., Jr., and Serafin, W.E. Histamine, bradykinin, and their antagonists. Chapter 25 in *Goodman and Gilman's The Pharmacological Basis of Therapeutics* (9th ed.), J.G. Hardman and L.E. Limbird, eds. New York: McGraw-Hill, 1996. Pp. 588–591.

Erez, S., Schifrin, B.S., and Dirim, O. Double-blind evaluation of hydroxyzine as an antiemetic in pregnancy. *J. Reprod. Med.* 7:57, 1971.

Heinonen, O.P., Slone, D., and Shapiro, S. *Birth Defects and Drugs in Pregnancy.* Boston: Wright-PSG, 1977. Pp. 335–337.

Petrie, R.H., et al. The effect of drugs on fetal heart rate variability. *Am. J. Obstet. Gynecol.* 130:294, 1978.

Prenner, B.M. Neonatal withdrawal syndrome associated with hydroxyzine hydrochloride. *Am. J. Dis. Child.* 131:529, 1977.

Walker, B.E., and Patterson, A. Induction of cleft palate in mice by tranquilizers and barbiturates. *Teratology* 10:159, 1974.

Idoxuridine (Herplex®)

INDICATIONS AND RECOMMENDATIONS

Idoxuridine (IDUR) is relatively contraindicated in pregnancy because other therapeutic modalities are preferable. It is a topical ophthalmic preparation used in the treatment of herpes simplex keratitis. These infections are usually not associated with grave prognoses; they are most often limited to the eye and resolve completely. Idoxuridine will often control the infection but will have no effect on accumulated scarring, vascularization, or resultant progressive loss of vision. It alters herpes simplex virus reproduction by replacing thymidine during viral DNA synthesis.

Experience with IDUR in pregnant women is lacking, and its effects on the fetus are unknown. In rabbits, however, dosages similar to those used clinically are associated with fetal malformation, including exophthalmos and clubbing of the forelegs.

Should treatment be required, mechanical debridement is preferred over IDUR therapy.

RECOMMENDED READING

Garner, A., and Klintworth, G.K. *Pathobiology of Ocular Disease.* New York: Marcel Dekker, 1982. Pp. 258–262.

Gittinger, J.W. *Ophthalmology: A Clinical Introduction.* Boston: Little, Brown, 1984. Pp. 75–76.

Itoi, M., et al. Teratogenicities of ophthalmic drugs. I. Antiviral ophthalmic drugs. *Arch. Ophthalmol.* 93:46, 1975.

Indigo Carmine

INDICATIONS AND RECOMMENDATIONS

Indigo carmine may be introduced into the amniotic fluid for documentation of ruptured membranes and for identification of individual amniotic sacs in multiple gestations. Inadequate data are available to evaluate its safety when administered intravenously during urologic procedures in pregnant women.

SPECIAL CONSIDERATIONS IN PREGNANCY

Indigo carmine has replaced methylene blue as a marker dye for amniotic fluid because of the risks of fetal methemoglobinemia with the latter. There are no data available to suggest fetal risk from this substance when it is injected intraamniotically. In addition, a number of case reports suggested an association between methylene blue instillation in the amniotic fluid and intestinal atresia. There is a case report of small bowel atresia in one of twins, in which indigo carmine was injected during amniocentesis at 16 weeks. However, no large series have suggested an excess risk with this dye.

When indigo carmine is used to identify the fluid from multiple sacs during amniocentesis for diagnosis of fetal hemolytic disease, its presence may obfuscate measurement of the delta optical density at 450 nm. The dye should therefore not be injected until a sample of fluid has been aspirated. If, however, the amniotic fluid is contaminated with dye, a chloroform extraction procedure can be performed to permit more accurate measurements.

DOSAGE

When indigo carmine is used for amniocentesis, 0.5–1.0 ml of 0.8% solution is diluted to a 10 ml volume.

ADVERSE EFFECTS

Intravenously injected indigo carmine has been associated with increased peripheral resistance, increased blood pressure, increased central venous pressure, and lowered cardiac output with reflex-diminished stroke volume and pulse rate. These results resemble those associated with α-adrenergic stimulation. There is also a single case report of hypertension and tachycardia with ectopic ventricular beats in a patient given 5 ml of 0.8% indigo carmine while under halothane anesthesia. Thus, care should be exercised in administering this dye intravenously to patients with cardiovascular disease.

MECHANISM OF ACTION

When indigo carmine is instilled at amniocentesis, it colors the amniotic fluid blue. In the case of a multiple gestation, subsequent taps may be performed, with the absence of blue discoloration in the aspirated samples indicating success at puncturing the remaining sac(s). In the case of ruptured membranes, the appearance of blue fluid in the vagina confirms the diagnosis. However, since the dye can be absorbed into the maternal circulation and enter the urine, a sterile sponge or tampon placed in the vagina will help to differentiate between true amniotic fluid and maternal urine contamination.

ABSORPTION AND BIOTRANSFORMATION

Indigo carmine is injected into the amniotic fluid directly. It is absorbed into the maternal bloodstream and excreted in the urine. Thus, the urine may be stained.

RECOMMENDED READING

Cragan, J.D., Martin, M.L., Khoury, M.J., et al. Dye use during amniocentesis and birth defects. *Lancet* 341:1352, 1993.

Elias, S., et al. Genetic amniocentesis in twin gestations. *Am. J. Obstet. Gynecol.* 138:169, 1980.

Erickson, J.C., and Widmer, B.A. The vasopressor effect of indigo carmine. *Anesthesiology* 29:188, 1968.

Fribourg, S. Safety of intra-amniotic injection of indigo carmine. *Am. J. Obstet. Gynecol.* 140:350, 1981.

Glüer, S. Intestinal atresia following intraamniotic use of dyes. *Eur. J. Pediatr. Surg.* 5:240–242, 1994.

Horger, E.O., and Moody, L.O. Use of indigo carmine for twin amniocentesis and its effect on bilirubin analysis. *Am. J. Obstet. Gynecol.* 150:858, 1984.

Kennedy, W.F., Jr., et al. Cardiovascular and respiratory effects of indigo carmine. *J. Urol.* 100:775, 1968.

Knuppel, R.A., et al. Rhesus isoimmunization in twin gestation. *Am. J. Obstet. Gynecol.* 150:136, 1984.

Ng, T.Y., Datta, T.D., and Kirimli, B.I. Reaction to indigo carmine. *J. Urol.* 116:132, 1976.

Schwerin, G.S. Severe reaction to indigo-carmine. Illinois. *Med. J.* 101:48, 1952.

Indomethacin (Indocin®) and Sulindac (Clinoril®)

INDICATIONS AND RECOMMENDATIONS

Indomethacin is a nonsteroidal antiinflammatory drug that may be used to arrest and prevent preterm labor and delivery. Although comparative trials have shown it to be more effective than other tocolytic agents, there have been more frequent and serious adverse fetal and neonatal effects associated with its use. It should be used during pregnancy in situations where other tocolytic agents are contraindicated or unsuccessful, and for no more than 48 hours if possible. It is best avoided after 32 weeks gestation. Experience with sulindac as a tocolytic agent is limited but promising.

Indomethacin and sulindac are generally used as antiinflammatory and analgesic agents in the treatment of rheumatic and nonrheumatic inflammatory disease. Indomethacin has been shown to be effective as an antipyretic in Hodgkin's disease when the fever is refractory to other therapy. It is relatively contraindicated as an antiinflammatory, analgesic, and antipyretic agent in pregnancy because other agents with fewer undesirable effects are available.

Because of its inhibition of prostaglandin synthetase with consequent tocolytic effect, indomethacin has become widely prescribed in the treatment of preterm labor. Use during pregnancy has been associated with premature closure of the ductus arteriosus, and an increased frequency of necrotizing enterocolitis and intracranial hemorrhage among very premature babies delivering prior to 30 weeks, soon after treatment. In addition, because of its renal side effects which can reduce fetal urine production, indomethacin has been used for the management of symptomatic hydramnios.

SPECIAL CONSIDERATIONS IN PREGNANCY

Animal studies of indomethacin have demonstrated teratogenicity inconsistently and at high dosages. Sulindac and other prostaglandin synthesis inhibitors were shown to cause cleft palate in mice. First- trimester human exposure to indomethacin has not been linked to congenital anomalies thus far. Experience with sulindac has been extremely limited. Indomethacin has been shown to cross the placenta in the second and third trimesters, with fetal serum levels measured at cordocentesis being similar to maternal levels. Sulindac has been demonstrated to cross the placenta by virtue of its fetal effects. In addition, sulindac levels have been shown to be similar in mother and fetus, although the active sulfide metabolite was significantly lower in the fetal than the maternal compartment. Constriction of the ductus arteriosus of the fetus, which may be transient or intermittent, has been detected by fetal echocardiography in a number of studies of maternal indomethacin treatment. This same phenomenon is useful to pediatricians who may treat neonates with patent ductus arteriosus with indomethacin in order to close the ductus. In one series, the likelihood of fetal ductal constriction induced by maternal indomethacin treatment increased with increasing gestational age, with 50% manifesting constriction at or beyond 32 weeks gestation. On the other hand, as gestational age increases beyond 32 weeks the need for tocolysis is likely to diminish. When indomethacin and sulindac were compared in a randomized trial, Doppler flow studies suggested a more significant effect on the fetal ductus arteriosus with indomethacin than with sulindac, although both caused some degree of ductal constriction.

A number of comparative trials have suggested that indomethacin is as effective or more effective as a first-line tocolytic agent compared to β-adrenergic agonists and magnesium sulfate. Adverse perinatal outcomes, including necrotizing enterocolitis, intracranial hemorrhage, patent ductus arteriosus, and bronchopulmonary dysplasia, have been reported to occur with increased frequency after indomethacin was administered to the mother, particularly when delivery occurred soon after failed tocolysis and the gestational age was less than 30 or 32 weeks. Because indomethacin is often used as a second- or third-line tocolytic agent, when other drugs have failed, patients receiving indomethacin may be more likely to break through tocolysis and deliver, with greater risk of the above adverse effects.

In a randomized trial comparing long-term oral treatment with indomethacin versus terbutaline, constriction of the fetal ductus arteriosus and oligohydramnios were reported in close to a third of indomethacin-treated patients. Six neonatal deaths from renal failure, after prolonged maternal indomethacin treatment (2–11 weeks), have been reported. Pulmonary hypertension was reported in 3 of 25 neonates whose mothers received long-term indomethacin in a randomized trial. Findings of adverse neonatal outcomes have not been universal, however.

When 93 Swedish children exposed to indomethacin or a β-adrenergic agonist, as part of a randomized clinical trial, were followed to 12–18 months of age, adverse outcomes such as death, severe bronchopulmonary dysplasia, cerebral palsy, and severe retinopathy of prematurity were significantly more common in the group exposed to indomethacin (23% versus 5%). Neurologic assessment at 18 months was slightly, but not significantly, worse in the indomethacin- exposed children.

Sulindac was used in three cases of monoamniotic twins in the second trimester in order to reduce the likelihood of cord entanglement. Amniotic fluid volume and fetal urine production were reduced, without evidence of ductal constriction by Doppler ultrasound. A 48-hour course of oral sulindac was compared to indomethacin in a randomized trial treating preterm labor in 36 gravidas refractory to magnesium sulfate. Both drugs were similarly effective, but sulindac appeared to have less effect on fetal renal function and amniotic fluid volume, and possibly less effect on the ductus arteriosus. In a randomized trial of oral sulindac versus placebo for maintenance tocolysis, sulindac did not reduce the rate of preterm birth, although the time to readmission for recurrent preterm labor was lengthened.

DOSAGE

Both indomethacin and sulindac should be given with food in order to diminish the likelihood of gastric irritation. When used to treat preterm labor, indomethacin is generally administered as a 50 mg loading dose, by rectal suppository or orally, followed by 25 mg orally every 6 hours for 48 hours. The time limitation of 48 hours was rather arbitrarily chosen but is intended to limit the likelihood of fetal and neonatal adverse effects. When there is reason to continue indomethacin treatment for more than 48 hours, many centers utilize ultrasound and fetal echocardiography to rule out ductal constriction and oligohydramnios.

The most commonly described dose of indomethacin for treatment of hydramnios is 2.2–2.5 mg/kg/day, divided and given orally every 6 hours, although dosage as high as 3 mg/kg/day has been reported. In the study in which sulindac was used for this condition, the dose was 200 mg orally, twice daily. A similar dose of sulindac has been used for preterm labor.

ADVERSE EFFECTS

Adverse effects of indomethacin are common, resulting in discontinuation of the drug in approximately 20% of patients. Gastrointestinal problems include anorexia, nausea, abdominal pain, ulcers, and occult blood loss. Pancreatitis, hepatitis, and jaundice have been reported. Headache in the frontal area is quite common with prolonged usage, and other symptoms such as dizziness, vertigo, lightheadedness, and mental confusion are also common. Neutropenia, thrombocytopenia, platelet dysfunction, and aplastic anemia may occur. Allergic reactions are common, and aspirin-sensitive patients may also be sensitive to indomethacin. Renal prostaglandin production may be impaired with indomethacin treatment, leading to renal decompensation especially in patients with compromised or marginal renal blood flow.

Because indomethacin is a prostaglandin synthesis inhibitor, its effects on hemodynamics during pregnancy have been investigated. In healthy gravidas during the third trimester, three 6 hourly oral doses of 25 mg of indomethacin resulted in increased peripheral resistance and decreased stroke volume, without a change in blood pressure. Based on these results the authors urged caution in using indomethacin in hypertensive pregnant patients. Two cases of acute, severe hypertensive responses to indomethacin in women with preeclampsia receiving beta blockers have been reported. Acute renal insufficiency, accompanied by dyspnea and hypoxemia, has been reported in patients with preterm labor treated with indomethacin. In a study of 20 pregnant women at 24–32 weeks gestation, 48 hours of oral indomethacin

(50 mg loading dose and 25 mg every 6 hours) was associated with a significant prolongation of the maternal bleeding time, and no change in prothrombin time or partial thromboplastin time.

Sulindac appears to be less likely than indomethacin to cause adverse reactions, but the type of side effects are similar, including gastrointestinal, central nervous system, and allergic effects.

Prostaglandin synthesis inhibitors should be avoided in patients with asthma, coronary artery disease, and gastrointestinal bleeding and/or ulcers.

MECHANISM OF ACTION

Indomethacin and sulindac inhibit cyclooxygenase, an enzyme necessary for the formation of prostaglandins.

ABSORPTION AND BIOTRANSFORMATION

After an oral dose, indomethacin achieves peak serum levels in 2 hours and has a half-life of approximately 2–3 hours. Its absorption may be somewhat slower when taken on a full stomach. The drug is highly protein-bound. It is primarily converted to inactive metabolites, although 10% to 20% of an administered dose is excreted unchanged in the urine. There is significant enterohepatic recirculation.

Sulindac was developed as a substitute for indomethacin and is not an active compound but must first be bioactivated by conversion to a sulfide. This property is believed to be responsible for decreased gastrointestinal irritation compared to indomethacin, since the gastric mucosa is exposed to less of the active prostaglandin synthesis inhibitor. Peak plasma concentrations of sulindac are reached about an hour after oral administration, whereas the active sulfide metabolite does not reach peak levels for about 2 hours. The half-life of sulindac is about 7 hours, but that of the active metabolite is about 18 hours, accounting for the twice-daily dosing.

RECOMMENDED READING

Besinger, R.E., Niebyl, J.R., Keyes, W.G., et al. Randomized comparative trial of indomethacin and ritodrine for the long-term treatment of preterm labor. *Am. J. Obstet. Gynecol.* 164:981, 1991.

Bivins, H.A., Jr., Newman, R.B., Fyfe, D.A., et al. Randomized trial of oral indomethacin and terbutaline sulfate for the long-term suppression of preterm labor. *Am. J. Obstet. Gynecol.* 169:1065, 1993.

Cabrol, D., Jannet, D., and Pannier, E. Treatment of symptomatic polyhydramnios with indomethacin. *Eur. J. Obstet. Gynecol.* 66:11, 1996.

Carlan, S.J., O'Brien, W.F., O'Leary, T.D., et al. Randomized comparative trial of indomethacin and sulindac for the treatment of refractory preterm labor. *Obstet. Gynecol.* 79:223, 1992.

Carlan, S.J., O'Brien, W.F., Jones, M.H., et al. Outpatient oral sulindac to prevent recurrence of preterm labor. *Obstet. Gynecol.* 85:769, 1995.

Eronen, M., Pesonen, E., Kurki, T., et al. Increased incidence of bronchopulmonary dysplasia after antenatal administration of indomethacin to prevent preterm labor. *J. Pediatrics* 124:782, 1994.

Gardner, M.O., Owen, J., Skelly, S., et al. Preterm delivery after indomethacin: a risk factor for neonatal complications? *J. Reprod. Med.* 41:903, 1996.

Higby, K., Xenakis, E.M.-J., and Pauerstein, C.J. Do tocolytic agents stop preterm labor? A critical comprehensive review of efficacy and safety. *Am. J. Obstet. Gynecol.* 168:1247, 1993.

Insel, P.A. Analgesic-antipyretic and antiinflammatory agents and drugs employed in the treatment of gout. Chapter 27 in *Goodman and Gilman's The Pharmacological Basis of Therapeutics* (9th ed.), J.G. Hardman and L.E. Limbard, eds. New York: McGraw-Hill, 1996. Pp. 633–635.

Kramer, W.B., Sade, G., Ou, C.-N., et al. Placental transfer of sulindac and its active sulfide metabolite in humans. *Am. J. Obstet. Gynecol.* 172:886, 1995.

Kurki, T., Eronen, M., Lumme, R., et al. A randomized double-dummy comparison between indomethacin and nylidrin in threatened preterm labor. *Obstet. Gynecol.* 78:1093–1097, 1991.

Lione, A., and Scialli, A. The developmental toxicity of indomethacin and sulindac. *Reprod. Toxicol.* 9:7, 1995.

Lunt, C.C., Satin, A.J., Barth, W.H. Jr., et al. The effect of indomethacin tocolysis on maternal coagulation status. *Obstet. Gynecol.* 84:820, 1994.

Major, C.A., Lewis, D.F., Harding, J.A., et al. Tocolysis with indomethacin increases the incidence of necrotizing enterocolitis in the low-birth-weight neonate. *Am. J. Obstet. Gynecol.* 170:102, 1994.

Manchester, D., Margolis, H.S., and Sheldon, R.E. Possible association between maternal indomethacin therapy and primary pulmonary hypertension of the newborn. *Am. J. Obstet. Gynecol.* 126:467, 1976.

Merrill, J.D., Clyman, R.I., and Norton, M.E. Indomethacin as a tocolytic agent: the controversy continues. *J. Pediatrics* 124:734, 1994.

Moise, K.J., Jr., Ou, C.-N., Kirshon, B., et al. Placental transfer of indomethacin in the human pregnancy. *Am. J. Obstet. Gynecol.* 162:549, 1990.

Moise, K.J., Jr. Effect of advancing gestational age on the frequency of fetal ductal constriction in association with maternal indomethacin use. *Am. J. Obstet. Gynecol.* 168:1350, 1993.

Morales, W.J., and Madhav, H. Efficacy and safety of indomethacin compared with magnesium sulfate in the management of preterm labor: a randomized study. *Am. J. Obstet. Gynecol.* 169:97, 1993.

Norton, M.E., Merrill, J., Cooper, B.A.B., et al. Neonatal complications after the administration of indomethacin for preterm labor. *N. Engl. J. Med.* 329:1602, 1993.

Peek, M.J., McCarthy, A., Kyle, P., et al. Medical amnioreduction with sulindac to reduce cord complications in monoamniotic twins. *Am. J. Obstet. Gynecol.* 176:334, 1997.

Räsänen, J., and Jouppila, P. Fetal cardiac function and ductus arteriosus during indomethacin and sulindac therapy for threatened preterm labor: a randomized study. *Am. J. Obstet. Gynecol.* 173:20, 1995.

Rubaltelli, F.F., et al. Effect on neonate of maternal treatment with indomethacin. *J. Pediatrics* 94:161, 1979.

Salokorpi, T., Eronen, M., von Wendt, L. Growth and development until 18 months of children exposed to tocolytics indomethacin or nylidrin. *Neuropediatrics* 27:174, 1996.

Schoenfeld, A., Freedman, S., and Hod, M. Antagonism of antihypertensive drug therapy in pregnancy by indomethacin? *Am. J. Obstet. Gynecol.* 161:1204, 1989.

Sorensen, T.K., Easterling, T.R., Carlson, K.L., et al. The maternal hemodynamic effect of indomethacin in normal pregnancy. *Obstet. Gynecol.* 79:661, 1992.

Steiger, R.M., Boyd, E.L., Powers, D.R., et al. Acute maternal renal insufficiency in premature labor treated with indomethacin. *Am. J. Perinatol.* 10:381, 1993.

Van der Heijden, B.J., Carlus, C., Narcy, F., et al. Persistent anuria, neonatal death, and renal microcystic lesions after prenatal exposure to indomethacin. *Am. J. Obstet. Gynecol.* 171:617–623, 1994.

Insulin

INDICATIONS AND RECOMMENDATIONS

Insulin is safe to use during pregnancy. It is a naturally occurring polypeptide hormone given parenterally to diabetic patients to lower the blood glucose and correct some of the other metabolic abnormalities related to diabetes. It is the treatment of choice for management of pregnancy in the diabetic. Careful attention to diet is equally important. Frequent blood glucose monitoring is mandatory for any patient taking insulin.

SPECIAL CONSIDERATIONS IN PREGNANCY

Insulin administered exogenously to the mother does not cross the placenta in any appreciable amount. Fetal endogenous insulin, presumably increased due to the effect of maternal hyperglycemia on the fetus, may be responsible for macrosomia and hypoglycemia in the newborn. Fetal hypoglycemia accompanies maternal hypoglycemia. As yet, there is no convincing evidence that insulin-induced maternal-fetal hypoglycemia has a detrimental effect on the developing fetus. Lispro insulin has not been evaluated during pregnancy to date and so its safety in pregnancy is unknown.

DOSAGE

The dosage of insulin given to a pregnant woman with diabetes must be individually tailored to that patient's needs. In general, insulin requirements may decrease slightly during the first one-third to one-half of pregnancy, and rapid swings of blood sugar with episodes of hypoglycemia are frequently observed. During the second half of pregnancy, insulin requirements often increase to 2–3 times the prepregnancy dose. There is a tendency toward diabetic ketoacidosis, and hypoglycemia is less common.

Most authorities agree that strict control of circulating glucose is extremely important in managing the pregnancy of a diabetic woman. It is well documented that diabetic ketoacidosis is associated with an extremely high perinatal mortality (in some studies as high as 50%). There is some controversy over how low the circulating glucose level should be allowed to fall. At most centers caring for large numbers of diabetic pregnancies, the aim is to render the patient euglycemic; that is, glucose should be maintained at levels comparable to those in normal nondiabetic pregnant women. Fasting blood glucose is kept in the range of 50–100 mg/dl, 1-hour postprandial values are kept below 130–140 mg/dl, and 2-hour postprandial values are kept below 120 mg/dl. Although transient hypoglycemia occurs in some patients, it is believed safer to have to treat this complication occasionally (with a high-protein snack) than to allow continuous hyperglycemia.

There are numerous schemata for the administration of insulin during pregnancy. Some involve split doses of mixed short- and intermediate-acting insulin, some involve multiple doses of short-acting insulin throughout the day, whereas others utilize the insulin pump. None has been proved superior to the others. The detailed description of these protocols is beyond the scope of this book.

The use of low doses of insulin (10 units neutral protamine Hagedorn [NPH] or 20 units NPH with 10 units regular) has been investigated and found to be effective in reducing the incidence of macrosomia in the infants of mild gestational diabetics. These patients would not generally require insulin to maintain euglycemia, but it may be used prophylactically to prevent macrosomia.

In 1996 lispro insulin (Humalog), an analogue of human insulin produced by recombinant DNA technology, was approved in the United States. Lispro insulin is absorbed more rapidly from its injection site and has a shorter duration of action than regular insulin. Consequently, patients with diabetes can inject their premeal insulin just before eating, allowing for greater flexibility, and there appear to be lower postprandial glucose excursions when this form of insulin is used.

ADVERSE EFFECTS

An overdose of insulin can obviously create the side effect of hypoglycemia. Another side effect, not necessarily related to overdosing, is hypertrophy or atrophy of subcutaneous fat at injection sites. Allergic reactions to the impurities contained in insulin derived from animals are commonly reported. These symptoms often disappear when the patient is switched to highly purified animal species insulin or to human insulin. Circulating antibodies to exogenous insulin are consistently found in patients treated with animal species insulins, but their clinical significance is controversial. Theoretically, patients taking insulin intermittently are most likely to be placed at a disadvantage by the presence of these antibodies. Women who require insulin for the first time during pregnancy, either because their hyperglycemia has intensified or because they have gestational diabetes, are likely to discontinue this therapy after delivery. We therefore recommend that such patients be treated with human rather than pork or beef insulin.

MECHANISM OF ACTION

In the past, insulin was generally derived from pigs (pork insulin), cattle (beef insulin), or a mixture of the two. Of the 51 amino acids in chains comprising the insulin protein structure, pork insulin and human insulin differ by a single amino acid, whereas beef insulin contains three amino acid differences. Subsequently, human insulin (produced by recombinant DNA technology or by a chemical substitution in the pork insulin B chain) became widely available.

Insulin consists of 51 amino acids in the form of a 21-amino-acid A chain and a 30-amino-acid B chain connected by disulfide linkages. It is produced as a single 84-amino-acid proinsulin chain, but the C chain of 33 amino acids (known as connecting peptide) must be cleaved from between the A and B chains in order for the insulin to become metabolically active.

Insulin is necessary for the efficient transport of glucose from blood to tissues other than those of the central nervous system, renal medulla, pancreatic β cells, and gut epithelium. It also favors hepatic glycogen synthesis and storage of glucose in adipose tissue as triglyceride. Insulin facilitates the transport of ingested amino acids into cells, thus increasing protein synthesis. It inhibits lipolysis and is therefore antiketogenic.

Exogenous insulin can reverse the symptoms of diabetes, i.e., polyuria and polydipsia, by lowering the blood glucose level. It can also reverse diabetic ketoacidosis. Good diabetic control using exogenous insulin reverses or slows the vascular complications of diabetes.

Diabetes is characterized as a disease state in which there is a deficiency of insulin that can be either relative or absolute. Many long-standing overt diabetics have virtually undetectable endogenous insulin secretion as measured by C-peptide assay. On the other hand, mild gestational diabetics can have elevated levels of endogenous insulin. In these cases, the metabolic abnormality is presumably caused by peripheral resistance to insulin and its increased degradation. This is probably related to the effects of insulinase activity as well as placental steroid and polypeptide hormone production.

ABSORPTION AND BIOTRANSFORMATION

Controversy exists as to the fate of different forms of insulin in humans. A detailed exploration of this subject is beyond the scope of this book. It is known that insulin is degraded in the liver, kidneys, lungs, and placenta and that some insulin is excreted in the urine. Although some dispute exists, most investigators agree that insulin administered to the mother does not cross the placenta into the fetal circulation to a clinically relevant extent.

The duration of action of exogenously administered insulin varies according to the preparation. The action of purified crystalline zinc insulin (CZI), "regular" insulin, peaks at 1–2 hours and has a duration of 5–6 hours when administered subcutaneously. Semilente insulin, another rapid-acting form, has a peak similar to CZI, but a longer duration (12–16 hours). An intermediate-acting insulin, NPH, is a combination of regular insulin and protamine zinc insulin, and has a peak of action at 2–8 hours and a duration of approximately 24 hours. Lente insulin has a similar time course. These peaks and durations of action are related more to absorption than to metabolic rate.

Lispro insulin is human insulin with a reversal of a proline and lysine residue at positions B28 and B29 on the B chain. This structural change interferes with dimer formation, leading to more rapid and complete absorption. The peak (approximately 40 minutes) and duration of action (approximately 3 hours) of lispro insulin are shorter than those of regular (CZI) insulin.

RECOMMENDED READING

Anderson, J.H., Jr., Brunelle, R.L., Koivisto, V.A., et al. Reduction of postprandial hyperglycemia and frequency of hypoglycemia in IDDM patients on insulin-analog treatment. *Diabetes* 46:265, 1997.

Holleman, F., and Hoekstra, J.B.L. Insulin lispro. *N. Engl. J. Med.* 337:176, 1997.

Landon, M.B., and Gabbe, S.G. Insulin treatment. Chapter 11 in *Diabetes Mellitus in Pregnancy* (2nd ed.), E.A. Reece and D.R. Coustan, eds. New York: Churchill Livingstone, 1995. Pp. 173–190.

Isoniazid (INH)

INDICATIONS AND RECOMMENDATIONS

Isoniazid (INH) is recommended for the treatment of active tuberculosis during pregnancy. It is generally considered to be the primary drug used for chemotherapy of tuberculosis and appears to be the safest antitubercular agent available for use during pregnancy. Although the need for antibiotic prophylaxis in patients whose skin tests are first reactive during pregnancy is controversial, fear of exposing the fetus to isoniazid, particularly after the first trimester, should not be a determining factor.

SPECIAL CONSIDERATIONS IN PREGNANCY

There appear to be no unusual maternal effects of isoniazid use during pregnancy. Isoniazid is known to cross the placenta. Several large-scale studies of women who received isoniazid therapy during all trimesters of pregnancy have shown no significant increase in congenital malformations and no detectable patterns in the malformations that did occur. The authors of a review of 1480 pregnancies in which isoniazid was used report that 95% of the patients delivered normal infants at term. Approximately 1% of the infants or fetuses were found to be abnormal. There is a single case report of a child who was exposed to isoniazid in utero who developed malignant mesothelioma at 9 years of age. Because of the rareness of the disease, the author suggests that INH may be a causative factor. However, one-large scale study has found no association between INH and carcinogenic effect.

Isoniazid is excreted in breast milk and should be used with caution in women who are breast-feeding, as the infant is at risk for hepatic toxicity. If INH is also being given to the neonate, its dosage may have to be reduced.

DOSAGE

The usual dose for treatment of active tuberculosis is 300 mg/day (5 mg/kg). This dose is usually given in combination with other antitubercular medications for 18–24 months. When isoniazid is administered to skin test reactors without active disease, it is given without other antitubercular drugs at the dose specified above for 12 months. Pyridoxine, 50 mg/day, is usually given prophylactically whenever isoniazid is prescribed.

ADVERSE EFFECTS

The most common treatable side effect is a pyridoxine-responsive peripheral neuropathy, which occurs most commonly in malnourished patients receiving more than 5 mg/kg/day. Other common side effects include rash, fever, and jaundice. Subclinical hepatitis characterized by reversible, usually asymptomatic elevation of serum glutamic oxaloacetic transaminase (SGOT) and serum glutamic pyruvic transaminase (SGPT) is common. Clinical hepatitis is age-dependent and is rare in patients under 35 years old.

MECHANISM OF ACTION

The exact mechanism of action of isoniazid is unknown. It inhibits the synthesis of mycolic acid, a component of mycobacterial cell walls, and probably has other actions. Its bactericidal effects are seen only in actively growing bacilli, and "resting" organisms resume normal growth when removed from contact with the drug.

ABSORPTION AND BIOTRANSFORMATION

Isoniazid is rapidly and completely absorbed after oral administration. It is widely distributed into all body fluids and cells including the cerebral spinal fluid. Elimination is primarily by hepatic acetylation and urinary excretion of the metabolites. The specific pattern of elimination depends on the acetylator phenotype of the individual. In rapid acetylators, the half-life is 0.5–1.5 hours; in slow acetylators, it is 2–4 hours. The half-life is significantly increased in patients with liver disease.

RECOMMENDED READING

Good, J.T., et al. Tuberculosis in association with pregnancy. *Am. J. Obstet. Gynecol.* 140:492, 1981.

Mandell, G.L. and Petri, Jr., W.A. Antimicrobial agents: drugs used in the chemotherapy of tubercolosis and leprosy. Chapter 44 in *Goodman and Gilman's The Pharmacological Basis of Therapeutics* (9th ed.), J.G. Hardman and L.E. Limbird, eds. New York: McGraw-Hill, 1996. Pp. 1155–1159.

Medchill, M.T., and Gillum, M. Diagnosis and management of tuberculosis during pregnancy. *Obstet. Gynecol. Surv.* 44:81, 1989.

Scheinhorn, D.J., and Angelillo, V.A. Antituberculosis therapy in pregnancy: risks to the fetus. *West. J. Med.* 127:195, 1977.

Snider, D.E., et al. Treatment of tuberculosis during pregnancy. *Am. Rev. Resp. Dis.* 122:65, 1980.

Snider, D. Pregnancy and tuberculosis. *Chest* 86:10S, 1985.

Isoproterenol (Isuprel®)

INDICATIONS AND RECOMMENDATIONS

Isoproterenol is used as a medical therapy of heart block, as a cardiac stimulant to raise systemic blood pressure, and in inhaled form as a bronchodilator in the treatment of bronchospasm. It is relatively contraindicated during pregnancy because other, more selective agents with fewer cardiovascular side effects are available for treatment of asthma. One study has demonstrated marked hepatotoxicity caused by isoproterenol in chick embryos, but to date this has not been reported in humans. Another study used isoproterenol in rat pregnancy to experimentally induce hypertrophic cardiomyopathy in the fetuses. Although this was accomplished, it was with chronic doses, and was reversed after cessation of the drug. In a recent report, isoproterenol was used in an attempt to treat fetal complete heart block in three patients and was ineffective in increasing the heart rate or improving fetal cardiac function.

Isoproterenol is a pure β-adrenergic agonist that increases myocardial strength while relaxing arteriolar and bronchiolar smooth muscle tone. It therefore has positive cardiac inotropic and chronotropic effects and causes peripheral vascular relaxation and bronchodilatation. In late pregnancy, the chronotropic effect of isoproterenol is reduced, with a fivefold increase in dose required to elicit a 25 beat/minute increase in heart rate, compared to the dose required in nonpregnant women.

Sympathomimetics seem to influence the fetus indirectly by altering uterine blood flow. Uterine vessels only have α-adrenergic receptors, and under baseline conditions during pregnancy they are thought to be maximally dilated. Peripheral vasodilatation may therefore shunt blood away from the uterus. This decrease in uterine blood flow may adversely affect the fetus.

RECOMMENDED READING

DeSimone, C.A., Leighton, B.L., Norris, M.C., Chayen, B., and Menduke, H. The chronotropic effect of isoproterenol is reduced in term pregnant women. *Anesthesiology* 69:626, 1988.

Dusek, J., and Ostadal, B. Isoproterenol-induced damage to the liver of chick embryos. *Physiol. Bohemoslov.* 33:67, 1984.

Groves, A.M.M., Allan, L.D., and Rosenthal E. Therapeutic trial of sympathomimetics in three cases of complete heart block in the fetus. *Circulation* 92:3394, 1995.

Hoffman, B.B., and Lefkowitz, R.J. Catecholamines, sympathomimetic drugs, and adrenergic receptor agonists. Chapter 10 in *Goodman and Gilman's The Pharmacological Basis of Therapeutics*(9thed.),J.G. Hardman and L.E. Limbird, eds. New York: McGraw-Hill, 1996. Pp. 199–212.

Iwasaki, T., Takino, Y., and Suzuki, T. Effects of isoproterenol on the developing heart in rats. *Jpn. Circ. J.* 54:109, 1990.

Smith, N.T., and Corbasciao, A.N. The use and misuse of pressor agents. *Anesthesiology* 33:58, 1970.

Isotretinoin (Accutane®)

INDICATIONS AND RECOMMENDATIONS

Isotretinoin, a synthetic vitamin A derivative used in the treatment of severe cystic acne, is contraindicated during pregnancy. It is a known human teratogen. A pregnancy test should be documented as being negative before any woman begins therapy with isotretinoin, and effective contraception should be maintained throughout the treatment course.

When nonhuman primates were exposed to retinoic acid at appropriate stages of pregnancy, a high incidence of major structural abnormalities (craniofacial, limb reduction, ear) occurred. Among 21 abnormal children exposed to isotretinoin in utero and reported to the FDA over 2 years, all had small or absent ears, neurologic injuries, and cardiac defects. Some had facial dysmorphia as well. An additional 26 normal pregnancies and 12 spontaneous abortions were reported. Another 95 patients elected to terminate their pregnancies. Whether the women with normal pregnancies were exposed during the critical period in embryogenesis (28–70 days menstrual age) is unknown. The true denominator (i.e., number of exposed pregnancies) is also unknown. A subgroup of 36 exposed pregnancies that were followed prospectively yielded 5 malformed infants, 23 normal infants, and 8 spontaneous abortions. Because these anomalies followed a similar pattern and this pattern resembles the anomalies produced by the drug in laboratory animals, isotretinoin should be considered a human teratogen and avoided during pregnancy.

Despite the admonition to avoid pregnancy during treatment with isotretinoin, between 1982, when the drug was introduced, and 1989 there were 78 accumulated cases of birth defects associated with the drug. In 1988 the manufacturer of isotretinoin implemented a program aimed at preventing pregnancy in women using the drug. The program included guidelines for prescribers, an information booklet for patients, and a contraception referral program in which the patient would be reimbursed for a contraceptive counseling visit. The packaging was changed so that warnings about pregnancy were prominently displayed. A follow-up survey of more than 23,000 women of childbearing age who were prescribed isotretinoin between 1989 and 1993 was published in 1995. This study found that 99% reported being told by their doctor of the importance of avoiding pregnancy, but only two-thirds reported having a pregnancy test before starting the drug. Approximately 96% reported that they were either using contraception or were not sexually active. The reported pregnancy rate among 122,582 women prescribed isotretinoin in the years 1989–1993 was 3.4 per 1000 20-week courses of the drug, or a total of 402 pregnan-

cies. Of these, 290 had elective terminations and 76 had spontaneous abortions or ectopic pregnancies, leaving 32 live births
and 4 lost to follow-up. Among the 32 liveborn infants there
were 5 with known birth defects possibly attributable to the
drug, and a sixth with parental report of congenital anomalies
incompatible with life, for a known anomaly rate that could be
as low as 19% or as high as 38%, depending on whether the denominator used is all births or just those who were examined
by the survey teratologist. Either way, isotretinoin remains the
most potent known human teratogen.

The manufacturer of isotretinoin reported outcomes of 88
prospectively ascertained pregnancies in which conception occurred within 2–60+ days after discontinuance of the drug. The
malformation rate was 4.5% and the spontaneous abortion rate
was 9.1%. These did not differ significantly from background
risks, perhaps because of small numbers. However, it is reassuring that none of the four cases with congenital malformations had defects typically described as isotretinoin-induced.

There is no evidence available at the present time to support
an association between the topical use of tretinoin (Retin-A®)
and teratogenicity. The total dose absorbed systemically is
small enough to make fetal effects unlikely.

RECOMMENDED READING

Benke, P.J. The isotretinoin teratogen syndrome. *J.A.M.A.* 251:
3267, 1984.

Dai, W.S., Hsu, M.-A., and Itri, L.M. Safety of pregnancy after discontinuation of isotretinoin. *Arch. Dermatol.* 125:362, 1989.

De La Cruz, E., Vangvanichyakorn, K., and Desposito, F. Multiple
congenital malformations associated with maternal isotretinoin
therapy. *Pediatrics* 74:428, 1984.

Lammer, E.J., et al. Retinoic acid embryopathy. *N. Engl. J. Med.*
313:837, 1985.

McBride, W.G. Limb reduction deformities in child exposed to
isotretinoin in utero on gestation days 26–40 only. *Lancet* 1:1276,
1985.

Mitchell, A.A., van Bennekom, C.M., and Louik, C. A pregnancy-
prevention program in women of childbearing age receiving isotretinoin. *N. Engl. J. Med.* 333:101, 1995.

Tremblay, M., Voyer, P., and Aubin, G. Malformations congenitales
dues a l'Accutane. *Can. Med. Assoc. J.* 133:208, 1983.

Isoxsuprine (Vasodilan®)

INDICATIONS AND RECOMMENDATIONS

Isoxsuprine, which is a β_2-adrenergic agonist and peripheral
vasodilator, has been administered to pregnant women to stop
premature labor. Although isoxsuprine once was widely used as
a tocolytic agent in the United States, the relatively higher incidence of cardiovascular side effects associated with this drug
has made other β agonists more popular choices for the treatment of premature labor, and isoxsuprine is seldom used in current practice.

SPECIAL CONSIDERATIONS IN PREGNANCY

Hypotension is the major threat to fetal well-being. This complication is usually mild, especially when the maternal intravascular volume is adequate. Some recent data suggest an acceleration of maturity of the fetus's pulmonary system when β_2 agonists are administered to the mother.

A retrospective study of outcome for the neonate when the mother was treated with isoxsuprine before giving birth caused concern. Twenty babies whose mothers were treated with isoxsuprine and delivered prior to 32 weeks were compared with 20 nontreated controls. Seven babies in the treated group died in the neonatal period, as compared with two in the control group (not statistically significant). All of the isoxsuprine-exposed babies manifested some degree of hypotension during the first 6 hours of life, as compared to 75% of the babies in the control group ($p < 0.05$). Half of the treated babies developed clinically evident ileus, as opposed to 15% of the untreated babies ($p < 0.05$). These effects on the newborn were most likely to be seen if the interval between the administration of the loading dose of isoxsuprine and the delivery of the baby was short. There have been reports of fetal tachycardia, hypocalcemia, hypoglycemia, ileus, and hypotension severe enough to lead to fetal demise. Although reports of adverse outcomes in the newborn period are limited in scope and retrospective, they do point out the necessity of being as certain as possible that a woman is truly in premature labor before administering isoxsuprine or any other β_2 agonist.

DOSAGE

When used for tocolysis, the usual dose was 0.25–0.5 mg/min IV for 8–12 hours. This was followed by intramuscular or oral isoxsuprine at 5–20 mg every 3–6 hours. The intravenous infusion was stopped and considered a failure if labor-like activity persisted beyond 1 hour. To prevent hypotension, the dose was carefully titrated and the patient placed in the left lateral position.

ADVERSE EFFECTS

Because β_2 receptors are not confined to the uterine muscle but are also responsible for smooth muscle relaxation in arterioles and bronchi as well as being involved in glycogenolysis, the side effects of isoxsuprine may involve any of these systems. Thus, overdosage or rapid infusion may cause hypotension and tachycardia in the mother. Hyperglycemia has also been reported with this drug. The most common side effects are tremor, palpitations, and restlessness. Allergic dermatitis has also been reported.

Case reports of pulmonary edema occurring in women receiving the combination of a β_2 agonist and glucocorticoid therapy (in an attempt to enhance the maturity of the pulmonary system in the fetus) suggest that caution be exercised when these classes of agents are combined.

MECHANISM OF ACTION

Isoxsuprine interacts with β_2 receptors on the myometrial cell membrane to release adenyl cyclase within the cell. This catalyzes the intracellular formation of cAMP, which subsequently leads to relaxation of the uterine musculature, presumably through changes in calcium availability. In addition, isoxsuprine may act directly on smooth muscle because the vasodilatation caused by this drug is not blocked by propranolol.

ABSORPTION AND BIOTRANSFORMATION

Isoxsuprine is largely metabolized by monoamine oxidase. Some is excreted by the kidneys, with the rate of excretion being higher in acidic urine.

RECOMMENDED READING

Brazy, J.E., and Pupkin, M.J. Effects of maternal isoxsuprine administration on preterm infants. *J. Pediatrics* 94:444, 1979.

Brazy, J.E., et al. Isoxsuprine in the neonatal period. II. Relationships between neonatal symptoms, drug exposure, and drug concentrations at the time of birth. *J. Pediatrics* 98:146, 1981.

Casten, O., Gummerus, M., and Saarikoski, S. Treatment of imminent premature labour. *Acta Obstet. Gynecol. Scand.* 54:95, 1975.

Manley, E.S., and Lawson, J.W. Effect of beta adrenergic receptor blockade on skeletal muscle vasodilation produced by isoxsuprine and nylidrin. *Arch. Int. Pharmacodyn. Ther.* 175:239, 1968.

Stubblefield, P.G. Pulmonary edema occurring after therapy with dexamethasone and terbutaline for premature labor: a case report. *Am. J. Obstet. Gynecol.* 132:341, 1978.

Ketoconazole (Nizoral®)

INDICATIONS AND RECOMMENDATIONS

Ketoconazole is relatively contraindicated during pregnancy because other therapeutic agents are preferable. Use of the systemic preparation should be reserved for the treatment of life-threatening systemic fungal infections or Cushing's syndrome. It is an antifungal agent useful in the treatment of a number of superficial and systemic fungal infections.

In animals, teratogenic effects (syndactylia and oligodactylia), embryotoxic effects, and dystocia have been seen. There are no well-controlled studies of the use of ketoconazole in pregnant women and, in light of the experience in animals, it is not recommended for use.

Ketoconazole is known to block androgen and corticosteroid synthesis in vivo and in vitro. Because morphologic and functional differentiation of embryonic and fetal organ systems is influenced by both androgens and corticosteroids, ketoconazole use should be avoided especially in the first trimester.

Ketoconazole's ability to inhibit adrenal steroidogenesis has been used to treat Cushing's syndrome. There is one report of its use in the treatment of Cushing's syndrome during pregnancy. The drug was begun at 32 weeks gestation after the mother's clinical deterioration and a documented pattern of slow fetal growth. Upon treatment, the patient's clinical status improved quickly and the drug was discontinued at 37 weeks, 36 hours prior to delivery. The woman gave birth to a normally formed infant with no evidence of adrenal insufficiency. The infant was growing normally at 18 months of age. The authors concluded that low-dose ketoconazole therapy may be used during the last period of pregnancy in Cushing's syndrome if the patient's clinical course deteriorates and the fetus is female. Should a pregnant woman require topical antifungal therapy, miconazole may be used.

RECOMMENDED READING

Amado, J.A. Successful treatment with ketoconazole of Cushing's syndrome in pregnancy. *Postgrad. Med. J.* 66:221, 1990.

Aron, D.C., et al. Cushing's syndrome and pregnancy. *Am. J. Obstet. Gynecol.* 162:244, 1990.

Bennett, J.E. Antimicrobial agents: antifungal agents. Chapter 49 in *Goodman and Gilman's The Pharmacological Basis of Therapeutics* (9th ed.), J.G. Hardman and L.E. Limbird, eds. New York: McGraw-Hill, 1996. Pp. 1180–1182.

Guaschino, S., et al. Mycotic vaginitis in pregnancy: a double evaluation of the susceptibility to the main antimycotic drugs of isolated species. *Biol. Res. Preg. Perinatol.* 7:20, 1986.

Latanoprost (Xalatan®)

INDICATIONS AND RECOMMENDATIONS

Latanoprost, an analog of prostaglandin $F_{2\alpha}$, is contraindicated in pregnancy because other drugs are preferable. It is indicated for the reduction of elevated intraocular pressure in patients with open angle glaucoma and ocular hypertension. Agents applied topically to the eye can enter the systemic circulation via the nasolacrimal duct and absorption through the nasopharyngeal mucosa. Prostaglandins of the F series are known to increase uterine activity and carbaprost, 15-methyl-prostaglandin $F_{2\alpha}$, is used therapeutically as an abortifacient. Latanoprost, therefore, should not be used during pregnancy.

REFERENCES

O'Brien, W.F. The role of prostaglandins in labor and delivery. *Clin. Perinatol.* 22:973, 1995.

Patel, S.S., and Spencer, C.M. Latanoprost. A review of its pharmacological properties, clinical efficacy and tolerability in the management of primary open angle glaucoma and ocular hypertension. *Drugs Aging* 9:363, 1996.

Levodopa (Bendopa®, Dopar®, Larodopa®)

INDICATIONS AND RECOMMENDATIONS

Levodopa (l-3,4-dihydroxyphenylalanine) is a drug used in the treatment of Parkinson's disease. Although insufficient data exist to comment on its safety during human pregnancy, reports of animal teratogenicity support withholding this drug in all but the most serious clinical situations.

SPECIAL CONSIDERATIONS IN PREGNANCY

Only one report has been published to date describing the outcome of pregnancies in which levodopa was taken throughout gestation. In that small series, two women were treated during three pregnancies, all of which resulted in the birth of healthy neonates at term. Follow-up study at 1.5, 5.0, and 7.0 years, respectively, revealed the infants to be developing normally. In one of these cases, the patient was taking amantadine hydrochloride for her Parkinson's disease at the time of conception. The authors chose to discontinue that drug because of reports of animal teratogenicity, as well as a single case of an infant who was born with a complex congenital cardiovascular lesion after exposure to amantadine in utero.

One other case has been reported in which levodopa was given to improve the level of consciousness during an episode of acute hepatic failure occurring in the fifth month of pregnancy. That patient also delivered a healthy infant at term.

In rodents and some other laboratory animals, levodopa has been found to cause skeletal malformations, stunting, and increased numbers of stillborns. Although the data are very sparse, there are no reports of teratogenicity in humans.

Levodopa inhibits lactation by blocking the neurohumoral secretion of prolactin. This, as well as the major pharmacologic effects of levodopa, is due to the action of dopamine, which is the drug's principal decarboxylation product.

DOSAGE

The usual initial dose is 0.5–1.0 g/day in 3–4 divided doses. The total daily dosage must then be titrated for optimal therapeutic effectiveness. The usual daily maintenance dose ranges from 3 to 8 g, and this is reached by gradual incremental increases of 100–750 mg every 3–7 days. A good therapeutic effect may not be reached in some patients for as long as 1–6 months.

ADVERSE EFFECTS

Eighty percent of patients experience anorexia, nausea, vomiting, or epigastric distress, and these symptoms often occur early in therapy. Mild and asymptomatic orthostatic hypotension is frequently present, and some patients may develop cardiac arrhythmias. Long-term effects include abnormal involuntary movements and psychiatric disturbances. All of these side effects are reversible and can usually be controlled by a reduction in dosage.

MECHANISM OF ACTION

Levodopa itself is practically inert pharmacologically. Its principal effects are produced by dopamine, which is the product of its decarboxylation. About 95% of orally administered levodopa is rapidly converted in the periphery to dopamine, which, unlike the parent compound, does not cross the blood–brain barrier. Therefore, large doses of levodopa must be taken in order to allow sufficient accumulation of this drug in the brain, where its decarboxylation raises the central dopamine concentration. Although levodopa's mechanism of action in patients with Parkinson's disease is not completely clear, it acts, at least in part, by replenishing depleted striatal dopamine stores in the central nervous system (CNS).

ABSORPTION AND BIOTRANSFORMATION

Levodopa is rapidly absorbed from the small intestine after oral administration. Peak plasma concentrations occur 0.5–2.0 hours after a single oral dose. The half-life is between 1 and 3 hours.

Ninety-five percent of levodopa is decarboxylated peripherally by widely distributed extracerebral aromatic *l*-aminodecarboxylase. An extensive first-pass effect occurs in the liver, so that little unchanged drug reaches the cerebral circulation, and less than 1% penetrates the CNS.

Most levodopa is converted to dopamine, small amounts of which are in turn metabolized to norepinephrine and epinephrine. Biotransformation of dopamine results in the formation of its principal excretion products, 3,4-dihydroxyphenylacetic acid (DOPAC) and 3-methoxy-4-hydroxyphenylacetic acid [homovanillic acid (HVA)], but at least 30 metabolites of levodopa have been identified. The metabolites of dopamine are rapidly excreted through the kidneys, and 80% of a radioactively labeled dose can be recovered in the urine within 24 hours.

RECOMMENDED READING

Chajek, T., et al. Treatment of acute hepatic encephalopathy with *l*-dopa. *Postgrad. Med. J.* 53:262, 1977.

Cook, D.G., and Klawans, H.L. Levodopa during pregnancy. *Clin. Neuropharmacol.* 8:93, 1985.

Standaert, D.G., and Young, A.B. Treatment of central nervous system degenerative disorders. Chapter 22 in *Goodman and Gilman's The Pharmacological Basis of Therapeutics* (9th ed.), J.G. Hardman and L.E. Limbird, eds. New York: McGraw-Hill, 1996. Pp 506–513.

Stone, S.C., and Dickey, R.P. Management of nursing and non-nursing mothers. *Clin. Obstet. Gynecol.* 18:139, 1975.

Lidocaine (Xylocaine®) and Its Analogs (Mexiletine [Mexitil®] and Tocainide [Tonocard®])

INDICATIONS AND RECOMMENDATIONS

Lidocaine may be administered to pregnant women as an antiarrhythmic agent. It is used primarily in the emergency treatment of ventricular arrhythmias. Its use as an anesthetic agent will not be considered in this discussion. Mexiletine and tocainide are lidocaine analogs developed to resist first-pass hepatic metabolism and thus allow oral maintenance therapy. Because of its potential for bone marrow aplasia and pulmonary fibrosis, tocainide is used less often than mexiletine. Long-term maintenance therapy with these drugs is generally prescribed only for significant, life-threatening arrhythmias.

SPECIAL CONSIDERATIONS IN PREGNANCY

Lidocaine crosses the placenta, and high blood levels in the mother may be associated with neonatal depression and neurobehavioral changes in the first few days of life. Fortunately, blood levels that are in the therapeutic range for treatment of arrhythmias (2–5 µg/ml) are somewhat lower than the levels found to be associated with these adverse neonatal effects. Very high blood levels in sheep, as well as in experimentally isolated uterine artery segments, may be associated with a transient decrease in uterine blood flow. This has not been reported in humans given lidocaine in therapeutic dosages. Studies of drug levels have been conducted in sheep and humans. The administration of intravenous lidocaine to healthy pregnant ewes at therapeutic doses did not result in significantly different lidocaine levels in term versus preterm fetuses. The cardiovascular and acid–base status of the healthy preterm lambs were not adversely affected by the drug. In one case report describing continuous maternal lidocaine infusion over 12 days in a twin pregnancy complicated by twin–twin transfusion and preterm labor, drug levels were obtained from the mother, fetuses, and amniotic fluid. Concentrations were highest in maternal serum, followed by amniotic fluid, and lowest in fetal serum. The umbilical vein/maternal vein ratios were approximately 50%, and the drug did not appear to accumulate in the amniotic fluid despite prolonged administration. Fetal gastric fluid lidocaine levels are reportedly higher than serum levels, possibly related to swallowing of amniotic fluid. Fetal drug levels may increase in the presence of acidosis.

Very little information is available concerning the use of mexiletine and tocainide during pregnancy. In a published case report of mexiletine exposure throughout pregnancy and lactation, there were no obvious adverse effects on the fetus. However, the serum mexiletine level in the newborn 9 hours post partum was 0.4 µg/ml, near the recommended therapeutic level of more than 0.5 µg/ml.

Lidocaine is excreted into breast milk in small amounts. The American Academy of Pediatrics considers lidocaine to be compatible with breast-feeding. Mexiletine is excreted in breast milk with a milk/plasma ratio of 1.45.

DOSAGE

In the emergency management of ventricular arrhythmias, lidocaine is administered intravenously at a dose of 1–1.5 mg/kg. Subsequent doses of 0.5–0.75 mg/kg may be repeated every 8–10 minutes for a total dose of 3 mg/kg. The maintenance dose is 1–4 mg/min by continuous infusion. Measurement of plasma levels may be helpful in adjusting the maintenance rate. The therapeutic range is 1.5–5 µg/ml.

Mexiletine is supplied as 150 mg, 200 mg, and 250 mg capsules. It is to be taken with food or antacid, and when rapid control of arrhythmia is not necessary the starting dose is 200 mg every 8 hours. Dosage is adjusted every 2–3 days or more, in increments of 50–100 mg, based on response and side effects.

ADVERSE EFFECTS

Toxic effects of lidocaine occur in the cardiovascular and central nervous systems. One of the earliest signs of toxicity is nystagmus. Central nervous system effects include lightheadedness, drowsiness, tremors, convulsions, and respiratory depression and arrest. Cardiovascular effects include hypotension, cardiovascular collapse, and bradycardia, which may lead to cardiac arrest. These toxic effects are usually seen at serum levels above 5 μg/ml. Side effects of mexiletine and tocainide include tremor and nausea. Both drugs have been associated with bone marrow depression, with tocainide more likely to cause this problem.

MECHANISM OF ACTION

Lidocaine's antiarrhythmic activity is related to a depression in the automaticity of Purkinje cells and a decrease in membrane responsiveness. It blocks open and deactivated sodium channels in cardiac muscle. There is little electrophysiologic effect on atrial muscle, probably due to the relatively short atrial actions potentials. There is little or no effect on the PR or QRS length, although the QT interval may be slightly shortened. Lidocaine can eliminate premature ventricular contractions and convert a ventricular arrhythmia to normal sinus rhythm. It is not recommended for treatment of supraventricular arrhythmias.

ABSORPTION AND BIOTRANSFORMATION

Lidocaine is not effective when given orally and should be given by the intravenous route. It is primarily metabolized in the liver. The initial half-life after intravenous administration is 8 minutes, increasing to 1–3 hours with continuous infusion. Steady-state concentrations require 8–10 hours.

RECOMMENDED READING

Banzai, M., Sato, S., Tezuka, N., et al. Placental transfer of lidocaine hydrochloride after prolonged continuous maternal intravenous administration. *Can. J. Anaesth.* 42:338, 1995.

Boehringer Igelheim Company. Mexitil (mexiletine hydrochloride). Entry in *Physicians Desk Reference* (52nd ed.). Montvale, NJ: Medical Economics, 1998. Pp. 720–723.

Committee on Drugs of the American Academy of Pediatrics. The transfer of drugs and other chemicals into human milk. *Pediatrics* 93:137, 1994.

Finster, M., Morishima, H.O., Boyes, R.N., and Covino, B.G. The placental transfer of lidocaine and its uptake by fetal tissues. *Anesthesiology* 36:159, 1972.

Gregg, A.R., and Tomich, P.G. Mexiletine use in pregnancy. *J. Perinatol.* 8:33, 1988.

Heymann, M.A. Correlations of fetal circulation and the placental transfer of drugs. *Fed. Proc.* 31:44, 1972.

Lewis, A.M., Patel, L., Johnston, A., et al. Mexiletine in human blood and breast milk. *Postgrad. Med.* 57:546, 1981.

Lownes, H.E., and Ives, T.J. Mexiletine use in pregnancy and lactation. *Am. J. Obstet. Gynecol.* 157:446, 1987.

Mann, L.I., Bailey, C., Carmichael, A., and Duchin, S. Effect of lidocaine on fetal heart rate and fetal brain metabolism and function. *Am. J. Obstet. Gynecol.* 112:789, 1972.

Pedersen, H., Santos, A.C., Morishima, H.O., et al. Does gestational age affect the pharmacokinetics and pharmacodynamics of lidocaine in mother and fetus? *Anesthesiology* 68:367, 1988.

Recchia, D. Cardiopulmonary resuscitation and advanced cardiac life support. In Chapter 8 of *Washington University Manual of Medical Therapeutics* (28th ed.), G.A. Ewald and C.R. McKenzie, eds. Boston: Little, Brown. Pp. 170–183.

Roden, D.M. Antiarrhythmic drugs. In Chapter 35 of *Goodman and Gilman's The Pharmacological Basis of Therapeutics* (9th ed.), J.G. Hardman and L.E. Limbird, eds. New York: McGraw-Hill, 1996. Pp. 865–867.

Teramo, K., et al. Effects of lidocaine on heart rate, blood pressure, and electrocortigram in fetal sheep. *Am. J. Obstet. Gynecol.* 118:935, 1974.

Lithium Carbonate (Eskalith®, Lithane®, Lithonate®, Lithobid®, Lithotabs®)

INDICATIONS AND RECOMMENDATIONS

Lithium carbonate may be administered to pregnant women for treatment of the manic phase of manic-depressive illness. However, it should be discontinued during the first trimester of pregnancy unless withdrawal would seriously jeopardize the woman or the pregnancy. During pregnancy, the smallest dosage possible for acceptable therapeutic effects should be used and plasma lithium levels should be monitored frequently. Frequent, small dosages should be used to avoid large fluctuations in maternal plasma concentrations. Individual doses should not exceed 300 mg and should be spaced evenly throughout the day. Major changes in maternal dietary intake or excretion of sodium, especially those causing hyponatremia, should be avoided. The fetus should be screened for cardiac anomalies.

Whenever possible, it is advisable to reduce the daily lithium dose by 50% in the last week of gestation and to discontinue it entirely at the onset of labor. When lithium therapy is restarted at prepregnancy dosage immediately after delivery, it is effective in preventing relapse during the postpartum period.

SPECIAL CONSIDERATIONS IN PREGNANCY

Lithium is not known to have any unusual maternal effects. It is cleared more quickly than it is in the nonpregnant state. Lithium clearance normally ranges from 15–30 ml/min and increases by 50% to 100% during the course of pregnancy. This value drops to prepregnancy levels at the time of delivery.

Lithium is known to cross the placenta, with concentrations being equal on both sides. It can be teratogenic in rodents if even transiently high lithium concentrations are delivered. However, when given in divided daily doses and maintained at steady serum concentrations in the human therapeutic range, lithium has been found to be without any deleterious effects on either mother or fetus in rodents, rabbits, and monkeys.

Early anecdotal data implicated lithium as causing a 400-fold increase in the risk of congenital anomalies including Ebstein's malformation. While it is now generally accepted that there is an association between lithium exposure in utero (particularly at high blood levels) and this cardiac defect, later studies indicate that the risk of first-trimester exposure is much lower than previously thought. In addition to heart defects, malformations of the central nervous system, external ear, ureters, and endocrine system have been reported. Children exposed to lithium in utero and born without malformation appear to be at no greater risk than other children for developing abnormalities later in life.

Maternal lithium therapy has been associated with an increase in the incidence of premature birth as well as an increased incidence of large-for-gestational-age births.

Infants born to mothers whose lithium plasma concentrations are in the therapeutic range may exhibit neonatal intoxication. Symptoms include cyanosis, lethargy, hypotonia, jaundice, hypothermia, duskiness, poor sucking, poor respiratory effort, low Apgar scores, absent Moro reflex, diabetes insipidus, and altered thyroid and cardiac function. Most of these toxic effects are self-limiting and resolve in 1 or 2 weeks. There are case reports of neonatal goiters in babies born to mothers taking lithium who themselves had goiters. These babies were euthyroid and their goiters transient. The half-life of lithium in the newborn is 68–96 hours.

Lithium is secreted in breast milk and has been measured at levels of about 40% of those found in the mother's serum. Infants breast-fed by mothers taking lithium have been reported to be hypotonic, hypothermic, and cyanotic, and to have electrocardiographic changes. However, drug intoxication does not always occur in the suckling infants of women taking lithium. Therefore, some authorities recommend that nursing be permitted but that these mothers be instructed to watch for signs of toxicity.

DOSAGE

Lithium carbonate is available in capsules and tablets of 150, 300, and 600 mg. Lithium is also available in liquid form as lithium citrate 8 mEq (equivalent of 300 mg lithium carbonate) per 5 ml. Dosage is determined by the severity of the illness and the patient's physical state, body weight, and age. In the treatment of acute mania, the usual dose range is 600 mg tid or 900 mg bid to achieve a therapeutic serum concentration in the range of 0.9–1.4 mEq/L. Plasma concentrations greater than 1.5 mEq/L produce no clinical advantage and increase the incidence of side effects. As the manic episode subsides, the lithium requirement decreases; the dosage therefore should be decreased fairly rapidly to about

600–1200 mg/day to achieve plasma levels of 0.7–1.2 mEq/L. This maintenance dosage must be individually adjusted according to symptoms and side effects.

There is a 4- to 10-day lag period in the onset of therapeutic effect due to the slow rate at which lithium crosses cell boundaries.

ADVERSE EFFECTS

Initial lithium therapy is associated with a transient increase in the excretion of 17-hydroxycorticosteroids, sodium, potassium, and water. Patients must maintain salt and fluid intake, especially during the initial stabilization period. Polydipsia and polyuria frequently occur, and the drug has been implicated in cases of nephrogenic diabetes insipidus. Circulating thyroid hormone levels fall, thyroid ^{131}I uptake is elevated, and plasma protein-bound iodine and free thyroxine levels are reduced. Patients usually remain euthyroid, although some may develop a goiter and become clinically hypothyroid. Reversible electrocardiographic changes can occur. Patients may also develop a fine tremor of the hands.

At toxic levels (more than 2.0 mEq/L), severe persistent nausea, vomiting, and diarrhea, gross hand tremor, slurred speech, muscle twitching, lethargy, seizures, and stupor progressing to coma may appear.

MECHANISM OF ACTION

The precise mechanism of lithium's action is unknown. Lithium alters sodium transport in nerve and muscle cells and causes a shift to intraneuronal catecholamine metabolism. It affects norepinephrine and serotonin, the neurotransmitters associated with affective disorders. It also affects the distribution of sodium, calcium, and magnesium ions.

ABSORPTION AND BIOTRANSFORMATION

Lithium is completely absorbed from the gastrointestinal tract within 8 hours, with peak plasma levels occurring in 1–4 hours. Distribution approximates total body water. It is not protein-bound. About 95% of a lithium dose is excreted unchanged in the urine, 4% to 5% in perspiration, and less than 1% in feces. Approximately 80% of filtered lithium is actively reabsorbed and is competitive with sodium. Sodium depletion will result in a greater reabsorption of lithium and possible toxicity. The plasma half-life in the average adult is 24 hours, with steady-state blood levels being reached in 56 days.

RECOMMENDED READING

Ananth, J. Side effects in the neonate from psychotropic agents excreted through breast feeding. *Am. J. Psychiatry* 135:801, 1978.

Baldessarini, R.J. Drugs and the treatment of psychiatric disorders: depression and mania. Chapter 19 in *Goodman and Gilman's The Pharmacological Basis of Therapeutics* (9th ed.), J.G. Hardman and L.E. Limbird, eds. New York: McGraw-Hill, 1996. Pp. 446–449.

Goldberg, H.L., and Nissim, R. Psychotropic drugs in pregnancy and lactation. *Int. J. Psychiatry Med.* 24:129, 1994.

Jacobson, S.J., et al. Prospective multicentre study of pregnancy outcome after lithium exposure during first trimester. *Lancet* 339:530, 1992.

Kallen, B., and Tandberg, A. Lithium and pregnancy. A cohort study on manic-depressive women. *Acta Psychiatr. Scand.* 68:134, 1983.

Schou, M., and Amdisen, A. Lithium and pregnancy—III. Lithium ingestion by children breast fed by women on lithium treatment. *Br. Med. J.* 2:138, 1973.

Troyer, W.A., et al. Association of maternal lithium exposure and premature delivery. *J. Perinatol.* 13:123, 1993.

Tunnessen, W.W., and Hertz, C.G. Toxic effects of lithium in newborn infants: a commentary. *J. Pediatrics* 81:804, 1972.

Weinstein, M.R., and Goldfield, M.D. Cardiovascular malformations with lithium use during pregnancy. *Am. J. Psychiatry* 132: 529, 1975.

Zalstein, E., et al. A case-control study on the association between first trimester exposure to lithium and Ebstein's anomaly. *Am. J. Cardiol.* 65:817, 1990.

Local Anesthetics: Bupivacaine (Marcaine®), Chloroprocaine (Nesacaine®), Etidocaine (Duranest®), Lidocaine (Xylocaine®), Mepivacaine (Carbocaine®), Ropivacaine (Naropin®), Tetracaine (Pontocaine®)

INDICATIONS AND RECOMMENDATIONS

Local anesthetics are generally safe to use for local infiltration and regional block for pain relief during labor and delivery as well as for cesarean section. Paracervical block is no longer recommended because of the high incidence of associated fetal bradycardias. Bupivacaine in a concentration of 0.75% has been found to have maternal cardiac toxicity when used as an epidural anesthetic, and therefore this concentration is no longer used in obstetric patients. In general, however, local anesthetics are highly selective with only minor systemic effects, making them ideal agents for use in pregnant women.

The use of lidocaine as an antiarrhythmic agent is discussed elsewhere in this book (see "Lidocaine").

SPECIAL CONSIDERATIONS IN PREGNANCY

Bupivacaine and ropivacaine appear to be the agents of choice for epidural analgesia in labor, due to limited motor blockade. Ropivacaine is slightly less potent than bupivacaine, but it also has less cardiotoxicity and fewer motor effects and is becoming more widely used in obstetric anesthesia. These agents are often combined with a narcotic to enable usage of lower dosages of the local anesthetic while achieving adequate analgesia. Lidocaine and chloroprocaine result in a dense motor block that is useful for cesarean delivery. Chloroprocaine use is limited by its short duration, but it has the advantage of increased safety for the fetus due to limited transfer. When used for epidural anesthesia, etidocaine and tetracaine produce profound motor block but suboptimal sensory blockade. Tetracaine, however, is one of the most effective drugs for subarachnoid block. Mepivacaine is not frequently used in obstetric anesthesia because of its greater propensity to reach the fetus as well as its long half-life in the neonate compared to other agents.

There are several reports of maternal deaths following ventricular arrhythmias and subsequent cardiac arrest after inadvertent intravascular injections of 0.75% bupivacaine during epidural anesthesia. Therefore, this concentration is no longer used in obstetric patients.

Paracervical blocks have been associated with a significant incidence of fetal bradycardias. An increased incidence of these fetal heart rate changes was observed in association with primiparity, prematurity, and preexisting fetal distress. Neonatal depression was significantly increased in those infants who had developed fetal heart rate changes following the paracervical block as compared to those infants whose heart rates had remained within the normal range. For these reasons, paracervical blocks are no longer commonly used in pregnancy, although low doses of bupivacaine have been administered with fewer apparent fetal cardiac effects.

Experiments in pregnant ewes and baboons have shown that local anesthetics administered intravenously or by paracervical block to produce clinically encountered blood levels stimulate myometrial contractility and vasoconstriction. This may result in a subsequent reduction in uteroplacental perfusion and decreased oxygen availability to the fetus. Other studies have shown that human uterine arteries constrict when exposed to lidocaine in vitro and that arteries from pregnant patients elicit significantly greater responses than those from nonpregnant women. Studies on bupivacaine given to pregnant sheep have demonstrated reversible fetal bradycardia and decreased umbilical blood flow. Human studies using Doppler measurements have not shown any decrease in umbilical or fetal blood flow; however, bupivacaine has been associated with occasional fetal bradycardia. Studies in preterm lambs have shown an impaired cardiovascular response to asphyxia after exposure to lidocaine, but there are no similar data available for preterm human fetuses. Ropivacaine has been studied in sheep and humans and has not been associated with any significant fetal toxicity.

Local anesthetics may affect the fetus directly via transplacental transfer of the drug or indirectly via maternal effects such as hypotension. The latter is likely to occur when vasodilatation secondary to sensory blockade occurs in a relatively dehydrated patient. It is therefore recommended that prophylactic intravenous hydration with at least 1 L of crystalloid solution be administered before an epidural or subarachnoid block is administered. Care should be taken, however, not to infuse an excessive glucose load. One study has shown that rapid infusions of 25 g or more of glucose into women prior to elective cesarean section was associated with fetal acidosis and neonatal hyperinsulinemia, hypoglycemia, and hyperbilirubinemia. These authors suggest that infusions be limited to 6 g dextrose per hour in preparation for elective cesarean section until a maximum safe level can be established. Additionally, when an epidural anesthetic is administered, a test dose should be delivered into the catheter before the full dose is injected in order to rule out the possibility that the drug is inadvertently being given intravenously.

All local anesthetics cross the placenta, but they do so at different rates. Transplacental diffusion is greater in those agents with the highest lipid solubility and the lowest maternal protein binding. The nonionized form of the drug is the most lipid-soluble. Clinically, this could be significant during fetal acidosis, at which time the agent becomes ionized and therefore "trapped" in the fetal circulation, making fetal toxicity of the drug more likely.

In animal studies, fetal convulsions have been produced with high fetal blood levels of these agents. In dosages used in humans, no such effects have been reported. Epidural analgesia using bupivacaine and lidocaine has been associated with fetal hyperthermia in prolonged labor.

Transient neonatal motor retardation during the first 8 hours of life has been reported by Scanlon et al. after epidural anesthesia using mepivacaine and lidocaine. However, no difference in Apgar scores was found between the epidural and control groups. Abboud and colleagues, in a later study, found no difference in neonatal neurobehavioral scores between epidural and control groups. The drugs used in this study were chloroprocaine, bupivacaine, and lidocaine. Epidural anesthesia is associated with higher maternal blood levels of anesthetic in the maternal blood than is spinal anesthesia. To reduce the risk of neonatal depression, dilute anesthetic solutions for epidural anesthesia are favored.

Case reports have described neonatal intoxication following maternal perineal and pudendal infiltration with lidocaine at delivery. While extremely rare, central nervous system (CNS) effects such as hypotonia, seizures, and respiratory arrest, as well as cardiac depression, may be seen shortly after birth.

As a group, these agents have not been associated with an increased risk of congenital malformations, as demonstrated by the Collaborative Perinatal Project. In the first trimester, local anesthetics are often used in the setting of assisted reproductive technology for ovarian follicle aspiration. Studies in the mouse suggest decreased fertilization and embryo development after exposure to local anesthetics. These findings have not been demonstrated in humans, and first-trimester use has not been associated with teratogenicity to date.

DOSAGE

The total dosage of local anesthetic to be used depends on the route of administration, the specific agent used, and the level as well as duration of blockade desired (Table 3).

For use in skin infiltration, maximum doses (in the absence of epinephrine) are as follows: lidocaine (0.5% to 1%), 4.5 mg/kg; bupivacaine (0.125% to 0.25%), 2 mg/kg; and procaine (0.5% to 1%), 7 mg/kg. These amounts can be increased by one-third in the presence of epinephrine.

In pregnancy, reduced doses of local anesthetics are required for spinal and epidural anesthesia, and their onset of action is more rapid.

TABLE 3. Dosages for local anesthetics

Agent	Concentration	Protein binding (%)	Approximate lipid solubility	Maximum dose (mg)	Duration (min)
Chloroprocaine	2.0–3.0	≈5	<1	1000	45–69
Mepivacaine	1.0–2.0	75	1	500	120–140
Lidocaine	1.0–2.0	65	4	500	90–200
Tetracaine	0.15–0.25	85	80	200	180–600
Bupivacaine	0.25–0.75	95	30	300	180–600
Etidocaine	0.5–1.5	94	140	300	180–600
Ropivacaine	0.5	94	1–30?	150	120–240

Source: *J. Obstet. Gynecol. Reprod. Biol.* 59:S17, 1995.

ADVERSE EFFECTS

High maternal blood levels of local anesthetics may cause CNS toxicity. They can initially stimulate the CNS, causing restlessness, nervousness, tremors, and convulsions. This stimulation is followed by depression and respiratory failure. The reported incidence of convulsions during obstetric regional anesthesia is low, varying from 0.03% to 0.50%. Horner's syndrome and trigeminal palsy have been reported following epidural anesthesia with local anesthetics. Reversible hearing loss also has been described following spinal anesthesia with bupivacaine.

Local anesthetics may affect the cardiovascular system by acting directly on the heart and peripheral vasculature, as well as indirectly by sympathetic blockade. In the myocardium, local anesthetics decrease electrical excitability, rate of conduction, and force of contractility. Arterial hypotension is the most common complication of spinal or epidural anesthesia. This is secondary to the sympathetic blockade as well as a direct effect on the arterioles when the drug is absorbed into the bloodstream. Generally, cardiotoxicity does not occur unless high systemic concentrations are achieved, usually after CNS toxicity is present. On rare occasions, lower doses (particularly of bupivacaine) can result in cardiovascular collapse secondary to arrhythmias. Pregnancy does not appear to increase the risk of lidocaine or ropivacaine toxicity.

Allergic reactions to local anesthetics are rare and more likely to be associated with the ester derivatives. These reactions include localized edema, urticaria, bronchospasm, and pruritus and are related to breakdown products of metabolized esters. Anaphylactic reactions are extremely uncommon.

MECHANISM OF ACTION

Local anesthetics reduce pain by inhibiting neural excitation via a direct effect on the nerve cell membrane. They are thought to obstruct the inward surge of sodium ions associated with depolarization. They do not affect either the resting membrane or threshold potentials of nerve cells. The predominant effect of these agents is to decrease the maximum rate of rise of the action potential. As a result, threshold cannot be achieved and a propagated action potential fails to develop. The effects of individual local anesthetics are mediated by their lipid solubility, molecular size, and pK_a. They affect all nerve fibers but block small sensory fibers most rapidly.

ABSORPTION AND BIOTRANSFORMATION

The absorption of local anesthetics depends on the site of injection, the dosage, the addition of a vasoconstrictor agent, serum protein levels, and the specific agent employed. Comparison of blood levels of local anesthetics after various types of obstetric regional anesthesia reveals that the most rapid rate of absorption occurs after paracervical blocks. This is followed, in order of diminishing blood levels, by administration of the agent into the caudal canal, lumbar epidural space, and subarachnoid space. The blood level of local anesthetic agents is related to the total dosage of drug given rather than the volume or concentration.

The rate of absorption of these drugs can be reduced considerably by the incorporation of a vasoconstrictor agent such as epinephrine. However, absorbed epinephrine may cause reduction of uterine blood flow and inhibition of uterine activity, making its use in obstetric anesthesia controversial.

Local anesthetics are divided into two groups, depending on their molecular structure: those with ester-type linkage in the molecule and those with an amide linkage. The esters include chloroprocaine and tetracaine. The amide-linked agents include lidocaine, mepivacaine, bupivacaine, and etidocaine.

The esters are broken down in the bloodstream by plasma pseudocholinesterase at different rates, with chloroprocaine having the fastest rate of hydrolysis. Since the amide-linked agents are metabolized in the liver, their half-lives are longer. The half-life of bupivacaine is much longer in pregnant than nonpregnant adults.

All local anesthetics employed for obstetric anesthesia diffuse across the placenta. Peak fetal levels usually are reached 20–90 minutes after administration. Lidocaine and its metabolites have been detected in neonatal urine as late as 48 hours after delivery following perineal infiltration. The rate of placental diffusion is related to the degree of plasma protein binding in maternal blood and the rate of fetal tissue uptake. Fetal tissue uptake in turn is higher with the more lipid-soluble agents. Fetal plasma binding of local anesthetic agents is approximately 50% less than binding in maternal plasma, so that more unbound drug is present in the fetus. The main binding protein in both maternal and fetal plasma is α_1-acid glycoprotein, which is found in lesser concentration in the fetus. Those drugs that have the highest degree of protein binding also tend to be more lipid-soluble (see Table 3) so that the rate of tissue uptake of the unbound drug is enhanced. Therefore, maternal-fetal anesthetic blood concentrations can differ markedly between agents, but the total amount of drug transferred across the placenta may be similar for agents of higher and lower protein binding capacity. It was originally thought that agents such as bupivacaine, 95% of which is bound to maternal protein, did not cross the placenta in significant amounts. It is now believed, however, that this agent's high lipid solubility increases the fetal tissue uptake of the drug that is transferred. The clinical significance of these findings is not certain, but it may be true that the potential for fetal toxicity is similar for all local anesthetic agents. Free drug and tissue drug levels determine the likelihood of fetal toxicity. As the amide-type anesthetics are weak bases, free drug may accumulate in the fetus more readily in the setting of acidosis or an increased fetal–maternal pH gradient.

BREAST-FEEDING

Local anesthetics are found in breast milk. Lidocaine is listed as compatible with breast-feeding by the American Academy of Pediatrics.

RECOMMENDED READING

Abboud, T.K., et al. Maternal, fetal and neonatal responses after epidural anesthesia with bupivacaine, 2-chloroprocaine, or lidocaine. *Anesth. Analg.* 61:638, 1982.

Alahuhta, S., Rasanen, J., Jouppila, P., et al. The effects of epidural ropivacaine and bupivacaine for cesarean section on uteroplacental and fetal circulation. *Anesthesiology* 83:23, 1995.

Catterall, W., and Mackie, K. Local anesthetics. Chapter 15 in *Goodman and Gilman's The Pharmacological Basis of Therapeutics* (9th ed.),J.G. Hardman and L.E. Limbird, eds. New York: McGraw-Hill, 1996. Pp. 331–347.

Curran, M.J.A. Options for labor analgesia: techniques of epidural and spinal analgesia. *Semin. Perinatol.* 15:348, 1991.

Datta, S. Local anesthetic pharmacology. Chapter 2 in *The Obstetric Anesthesia Handbook*, S. Datta, ed. Boston: Mosby–Year Book, 1992. Pp. 13–21.

de Jong, R.H. Ropivacaine, white knight or dark horse? *Reg. Anesth.* 20:474, 1995.

Friedman, J.M. Teratogen update: anesthetic agents. *Teratology* 37: 69, 1988.

Halpern, S., Myhr, T., Fong, K., et al. Uterine and umbilical blood flow velocity during epidural anaesthesia for caesarean section. *Can. J. Anaesth.* 41:1057, 1994.

Johnson, R.F., Herman, N.L., Johnson, H.V., et al. Effects of fetal pH on local anesthetic transfer across the human placenta. *Anesthesiology* 85:608, 1996.

Kenepp, N.B., et al. Fetal and neonatal hazards of maternal hydration with 5% dextrose before cesarean section. *Lancet* 1:1150, 1982.

Morishima, H.O., Finster, M., Arthur, R., et al. Pregnancy does not alter lidocaine toxicity. *Am. J. Obstet. Gynecol.* 162:1320, 1990.

Nau, H. Clinical pharmacokinetics in pregnancy and perinatology. I. Placental transfer and fetal side effects of local anaesthetic agents. *Dev. Pharmacol. Ther.* 8:149, 1985.

Philipson, E.H., Kuhnert, B.R., and Syracuse, C.D. Maternal, fetal, and neonatal lidocaine levels following local perineal infiltration. *Am. J. Obstet. Gynecol.* 149:403, 1984.

Scherer, R., and Holzgreve, W. Influence of spinal analgesia on fetal and neonatal well-being. *Eur. J. Obstet. Gynecol. Reprod. Biol.* 59:S17, 1995.

Loperamide (Imodium®, Imodium AD®)

INDICATIONS AND RECOMMENDATIONS

Loperamide is relatively contraindicated during pregnancy because other therapeutic agents are preferable. It is a narcotic congener that is used as an antidiarrheal agent to provide symptomatic relief only. Primary treatment of diarrhea should be directed to the underlying condition, together with correcting fluid and electrolyte deletion.

While reproductive studies in rats and rabbits reveal no drug-induced embryotoxicity or teratogenicity, no data are available regarding its use in humans.

The American Academy of Pediatrics lists loperamide as being compatible with breast-feeding.

Because loperamide's effects on pregnancy and on the fetus have not been reported, its use should be avoided in favor of treating the underlying cause of diarrhea and, if necessary, treatment with diphenoxylate and atropine, which has been better studied in humans.

RECOMMENDED READING

Brunton, L.L. Agents affecting gastrointestinal water flux and motility; emesis and antiemetics; bile acids and pancreatic enzymes. Chapter 38 in *Goodman and Gilman's The Pharmacological Basis of Therapeutics* (9th ed.), J.G. Hardman and L.E. Limbird, eds. New York: McGraw-Hill, 1996. Pp. 926–927.

Committee on Drugs. The transfer of drugs and other chemicals into human milk. *Pediatrics* 93:137–150, 1994.

Marsboom, R., et al. Loperamide (R-18–553), a novel type of antidiarrheal agent. Part 4: studies on subacute and chronic toxicity and the effect on reproductive processes in rats, dogs and rabbits. *Arzneimittel-Forschung* 24:1645, 1974.

Losartan (Cozaar®)

INDICATIONS AND RECOMMENDATIONS

Losartan is contraindicated in pregnancy. It is a nonpeptide angiotensin II receptor antagonist, which selectively competes at the AT_1 receptor. Its use will reverse and prevent all known effects of angiotensin II. In the nonpregnant patient, it is indicated for the treatment of hypertension.

Losartan use in pregnant animals has been shown to cause decreased fetal body weight and an increase in pre- and post-weaning deaths. In rats, there is evidence of decreased pup cardiac weights as well as histopathologic changes of the kidneys.

No studies have been performed investigating its use during pregnancy in humans. This is at least partly because angiotensin-converting enzyme (ACE) inhibitors, which also act directly on the renin-angiotensin system and are also used as antihypertensives, are known to cause severe adverse fetal and neonatal effects, including hypotension, anuria, renal failure, and death.

In vitro studies of isolated human placental cotyledons have shown angiotensin II binding sites, specifically AT_1 receptors, which seem to contribute to the regulation of fetoplacental perfusion. The effect of losartan on fetoplacental blood flow, if any, has yet to be determined.

RECOMMENDED READING

Knock, G.A., et al. Angiotensin II (AT1) vascular binding sites in human placentae from normal-term, preeclamptic and growth retarded pregnancies. *J. Pharmacol. Exp. Ther.* 271:1007, 1994.

Lumbers, E.R. Functions of the renin-angiotensin system during development. *Clin. Exp. Pharmacol. Physiol.* 22:499, 1995.

Oates, J.A. Antihypertensive agents and the drug therapy of hypertension. Chapter 33 in *Goodman and Gilman's The Pharmacological Basis of Therapeutics* (9th ed.), J.G. Hardman and L.E. Limbird, eds. New York: McGraw-Hill, 1996. Pp. 751–753.

Spence, S.G., et al. Toxicokinetic analysis of losartan during gestation and lactation in the rat. *Teratology* 53:245, 1996.

Spence, S.G., et al. Evaluation of the reproductive and developmental toxicity of the AT1-selective angiotensin II receptor antagonist losartan in rats. *Teratology* 51:383, 1995.

Stevenson, K.M., Gibson, K.G., and Lumbers, E.R. Effects of losartan on the cardiovascular system, renal haemodynamics and function and lung liquid flow in fetal sheep. *Clin. Exp. Pharmacol. Physiol.* 23:125, 1996.

Magnesium Sulfate

INDICATIONS AND RECOMMENDATIONS

Magnesium sulfate is the drug of choice for the prevention of seizures in patients with preeclampsia. Women whose hypertensive disorder is severe enough to warrant administration of this drug should be delivered of their infants soon after stabilization has been accomplished.

When this drug is given, deep tendon reflexes should be elicited each hour, respirations should be 12/minute or more, and urinary output should exceed 30 ml/h. The administration of magnesium sulfate should be discontinued if respiratory depression is noted. A serum magnesium level should be obtained if deep tendon reflexes are lost but the urinary output and respiratory rate are normal. Because diminished urinary output may result in dangerously high serum levels, the rate of infusion should be decreased and serum magnesium levels checked frequently when this occurs. Although magnesium sulfate can be given by either the intramuscular or intravenous route, the latter is recommended both to ensure adequate therapeutic levels and to allow maximal control over administration.

The drug should be continued for approximately 24 hours following delivery as prophylaxis against postpartum seizures. If hyperreflexia persists, longer periods of administration may be necessary.

Magnesium sulfate has also been used as a tocolytic agent to arrest premature labor. In this setting, it is currently the drug of choice for patients with insulin-dependent diabetes, heart disease, or other relative contraindications to β-mimetic tocolytic therapy. Magnesium sulfate may also be given to patients who have failed a trial of β-mimetic therapy. It is administered intravenously when given for tocolysis.

SPECIAL CONSIDERATIONS IN PREGNANCY

Until 1995 there was a good deal of controversy surrounding the use of magnesium sulfate as an anticonvulsant in women with preeclampsia, particularly outside the United States. In that year, two randomized trials were published. One was an international collaborative study of 1680 women with eclamptic convulsions who were randomized to either magnesium sulfate, phenytoin, or diazepam. Magnesium sulfate was associated with a 52% lower risk of recurrent convulsions than diazepam, and a 67% lower risk than phenytoin. In the second study, which was from Dallas, 2138 women with pregnancy-induced hypertension were randomized to receive intramuscular or intravenous magnesium sulfate versus intravenous phenytoin followed by oral phenytoin. Eclamptic convulsions occurred in 1% of patients assigned to phenytoin versus none of the patients given magnesium ($p = 0.004$). Outcomes were otherwise similar in the two groups. Magnesium sulfate infusion has been associated with a small but significant increase in cerebrospinal fluid magnesium levels.

Short-term (2.5 hours) infusions of magnesium sulfate have been shown to decrease plasma renin activity in women with preeclampsia, with no sustained change in angiotensin-converting enzyme (ACE) concentrations. Longer infusions of magnesium sulfate (4–24 hours) have been associated with moderate (approx. 25%) declines in ACE concentrations in patients with pregnancy-induced hypertension. Central hemodynamic monitoring of patients with severe pregnancy-induced hypertension has demonstrated a transient hypotensive effect when the drug was administered as a bolus, but not as a constant infusion. However, there are case reports of profound hypotension in preeclamptic, hypovolemic patients receiving usual doses of magnesium sulfate. The drug can dilate human uterine arteries in vitro. Long- term intravenous followed by oral magnesium sulfate therapy (average duration of treatment 10 days) in subjects with moderate hypertensive disorders of pregnancy has been demonstrated to lower mean arterial pressure in a randomized trial from Denmark.

Magnesium sulfate may diminish the frequency and intensity of uterine contractions by direct action on the myometrium. In one study comparing the effectiveness of this drug with other agents, magnesium sulfate was successful in arresting premature labor in 77% of cases as opposed to 45% for intravenous ethanol and 44% for dextrose in water. However, as with other tocolytic agents, long-term benefits of magnesium sulfate tocolysis, such as prevention of preterm birth or lowering of perinatal mortality, have not been demonstrated. Despite its apparent tocolytic activity, one randomized trial of 54 patients with preeclampsia randomized to either magnesium sulfate or phenytoin found no impact of magnesium sulfate on the length of induced labor.

Magnesium crosses the placenta, and hypotonia, lethargy, weakness, and low Apgar scores have been attributed to fetal hypermagnesemia. A large number of published reports have addressed the possibility that therapeutic blood levels of magnesium sulfate in the mother may alter the characteristics of fetal heart rate recordings. While some studies have shown statistically significant reductions in beat-to-beat variability and other characteristics of reactivity, particularly when computerized analysis of the tracings was undertaken, most authors have concluded that these differences are not clinically significant and the fetus whose mother is treated with magnesium sulfate should be evaluated in a similar way to other fetuses. It should be noted, however, that the majority of the above studies were performed in healthy term fetuses, and once case series of five patients in preterm labor suggested a blunted fetal response to vibroacoustic stimulation when magnesium sulfate was administered.

A retrospective cohort study, published in 1996, raised the possibility that babies weighing less than 1500 g at birth who were exposed to magnesium sulfate in utero had a lower risk for cerebral palsy than did babies of similar weight and gestational age but not exposed to magnesium sulfate. There is considerable ongoing debate as to whether magnesium sulfate has some protective effect against cerebral palsy or whether conditions associated with preterm delivery not qualifying for magnesium tocolysis may have a higher risk. Prospective studies are in progress to address this issue.

When fetal blood samples were obtained by cordocentesis, fetal magnesium levels rose within an hour of maternal treatment, whereas amniotic fluid magnesium levels did not go up until 3 hours had passed. Magnesium levels in the cord blood of neonates have been shown to reflect those of their mothers. Magnesium levels in breast milk are mildly elevated for 24 hours after discontinuation of the drug. The Committee on Drugs of the American Academy of Pediatrics considers magnesium sulfate to be usually compatible with breast-feeding.

DOSAGE

When administered as seizure prophylaxis, magnesium sulfate may be given intravenously or intramuscularly as is shown below. The intravenous route is preferred in the treatment of hypertensive disorders of pregnancy and is always used when treating premature labor.

Intravenous administration via infusion pump:

Loading dose: 4–6 g in 250 ml 5% D/W over 20 minutes

Maintenance dose: 2–3 g/hour, titrated by deep tendon reflexes and serum levels

Intramuscular administration:

Loading dose: 5 g in 50% solution in each buttock (total–10 g) along with 4 g given intravenously as above

Maintenance dose: 5 g of a 50% solution q4h after checking deep tendon reflexes, respiratory rates, and urinary output

The presence or absence of deep tendon reflexes is not always a reliable predictor of the serum magnesium level and should not, by itself, lead to an increase in dosage or a cessation of the infusion. The only reliable indicator of adequate dosage is a serum magnesium level of 4–7 mEq/L or 5–8 mg/dl. Serum levels do not correlate particularly well with clinical success in stopping preterm labor and are most useful as an indicator that the dose can be safely increased without a high likelihood of toxicity.

Magnesium can be administered orally as the oxide, chloride, or gluconate salt. Available data do not support efficacy for oral magnesium tocolysis or prophylaxis against preterm labor.

Magnesium sulfate toxicity in the mother can be treated by administering 1 g calcium gluconate intravenously into a peripheral vein over 3 minutes.

ADVERSE EFFECTS

Toxic signs and symptoms associated with magnesium sulfate administration do not appear until blood levels exceed

8–10 mEq/L. At or near this level, knee jerks disappear. Between 10 and 12.5 mEq/L, heart block and peaked T waves on electrocardiogram may be noted, the patient can become obtunded, and respirations may cease. Above this level, cardiac arrest can occur.

Pulmonary edema has been reported with intravenous magnesium sulfate infusion for tocolysis. One group of investigators has attributed this phenomenon to volume overload. Another study found pulmonary edema in patients with preeclampsia but not those in preterm labor, and attributed the problem to lowered colloid osmotic pressure. A case of chest pain with transient subendocardial ischemia during magnesium sulfate therapy has been reported.

Short-term magnesium therapy of hypertensive women in labor and those with preterm labor has been demonstrated to cause elevations in vitamin D and parathormone levels, and declines in calcium levels. Long-term intravenous magnesium therapy (mean of 26 days) has been associated with marked urinary calcium loss, calcium depletion, and subsequent decreased bone density.

Magnesium sulfate therapy has been reported to cause allergic urticarial skin eruptions and maternal hypothermia.

Fetal hypermagnesemia is known to be associated with hypotonia, lethargy, and respiratory depression of the neonate. Some authors believe that this neonatal symptom complex is more severe when maternal administration of the drug has been intravenous, but to date there have been no prospective studies that have conclusively demonstrated this. A case-control study of neonates exposed to magnesium sulfate treatment in utero for more than 7 days revealed abnormal patterns of bone mineralization. The significance of these findings is not known.

MECHANISM OF ACTION

In pharmacologic dosages, magnesium sulfate is a CNS depressant. It also blocks neuromuscular impulse transmission by diminishing the amplitude of the end-plate potential and decreasing its sensitivity to the depolarizing action of acetylcholine. Furthermore, the excitability of muscle fibers to direct stimulation is diminished.

By its action on the CNS and peripheral neuromuscular functions, magnesium sulfate reduces the hyperreflexia associated with preeclampsia and is an effective prophylaxis against eclamptic seizures. By acting directly on blood vessel walls, this drug causes some vasodilatation. This may result in a modest decline in blood pressure and an increase in uterine blood flow in patients with preeclampsia.

ABSORPTION AND BIOTRANSFORMATION

When used for the treatment of preeclampsia, magnesium sulfate is administered either intravenously or intramuscularly. When given by the latter route, there is a lag of 90–120 minutes before plasma levels reach a plateau. Thirty-five percent of the drug is protein- bound, whereas the rest remains in the ionic form. Magnesium is excreted entirely in the urine, and elevated serum levels may accumulate when standard dosages of the drug are given to patients with diminished renal function.

RECOMMENDED READING

Armson, B.A., Samuels, P., Miller, F., et al. Evaluation of maternal fluid dynamics during tocolytic therapy with ritodrine hydrochloride and magnesium sulfate. *Am. J. Obstet. Gynecol.* 167:758, 1992.

Atkinson, M.W., Belfort, M.A., Saade, G.R., et al. The relation between magnesium sulfate therapy and fetal heart rate variability. *Obstet. Gynecol.* 83:967, 1994.

Atkinson, M.W., Guinn, D., Owen, J. et al. Does magnesium sulfate affect the length of labor induction in women with pregnancy-associated hypertension? *Am. J. Obstet. Gynecol.* 173:1219, 1995.

Bourgeois, F.J., Thiagarajah, S., Harbert, G.M., Jr., et al. Profound hypotension complicating magnesium therapy. *Am. J. Obstet. Gynecol.* 154:919, 1986.

Cañez, M.S., Reed, K.L., and Shenker, L. Effect of maternal magnesium sulfate treatment on fetal heart rate variability. *Am. J. Perinatol.* 4:167, 1987.

Carlan, S.J., and O'Brien, W.F. The effect of magnesium sulfate on the biophysical profile of normal term fetuses. *Obstet. Gynecol.* 77:681, 1991.

Cholst, I.N., Steinberg, S.F., Tropper, P.J., et al. The influence of hypermagnesemia on serum calcium and parathyroid hormone levels in human subjects. *N. Engl. J. Med.* 310:1221, 1984.

Committee on Drugs of the American Academy of Pediatrics. The transfer of drugs and other chemicals into human milk. *Pediatrics* 93:137, 1994.

Cotton, D.B., Gonik, B., and Dorman, K.F. Cardiovascular alterations in severe pregnancy-induced hypertension: acute effects of intravenous magnesium sulfate. *Am. J. Obstet. Gynecol.* 148:162, 1984.

Cox, S.M., Sherman, M.L., and Leveno, K.J. Randomized investigation of magnesium sulfate for prevention of preterm birth. *Am. J. Obstet. Gynecol.* 163:767, 1990.

Cruikshank, D.P., Varner, M.W., and Pitkin, R.M. Breast milk magnesium and calcium concentrations following magnesium sulfate treatment. *Am. J. Obstet. Gynecol.* 143:685, 1982.

Cruikshank, D.P., Chan, G.M., and Doerrfield, D. Alterations in vitamin D and calcium metabolism with magnesium sulfate treatment of preeclampsia. *Am. J. Obstet. Gynecol.* 168:1170, 1993.

Fuentes, A., and Goldkrand, J.W. Angiotensin-converting enzyme activity in hypertensive subjects after magnesium sulfate therapy. *Am. J. Obstet. Gynecol.* 156:1375, 1987.

Ghuzman, E.R., Conley, M., Stewart, R., et al. Phenytoin and magnesium sulfate effects on fetal heart rate tracings assessed by computer analysis. *Obstet. Gynecol.* 82:375, 1993.

Gray, S.E., Rodis, J.F., Lettieri, L., et al. Effect of intravenous magnesium sulfate on the biophysical profile of the healthy term fetus. *Am. J. Obstet. Gynecol.* 170:1131, 1994.

Green, K.W., Key, T.C., Coen, R., and Resnick, R. The effects of maternally administered magnesium sulfate on the neonate. *Am. J. Obstet. Gynecol.* 146:29, 1983.

Hallack, M., Berry, S.M., Madincea, F., et al. Fetal serum and amniotic fluid magnesium concentrations with maternal treatment. *Obstet. Gynecol.* 81:185, 1993.

Hiett, A.K., Devoe, L.D., Brown, H.L., et al. Effect of magnesium on fetal heart rate variability using computer analysis. *Am. J. Perinatol.* 12:259, 1995.

Lucas, M.J., Leveno, K.J., and Cunningham, F.G. A comparison of magnesium sulfate with phenytoin for the prevention of eclampsia. *N. Engl. J. Med.* 333:201, 1995.

Martin, R.W., Perry, K.G., Jr., Hess, L.W., et al. Oral magnesium and the prevention of preterm labor in a high-risk group of patients. *Am. J. Obstet. Gynecol.* 166:144, 1992.

Nelson, S.H., and Suresh, M.S. Magnesium sulfate induced relaxation of uterine arteries from pregnant and nonpregnant patients. *Am. J. Obstet. Gynecol.* 164:1344, 1991.

Pritchard, J.A. Standardized treatment of 154 consecutive cases of eclampsia. *Am. J. Obstet. Gynecol.* 123:545, 1975.

Ricci, J.M., Hariharan, S., Helfgott, A., et al. Oral tocolysis with magnesium chloride: a randomized controlled prospective clinical trial. *Am. J. Obstet. Gynecol.* 165:603, 1991.

Rodis, J.F., Vintzileos, A.M., Campbell, W.A., et al. Maternal hypothermia: an unusual complication of magnesium sulfate. *Am. J. Obstet. Gynecol.* 156:436, 1987.

Rudnicki, M., Frölich, A., Rasmussen, W.F., et al. The effect of magnesium on maternal blood pressure in pregnancy-induced hypertension: a randomized double blind placebo controlled trial. *Acta Obstet. Gynecol. Scand.* 70:445, 1991.

Schendel, D.E., Berg, C.J., Yeargin-Allsopp, M., et al. Prenatal magnesium sulfate exposure and the risk for cerebral palsy or mental retardation among very low birth weight children aged 3 to 5 years. *J.A.M.A.* 276:1805, 1996.

Sherer, D.M., Cialone, P.R., Abramowicz, J.S., et al. Transient symptomatic subendocardial ischemia during intravenous magnesium sulfate tocolytic therapy. *Am. J. Obstet. Gynecol.* 166:33, 1992.

Sherer, D.M. Blunted fetal response to vibroacoustic stimulation associated with maternal intravenous magnesium sulfate therapy. *Am. J. Perinatol.* 11:401, 1994.

Sibai, B.M., Villar, M.A., and Bray, E. Magnesium supplementation during pregnancy: a double-blind randomized controlled trial. *Am. J. Obstet. Gynecol.* 161:115, 1989.

Sipes, S.L., Weiner, C.P., Gellhaus, T.M., et al. The plasma renin-angiotensin system in preeclampsia: effects of magnesium sulfate. *Obstet. Gynecol.* 73:934, 1989.

Smith, L.G., Burns, P.A., and Schanler, R.J. Calcium homeostasis in pregnant women receiving long-term magnesium sulfate therapy for preterm labor. *Am. J. Obstet. Gynecol.* 167:45, 1992.

Stallworth, J.C., Yeh, S.-Y., and Petrie, R.H. The effect of magnesium sulfate on fetal heart rate variability and uterine activity. *Am. J. Obstet. Gynecol.* 140:702, 1981.

Steer, C.H., and Petrie, R.H. A comparison of magnesium sulfate and alcohol for the prevention of premature labor. *Am. J. Obstet. Gynecol.* 129:1, 1977.

The Eclampsia Trial Collaborative Group. Which anticonvulsant for women with eclampsia? Evidence from the Collaborative Eclampsia Trial. *Lancet* 345:1455, 1995.

Thorpe, J.M., Jr., Katz, V.L., Campbell, D., et al. Hypersensitivity to magnesium sulfate. *Am. J. Obstet. Gynecol.* 161:889, 1989.

Thurnau, G.R., Kemp, D.B., and Jarvis, A. Cerebrospinal fluid levels of magnesium in patients with preeclampsia after treatment with intravenous magnesium sulfate: a preliminary report. *Am. J. Obstet. Gynecol.* 157:1435, 1997.

Wacker, W., and Parisi, A. Magnesium metabolism. *N. Engl. J. Med.* 278:712, 1968.

Yeast, J.D., Halberstadt, C., Meyer, B.A., et al. The risk of pulmonary edema and colloid osmotic pressure changes during magnesium sulfate infusion. *Am. J. Obstet. Gynecol.* 169:1566, 1993.

Mannitol (Osmitrol®)

INDICATIONS AND RECOMMENDATIONS

Mannitol may be administered to critically ill pregnant patients. It is used to promote diuresis and to reduce intracranial pressure. The effect that changes in fetal extracellular fluid volume and intravascular tonicity have on the fetus at various stages of gestation is unknown. For this reason, an osmotic diuretic such as mannitol should only be used for life-threatening conditions during pregnancy.

SPECIAL CONSIDERATIONS IN PREGNANCY

The administration of hypertonic solutions to a pregnant woman results in changes in the composition of the maternal extracellular fluid with similar effects on tonicity and blood volume in the fetus. Mannitol crosses the placenta and can result in fetal dehydration. Both of these factors may lead to oxygen and acid–base imbalances in the fetus. In addition, maternal cardiac decompensation could seriously hinder uterine blood flow and thus adversely affect the fetus.

In a study involving the intravenous administration of mannitol to nine normal pregnant women at term, the drug was detected in amniotic fluid within 5 minutes. The concentration of mannitol continued to increase in the amniotic fluid up to 240 minutes after administration of the drug and reached values that were higher than those simultaneously obtained in maternal plasma. In one woman with a dead fetus at 29 weeks, however, intravenously administered mannitol appeared in amniotic fluid but increased very little over time and never reached values higher than those of the maternal plasma. When intravenous mannitol was given to pregnant sheep, it was found that drug concentrations in fetal urine were 10–20 times higher than drug concentrations in the fetal plasma. There is one older report of the use of intraamniotic mannitol for the induction of abortion.

DOSAGE

Mannitol is available for intravenous administration as a 5%, 10%, 15%, 20%, or 25% solution. Specific dosages depend on the underlying disease as well as renal response and fluid balance in a particular patient. Usual adult doses range from 50 to 200 g/24 hours. A test dose of 0.2 g/kg should be given to a patient with marked oliguria or one believed to have inadequate renal function.

ADVERSE EFFECTS

Adverse effects are related to the load of solute administered and the effect of mannitol on fluids and electrolytes. The most serious side effect is cardiac decompensation secondary to circulatory overload. The patient's cardiovascular status, therefore, must be carefully monitored during administration. There is one report of hemorrhagic limbs in pregnant rats treated with concentrated mannitol, but there were no increases in birth defects in the offspring of treated dams.

MECHANISM OF ACTION

Mannitol is a nonelectrolyte, osmotically active solute that, when excreted by the kidneys, is accompanied by an obligatory osmotic diuresis. The solute prevents reabsorption of water, and urine volume thus can be maintained even in the presence of decreased glomerular function. The concentration of sodium in the tubular fluid is decreased and the amount of sodium that is reabsorbed is therefore decreased. The excretion of sodium and chloride is increased. In the treatment of elevated intracranial pressure, mannitol again acts osmotically to draw excess fluid across the blood–brain barrier into the intravascular space.

ABSORPTION AND BIOTRANSFORMATION

The drug is poorly absorbed from the gastrointestinal tract and must be administered intravenously. It is confined to the extracellular space, only slightly metabolized, and rapidly excreted in the urine. Approximately 80% of a 100 g dose appears unchanged in the urine in 3 hours.

RECOMMENDED READING

Basso, A., et al. Passage of mannitol from mother to amniotic fluid and fetus. *Obstet. Gynecol.* 49:628, 1977.

Craft, I.L., and Mus, B.D. Hypertonic solutions to induce abortions. *Br. Med. J.* 2:49, 1971.

Jackson, E.K. Diuretics. Chapter 19 in *Goodman and Gilman's The Pharmacological Basis of Therapeutics* (9th ed.), J.G. Hardman and L.E. Limbird, eds. New York: McGraw-Hill, 1996. Pp. 695–697.

Petter, C. Lesions des extremities provoquees chez le foetus de rat par des injections intraveineuses de mannitol hyertonique a la mere. *C. R. Soc. Biol.* 161:1010, 1967.

Pritchard, J.A. Standardized treatment of 154 consecutive cases of eclampsia. *Am. J. Obstet. Gynecol.* 123:543, 1975.

Ross, M.G., et al. Bulk flow of amniotic fluid water in response to maternal osmotic challenge. *Am. J. Obstet. Gynecol.* 147:697, 1983.

Ross, M.G., et al. Fetal lung fluid response to maternal hyperosmolality. *Pediatr. Pulmonol.* 2:40, 1986.

Marijuana

INDICATIONS AND RECOMMENDATIONS

Marijuana is contraindicated during pregnancy. A number of factors are responsible for this recommendation. First, the hazards of cigarette smoking (see "Tobacco") are, if anything, greater with marijuana because the smoke is generally inhaled deeply into the lungs and kept there for as long as possible. Second, there is no approved indication for its use, although research into its efficacy as an antiglaucoma agent, an antiemetic, and a tranquilizer is ongoing and in some localities it is used for these indications. Third, Δ9-tetrahydrocannabinol (THC), the active ingredient of marijuana, is known to cross the placenta, depressing the fetal heart rate and changing fetal electroencephalographic patterns. Finally, there are data to suggest an increased incidence of fetal wastage, prematurity, growth restriction, meconium passage, congenital anomalies, and possibly a predisposition to the dysmorphic features of the fetal alcohol syndrome among offspring of marijuana users. Maternal marijuana use was found to be more common in the histories of children with certain types of leukemias. Children exposed to marijuana in utero scored lower in verbal and memory testing at 48 months of age, compared to nonexposed children. Tetrahydrocannabinol has been demonstrated to accumulate in the breast milk of lactating women who use marijuana and to be absorbed by the nursing baby. For these reasons, it would seem judicious to abstain from marijuana use during pregnancy and lactation.

RECOMMENDED READING

Blackard, C., and Tennes, K. Human placental transfer of cannabinoids. *N. Engl. J. Med.* 311:797, 1984.

Fried, P.A., Watkinson, B., and Willan, A. Marijuana use during pregnancy and decreased length of gestation. *Am. J. Obstet. Gynecol.* 150:23, 1984.

Fried, B., and Watkinson, B. 36- and 48-month neurobehavioral follow-up of children prenatally exposed to marijuana, cigarettes and alcohol. *Dev. Behav. Pediatrics* 11:49, 1990.

Gibson, G.T., Baghurst, P.A., and Colley, D.P. *Aust. N. Z. J. Obstet. Gynaecol.* 23:15, 1983.

Greenland, S., Staisch, K.J., Brown, N., and Gross, S.J. The effects of marijuana use during pregnancy. I. A preliminary epidemiologic study. *Am. J. Obstet. Gynecol.* 143:408, 1982.

Hatch, E.E., and Bracken, M.B. Effect of marijuana use in pregnancy on fetal growth. *Am. J. Epidemiol.* 124:986, 1986.

Hingson, R., et al. Effects of maternal drinking and marijuana use on fetal growth and development. *Pediatrics* 70:539, 1982.

Mantilla-Plata, B., Clewe, G.L., and Harbison, R.D. Teratogenic and mutagenic studies of delta-9-tetrahydrocannabinol in mice. *Fed. Proc.* 32:746, 1973.

Nahas, G., and Latour, C. The human toxicity of marijuana. *Med. J. Aust.* 156:495, 1992.

Perez-Reyes, M. Presence of delta-9-tetrahydrocannabinol in human milk. *N. Engl. J. Med.* 307:819, 1982.

Robison, L.L., Buckley, J.D., Daigle, A.E., et al. Maternal drug use and risk of childhood nonlymphoblastic leukemia among offspring. *Cancer* 63:1904, 1989.

Mebendazole (Vermox®)

INDICATIONS AND RECOMMENDATIONS

Because of its teratogenicity in animal studies, mebendazole is relatively contraindicated during pregnancy. It should be used only when the particular parasitic infestation poses a significant threat to the mother or fetus, and other agents are not appropriate. It is a broad-spectrum antihelminthic agent that is effective in the treatment of ascariasis, enterobiasis, trichuriasis, and hookworm disease. Although mebendazole is poorly absorbed from the gastrointestinal tract and is used during pregnancy in some parts of the world, it has been found to be embryotoxic and teratogenic at single doses of 10 mg/kg body weight in rats. Human teratogenicity has not been reported; nevertheless, mebendazole should be avoided during pregnancy if possible. A case series of four lactating mothers reported that all breast-fed successfully while taking mebendazole.

RECOMMENDED READING

Atukorala, T.M.S., de Silva, L.P.R., Dechering, W.H.J.C., et al. Evaluation of effectiveness of iron-folate supplementation and antihelminthic therapy against anemia in pregnancy: a study in the plantation sector of Sri Lanka. *Am. J. Clin. Nutr.* 60:286, 1994.

Brugmans, J.P., et al. Mebendazole in enterobiasis. *J.A.M.A.* 217:313, 1971.

Keystone, J.S., and Murdoch, J.K. Mebendazole. *Ann. Intern. Med.* 91:582, 1979.

Kurzel, R.B., Toot, P.J., Lambert, L.V., et al. Mebendazole and postpartum lactation. *N. Z. J. Med.* 107:439, 1994.

Leach, F.N. Management of threadworm infestation during pregnancy. *Arch. Dis. Child.* 65:399, 1990.

Leah, S.K.K. Mebendazole in the treatment of helminthiasis. *Can. Med. Assoc. J.* 115:777, 1976.

Liu, L.X., and Weller, P.F. Antiparasitic drugs. *N. Engl. J. Med.* 334:1178, 1996.

Pawlowski, Z.S. Letter and comment: antihelminthic therapy and iron supplementation of pregnant women. *Am. J. Clin. Nutr.* 62:1023, 1995.

Sargent, R.G., et al. A clinical evaluation of the efficacy of mebendazole in the treatment of trichuriasis. *South. Med. J.* 68:38, 1975.

Meclizine (Antivert®, Antrizine®, Bonine®, Dramamine II®)

INDICATIONS AND RECOMMENDATIONS

Meclizine is safe to use during pregnancy. It is used for the prevention and treatment of the nausea, vomiting, and dizziness associated with motion sickness, and it may be effective for the relief of vertigo associated with diseases affecting the vestibular system.

SPECIAL CONSIDERATIONS IN PREGNANCY

Meclizine has been shown to be teratogenic in rodents. It is known to cross the placenta. In the early 1960s, meclizine, widely used as an antinauseant during pregnancy, was suspected to be a possible cause of fetal anomalies such as cleft palate and cleft lip. Subsequently, at least seven well-documented prospective trials have found no evidence of teratogenic effects of meclizine in humans.

DOSAGE

For prevention of motion sickness, meclizine is given in a dose of 25–50 mg 1 hour prior to departure. It may be repeated every 24 hours as needed for the duration of the journey.

For the control of vertigo it is given 25–100 mg/day in divided doses.

ADVERSE EFFECTS

The most common side effects of meclizine include drowsiness, dry mouth, and, rarely, blurred vision.

MECHANISM OF ACTION

Meclizine is a piperazine antihistamine that depresses labyrinth excitability and vestibular-cerebellar pathway conduction. It inhibits the effects of histamine on capillary permeability and on smooth muscle by competitive inhibition at H_1 receptors. Either stimulation or depression of the central nervous system may occur through an unknown mechanism. It has anticholinergic activity, although no significant effects on the cardiovascular system occur at normal therapeutic dosages.

ABSORPTION AND BIOTRANSFORMATION

Meclizine is readily absorbed from the gastrointestinal tract and is widely distributed to body tissues. The exact nature of elimination in humans is unknown, but it appears to be extensively metabolized in the liver and excreted in the urine. Its duration of action is 12–24 hours.

RECOMMENDED READING

Babe, K.S., and Serafin, W.E. Histamine, bradykinin, and their antagonists. Chapter 25 in *Goodman and Gilman's The Pharmacological Basis of Therapeutics* (9th ed.), J.G. Hardman and L.E. Limbird, eds. New York: McGraw-Hill, 1996. P. 591.

Biggs, J.S.G. Vomiting in pregnancy: causes and management. *Drugs* 9:299, 1975.

Heinonen, O.P., Slone, D., and Shapiro, S. *Birth Defects and Drugs in Pregnancy*. Littleton, MA: PSG, 1977. Pp. 322–327.

Leathem, A.M. Safety and efficacy of antiemetics used to treat nausea and vomiting in pregnancy. *Clin. Pharm.* 5:660, 1986.

Milkovich, L., and VandenBerg, B.J. An evaluation of the teratogenicity of certain antinauseant drugs. *Am. J. Obstet. Gynecol.* 125:244, 1976.

Nishimura, H., and Tanimura, T. *Clinical Aspects of the Teratogenicity of Drugs*. Amsterdam: Excerpta Medica, 1976.

Mefloquine (Lariam®)

INDICATIONS AND RECOMMENDATIONS

Mefloquine is a quinolone-methanol antimalarial that is effective as prophylaxis against and treatment of falciparum malaria that is resistant to chloroquine and quinine. Although human teratogenesis has not been evaluated, this drug is teratogenic in laboratory animals. Therefore, it would be preferable for pregnant women in the first trimester to avoid entering areas in which resistant falciparum malaria is endemic rather than taking mefloquine for prophylaxis. However, the use of mefloquine as prophylaxis, and as treatment of resistant malaria during pregnancy, may be justified, provided the patient is counseled appropriately about potential and possibly unknown risks.

The U.S. Centers for Disease Control (CDC) has issued the following statement:

A review of mefloquine use in pregnancy from clinical trials and reports of inadvertent use of mefloquine during pregnancy, suggest its use during the second and third trimester of pregnancy is not associated with adverse fetal or pregnancy outcome. Limited data suggest it is also safe during the first trimester. Consequently, mefloquine may be considered for use by health care providers for prophylaxis in women who are pregnant or likely to become so, when exposure to chloroquine-resistant P. falciparum is unavoidable. Because information on the use of mefloquine in the first trimester is limited, women who elect to use mefloquine during the first trimester of pregnancy or their health care providers are asked to report the exposure to the Malaria Section, CDC, telephone 770–488–7760, for inclusion in a registry to assess pregnancy outcomes.

Health Canada, the Canadian equivalent of the CDC, makes a similar recommendation except that prophylaxis with mefloquine is recommended only after 16 weeks of gestation.

SPECIAL CONSIDERATIONS IN PREGNANCY

According to the manufacturer, mefloquine was teratogenic in mice and rats at a dose of 100 mg/kg/day and in rabbits at 80 mg/kg/day. These are considerably higher than the dose typically given to a pregnant woman. There have been case reports of 6 fetal anomalies in 66 human pregnancies, but no consistent pattern was present and further studies have not confirmed human teratogenesis.

A randomized, controlled study in Thailand demonstrated that mefloquine was superior to placebo in preventing multidrug-resistant malaria transmission in the second half of pregnancy. Although there appeared to be an excess of stillbirths among mefloquine-treated mothers in the first phase of the study, this could not be confirmed with larger numbers in the second phase of the study and was not statistically significant.

A treatment study in Nigeria found that a single oral dose of mefloquine, 12.5 mg/kg body weight, was 100% effective in eradicating parasitemia in 33 pregnant women with *P. falciparum* malaria. Side effects were described as mild and transient.

DOSAGE

Mefloquine is available as 250 mg tablets. The recommended prophylactic dose is 250 mg, beginning 1 week prior to entering an endemic area and continuing for 4 weeks after leaving the endemic area. The usual dose for treatment of resistant malaria is 1250 mg given as a single dose, accompanied by at least 8 oz of water, not on an empty stomach. Because of the long half-life of mefloquine, quinine should not be taken within 12h of ingestion of mefloquine. To avoid toxicity, mefloquine should not be taken concurrently with quinine, quinidine, or chloroquine.

ADVERSE EFFECTS

Central nervous system signs and symptoms are particularly frequent, being reported in about half of patients taking the drug. They include dizziness, ataxia, headache, alterations in motor function or consciousness, and visual or auditory disturbances. Other frequently reported side effects include nausea, vomiting, abdominal pain, and diarrhea. These are described as dose-related and self-limited. Severe psychiatric manifestations occur rarely and include disorientation, seizures, psychosis, and encephalopathy. These usually ameliorate when the drug is discontinued. Mefloquine should not be given to patients with a history of seizures, severe psychiatric disturbances, or adverse reactions to quinoline antimalarials in the past. Such patients have an increased likelihood of convulsions and cardiotoxicity. Mefloquine may increase the risk of seizures in patients whose epilepsy is controlled by valproic acid.

MECHANISM OF ACTION

Mefloquine is effective against mature trophozoites and schizont forms of malarial parasites found in the blood, but not against hepatic stages of *P. falciparum* or latent tissue forms of *P. vivax*. The mechanism of action is not completely understood. Some isolates of *P. falciparum* are resistant to mefloquine and require higher than usual dosages for efficacy.

ABSORPTION AND BIOTRANSFORMATION

Kinetic studies in perfused human placentas have demonstrated that mefloquine is preferentially concentrated in placental tissue, with fetal concentrations reaching only 10% of maternal concentrations. A pharmacokinetic study in 20 pregnant women in the third trimester determined that the median time to peak blood level after oral administration was 6 hours (range 3–24 hours). Peak and trough blood levels were lower than in nonpregnant individuals. The apparent elimination half-life was 11.6 ± 8 days. The drug is highly protein-bound, and clearance is primarily by the liver.

RECOMMENDED READING

Bangchang, K.N., Davis, T.M.E., Looareesuwan, N.J., et al. Mefloquine pharmacokinetics in pregnant women with acute falciparum malaria. *Transactions of the Royal Soc. Trop. Med. Hyg.* 88:321–323, 1994.

Bargazo, M.M., Omarini, D., Bortolotti, A., et al. Mefloquine transfer during in vitro human placenta perfusion. *J. Pharm. Exp. Ther.* 269:28, 1994.

Centers for Disease Control. *Health Information for International Travel 1996–1997.* Atlanta: Public Health Service, 1997. P. 136.

Cook, G.C. Editorial: Use of antiprotozoan and antihelminthic drugs during pregnancy: side-effects and contraindications. *J. Infect.* 25:1, 1992.

Health Canada. Canadian recommendations for the prevention and treatment of malaria among international travelers 1997. *Can. Commun. Dis. Rep. Suppl.* Vol 23S5, October 1997.

Nosten, F., Karbwang, J., White, N.J., et al. Mefloquine antimalarial prophylaxis in pregnancy: dose finding and pharmacokinetic study. *Br. J. Clin. Pharmacol.* 30:79, 1990.

Nosten, F., ter Kuile, F., Maelankiri, L., et al. Mefloquine prophylaxis prevents malaria during pregnancy: a double-blind, placebo-controlled study. *J. Infect. Dis.* 169:595, 1994.

Okeyeh, J.N., Lege-Oguntoye, L., Emembolu, J.O., et al. Malaria in pregnancy: efficacy of a low dose of mefloquine in an area holoendemic for multi-drug resistant Plasmodium falciparum. *Ann. Trop. Med. Parasitol.* 90:265, 1996.

Roche Laboratories. Lariam (mefloquine hydrochloride). Entry in *Physicians Desk Reference* (52nd ed.). Montvale, NJ: Medical Economics, 1998. Pp. 2478–2479.

Tracy, J.W., and Webster, L.T., Jr. Drugs used in the chemotherapy of protozoal infections. Chapter 40 in *Goodman and Gilman's The Pharmacological Basis of Therapeutics* (9th ed.), J.G. Hardman and L.E. Limbird, eds. New York: McGraw-Hill, 1996. Pp. 975–977.

Meperidine (Demerol®)

INDICATIONS AND RECOMMENDATIONS

Meperidine may be used as a short-term analgesic throughout pregnancy and may be used for the relief of pain during labor at term. A narcotic indicated for the relief of moderate to severe pain, it is commonly used in laboring patients, often in combination with a tranquilizer. A study of cord blood samples from all liveborn infants in Finland over a 1 week interval in 1991 found that 22% were exposed to meperidine prior to delivery.

It is recommended that if this drug is used in pregnant women, the lowest effective dosage should be administered. Infants born to mothers who received meperidine as antepartum analgesia should be observed for respiratory depression. This can be reversed by naloxone. The degree of neonatal respiratory depression produced by any narcotic administered during labor depends on the gestational age and condition of the infant. The magnitude of this effect is inversely proportional to gestational age and may be made greater by hypoxemia and acidemia.

A number of randomized trials have compared intravenous or intramuscular meperidine with other forms of analgesia during labor. Results have been mixed, regarding both efficacy and side effects, and appear to depend on dosage, among other variables. Regional analgesia such as epidural block clearly is more effective than parenteral meperidine but may arguably be associated with a greater likelihood of operative delivery and a prolonged second stage. Patient preference and individualization are important contributors to decision making regarding labor analgesia.

SPECIAL CONSIDERATIONS IN PREGNANCY

Teratogenicity has not been associated with the use of meperidine during human pregnancies. When given before delivery, this drug does not appear to delay labor or to decrease uterine motility. It does not increase the incidence of postpartum hemorrhage, nor does it interfere with postpartum contractions or involution of the uterus.

Placental transfer of meperidine is very rapid, with fetal blood levels reaching approximately 80% of maternal levels. There may be a dose-related decrease in fetal beat-to-beat heart rate variability when meperidine is administered to the laboring mother, as well as a decrease in fetal movements. One study found no change in fetal heart rate patterns with a moderate dose (50 mg intravenously) of meperidine. At least one study has demonstrated an increase in uterine activity with meperidine administration during active labor, but there were no concomitant controls. Administering meperidine to the mother before delivery has been associated with neonatal respiratory depression and lower psychophysiologic test scores. Both of these effects appear to be more marked when the dose is administered more than 1 hour and up to 4 hours before birth. These are relatively short-term effects, lasting days to weeks, and seem to have no long-lasting impact on the infant. These effects may be related to the presence of normeperidine, an active metabolite with a long half-life, in the fetus. One small study of infant Rhesus monkeys at 3–12 months of age demonstrated subtle behavioral changes in those whose dams received meperidine (2–3 mg/kg intravenously) during labor. Multiple dosages of both meperidine and normeperidine to the mother may create a continued diffusion gradient resulting in maximum fetal exposure. If neonatal respiratory depression does occur in a meperidine-exposed newborn, naloxone should be administered to the baby. One observational study noted that meperidine-exposed infants demonstrated delayed breast-feeding behavior in the immediate neonatal period. The investigators suggested that meperidine-exposed mother–newborn pairs be allowed sufficient time together after birth to establish nursing behavior.

As with all narcotic analgesics, infants born to meperidine-addicted mothers are addicted at birth and will experience withdrawal.

Meperidine is secreted into breast milk, but only in small amounts. It does not appear to have significant effects on the infant at dosages normally prescribed for analgesia.

DOSAGE

Meperidine may be administered orally, intravenously, or intramuscularly. Best documented in nonpregnant individuals, the plasma meperidine concentration necessary for analgesia averages 500 ng/ml, a level usually achieved with the administration of 25 mg/h. The effective meperidine level tends to be constant for a given individual, but there is wide interindividual variation. The usual analgesic dose is 50–100 mg intramuscularly every 3–4 hours, although doses as high as 150 mg have been administered to patients with a larger volume of distribution. The dose must be increased if the oral route is used. When intravenous meperidine is given, the usual dose is 25–50 mg every 2–3 hours. Subcutaneous administration causes local irritation and tissue induration.

ADVERSE EFFECTS

The most frequently observed side effects seen with meperidine use include light-headedness, nausea, vomiting, dizziness, and sedation. Other less common side effects include euphoria, dysphoria, dry mouth, flushing, syncope, and palpitations. Meperidine produces less constipation and urinary retention than other narcotic analgesics. Excitation and convulsions may occur at higher dosages. Overdosage is characterized by respiratory depression; cold, clammy skin; and extreme somnolence progressing to coma. Death may result from respiratory arrest and cardiovascular failure.

MECHANISM OF ACTION

Meperidine exerts its analgesic effect on the central nervous system. Like morphine, meperidine primarily stimulates μ receptors in the central nervous system. Analgesia is thought to occur through effects on the sensory cortex of the frontal lobes and the diencephalon. In addition, meperidine may interfere with pain conduction or may affect the patient's emotional response to pain.

Meperidine's physiologic effects are similar to those of all the narcotic analgesics. It produces prompt relief of moderate to severe pain, and the duration of its analgesia is between 2 and 4 hours. Meperidine has little or no antitussive activity in analgesic dosages.

One group of investigators has demonstrated that meperidine, in vitro, stimulates the activity of a number of enzymes, that could enhance the degradation of cervical collagen and elastin, suggesting that this drug may enhance cervical changes during labor by such a mechanism.

ABSORPTION AND BIOTRANSFORMATION

Meperidine is poorly absorbed when given orally; an oral dose is less than half as effective as an identical parenteral dose. Following oral administration, peak analgesia occurs within 1 hour, and its duration is between 2 and 4 hours. After intramuscular injection, peak analgesia occurs within 40–60 minutes and subsides after 2–4 hours. One study has demonstrated better absorption from the injection into the deltoid than the gluteus muscle during labor. Intravenous administration leads to instantaneous peak plasma levels, with higher plasma levels measured over the ensuing 2.5 hours. Meperidine is primarily metabolized in the liver by hydrolysis and *N*-demethylation. One metabolite, normeperidine, is active, although less so than meperidine. Normeperidine has a half-life of 15–20 hours. Five percent of a dose is excreted unchanged.

RECOMMENDED READING

Adams, R.J. Obstetrical medication and the newborn infant. II: The influence of meperidine (pethidine) on visual behavior. *Dev. Med. Child. Neurol.* 34:247, 1992.

Bardy, A.H., Lillsunde, P., and Hiilesmaa, V.K. Objectively measured perinatal exposure to meperidine and benzodiazepines in Finland. *Clin. Pharmacol. Ther.* 55:471, 1994.

Dan, U., Rabinovici, Y., Barkai, G., et al. Intravenous pethidine and nalbuphine during labor: a prospective double-blind comparative study. *Gynecol. Obstet. Invest.* 32:39, 1991.

Giannina, G., Guzman, E.R., Lai, Y.-L., et al. Comparison of the effects of meperidine and nalbuphine on intrapartum fetal heart rate tracings. *Obstet. Gynecol.* 86:441, 1995.

Golub, M.S., and Donald, J.M. Effect of intrapartum meperidine on behavior of 3- to 12-month-old infant Rhesus monkeys. *Biol. Neonate* 67:140, 1995.

Hodgkinson, R., and Husain, F.J. The duration of effect of maternally administered meperidine on neonatal behavior. *Anesthesiology* 56:51, 1982.

Kuhnert, B.R., et al. Meperidine and normeperidine levels following meperidine administration during labor. I. Mother. *Am. J. Obstet. Gynecol.* 133:904, 1979.

Kuhnert, B.R., et al. Meperidine and normeperidine levels following meperidine administration during labor. II. Fetus and neonate. *Am. J. Obstet. Gynecol.* 133:909, 1979.

Kuhnert, B.R., et al. Meperidine disposition in mother, neonate and non-pregnant females. *Clin. Pharmacol. Ther.* 27:486, 1980.

Kuhnert, B.R., et al. Disposition of meperidine and normeperidine following multiple doses during labor. 1. Mother. *Am. J. Obstet. Gynecol.* 151:406, 1985.

Kuhnert, B.R., et al. Disposition of meperidine and normeperidine following multiple doses during labor. II. Fetus and neonate. *Am. J. Obstet. Gynecol.* 151:410, 1985.

Lazebnik, N., Kuhnert, B.R., Carr, P.C., et al. Intravenous, deltoid, or gluteus administration of meperidine during labor? *Am. J. Obstet. Gynecol.* 160:1184, 1989.

Milwidsky, A., Finci-Yeheskel, Z., and Mayer, M. Direct stimulation of urokinase, plasmin, and collagenase by meperidine: a possible mechanism for the ability of meperidine to enhance cervical effacement and dilation. *Am. J. Perinatol.* 10:130–134. 1993.

Morrison, C.E., Dutton, D., Howie, H., et al. Pethidine compared with meptazinol during labor. *Anaesthesia* 42:7–14, 1987.

Morrison, J.C., et al. Meperidine metabolism in the parturient. *Obstet. Gynecol.* 59:359, 1982.

Nissen, E., Lilja, G., Matthiesen, A.-S., et al. Effects of pethidine on infants developing breast feeding behavior. *Acta Pediatr*.84:140, 1995.

Petrie, R.H. Dose/response effects of intravenous meperidine on fetal heart rate variability. *J. Maternal-Fetal Med.* 2:215, 1993.

Rayburn, W.F., Smith, C.V., Parriott, J.E., et al. Randomized comparison of meperidine and fentanyl during labor. *Obstet. Gynecol.* 74:604, 1989.

Reisine, T., and Pasternak, G. Opioid analgesics and antagonists. Chapter 23 in *Goodman and Gilman's The Pharmacological Basis of Therapeutics* (9th ed.), J.G. Hardman and L.E. Limbird, eds. New York: McGraw-Hill, 1996. Pp. 521–543.

Szeto, H.H., et al. Amniotic fluid transfer of meperidine from maternal plasma in early pregnancy. *Obstet. Gynecol.* 52:59, 1978.

Tomson, G., et al. Maternal kinetics and transplacental passage of pethidine during labour. *Br. J. Clin. Pharmacol.* 13:653, 1982.

Zimmer, E.T., Divon, M.Y., and Vadasz, A. Influence of meperidine on fetal movements and heart rate beat-to-beat variability in the active phase of labor. *Am. J. Perinatol.* 5:197, 1988.

Mephobarbital (Mebaral®)

INDICATIONS AND RECOMMENDATIONS

Mephobarbital is relatively contraindicated during pregnancy because other therapeutic agents are preferable. This drug is metabolized to phenobarbital. It has properties and uses similar to those of phenobarbital, but larger dosages must be given. Mephobarbital may be prescribed for routine sedation as well as therapy for various forms of epilepsy. If a long-acting barbiturate is necessary during pregnancy, however, phenobarbital is preferable to mephobarbital because it is as effective and much better studied.

RECOMMENDED READING

Hobbs, W.R., Rall, T.W., and Verdoorn, T.A. Hypnotics and sedatives; ethanol. Chapter 17 in *Goodman and Gilman's The Pharmacological Basis of Therapeutics* (9th ed.). J.G. Hardman and L.E. Limbird, eds. New York: McGraw-Hill, 1996. Pp. 375, 380.

Metaproterenol (Alupent®, Orciprenaline)

INDICATIONS AND RECOMMENDATIONS

Metaproterenol may be administered to pregnant patients in aerosol form in the treatment of infrequent, mild episodes of bronchospasm. If the patient remains symptomatic, an oral bronchodilator should be used. Oral metaproterenol may be used as an adjunctive bronchodilator in a pregnant asthmatic.

Although no reports of adverse effects have been published thus far, there have not been any large series that have studied the effect of this drug on the human fetus.

The drug must be administered with caution to patients with hyperthyroidism, hypertension, diabetes, congestive heart failure, and coronary artery disease. Furthermore, if it is administered along with another sympathomimetic drug, the potential for adverse side effects may be significantly increased.

SPECIAL CONSIDERATIONS IN PREGNANCY

Metaproterenol has been used to arrest premature labor, although it has not been approved for that use in this country. No information is available regarding the passage of metaproterenol across the placenta or into breast milk.

Rabbit studies have produced conflicting results, with no consistent proof of teratogenesis. There is one report of increased incidence of cleft palate in the offspring of metaproterenol-treated mice, presumably due to increased corticosterone, but this pathway would not be expected in humans. No increases in perinatal mortality or congenital malformations were seen in offspring of 259 women with asthma who used inhaled bronchodilators (primarily metaproterenol) during pregnancy. There are no controlled studies available to establish metaproterenol's safety during pregnancy.

DOSAGE

For oral administration, the dose is 20 mg q6–8h. The onset of action is about 30 minutes. Peak effect occurs in 2 hours, and the duration of action is 4–6 hours.

For aerosol administration, the dose is 1–3 puffs (0.65 mg/puff) q3–4h. The onset of action is about 2–10 minutes. Peak effect occurs within 30–90 minutes, and the duration of action is 1–5 hours.

ADVERSE EFFECTS

In addition to causing bronchodilatation, metaproterenol increases heart rate, stroke volume, and pulse pressure. It also may cause hyperglycemia and an increase in free fatty acids and glycerol. Metaproterenol may also reduce gastrointestinal tone and motility and cause mild general central nervous system stimulation.

Side effects include tachycardia, hypertension, palpitation, nervousness, tremor, nausea, and vomiting. The incidence of side effects is greater when the drug is given orally as opposed to by the aerosol route.

MECHANISM OF ACTION

Metaproterenol is a β-sympathomimetic agonist with predominantly β_2 activity. It seems to work by stimulating adenyl cyclase, the enzyme that catalyzes the conversion of adenosine triphosphate (ATP) to cyclic AMP. Cyclic AMP acts locally as a bronchodilator.

ABSORPTION AND BIOTRANSFORMATION

An average of 40% of an oral dose of metaproterenol is absorbed. This is primarily excreted in the urine as glucuronic acid conjugates. Metaproterenol's prolonged duration of action when compared to catecholamine β-sympathomimetic agonists is due to the fact that it is not metabolized by catechol-*O*-methyltransferase.

RECOMMENDED READING

Drewitt, A.H. First clinical experience with Alupent: a new bronchodilator. *Br. J. Clin. Pract.* 16:549, 1962.

Freedman, B.J., and Hill, G.B. Comparative study of duration of action and cardiovascular effect of bronchodilator aerosols. *Thorax* 26:46, 1970.

Holmes, T.H. A comparative clinical trial of metaproterenol and isoproterenol as bronchodilator aerosols. *Clin. Pharmacol. Ther.* 9: 615, 1968.

Hurst, A. Metaproterenol: a potent and safe bronchodilator. *Ann. Allergy* 31:460, 1973.

Iida, H., et al. Corticosterone induction of cleft palate in mice dosed with ociprenaline sulfate. *Teratology* 38:15, 1988.

Rebuck, A.S., and Real, J. Oral Orciprenaline in the treatment of chronic asthma. *Med. J. Aust.* 1:445, 1965.

Schatz, M., et al. The safety of inhaled beta-agonist bronchodilators during pregnancy. *J. Allergy Clin. Immunol.* 82:686–695, 1988.

Zilianti, A. Action of Orciprenaline on uterine contractility during labor, maternal cardiovascular system, fetal heart rate and acid–base balance. *Am. J. Obstet. Gynecol.* 109:1073, 1971.

Metaraminol (Aramine®)

INDICATIONS AND RECOMMENDATIONS

Metaraminol, an α-adrenergic agent used to increase systemic blood pressure, is relatively contraindicated during pregnancy because other therapeutic agents are preferable. Uterine vessels have only α-adrenergic receptors and react to adrenergic stimulus solely by contracting. Such decrease in uterine blood flow may adversely affect the fetus. Should a pressor be needed to treat hypotension associated with conduction anesthesia in a pregnant woman, ephedrine is the agent of choice.

RECOMMENDED READING

Avery, G.S. *Drug Treatment: Principles and Practice of Clinical Pharmacology and Therapeutics.* Sydney, Aust.: Adis, 1976.

Hoffman, B.B., and Lefkowitz, R.J. Catecholamines. sympathomimetic drugs, and adrenergic receptor antagonists. Chapter 10 in *Goodman and Gilman's The Pharmacological Basis of Therapeutics* (9th ed.), J.G. Hardman and L.E. Limbird, eds. New York: McGraw-Hill, 1996. P. 217.

Smith, N.T., and Corbascio, A. The use and misuse of pressor agents. *Anesthesiology* 33:58, 1970.

Methadone

INDICATIONS AND RECOMMENDATIONS

Methadone may be used during pregnancy. It is a long-acting narcotic analgesic that is effective when given orally. Its principal use in women of childbearing age is in the treatment of heroin addiction. Heroin itself might be a more appropriate maintenance drug because the withdrawal symptoms are not as prolonged, but it is not available for therapeutic use in the United States. Patients who are maintained on methadone for treatment of heroin addiction should not be detoxified during pregnancy.

SPECIAL CONSIDERATIONS IN PREGNANCY

Teratogenicity has not been associated with the use of methadone during pregnancy. The primary problems associated with the administration of methadone for treatment of pregnant heroin addicts are low birth weight and neonatal withdrawal. Methadone-specific effects are difficult to evaluate, however, because patients in maintenance programs often consume a wide variety of drugs.

The neonatal withdrawal syndrome is seen in the majority of infants born to methadone-maintained mothers. It usually begins within 48 hours of delivery, but its onset can be delayed for up to 2 weeks. The phenomenon of late onset of symptoms has led to the widespread but mistaken belief that there is minimal effect of methadone on the newborn. The intensity of the symptoms increases in proportion to the maternal dosage, infant blood level of methadone at delivery, and the rapidity of the fall in infant blood levels after delivery, and may last for up to 6 months. In addition, infants born to addicted mothers are frequently premature and suffer from intrauterine growth restriction. The long-term effects on the infant are unknown.

Complete maternal narcotic withdrawal during pregnancy is not recommended. It may cause a marked response of the fetal adrenal gland and sympathetic nervous system. It is also associated with increased stillborn rates and neonatal mortality.

Methadone enters the breast milk in concentrations approaching maternal plasma levels and may prevent or ameliorate withdrawal symptoms in addicted infants.

DOSAGE

The usual oral analgesic dose is 2.5–15 mg q6–8h. The usual parenteral analgesic dose is 2.5–10 mg. Doses for the treatment of heroin addiction are titrated according to individual patient need and usually range from 10 to 80 or more mg/day. One study demonstrated an apparent lessening in sedation of the fetus when the daily dose was divided in half and given every 12 hours. Another study showed improved compliance with narcotic avoidance when split-dose methadone was utilized. However, the use of split-dose methadone can lead to administrative problems in either (1) giving clients the second dose to take home or (2) keeping the methadone facility open for longer hours in order to administer the second dose "in person." There is controversy as to whether the lowest possible dose of methadone should be utilized late in pregnancy in order to lessen neonatal withdrawal or whether a higher dose of methadone may help to ensure fetal well- being by preventing intermittent fetal withdrawal. In one case series, higher doses of methadone were associated with increased fetal weight and greater gestational age at delivery. In most case series of pregnant women methadone dosage has been maintained at or above 40 mg/day.

ADVERSE EFFECTS

The side effects of methadone are similar to those of other narcotic analgesics and include euphoria, light-headedness, dizziness, sedation, dry mouth, constipation, and urinary retention. Overdosage is characterized by respiratory depression. With chronic administration, additional side effects including excessive sweating, lymphocytosis, and increased concentrations of prolactin, albumin, and globulins in plasma can occur.

MECHANISM OF ACTION

As with morphine and meperidine, methadone appears to stimulate primarily μ receptors. It acts on the central nervous system to alter the response of several systems of neurotransmitters. Methadone is a potent antitussive in analgesic dosages. Because of its extended half- life and duration of action, methadone is useful as a substitute for morphine and other narcotics in addicted individuals, its withdrawal syndrome being milder but lasting longer.

ABSORPTION AND BIOTRANSFORMATION

Methadone is well absorbed from the gastrointestinal tract, reaching peak concentrations approximately 4 hours after an oral dose. Onset of analgesia occurs 30–60 minutes after oral administration. Approximately 90% of circulating methadone is bound to plasma proteins. With repeated administration, it gradually accumulates in tissues and is slowly released into the bloodstream after the drug is discontinued. It is extensively metabolized in the liver, and the metabolites as well as small amounts of unchanged drug are excreted in the urine and bile. In nontolerant patients, the half-life is 15 hours, but this increases to 22 hours in tolerant patients.

RECOMMENDED READING

Cejtin, H.E., Mills, A., and Swift, E.L. Effect of methadone on the biophysical profile. *J. Reprod. Med.* 41:819, 1996.

Chasnoff, I.J., Hatcher, R., and Burns, W.J. Early growth patterns of methadone-addicted infants. *Am. J. Dis. Child.* 134:1049, 1980.

DePetrillo, P.B., and Rice, J.-M. Methadone dosing and pregnancy: impact on program compliance. *Int. J. Addict.* 30:207–217, 1995.

Doberczak, T.M., Kandall, S.R., and Friedmann, P. Relationships between maternal methadone dosage, maternal-neonatal methadone levels, and neonatal withdrawal. *Obstet. Gynecol.* 81:936, 1993.

Finnegan, L.P. The effects of narcotics and alcohol on pregnancy and the newborn. *Ann. N. Y. Acad. Sci.* 362:136, 1981.

Hagopian, G.S., Wolfe, H.M., Sokol, R.J., et al. Neonatal outcome following methadone exposure in utero. *J. Maternal-Fetal Med.* 5:348, 1996.

Levine, A.B., and Rebarber, A. Methadone maintenance treatment and the nonstress test. *J. Perinatol.* 15:229, 1995.

Malpas, T.J., Darlow, B.A., Lennox, R., et al. Maternal methadone dosage and neonatal withdrawal. *Aust. N. Z. J. Obstet. Gynaecol.* 35:175, 1995.

Reisine, T., and Pasternak, G. Opioid analgesics and antagonists. Chapter 23 in *Goodman and Gilman's The Pharmacological Basis of Therapeutics* (9th ed.), J.G. Hardman and L.E. Limbird, eds. New York: McGraw-Hill, 1996. Pp. 544–545.

Rementeria, J.L., and Nunag, N.N. Narcotic withdrawal in pregnancy: stillbirth incidence with a case report. *Am. J. Obstet. Gynecol.* 116:1152, 1973.

Rosen, T.S., and Johnson, H.L. Children of methadone-maintained mothers: follow-up to 18 months of age. *J. Pediatrics* 101:192, 1982.

Strauss, M.E., Andresko, M., and Stryker, J.C. Methadone maintenance during pregnancy: pregnancy, birth and neonate characteristics. *Am. J. Obstet. Gynecol.* 121:233, 1975.

Wilson, G.S., Desmond, M.M., and Wait, R.B. Follow-up of methadone-treated and untreated narcotic-dependent women and their infants: health, developmental and societal implications. *J. Pediatrics* 98:716, 1981.

Wittman, B.K., Segal, S.: A comparison of the effects of single- and split-dose methadone administration on the fetus: ultrasound evaluation. *Int. J. Addict. 26:213–218, 1991.*

Methenamine Hippurate (Hiprex®, Urex®) and Methenamine Mandelate (Mandelamine®)

INDICATIONS AND RECOMMENDATIONS

Methenamine hippurate and methenamine mandelate are relatively contraindicated during pregnancy because other therapeutic agents are preferable. They are used for chronic suppressive treatment of urinary tract infections and are not treatments of choice for an acute urinary tract infection.

Methenamine hippurate crosses the placenta; levels measured in umbilical cord plasma approximate those of maternal plasma. Levels in amniotic fluid vary, probably depending on the frequency of fetal micturition.

Prior to the availability of nitrofurantoin, methenamine was used to treat asymptomatic bacteriuria of pregnancy. In a study comparing 51 women who received methenamine mandelate and 53 women who received nitrofurantoin macrocrystals to treat asymptomatic bacteriuria of pregnancy, there was no difference in fetal outcome in either group when compared to untreated controls. Methenamine was, however, significantly less effective at sterilizing the urine than was nitrofurantoin.

Another study of methenamine mandelate and methenamine hippurate to treat asymptomatic bacteriuria of pregnancy found that there was no statistically significant effect on reducing the incidence of pyelonephritis. While the incidence of fetal abnormality and morbidity was no higher in the treated population than the control population, the authors could not recommend treatment with either drug for this indication.

Methenamine passes into breast milk with levels about equivalent to maternal serum levels. One author estimates that an infant would receive about 0.15 to 0.4 mg methenamine per feeding. No adverse effects to the nursing infant have been reported.

RECOMMENDED READING

Allgen, L.G., et al. Biological fate of methenamine in man. Absorption, renal excretion and passage to umbilical cord blood, amniotic fluid and breast milk. *Acta Obstet. Gynecol. Scand.* 58:287, 1979.

Furness, E.T., McDonald, P.J., and Beasley, N.V. Urinary antiseptics in asymptomatic bacteriuria of pregnancy. *N. Z. Med. J.* 81:417, 1975.

Gordon, S.F. Asymptomatic bacteriuria of pregnancy. *Clin. Med.* 79: 22, 1972.

Mandell, G.L., and Petri, Jr., W.A. Antimicrobial agents: sulfonamides, trimethoprim-sulfamethoxazole, quinolones, and agents for urinary tract infections. Chapter 44 in *Goodman and Gilman's The Pharmacological Basis of Therapeutics* (9th ed.), Hardman, J.G., and Limbird, L.E., eds. New York: McGraw-Hill, 1996. P. 1069.

Methsuximide (Celontin®)

INDICATIONS AND RECOMMENDATIONS

Methsuximide is contraindicated for use during pregnancy because other therapeutic agents are preferable. It is one of the succinimide group of anticonvulsants used in the treatment of absence, or petit mal, seizures. Experience with this drug in pregnancy is limited. First-trimester exposure to methsuximide has been reported in five pregnancies, with no adverse fetal outcomes reported. Nevertheless, because this drug is known to be less effective than ethosuximide, the latter is the anticonvulsant of choice when absence seizures must be treated in obstetric patients. Because of the limited use, data regarding breast-feeding are not currently available.

RECOMMENDED READING

Annegers, J.F., Elveback, L.R., Hauser, W.A., and Kurland, L.T. Do anticonvulsants have a teratogenic effect? *Arch. Neurol.* 31:364, 1974.

Fabro, S., and Brown, N.A. Teratogenic potential of anticonvulsants. *N. Engl. J. Med.* 300:1280, 1979.

Fedrick, J. Epilepsy and pregnancy: a report from the Oxford record linkage study. *Br. Med. J.* 2:442, 1973.

Heinonen, O.P., Slone, D., and Shapiro, S. *Birth Defects and Drugs in Pregnancy.* Littleton, MA: PSG, 1977. Pp. 358–359.

McMullin, G.P. Teratogenic effects of anticonvulsants. *Br. Med. J.* 2:430, 1971.

McNamara, J.O. Drugs effective in the therapy of the epilepsies. Chapter 20 in *Goodman and Gilman's The Pharmacological Basis of Therapeutics* (9th ed.), J.G. Hardman and L.E. Limbird, eds. New York: McGraw-Hill, 1996. P. 475.

National Institutes of Health. Anticonvulsants found to have teratogenic potential. *J.A.M.A.* 241:36, 1981.

Methyldopa (Aldomet®)

INDICATIONS AND RECOMMENDATIONS

Methyldopa is currently the drug of choice for pregnant women with moderate to severe chronic hypertension because of the extensive and long-term safety data describing lack of significant fetal and developmental effects. As a single agent, methyldopa is limited by its modest efficacy in treatment of hypertension, and its action may be potentiated by adding hydralazine or a beta blocker to the regimen. While a concomitant diuretic agent is frequently recommended for use in the nonpregnant patient, other second agents are preferable during pregnancy, as chronic diuretic use may impair maternal plasma volume expansion. Methyldopa should not be used as primary therapy in a hypertensive crisis due to its slow onset of action.

SPECIAL CONSIDERATIONS IN PREGNANCY

A study of 24 full-term neonates born to mothers treated with methyldopa compared with 50 full-term control neonates matched for birth weight and gestational age revealed mean systolic pressure in the treated infants to be 4.5 mm Hg lower on the first day and 4.3 mm Hg lower on the second. No differences were apparent thereafter. Furthermore, there were no episodes of bradycardia in the neonates of treated mothers. An investigation of 200 infants born to methyldopa-treated mothers revealed a reduction in neonatal head circumference when compared to matched controls. This difference, however, was confined to neonates whose mothers were initially treated between 16 and 20 weeks gestation. By age 4, no significant differences were seen in height, weight, general health, or frequency of visual and hearing problems between the two groups, but male children of the treated women had smaller heads. Mean intelligence quotients and growth did not differ in follow-up study at 7.5 years.

As methyldopa alters catecholamine balance in the central nervous system, there has been concern regarding potential effects on the developing fetal brain in the first trimester. One study compared norepinephrine levels in the cerebrospinal fluid of neonates exposed to methyldopa in utero and found that they were decreased in comparison to unexposed neonates, confirming an alteration in CNS catecholamines. In animal studies, impairment of neurotransmitters during early brain development leads to sleep and behavioral disturbances. There is a case report documenting sleep disturbance in a child exposed to methyldopa in utero; however, the child was exposed to multiple drugs.

Although methyldopa crosses the placental barrier, it is not known as to whether the Coombs test can be made positive in neonates of mothers who take this drug during pregnancy. This neonatal complication seems unlikely because of the duration of therapy necessary before its occurrence in adults. In a series of 117 women given methyldopa during their pregnancies, one mother and none of the neonates developed a positive Coombs test. The same series showed no effect on birth weight and maturity when offspring of patients given the drug were compared to offspring of untreated controls. The authors of this study believed that methyldopa had been demonstrated to be a safe drug for both mother and fetus.

Doppler studies of the uteroplacental or fetal circulation show no decrease in flow despite decreased systemic maternal blood pressure.

Methyldopa has been found in breast milk in small quantities, and blood levels were demonstrated in one of three infants tested. There is no contraindication to breast-feeding while taking methyldopa.

DOSAGE

When given orally, the dose is 250–1000 mg q12–24h. The onset of action is 2–4 hours, and the maximum effect is seen in 6–8hours. The duration of action is 24 hours. At fixed dosage levels, 2–3 days of therapy is required before the full effect of the drug is achieved; therefore, dosage increases should be made at intervals of no less than 48 hours. After discontinuation of the drug, there is a return to pretreatment blood pressure levels in 48 hours.

When given intravenously, the dose is 500–1000 mg q6–12h. The onset of action is 1–2 hours. Because of its relatively slow onset of action, this is not the drug of choice for a hypertensive emergency. Given intravenously, this drug may cause enough drowsiness to interfere with the patient's sensorium.

ADVERSE EFFECTS

Cardiac output is reduced by this drug but rarely to a significant degree. Renal and uterine blood flows are maintained in the presence of its hypotensive action, and in fact, there may be selective renal vasodilatation.

Side effects include sedation and drowsiness, depression, mild postural hypotension, sodium retention, dry mouth, and nasal stuffiness. A positive Coombs test will develop in 20% of patients who take this drug for more than 6 months, and this effect is dose- related. The positive Coombs test is rarely clinically significant as it is only occasionally associated with hemolytic anemia. Allergic reactions manifested as drug fever may also be seen. It may cause liver enzyme changes in up to 5%; therefore, its use is contraindicated in patients with active liver disease. The hepatitis is usually reversible with discontinuation of drug and will recur with repeat use. A case of reversible, severe hepatitis in pregnancy has been reported. A few cases of fulminant, fatal hepatitis have been reported in nonpregnant patients.

MECHANISM OF ACTION

Methyldopa is metabolized to α-methylnorepinephrine, which functions as a "false neurohumoral transmitter" by replacing active norepinephrine at α-adrenergic nerve endings, thereby preventing norepinephrine release. In the central nervous system, methylnorepinephrine release inhibits adrenergic neuronal output from the brainstem. In the peripheral nervous system, release of the metabolite causes vasoconstriction; therefore, it is believed that the antihypertensive action is centrally-mediated. It also suppresses the release of renal renin, but this is not a primary effect and contributes little to antihypertensive action.

ABSORPTION AND BIOTRANSFORMATION

When methyldopa is administered orally, only 50% or less is absorbed. Methyldopa and its metabolites are weakly bound to plasma proteins. It is metabolized in the gastrointestinal tract and liver and is excreted in the urine largely by glomerular filtration. Unabsorbed drug is eliminated in the feces unchanged. The usual half- life is about 2 hours. It can be used in patients with impaired renal function but in smaller-than-usual dosages and given at longer than usual intervals.

In a study of nine neonates born to hypertensive mothers who received methyldopa for several weeks before delivery, blood levels present in the infants at birth were comparable to those in the mother, and these levels persisted for several days. Elimination of the drug in the neonate is primarily controlled by the rate of the renal excretion of its conjugated product. Methyldopa is eliminated slowly from the neonate and its half-life seems to be 3–4 times that reported for adults.

RECOMMENDED READINGS

Cockburn, J., et al. Final report of study on hypertension during pregnancy: the effects of specific treatment on the growth and development of the children. *Lancet* 1:647, 1982.

Cummings, A.J., and Whitelaw, A.G. A study of conjugation and drug elimination in the human neonate. *Br. J. Clin. Pharmacol.* 12:511, 1981.

Frohlich, E.D. The sympathetic depressant antihypertensives. *Drug Ther.* 5:24, 1975.

Jones, H.M., and Cummings, A.J. A study of the transfer of alpha-methyldopa to the human foetus and newborn infant. *Br. J. Clin. Pharmacol.* 6:432, 1978.

Moar, V.A., et al. Neonatal head circumference and the treatment of maternal hypertension. *Br. J. Obstet. Gynaecol.* 85:933, 1978.

Montan, S., Anandakumar, C., Arulkumaran, S., Ingemarsson, I., and Ratnam, S.S. Effects of methyldopa on uteroplacental and fetal hemodynamics in pregnancy-induced hypertension. *Am. J. Obstet. Gynecol.* 168:152, 1993.

Oates, J.A. Antihypertensive agents and the drug therapy of hypertension. Chapter 33 in *Goodman and Gilman's The Pharmacological Basis of Therapeutics* (9th ed.), J.G. Hardman and L.E. Limbird, eds. New York: McGraw-Hill, 1996. Pp. 786–788.

Redman, C.W.G., et al. Fetal outcome in trial of antihypertensive treatment in pregnancy. *Lancet* 2:753, 756, 1976.

Shimohira, M., Kohyama, J., Kawano, Y., Suzuki, H., Ogiso, M., and Iwakawa, Y. Effect of alpha-methyldopa administration during pregnancy on the development of a child's sleep. *Brain Dev.* 8:416, 1986.

Smith, G.N., and Piercy, W.N. Methyldopa hepatotoxicity in pregnancy: a case report. *Am. J. Obstet. Gynecol.* 172:222, 1995.

Sulyok, E., Bodis, J., Hartman, G., and Ertl, T. Neonatal effects of methyldopa therapy in pregnancy hypertension. *Acta Paediatrica Hung.* 31:53, 1991.

White W.B., Andreoli, J.W., and Cohn R.D. Alpha-methyldopa disposition in mothers with hypertension and in their breast-fed infants. *Clin. Pharm. Ther.* 37:387, 1985.

Whitelaw, A. Maternal methyldopa treatment and neonatal blood pressure. *Br. Med. J. Clin. Res.* 283:471, 1981.

Methylene Blue

INDICATIONS AND RECOMMENDATIONS

Methylene blue is contraindicated in pregnancy, as safer agents are available. This dye, whose chemical name is tetramethylthionine chloride, has been utilized for intraamniotic injection to aid in the diagnosis of ruptured membranes. Evans blue dye was originally proposed for diagnosing ruptured membranes and as a marker when amniocentesis is performed on patients with multiple gestation; it is apparently harmless, but methylene blue was frequently substituted, presumably because of its wide availability on gynecologic services. Indigo carmine is now widely used for this purpose.

Methylene blue and its colorless reduced derivative, leukomethylene blue, form a reversible oxidation–reduction system. In low concentrations, methylene blue hastens the reduction of methemoglobin to hemoglobin, acting as an electron acceptor from reduced pyridine necleotides, than passing the electron along to methemoglobin. It is used in the treatment of both idiopathic and drug-induced methemoglobinemia. However, in higher concentrations it acts as an oxidant, producing methemoglobin by oxidizing the iron of reduced hemoglobin from the ferrous to the ferric form.

In addition, methylene blue may produce Heinz body hemolytic anemia in the fetus and newborn. The mechanism of this effect appears to be the production of leukomethylene blue, which reduces oxygen to hydrogen peroxide. When normal detoxification mechanisms are overwhelmed, the excess hydrogen peroxide oxidizes hemoglobin to produce sulfhemoglobin and, consequently, Heinz bodies. The lipid membrane of the red cell is damaged and hemolysis results.

There have been numerous case reports of hemolytic anemia and hyperbilirubinemia in neonates whose mothers had methylene blue instilled in the amniotic fluid. When looked for, Heinz bodies have been present and methemoglobin levels have been high. In one case, severe fetal tachycardia occurred immediately after the intraamniotic injection of 2 ml of 1%

methylene blue, and it was believed that a fetal intravascular injection caused immediate methemoglobinemia with resultant tissue hypoxia.

Since 1990 there have been a number of case reports and case series suggesting a relationship between intraamniotic injection of methylene blue during the middle trimester in twin gestations and small bowel atresia. The EUROCAT Working Group registry evaluated outcomes in over 1.3 million pregnancies at 11 centers and found a slightly increased likelihood of gastrointestinal atresias among twin pregnancies, as did the Centers for Disease Control in another registry-based study. While 5% of 19 gastrointestinal atresias involved twins, none had been exposed to methylene blue. A retrospective cohort study of 303 Australian twin pregnancies in which amniocentesis was performed over an 11 year interval found that fetal death was significantly more likely (32%) in cases exposed to high concentrations of methylene blue (1% solution in normal saline) as compared to those exposed to no methylene blue (4%) or a low concentration (0.125% to 0.25% in normal saline) of methylene blue (15%).

Methylene blue has been inadvertently injected into the uterus during the first trimester without apparent untoward effect. However, because of the previously mentioned problems, it is recommended that this dye not be utilized for amniotic injection for the diagnosis of ruptured membranes or in diagnostic amniocentesis for the identification of amniotic sacs in multiple gestations.

RECOMMENDED READING

Atlay, R.D., and Sutherst, J.R. Premature rupture of the fetal membranes confirmed by intraamniotic injection of dye (Evans blue T-1824). *Am. J. Obstet. Gynecol.* 108:993, 1970.

Cowett, R.M., et al. Untoward neonatal effect of intraamniotic administration of methylene blue. *Obstet. Gynecol.* 48:74s, 1976.

Cragan, J.D., Martin, M.L., Waters, G.D., et al. Increased risk of small intestinal atresia among twins in the United States. *Arch. Pediatr. Adol. Med.* 148:733, 1994.

Crooks, J. Haemolytic jaundice in a neonate after intra-amniotic injection of methylene blue. *Arch. Dis. Child.* 57:872, 1982.

Dolk, H. Methylene blue and atresia or stenosis of ileum and jejunum. *Lancet* 338:1021, 1991.

Katz, Z., and Lancet, M. Inadvertent intrauterine injection of methylene blue in early pregnancy. *N. Engl. J. Med.* 304:1427, 1981.

Kidd, S.A., Lancaster, P.A.L., Anderson, J.C., et al. Fetal death after exposure to methylene blue dye during mid-trimester amniocentesis in twin pregnancy. *Prenatal Diag.* 16:39, 1996.

Kirsch, I.R., and Cohen, H.J. Heinz body hemolytic anemia from the use of methylene blue in neonates. *J. Pediatrics* 96:276, 1980.

McEnerney, J.K., and McEnerney, L.N. Unfavorable neonatal outcome after intraamniotic injection of methylene blue. *Obstet. Gynecol.* 61:35, 1983.

McFadyen, I. The dangers of intra-amniotic methylene blue. *Br. J. Obstet. Gynaecol.* 99:89, 1992.

Nicolini, U., and Monni, G. Intestinal obstruction in babies exposed in utero to methylene blue. *Lancet* 336:1258, 1990.

Plunkett, G.D. Neonatal complications. *Obstet. Gynecol.* 41:476, 1973.

Spahr, R.C., Salsburey, D.J., Krissberg, A., and Prin, W. Intraamniotic injection of methylene blue leading to methemoglobinemia in one of twins. *Int. J. Gynaecol. Obstet.* 17:477, 1980.

Methylphenidate Hydrochloride (Ritalin®, Ritalin SR®)

INDICATIONS AND RECOMMENDATIONS

Methylphenidate hydrochloride may be administered to pregnant women with severe narcolepsy when treatment is considered essential. Although this drug is also used for minimal brain dysfunction in children, as a mild sedative, and as treatment for apathetic or withdrawn senile behavior. Narcolepsy, a rare phenomenon, seems to be the only likely indication for its use in pregnant women.

SPECIAL CONSIDERATIONS IN PREGNANCY

The Collaborative Perinatal Project monitored 11 mother–child pairs exposed to methylphenidate and found no evidence that it causes fetal malformation.

DOSAGE

The usual adult dose is 10 mg PO 2 or 3 times a day. Because of the possibility of degradation in the acid medium of the postprandial gastric fluid, the drug is taken 30–45 minutes before meals. In the treatment of narcolepsy methylphenidate is usually administered before important activities.

ADVERSE EFFECTS

Side effects include tachycardia, hypertension, palpitations, anorexia, insomnia, dizziness, headache, dry mouth, and anxiety. It has abuse potential similar to the amphetamines.

MECHANISM OF ACTION

Methylphenidate is a sympathomimetic central nervous system stimulant. Effects on mental function are somewhat greater than on motor activity. Patients suffering from narcolepsy experience a reduced number of sleep attacks when methylphenidate is combined with changes in daily habits.

ABSORPTION AND BIOTRANSFORMATION

Methylphenidate is rapidly and well absorbed from the gastrointestinal tract and has a half-life between 1 and 3 hours. Its pharmacologic effects last for 4–6 hours. The sustained release product is more slowly, but as extensively absorbed from the gastrointestinal tract. Its pharmacologic effects last for 8 hours. Methylphenidate is deesterified in plasma with less than 1% excreted in the urine unchanged.

RECOMMENDED READING

Debooy, V.D., et al. Intravenous pentazocine and methylphenidate abuse during pregnancy. Maternal lifestyle and infant outcome. *Am. J. Dis. Child.* 147:1062, 1993.

Heinonen, O.P., Slone, D., et al. *Birth Defects and Drugs in Pregnancy.* Littleton, MA: PSG, 1977. Pp. 346–347.

Hoffman, B.B., and Lefkowitz, R.J. Catecholamines, sympathomimetic drugs, and adrenergic receptor antagonists. Chapter 11 in *Goodman and Gilman's The Pharmacological Basis of Therapeutics* (9th ed.), J.G. Hardman, and L.E. Limbird, eds. New York: McGraw-Hill, 1996. Pp. 221, 224.

Methysergide Maleate (Sansert®)

INDICATIONS AND RECOMMENDATIONS

Methysergide maleate is contraindicated during pregnancy. It is a semisynthetic derivative of the ergot alkaloids that has complex effects on serotonergic and other neurotransmitter systems. Its in vitro effects on contraction of the umbilical artery, placental chorionic arteries and veins, and the myometrium are currently being studied. Methysergide also possesses weak oxytocic activity, and a theoretical risk of abortion or premature labor exists. The effects of the drug on the fetus are unknown.

This drug is effective in the prophylaxis of all types of migraine headaches. It is of no value in the treatment of acute attacks or prevention or management of tension headaches. Methysergide has also been of some value in combating intestinal hypermotility in patients with carcinoid and in the postgastrectomy dumping syndrome. Uninterrupted, long-term therapy with methysergide is contraindicated since it may induce fibrotic conditions, including retroperitoneal fibrosis, pleuropulmonary fibrosis, and endocardial fibrosis. Cardiovascular complications include cardiac murmurs; cold, numb, and painful extremities with or without paresthesias; and diminished or absent pulses.

RECOMMENDED READING

Cruz, M.A., et al. Effects of histamine and serotonin on the contractility of isolated pregnant and non-pregnant human myometrium. *Gynecol. Obstet. Invest.* 28:1, 1989.

Graves, C.R. Agents that cause contraction or relaxation of the uterus. Chapter 39 in *Goodman and Gilman's The Pharmacological Basis of Therapeutics* (9th ed.), J.G. Hardman and L.E. Limbird, eds. New York: McGraw-Hill, 1996. P. 943.

MacLennan, S.J., Whittle, M.J., and McGrath, J.C. 5-HT1-like receptors requiring functional cyclo-oxygenase and 5-HT2 receptors independent of cyclo-oxygenase mediate contraction of the human umbilical artery. *Br. J. Pharmacol.* 97:921, 1989.

Peroutka, S.J. Drugs effective in the therapy of migraine. Chapter 21 in *Goodman and Gilman's The Pharmacological Basis of Therapeutics* (9th ed.), J.G. Hardman and L.E. Limbird, eds. New York: McGraw-Hill, 1996. P. 499.

Revirego, J., and Marin, J. Effects of 5-hydroxytryptamn on human isolated placental chorionic arteries and veins. *Br. J. Pharmacol.* 96:961, 1989.

Sanders-Bush, E., and Mayer, S.E. 5-hydroxytryptamine (serotonin) receptor agonists and antagonists. Chapter 11 in *Goodman and Gilman's The Pharmacological Basis of Therapeutics* (9th ed.), J.G. Hardman and L.E. Limbird, eds. New York: McGraw-Hill, 1996. P. 260.

Silberstein, S.D. Headaches and women: treatment of the pregnant and lactating migraneur. *Headache* 33:533, 1993.

Uknis, A., and Silberstein, S.D. Review article: migraine and pregnancy. *Headache* 31:372, 1991.

Metoclopramide (Reglan®)

INDICATIONS AND RECOMMENDATIONS

Metoclopramide, a blocker of dopaminergic receptors, appears to be safe to use in pregnancy. Approved indications include symptomatic gastroesophageal reflux, diabetic gastric stasis, the prevention of nausea and vomiting associated with cancer chemotherapy, and the facilitation of small bowel intubation and radiologic examination. Metoclopramide has been used as an antiemetic, as a preanesthetic medication to reduce gastric volume, and as a lactation-enhancing agent, although it has not been specifically approved for these indications.

SPECIAL CONSIDERATIONS IN PREGNANCY

Animal studies have not documented teratogenicity for this drug, and there have not been any reports suggesting human teratogenicity. Metoclopramide crosses the placenta in humans at term, with fetal plasma concentrations approximately half of maternal levels. Neonates exposed to this drug during labor did not exhibit differences in Apgar scores or cardiovascular or neurobehavioral effects when compared with placebo-treated control subjects. Studies in the first and third trimesters have demonstrated a rapid and significant increase in maternal serum prolactin, but not in growth hormone levels, after intravenous administration of metoclopramide. During the first trimester, the administration of this drug did not change maternal levels of progesterone, estradiol, human chorionic gonadotropin (HCG), or human placental lactogen (HPL). Fetal prolactin levels were not increased when laboring mothers were given the drug. Physiologic studies in all three trimesters have demonstrated a significant reduction in maternal gastric volume when metoclopramide was administered.

Metoclopramide administered prophylactically prior to epidural or spinal anesthesia for cesarean section reduces perioperative nausea and vomiting without causing side effects in the neonate.

Metoclopramide has been advocated for improvement of "defective lactation" in nursing mothers and has been shown to increase milk volume. However, one study has demonstrated milk/plasma ratios greater than 1 in 5 of 7 mothers tested during the first 2 weeks post partum, with detectable levels of the drug in the plasma of two infants. The estimated infants' doses derived from mothers' milk were as high as 24 μg/kg/day in some instances. The recommended therapeutic dose in children is 500 μg/kg/day. Of greatest concern was the finding that four in seven newborns had serum prolactin levels above the highest seen in untreated control infants. More information is needed before the safety of metoclopramide in lactating mothers can be determined.

DOSAGE

Metoclopramide is available as a tablet containing 10 mg, a syrup containing 5 mg/5 ml, and an intravenous solution containing 5 mg/ml. The oral dose is 5–15 mg, up to 4 times daily, 15–30 minutes before meals. This may be continued up to 12 weeks. An intravenous dose of 10–20 mg given over 2 minutes is administered when prevention of nausea and vomiting during chemotherapy is desired. The dose usually employed for improving milk production is 10 mg PO, 2–3 times daily. In studies of gastric volume reduction, the usual dose is 10 mg IV.

ADVERSE EFFECTS

The principal side effect has been sedation. However, dystonic-dyskinetic head and neck movements have been reported in two pregnant patients who took metoclopramide as an antiemetic. These extrapyramidal effects seem to be most common in young females, and the reactions resemble oculogyric crisis. These have been reported to occur in approximately 0.2% of patients taking doses greater than 30–40 mg/day. Diazepam or diphenhydramine (25–50 mg intravenously) can be used to reverse these problems.

Other side effects include occasional agitation, excitability, seizures, constipation or diarrhea, rash, and dry mouth. Methemoglobinemia and edema of the mouth, tongue, or orbital areas have occurred. There has been a case report of a postpartum patient developing supraventricular tachycardia immediately after intravenous metoclopramide administration.

Metoclopramide should not be used in patients with pheochromocytoma, as hypertensive crisis may be precipitated. It is also contraindicated in epileptics and in patients with gastrointestinal obstruction.

MECHANISM OF ACTION

Metoclopramide relieves nausea and vomiting by blocking dopaminergic stimuli at the chemoreceptor trigger zone. Peripherally, it acts as a cholinergic agonist to increase tone in the esophageal sphincter, increase the tone and amplitude of gastric contractions, relax the pyloric sphincter and duodenal bulb, and increase peristalsis in the duodenum and jejunum. Gastric emptying and intestinal transit time are diminished. As was previously mentioned, prolactin release is potentiated. Additionally, there is a transient rise in aldosterone levels, which may be associated with fluid retention.

ABSORPTION AND BIOTRANSFORMATION

The onset of action is 1–3 minutes after an intravenous dose and 30–60 minutes following an oral dose. Pharmacologic effects persist for 1–2 hours, with a plasma half-life of about 3 hours. The drug is metabolized by the liver. Approximately 85% of an orally administered dose (or its metabolites) appears in the urine within 72 hours.

RECOMMENDED READING

Bevacqua, B.K. Supraventricular tachycardia associated with postpartum metoclopramide administration. *Anesthesiology* 68:124, 1988.

Bohnet, H.G., and Kato, A.K. Prolactin secretion during pregnancy and puerperium: response to metoclopramide and interactions with placental hormones. *Obstet. Gynecol.* 65:789, 1985.

Brock-Utne, J.G., et al. The effect of metoclopramide on the lower oesophageal sphincter in late pregnancy. *Anaesth. Intensive Care* 6:26, 1978.

Bylsma-Howell, M., et al. Placental transport of metoclopramide: assessment of maternal and neonatal effects. *Can. Anaesth. Soc. J.* 30:487, 1983.

Cohen, S.E., et al. Does metoclopramide decrease the volume of gastric contents in patients undergoing cesarean section? *Anesthesiology* 61:604, 1984.

Kauppila, A., Kivinen, S., and Ylikorkala, O. A dose response relation between improved lactation and metoclopramide. *Lancet* 1:1175, 1981.

Kauppila, A., et al. Metoclopramide and breast feeding: transfer into milk and the newborn. *Eur. J. Pharmacol.* 25:819, 1983.

Lussos, S.A., Bader, A.M., Thornhill, M.L., and Datta, S. The antiemetic efficacy and safety of prophylactic metoclopramide for elective cesarean delivery during spinal anesthesia. *Reg. Anesth.* 17:126, 1992.

Metronidazole (Flagyl®, Metrogel®)

INDICATIONS AND RECOMMENDATIONS

The use of metronidazole during pregnancy is controversial and, if at all, should be restricted to very specific situations. Metronidazole is a broad-spectrum antiprotozoal, antibacterial agent that has been used in the treatment of amebiasis, anaerobic infections (especially *Bacteroides* species), giardiasis, trichomoniasis, and vaginitis caused by *Haemophilus vaginalis* and as a radiosensitizer in the treatment of various tumors.

In pregnant women, metronidazole should not be used when other therapeutic options exist. It passes freely through the placental barrier and reaches levels of 66% of maternal serum levels in the fetus and 26% of maternal serum levels in the placenta. There is abundant evidence that metronidazole is mutagenic in bacteria and carcinogenic in rodents. Meta-analysis of the published articles reporting on metronidazole use during pregnancy concluded that metronidazole use during the first trimester carried no risk of teratogenicity. The data used in the analysis were insufficient for analysis of rates of stillbirth or spontaneous abortion. Also, several investigators report that metronidazole has been used in all stages of pregnancy without apparent fetal sequelae. However, it would be most prudent to avoid its use, especially during the first trimester.

Recently, metronidazole has been used for the treatment of bacterial vaginosis during pregnancy. Its use in this setting is promising as it appears significantly to reduce the rate of preterm labor in women with bacterial vaginosis who have a history of delivering prematurely. Because bacterial vaginosis is linked to adverse pregnancy outcomes including prematurity, premature rupture of membranes, and puerperal endometriosis, the benefits of using metronidazole in this situation appear to outweigh the risks. However, further research should be performed before a definite recommendation can be made.

Although metronidazole is probably the single most effective agent available for treating *Trichomonas* infections, use of clotrimazole vaginal tablets or vaginal cream may offer relief from *Trichomonas* infections and is preferable during pregnancy.

Because metronidazole is excreted in breast milk, the same precautions should be kept in mind for the nursing mother as for the pregnant woman. Should treatment be necessary, a single 2 g dose should be administered and breast-feeding deferred for 48 hours.

RECOMMENDED READING

Burtin, P., et al. Safety of metronidazole in pregnancy: a meta-analysis. *Am. J. Obstet. Gynecol.* 172: 525, 1995.

Erickson, S.H., Oppenheim, G.L., and Smith, G.H. Metronidazole in breast milk. *Obstet. Gynecol.* 57:48, 1981.

Hauth, J.C., et al. Reduced incidence of preterm delivery with metronidazole and erythromycin in women with bacterial vaginosis. *N. Engl. J. Med.* 333:1732, 1995.

Morales, W.J., Schorr, S., and Albritton, J. Effect of metronidazole in patients with preterm birth in preceding pregnancy and bacterial vaginosis: a placebo-controlled, double blind study. *Am. J. Obstet. Gynecol.* 171:345, 1994.

Norman, K., et al. Ampicillin and metronizazole treatment in preterm labour: a multicentre randomised controlled trial. *Br. J. Obstet. Gynaecol.* 101:404, 1994.

Tracy, J.W., and Webster, Jr., L.T. Drugs used in the chemotherapy of protozoal infections: trypanosomiasis, leishmaniasis, amebiases, giardiasis, trichomoniasis, and other protozoal infections. Chapter 41 in *Goodman and Gilman's The Pharmacological Basis of Therapeutics* (9th ed.), J.G. Hardman and L.E. Limbird, eds. New York: McGraw-Hill, 1996, Pp. 995–998.

Miconazole (Micatin®, Monistat®, Monistat 3®, Monistat 7®)

INDICATIONS AND RECOMMENDATIONS

Miconazole may be administered topically to pregnant women for the treatment of candidal vulvovaginitis and fungal infections of the skin and nails. It is a broad-spectrum antifungal agent. It should not be used vaginally if membranes are ruptured. Use of the intravenous preparation should be reserved for the treatment of life-threatening systemic fungal infections.

SPECIAL CONSIDERATIONS IN PREGNANCY

In rats, doses of 30 mg/kg/day resulted in an increased incidence of stillbirths and deaths of dams due to difficult labor; no dysmorphic effects were seen. In rabbits, doses of up to 100 mg/kg/day are associated with an increased percentage of fetal resorptions.

Topical use of miconazole for the treatment of vulvovaginal candidiasis has not been associated with adverse fetal effects. In one study of pregnancy outcomes after first-trimester vaginitis drug therapy, no statistically significant association was observed for miconazole and the overall frequency of birth defects or for any specific birth defect analyzed. However, the estimated relative risk of spontaneous abortions in patients with first-trimester miconazole exposure was 1.4 compared with a control group of nonexposed patients. Large numbers of exposures to other therapeutic agents did not show this association and prompted the authors to suggest that the spontaneous abortions were caused by miconazole and clotrimazole.

DOSAGE

For the treatment of candidal vulvovaginitis, one applicator dose of the vaginal cream should be inserted high into the vagina at bedtime for 7 days. Alternatively, a 100 mg suppository may be inserted intravaginally once daily at bedtime for 7 consecutive days or one 200-mg suppository inserted daily for 3 consecutive days. For fungal infections of the skin and nails, the cream should be applied twice daily for 7 days. Recommended doses for intravenous management of systemic fungal infections range from 200 to 3600 mg/day for 1–20 weeks, depending on the pathogen.

ADVERSE EFFECTS

Untoward effects of topical miconazole therapy are uncommon and include vaginal burning and itching, pruritus, and cramps. Reported adverse effects of intravenous therapy include phlebitis, thrombocytosis, pruritus, vomiting, and hyperlipidemia.

MECHANISM OF ACTION

Miconazole is fungicidal against pathogenic yeast-like and filamental fungi. It acts to alter the permeability of the fungal cell membrane and may also alter RNA and DNA metabolism or allow intracellular accumulation of toxins.

ABSORPTION AND BIOTRANSFORMATION

Small amounts of miconazole are absorbed from the vaginal mucosa and can be detected in the serum and urine. After intravenous administration, it is rapidly metabolized in the liver and the inactive metabolites are excreted in the urine.

RECOMMENDED READING

Abrams, L.S., and Weintraub, H.S. Disposition of radioactivity following intravaginal administration of 3H-miconazole nitrate. *Am. J. Obstet. Gynecol.* 147:920, 1983.

Bennett, J.E. Antimicrobial agents: antifungal agents. Chapter 49 in *Goodman and Gilman's The Pharmacological Basis of Therapeutics* (9th ed.), J.G. Hardman and L.E. Limbird, eds. New York: McGraw-Hill, 1996. Pp. 1176, 1186.

Boelaert, J., et al. Pharmacokinetic profile of miconazole in man. *Eur. J. Pharmacol.* 10:49, 1976.

Heil, R.C., et al. Miconazole: a preliminary review of its therapeutic efficacy in systemic fungal infections. *Drugs* 19:7, 1980.

Rosa, F.W., Baum, C., and Shaw, M. Pregnancy outcomes after first-trimester vaginitis drug therapy. *Obstet. Gynecol.* 69:751, 1987.

Mineral Oil (Over-the-Counter)

INDICATIONS AND RECOMMENDATIONS

Mineral oil is relatively contraindicated during pregnancy because other therapeutic agents are preferable. This stool softener retards the reabsorption of water from the fecal mass. Because mineral oil may decrease the absorption of vitamin K, leading to a prolonged prothrombin time, docusates are preferable as stool softeners in pregnancy.

RECOMMENDED READING

Brunton, L.L. Agents affecting gastrointestinal water flux and motility; emesis and antiemetics; bile acids and pancreatic enzymes. Chapter 38 in *Goodman and Gilman's The Pharmacological Basis of Therapeutics* (9th ed.), J.G. Hardman and L.E. Limbird, eds. New York: McGraw-Hill, 1996. Pp. 924–925.

Nelson, M.M., and Forfar, J.O. Associations between drugs administered during pregnancy and congenital abnormalities of the fetus. *Br. Med. J.* 1:523, 1971.

Schenkel, B., and Vorherr, H. Non-prescription drugs during pregnancy: potential teratogenic and toxic effects upon embryo and fetus. *J. Reprod. Med.* 12:27, 1974.

Misoprostol (Cytotec®)

Misoprostol is contraindicated during pregnancy, except as a cervical ripening agent when labor is to be induced. It is a synthetic prostaglandin E_1 analog that inhibits gastric acid secretion in response to stimuli, and is used to prevent gastric ulcers induced by nonsteroidal antiinflammatory drugs (NSAIDs), including aspirin, in patients at high risk.

Misoprostol can produce uterine contractions and abortion. It has been used in combination with both methotrexate and mifepristone (RU-486) to induce abortion. In recent years misoprostol has been used as a cervical ripening agent in patients about to undergo induction of labor. Both oral (50 mg every

4 hours) and vaginal (25–50 µg every 2 to 4 hours) routes have been successful. Misoprostol is considerably less expensive than other forms of prostaglandin used for this purpose.

Its use during the first trimester by women trying without success to abort has been associated with limb defects with and without Möbius sequence in seven infants. Its use in similar circumstances has also been associated with congenital malformations of the cranium and overlying scalp in five infants. The doses used in the above reports ranged from 400 to 1600 µg over 1–4 days and were taken orally and/or vaginally. The usual oral dose is 200 µg qid. Women should be advised not to become pregnant while on misoprostol therapy. If a woman becomes pregnant while taking the drug, it should be discontinued and the patient apprised of the potential hazards to the fetus.

No information is available regarding misoprostol's passage into breast milk. The manufacturer's product literature recommends against administration to nursing mothers because of the potential for significant diarrhea in the nursing infant.

RECOMMENDED READING

Cytotec product information. G.D. Searle & Co. 1997.

Fonseca, W., et al. Misoprostol and congenital malformations (letter). *Lancet* 338:56, 1991.

Gonzalez, C.H., et al. Limb deficiency with or without Möbius sequence in seven Brazilian children associated with misoprostol use in the first trimester of pregnancy. *Am. J. Med. Genetics* 47: 59, 1993.

Methotrexate and misoprostol for abortion. *Med. Lett.* 38:39, 1996.

Mundle, W.R., Young, D.C. Vaginal misoprostol for induction of labor: a randomized controlled trial. *Obstet. Gynecol.* 88:521, 1996.

Schuler, L.S., Ashton, P.W., and Sanseverino, M.T. Teratogenicity of misoprostol (letter). *Lancet* 339:437, 1992.

Windrim, R., Bennett, K., Mundle, W., Young, D.C. Oral administration of misoprostol for labor induction. *Obstet. Gynecol.* 89:392, 1997.

Wing, D.A., Rahall, A., Jones, M.M., Goodwin, T.M., Paul, R.H. Misoprostol: an effective agent for cervical ripening and labor induction. *Amer. J. Obstet. Gynecol.* 172:1811, 1995.

Naloxone (Narcan®)

INDICATIONS AND RECOMMENDATIONS

Naloxone is the drug of choice for the treatment of narcotic-induced respiratory depression in either mother or neonate. It should be administered immediately after birth to any depressed neonate whose mother has been treated with narcotic analgesics. It should not, however, be used routinely in narcotic-exposed newborns, nor is it recommended for administration to a mother just before delivery to reverse fetal and neonatal effects of maternally administered narcotic analgesics. In addition, it should not be used to "normalize" fetal heart rates that exhibit low beat-to-beat variability.

Naloxone administration to an addicted mother or infant may precipitate withdrawal. It should, therefore, not be administered to a pregnant woman in order to diagnose narcotic addiction, as sudden withdrawal may be deleterious to the fetus. Similarly, it should not be administered to asymptomatic infants of narcotic-addicted mothers, who may themselves be addicted.

SPECIAL CONSIDERATIONS IN PREGNANCY

Naloxone crosses the placenta and when given antenatally can reverse neonatal depression secondary to narcotic administration to the mother. Antenatal use for the prevention of neonatal respiratory depression is, however, contraindicated. It is hypothesized that enkephalins and endorphins play important regulatory functions in fetal physiology. Naloxone reversal of such functions may be deleterious. It should, therefore, be used only in the face of obvious neonatal depression.

Naloxone has been used to treat loss of fetal heart rate beat-to-beat variability unassociated with maternal narcotic use. In one reported case, such use was associated with fetal asphyxia with ensuing neonatal death. The authors hypothesize that fetal endorphins produce fetal tolerance to pain as well as abnormally "flat" heart rate patterns intrapartum and protect the fetus from asphyxia. The unopposed antagonism of fetal opioids in times of distress were, therefore, believed to be detrimental in this situation.

Naloxone has been shown to suppress enkephalin-mediated secretion of prolactin. Studies in nursing mothers, however, indicate that endogenous opioids do not play a major role in prolactin secretion during the puerperium. Lactation should, therefore, not be affected by naloxone use.

DOSAGE

For adults, the dose is 0.4 mg given intravenously, intramuscularly, or subcutaneously, repeated at 2- to 3-minute intervals. If no response is observed after 10 mg has been administered, the diagnosis of narcotic toxicity should be questioned. The intravenous route of administration produces the most rapid effect. Repeat doses may be required at 12-hour intervals, depending on the specific agent that is causing the depression. Supplemental intramuscular doses have a longer lasting effect.

The neonatal dose is 0.01 mg/kg given rapidly or intravenously via the endotracheal tube. That dose may need to be repeated in 30–90 minutes depending on the narcotic agent and dose to which the mother and newborn were exposed. It should be administered intravenously, as intramuscular or subcutaneous absorption may be delayed in the stressed and vasoconstricted infant.

ADVERSE EFFECTS

In opiate-dependent subjects, naloxone produces a moderate to severe withdrawal syndrome that appears within minutes and lasts for approximately 2 hours. Naloxone itself is devoid of narcotic agonist properties, and doses of up to 12 mg produce no discernible effect in the absence of a narcotic.

MECHANISM OF ACTION

Naloxone displaces morphine-like drugs from their specific receptor sites. It reverses narcotic-induced respiratory depression, analgesia, sedation, hypotension, and pupillary constriction. It also reverses the depressant effects of narcotic antagonists and congeners including nalorphine, levallorphan, pentazocine, and diphenoxylate.

ABSORPTION AND BIOTRANSFORMATION

Naloxone is readily absorbed from the gastrointestinal tract but is so quickly cleared by the liver that oral doses are for the most part ineffective. It is metabolized in the liver primarily by glucuronidation.

RECOMMENDED READING

Arduini, D., Rizzo, G., Dell Acqua, S., et al. Effect of naloxone on fetal behavior near term. *Am. J. Obstet. Gynecol.* 156:474, 1987.

Bloom, R.S., Cropley, C., AHA/AAP Neonatal Resuscitation Program Steering Committee. *Textbook of Neonatal Resuscitation.* American Heart Association, 1994. Pp. 6–51.

Chang, A., et al. The effects of nalorphine and naloxone on maternal and fetal blood gas and pH. *Med. J. Aust.* 1:263, 1976.

Gibbs, J., Newson, T., Williams, J., et al. Naloxone hazard in infant of opioid abuser. *Lancet* 2(8655):159, 1989.

Goodlin, R.C. Naloxone and its possible relationship to fetal endorphin levels and fetal distress. *Am. J. Obstet. Gynecol.* 139:16, 1981.

Kauffman, R.E. Why not use naloxone? (in Reply). *Pediatrics* 67:444, 1981.

Lodico, G., et al. Effects of naloxone infusion on basal and breast stimulation induced prolactin secretion in puerperal women. *Fertil. Steril.* 40:600, 1983.

Reisine, T., and Pasternak, G. Opioid analgesics and antagonists. Chapter 23 in *Goodman and Gilman's The Pharmacological Basis of Therapeutics* (9th ed.), J.G. Hardman and L.E. Limbird, eds. New York: McGraw-Hill, 1996. Pp. 549–551.

Segal, S., et al. Naloxone use in newborns. *Pediatrics* 65:667, 1980.

Narcotic Agonist-Antagonist Analgesics: Butorphanol (Stadol ®), Nalbuphine (Nubain®), Pentazocine (Talwin®)

INDICATIONS AND RECOMMENDATIONS

Narcotic agonist-antagonist analgesics may be used during pregnancy for short-term relief of severe pain. When used, however, they should be taken at the lowest effective dosage for the minimum required period. They should not be prescribed to mothers who are suspected of being addicted to narcotic agents, as use of these drugs may precipitate withdrawal and be detrimental to the fetus. Narcotic agonist-antagonists are also widely used for analgesia during labor and may be added to local anesthetics to enhance the efficacy of epidural analgesia.

SPECIAL CONSIDERATIONS IN PREGNANCY

Each of these agents crosses the placenta and reaches significant levels in the fetus. The abuse of pentazocine during pregnancy (often in combination with tripelennamine or methylphenidate) as a substitute for heroin is known to cause maternal and fetal dependence. Infants exposed chronically to pentazocine in utero experience withdrawal symptoms within 24 hours of birth. The use of pentazocine during pregnancy has not been associated with congenital malformation.

Some of these agents are used for analgesia during labor, either as intermittent intravenous injections or by patient-controlled pump administration. In one double-blind, randomized study patient-controlled analgesia with nalbuphine (up to 3 mg IV q10 minutes) was more effective than meperidine (up to 15 mg IV q10 minutes). Butorphanol added to epidural bupivacaine has been demonstrated to be equally effective as morphine, but with considerably less likelihood of pruritus. Butorphanol administered epidurally also may decrease shivering associated with epidural anesthesia. Nalbuphine administered intravenously has been associated with decreased fetal heart rate variability and spontaneous accelerations during early labor, as well as decreased fetal heart rate accelerations in response to vibroacoustic stimulation. In one study, cord plasma levels of nalbuphine measured 30 minutes to 2 hours after maternal intramuscular or intravenous injection averaged 74% of simultaneous maternal levels, and the calculated neonatal half-life was approximately 4 hours. Like the pure narcotic analgesics, the narcotic agonist-antagonist analgesics can produce severe neonatal respiratory depression and lower psychophysiologic test scores. Given the relatively long neonatal half-life, if neonatal respiratory depression occurs in an exposed newborn, naloxone should be administered immediately to the infant.

The Committee on Drugs of the American Academy of Pediatrics considers butorphanol to be usually compatible with breast-feeding.

DOSAGE

Drug	Route	Analgesic dosage
Butorphanol	IM	1–2 mg q3–4h
	epidural	1–2 mg as a supplement to loading dose of local anesthetic
Nalbuphine	SQ/IM/IV	10 mg q3–6h
	IV as PCA	2–4-mg loading dose, then up to 1 mg q6–10 min
Pentazocine	IM/IV	30–60 mg q3–4h
	PO	50–100 mg q3–4h

ADVERSE EFFECTS

The most frequent side effects are nausea, light-headedness and dizziness, and sedation. In addition, narcotic agonist-antagonist analgesics can produce euphoria, headache, nervousness, gastrointestinal cramping, and vomiting. Intramuscular use of pentazocine, but not butorphanol or nalbuphine, may cause soft tissue induration, nodules, and ulceration at the injection site. High dosages may produce marked respiratory depression and cardiovascular effects that are usually less severe than those produced by pure narcotic overdose.

MECHANISM OF ACTION

The narcotic agonist-antagonist analgesics are synthetic agents formulated to provide potent analgesia with a lower abuse potential than pure narcotic agonists. Like the pure narcotic analgesics, they appear to produce analgesia by acting at opiate receptors in the central nervous system. However, they also weakly antagonize narcotic effects at the receptor site and may precipitate withdrawal in patients who take narcotic agents regularly. These agents function as agonists at κ receptors but antagonists at μ receptors, although pentazocine has weaker μ antagonism.

ABSORPTION AND BIOTRANSFORMATION

Pentazocine is well absorbed from the gastrointestinal tract but undergoes extensive first-pass metabolism, which significantly lowers oral bioavailability. When given parenterally, all of these agents are well absorbed from injection sites. Nalbuphine and butorphanol have plasma half-lives of 2–3.5 hours, and their action lasts for approximately 4–6 hours. Pentazocine has a longer half-life of 4–5 hours, but a similar duration of action. They are primarily metabolized by the liver; metabolites are excreted in the urine.

RECOMMENDED READING

Abboud, T.K., Reyes, A., Richardson, M., et al. Epidural morphine or butorphanol augments bupivacaine analgesia during labor. *Reg. Anesthes.* 14:115, 1989.

Committee on Drugs of the American Academy of Pediatrics. The transfer of drugs and other chemicals into human milk. *Pediatrics* 93:137, 1994.

Frank, M., McAteer, E.J., Cattermole, R., et al. Nalbuphine for obstetric analgesia. *Anaesthesia* 42:697, 1987.

Giannina, G., Guzman, G., and Lai, Y.-L. Comparison of the effects of meperidine and nalbuphine on intrapartum fetal heart rate tracings. *Obstet. Gynecol.* 86:441, 1995.

Goetz, R.L., and Bain, R.V. Neonatal withdrawal symptoms associated with maternal use of pentazocine. *J. Pediatrics* 84:887, 1974.

Jujena, M., Ackerman, W.E. III, Heine, M.F., et al. Butorphanol for the relief of shivering associated with extradural anesthesia in parturients. *J. Clin. Anesth.* 4:390, 1992.

Lundquest, D.E., Young, W.K., and Edland, J.F. Maternal death associated with intravenous methylphenidate (Ritalin) and pentazocine (Talwin) abuse. *J. For. Sci.* 32:798, 1987.

Nicolle, E., Devillier, P., Delanoy, B., et al. Therapeutic monitoring of nalbuphine: transplacental transfer and estimated pharmacokinetics in the neonate. *Eur. J. Pharmacol.* 49:485, 1996.

Pittman, K.A., et al. Human perinatal distribution of butorphanol. *Am. J. Obstet. Gynecol.* 138:797, 1980.

Podlas, J., and Breland, B.D. Patient-controlled analgesia with nalbuphine during labor. *Obstet. Gynecol.* 70:202, 1987.

Poehlmann, S., Pinette, M., and Stubblefield, P. Effect of labor analgesia with nalbuphine hydrochloride on fetal response to vibroacoustic stimulation. *J. Reprod. Med.* 40:707, 1995.

Reisine, T., and Pasternak, G. Opioid analgesics and antagonists. Chapter 23 in *Goodman and Gilman's The Pharmacological Basis of Therapeutics* (9th ed.), J.G. Hardman and L.E. Limbird, eds. New York: McGraw-Hill, 1996. Pp. 521–555.

Narcotic Analgesics: Codeine, Dihydrocodeine (Synalgos®), Fentanyl (Sublimaze®), Hydrocodone, Hydromorphone (Dilaudid®), Levorphanol (Levo-Dromoran®), Morphine, Oxycodone (Percocet®, Percodan®)

INDICATIONS AND RECOMMENDATIONS

These various narcotic analgesics may be used during pregnancy for short-term relief of severe pain. When used, however, they should be taken at the lowest effective dosage for the minimum required duration. Fixed combinations of narcotics and aspirin or acetaminophen are not recommended as they do not allow independent adjustment of dosages. For analgesia during labor, however, butorphanol and meperidine are recommended, as they have been intensively studied in this setting. They are each discussed separately elsewhere in this handbook. It should be noted that a small randomized trial of morphine and meperidine in labor was unable to detect an effect of either drug on pain perception scores, although both caused sedation.

The use of intrathecal and epidural narcotics for labor or postoperative analgesia, in combination with local anesthetic agents, has become increasingly popular in recent years. Similarly, narcotics are often injected into the epidural space after cesarean section, just before the epidural catheter is removed, in order to provide postpartum analgesia.

SPECIAL CONSIDERATIONS IN PREGNANCY

With the exception of codeine, use of these agents during pregnancy has not been associated with teratogenicity. There have been no large-scale prospective studies of their use during pregnancy, however. In several retrospective studies, the use of codeine during the first trimester has been associated with such diverse anomalies as respiratory tract malformation, pyloric stenosis, inguinal hernia, cardiac and circulatory system defects, and cleft lip and palate. Although none of the studies clearly implicate codeine as a causative factor, they do suggest that codeine and the other narcotic analgesics should not be used indiscriminately during pregnancy, especially in the first trimester. Opiates have also been demonstrated to decrease maternal plasma oxytocin concentrations. The clinical significance of this finding is not yet clear.

All of these drugs readily cross the placenta and reach significant fetal levels. The use of fentanyl during general anesthesia has been associated with loss of fetal heart rate variability without fetal hypoxia. In addition, these drugs readily cross the immature blood–brain barrier and can produce severe neonatal respiratory depression and lower psychophysiologic test scores. If neonatal respiratory depression occurs in a narcotic-exposed newborn, naloxone should be administered immediately to the infant.

Infants born to narcotic-addicted mothers are addicted at birth and will experience withdrawal symptoms. The severity and duration of symptoms vary with the specific agent, dosage, and duration of maternal exposure. Withdrawal symptoms have been reported in infants whose mothers had taken antitussive doses of codeine for as little as 10 days before delivery.

Analgesic doses of narcotics appear in breast milk in small amounts, which appear to be insignificant. The Committee on Drugs of the American Academy of Pediatrics considers codeine, morphine, and fentanyl to be usually compatible with breast-feeding.

DOSAGE

Narcotic analgesics may be given orally, intramuscularly, subcutaneously, intravenously, and intrathecally. The following table lists common dosages:

Drug	Route	Analgesic dosage
Codeine	PO/IM/SQ	15–60 mg q4–6h
Dihydrocodeine	PO	Available in combination with aspirin and acetaminophen
Fentanyl	IM	0.05–0.10 mg given as a single dose pre- or intraoperatively
	Epidural	50–100 µg as initial bolus, then 1–2 µg/ml with local anesthetic via pump
	Intrathecal	One tenth of epidural dose
Hydrocodone	PO	Available in combination with aspirin and acetaminophen
Hydromorphone	PO	2 mg q4–6h
	IM/SQ	1–2 mg q4–6h
Levorphanol	PO/SQ	2 mg given in a single dose as an adjunct to anesthesia
Morphine	PO	10–30 mg q4h
	IM	10 mg q4–6h
	IV	2–10 mg
	Intrathecal	0.2–0.5 mg
	Epidural	5 mg postoperatively
Oxycodone	PO	5–10 mg q6h

ADVERSE EFFECTS

The major hazards of narcotic use occur primarily with overdose and include respiratory depression, apnea, and circulatory depression. The most common side effects are light-headedness, sedation, nausea, vomiting, and sweating. In addition, narcotics can produce euphoria, dysphoria, dry mouth, constipation, and urinary retention. Intrathecal and epidural narcotics, particularly morphine, have been associated with generalized or localized pruritus, in some studies affecting up to 50% or 60% of patients, often in the distribution of the maxillary division of the trigeminal nerve. One randomized study demonstrated that intravenous droperidol 2.5 mg, just after delivery, significantly reduced the likelihood of severe pruritus in such patients. Naloxone, a narcotic antagonist, may also be effective in treating or preventing pruritus after epidural or intrathecal morphine. However, reversal of the narcotic analgesic effect may make such treatment less desirable. Reactivation of labial herpes simplex has been reported to occur with increased frequency after the administration of epidural morphine compared to parenteral morphine, in at least one randomized trial.

MECHANISM OF ACTION

The narcotic analgesics act at opiate receptors in the central nervous system to mediate analgesic activity. Narcotic analgesia is potentiated by the analgesia of aspirin and acetaminophen. In addition to analgesia, these agents possess antitussive, antiemetic, and antidiarrheal properties.

ABSORPTION AND BIOTRANSFORMATION

The narcotic analgesics are absorbed from the gastrointestinal tract at differing rates; codeine, hydromorphone, and oxycodone are relatively better absorbed than the other agents of this category. Intravenous administration is most reliable and rapid. Intramuscular and subcutaneous administration may delay absorption and effect. All are metabolized by the liver and excreted primarily in the urine. About 10% of administered codeine is metabolized to morphine.

RECOMMENDED READING

Ackerman, W.E., Juneja, M.M., Kaczorowski, D.M., et al. A comparison of the incidence of pruritus following epidural opioid administration in the parturient. *Can. J. Anaesth.* 36:388, 1989.

Boyle, R.K. A review of anatomical and immunological links between epidural morphine and herpes simplex labialis in obstetric patients. *Anaesth. Intensive Care* 23:425, 1995.

Boyle, R.K. Herpes simplex labialis after epidural or parenteral morphine: a randomized prospective trial in an Australian obstetric population. *Anaesth. Intensive Care* 23:433–437, 1995.

Bracken, M.B., and Holford, T.R. Exposure to prescribed drugs in pregnancy and association with congenital malformations. *Obstet. Gynecol.* 58:336, 1981.

Committee on Drugs of the American Academy of Pediatrics. The transfer of drugs and other chemicals into human milk. *Pediatrics* 93:137, 1994.

Heinonen, O.P., Slone, D., and Shapiro, S. *Birth Defects and Drugs in Pregnancy.* Littleton, MA: PSG, 1977. Pp. 287–295.

Horta, M.L., Horta, B.L. Inhibition of epidural morphine-induced pruritus by intravenous droperidol. *Reg. Anesthesia* 18:118, 1993.

Johnson, E.S., and Colley, P.S. Effects of nitrous oxide and fentanyl anesthesia on fetal heart-rate variability intra- and postoperatively. *Anesthesiology* 52:429, 1980.

Kahn, K., and Chang, J. Neonatal abstinence syndrome due to codeine. *Arch. Dis. Child.* 76:F59, 1997.

Lindow, S.W., van der Spuy, Z.M., Hendricks, M.S., et al. The effect of morphine and naloxone administration on plasma oxytocin concentrations in the first stage of labour. *Clin. Endocrinol.* 37:349, 1992.

Mangurten, H.H., and Benawra, R. Neonatal codeine withdrawal in infants of nonaddicted mothers. *Pediatrics* 65:159, 1980.

Meny, R.G., Naumburg, E.G., Alger, L.S., et al. Codeine and the breastfed neonate. *J. Hum. Lact.* 9:237, 1993.

Nelson, T.W., Lilly, J.K. III, Baker, J.D., and Ackerly, J.A. Treatment of pruritus secondary to epidural morphine. *W. Virg. Med. J.* 84:183, 1988.

Olofsson, C., Ekblom, A., Ekman-Ordeberg, G., et al. Lack of analgesic effect of systemically administered morphine or pethidine on labour pain. *Br. J. Obstet. Gynaecol.* 103:968, 1996.

Ransom, S. Oxymorphone as an obstetric analgesic—a clinical trial. *Anesthesia* 21:464, 1966.

Reisine, T., and Pasternak, G. Opioid analgesics and antagonists. Chapter 23 in *Goodman and Gilman's The Pharmacological Basis of Therapeutics* (9th ed.), J.G. Hardman and L.E. Limbird, eds. New York: McGraw-Hill, 1996. Pp. 521–555.

Russell, J.A., Gosden, R.G., Humphreys, E.M., et al. Interruption of parturition in rats by morphine: a result of inhibition of oxytocin secretion. *J. Endocrinol.* 121:521, 1989.

Saxen, I. Epidemiology of cleft lip and palate: an attempt to rule out chance correlations. *Br. J. Prev. Soc. Med.* 29:103, 1975.

Nitrofurantoin (Furadantin®, Macrodantin®)

INDICATIONS AND RECOMMENDATIONS

Nitrofurantoin may be administered to pregnant patients to treat asymptomatic or symptomatic bacteriuria caused by sensitive organisms, but should be avoided near term. It is an antimicrobial agent used in the treatment of acute, uncomplicated, lower urinary tract infections as well as for long-term suppression in patients with chronic bacteriuria. It is contraindicated when there is a possibility of bacteremia, as oral nitrofurantoin does not achieve therapeutic serum levels. It is effective against *Escherichia coli, Enterococcus,* and *Staphylococcus,* but ineffective against *Pseudomonas* and *Proteus* as well as many species of *Enterobacter* and *Klebsiella.* Nitrofurantoin should not be used in patients with compromised renal function, including those with hypertensive, toxic, or diabetic nephropathy, and it may cause hemolysis in patients who have glucose 6-phosphate dehydrogenase (G6PD) deficiency.

SPECIAL CONSIDERATIONS IN PREGNANCY

Nitrofurantoin crosses the placenta rapidly but in small quantity and disappears rapidly from the fetal circulation. There are no unique maternal problems when nitrofurantoin is taken during pregnancy. Pregnant women who experience hemolytic anemia when treated with nitrofurantoin generally recover without sequelae after discontinuation of therapy. Because of its low levels of glutathione, an infant is theoretically predisposed to hemolytic anemia if exposed to nitrofurantoin shortly before birth. Therefore, it has been recommended that another antibiotic be used during the third trimester of pregnancy. However, a review of one manufacturer's database of known adverse reactions identified no well-documented cases of drug-induced hemolytic reactions in neonates whose mothers received nitrofurantoin late in pregnancy.

Nitrofurantoin is excreted into breast milk within 3 hours of drug administration. A neonate may receive up to 81 µg/kg in one nursing when its mother takes 100 mg nitrofurantoin tid. Because only a very small amount of the drug may be sufficient to trigger a hemolytic reaction in G6PD-deficient infants, the authors suggest that nitrofurantoin not be used by nursing mothers in populations with a high incidence of G6PD deficiency.

DOSAGE

The dose of nitrofurantoin for treatment of acute urinary tract infections is 50–100 mg PO qid. The dose used for long-term suppressive therapy is 50–100 mg PO at bedtime.

ADVERSE EFFECTS

Nausea and vomiting frequently occur but are less common with use of the macrocrystalline form. Occasional hypersensitivity reactions include chills, fever, leukopenia, granulocytopenia, hemolytic anemia (associated with G6PD deficiency), cholestatic jaundice, and hepatocellular damage. Acute pneumonitis may occur within hours to days of initiation of therapy and usually resolves after discontinuation of the drug. Interstitial pulmonary fibrosis can occur with long-term therapy.

MECHANISM OF ACTION

It is believed that bacteria reduce nitrofurantoin to highly reactive intermediates that, in turn, damage bacterial DNA. Because mammalian cells do not reduce the drug as quickly, they are thought to be relatively resistant to its effects.

ABSORPTION AND BIOTRANSFORMATION

Nitrofurantoin is absorbed rapidly and completely from the gastrointestinal tract. The macrocrystalline form is absorbed and excreted more slowly than the crystalline form and is associated with less gastrointestinal intolerance. Because of rapid elimination, the serum half-life is 20–60 minutes; therapeutically effective serum levels are not achieved with oral dosing. About 40% of an oral dose is excreted unchanged in the urine, reaching levels of 200 μg/ml. Uremic patients excrete very little drug in the urine, making it useless in such patients.

RECOMMENDED READING

Ben David, S., et al. The safety of nitrofurantoin during the first trimester of pregnancy: meta-analysis. *Fund. Clin. Pharmacol.* 9:503, 1995.

Bint, A.J., and Hill, D. Bacteriuria of pregnancy: an update on significance, diagnosis and management. *J. Antimicrob. Chemother.* 33 (Suppl. A):93, 1994.

Boggess, K.A., Benedetti, T.J., and Raghu, G. Nitrofurantoin-induced pulmonary toxicity during pregnancy: a report of a case and review of the literature. *Obstet. Gynecol. Surv.* 51:367, 1996

Gait, J.E. Hemolytic reactions to nitrofurantoin in patients with glucose-6-phosphate dehydrogenase deficiency: theory and practice. *Dicp* 24:1210, 1990.

Lenke, R.R., Van Dorsten, J.P., and Schiffrin, B.S. Pyelonephritis in pregnancy: a prospective randomized trial to prevent recurrent disease evaluating suppressive therapy with nitrofurantoin and dose surveillance. *Am. J. Obstet. Gynecol.* 146:953, 1983.

Mandell, G.L., and Petri, Jr., W.A. Antimicrobial agents: sulfonamides, trimethoprim-sulfamethoxazole, quinolones, and agents for urinary tract infections. Chapter 44 in *Goodman and Gilman's The Pharmacological Basis of Therapeutics* (9th ed.), J.G. Hardman and L.E. Limbird, eds. New York: McGraw-Hill, 1996. Pp. 1069–1070.

Perry, J.E., and LeBlanc, A.L. Transfer of nitrofurantoin across the human placenta. *Tex. Rep. Biol. Med.* 25:270, 1967.

Pons, G., et al. Nitrofurantoin excretion in human milk. *Dev. Pharmacol. Ther.* 14:148, 1990.

Nitrovasodilators: Amyl Nitrite, Isosorbide Dinitrate (Isordil®, Sorbitrate®), Nitroglycerin or Glyceryl Trinitrate, (Nitro-Bid®, Nitrol®, Nitrostat®, Nitro-Dur®)

INDICATIONS AND RECOMMENDATIONS

Nitrovasodilators may be administered to pregnant women with angina pectoris. They should be given in the lowest effective dosage and for treatment of acute attacks. Recently, there has been a good deal of interest in, and experience with, the use of nitric oxide donors to achieve uterine relaxation in clinical situations such as external version, facilitation of reduction of bulging membranes prior to emergency cerclage, extraction of retained placenta, management of uterine inversion, and treatment of preterm labor. Although case reports and case series have suggested efficacy, no prospective controlled trials have evaluated such uses. Nevertheless, in a survey of obstetric anesthesiologists in 1993, 39% reported that nitroglycerin was their drug of choice for intrapartum and intraoperative tocolysis.

SPECIAL CONSIDERATIONS IN PREGNANCY

Snyder et al. reported the use of nitroglycerin in six severely hypertensive women given general anesthesia for cesarean section. The drug was successful in rapidly providing control of the hypertension and blunting the response to endotracheal intubation. No adverse effects on the neonates were detected. Writer et al., however, demonstrated that nitroglycerin infusion diminishes autoregulation of cerebral blood flow in hypertensive dogs, with an increase in blood flow to the brain occurring despite a reduction in mean arterial pressure (MAP). They caution that any further increase in MAP, such as occurs during endotracheal intubation, could significantly increase intracranial pressure. Since the intracranial dynamics of women with severe preeclampsia-toxemia (PET) may already be disturbed, a sudden increase in MAP could potentially have drastic consequences if nitroglycerin were being used. Longmire et al. found that nitroglycerin was ineffective in preventing intubation-associated hypertension in primigravidas with preeclampsia who had previously received volume expansion, but speculated that the drug might be useful in volume-contracted hypertensive patients. This issue should be further investigated before the use of nitroglycerin can be recommended for the treatment of hypertensive crises in women with PET.

Nitroglycerin, with a molecular weight of 227, is expected to readily cross the placenta. However, significant hypotensive effects were not observed in the first 10 minutes of life in neonates delivered by cesarean section to preeclamptic mothers who received nitroglycerin intravenously during induction of anesthesia. This may be due to the extremely rapid rate of maternal hepatic metabolism of the drug via glutathione reductase.

Nitroglycerin has been demonstrated to cause vasodilatation in the fetal umbilical vasculature, as reflected by reduction in the systolic/diastolic ratio and pulsatility index measured by Doppler, particularly in patients with hypertensive disorders of pregnancy. Whether this phenomenon will have any practical application in the management of such disorders remains an open question.

DOSAGE

The dosages of various nitrovasodilators used for the acute treatment of angina pectoris depend on the preparation. Reports describing the use of intravenous nitroglycerin for uterine relaxation usually describe dosages in the range of 50–100 µg as a bolus; the effect is evanescent, and repeated dosage within minutes of the initial dose has sometimes been necessary. Sublingual nitroglycerin spray (0.4–0.8 mg) and inhaled amyl nitrate (one ampule of 0.33 ml via the anesthetic apparatus) have also been utilized. One uncontrolled case series described the use of glyceryl trinitrate patches to treat premature labor, with each patch delivering 10 mg of glyceryl trinitrate over 24 hours. If there was no response to the first patch, a second was added an hour later, and both were changed every 24 hours.

ADVERSE EFFECTS

The most common side effects of nitrites are headache, dizziness, weakness, postural hypotension, and a typical flush on the head, neck, and clavicular area. In very high dosages, the nitrite ion can significantly oxidize hemoglobin to methemoglobin. In one non-randomized case series of nine external versions attempted after 0.8 mg of nitroglycerin administered sublingually by aerosol spray, four patients manifested significant hypotension, with one requiring intravenous ephedrine. There is a single case report of maternal pulmonary edema following treatment with continuous intravenous nitroglycerin for postoperative tocolysis after fetal surgery. The authors speculated that the nitroglycerin may have combined with exogenous oxygen to form peroxynitrite, which could have adversely impacted on alveolar epithelial cell function. However, the patient also received numerous other agents and the precise etiology of the pulmonary edema is unclear.

MECHANISM OF ACTION

These drugs are thought to act through liberation of free radical nitric oxide, which activates guanylyl cyclase and increases the synthesis of cyclic GMP. This leads to stimulation of a protein kinase which leads to the dephosphorylation of the light chain of myosin, causing relaxation of smooth muscle. Their predominant therapeutic actions are on vascular smooth muscle. Generalized vasodilatation occurs, but venous dilatation is a prominent factor in the blood pressure response to nitroglycerin. Blood pressure is decreased secondarily to generalized vasodilatation, but, since the sympathetic nervous system is not blocked, tachycardia may occur. The extent of the hypotension depends on the patient's position. In people with angina, venous dilatation presumably causes peripheral pooling of blood, with a decrease in cardiac output and work load. In addition there may be a redistribution of coronary blood flow.

The nitrites are effective in the treatment of acute attacks of angina. They also can prevent these attacks when taken shortly before periods of stress. The studies on the long-acting nitrates used for chronic prophylaxis of angina are difficult to assess. The lack of correlation between some clinical findings and pharmacologic data is difficult to explain. Chronic administration of long-acting nitrates may lead to the development of tolerance, thus making nitroglycerin ineffective in acute situations.

ABSORPTION AND BIOTRANSFORMATION

Most organic nitrates (nitroglycerin and the long-acting compounds) are readily absorbed from the sublingual mucosa. When administered by this route, their effects are more intense and predictable than when they are administered orally. Peak plasma concentration occurs within 4 minutes of sublingual administration, and the half-life is 1–3 minutes. Degradation of these compounds takes place rapidly in the liver, so that even though they are well absorbed from the gastrointestinal tract, little drug reaches the systemic circulation in active form. Sustained release oral preparations have been formulated and may deliver enough drug to provide a prolongation in action. Nitroglycerin and other organic nitrates are also absorbed through the skin. These compounds are rapidly denitrated in the liver, and metabolites are excreted in the urine.

RECOMMENDED READING

Abouleish, A.E., and Corn, S.B. Intravenous nitroglycerin for intrapartum external version of the second twin. *Anesth. Analg.* 78: 808, 1994.

Altabef, K.M., Spencer, J.T., and Zinberg, S. Intravenous nitroglycerin for uterine relaxation of an inverted uterus. *Am. J. Obstet. Gynecol.* 166:1237, 1992.

Bell, E. Nitroglycerin and uterine relaxation. *Anesthesiology* 85: 683, 1996.

Cousins, L.M., and Pue, A. Nitroglycerin facilitates therapeutic cerclage placement. *J. Perinatol.* 16:127, 1996.

Dayan, S.S., and Schwalbe, S.S. The use of small-dose intravenous nitroglycerin in a case of uterine inversion. *Anesth. Analg.* 82: 1091, 1996.

DeSimone, C.A., Norris, M.C., and Leighton, B.L. Intravenous nitroglycerin aids manual extraction of a retained placenta. *Anesthesiology* 73:787, 1990.

Diaz, S.F., and Marx, G.F. Placental transfer of nitroglycerin. *Anesthesiology* 51:475, 1979.

DiFederico, E.M., Harrison, M., and Matthay, M.A. Pulmonary edema in a woman following fetal surgery. *Chest* 109:1114, 1996.

Giles, W., O'Callaghan, S., Boura, A., et al. Reduction in human fetal umbilical-placental vascular resistance by glyceryl trinitrate. *Lancet* 340:856, 1992.

Greenspoon, J.S., and Kovacic, A. Breech extraction facilitated by glyceryl trinitrate spray. *Lancet* 338:124, 1991.

Gruenwald, C., Kublickas, M., and Carlström, N.-O., et al. Effects of nitroglycerin on the uterine and umbilical circulation in severe preeclampsia. *Obstet. Gynecol.* 86:600, 1995.

Hendricks, S.K., Ross, B., Colvard, M.A., et al. Amyl nitrate: use as a smooth muscle relaxant in difficult preterm cesarean section. *Am. J. Perinatol.* 9:289, 1992.

Lees, C., Campbell, S., Jauniaux, E., et al. Arrest of preterm labour and prolongation of gestation with glyceryl trinitrate, a nitric oxide donor. *Lancet* 343:1325, 1994.

Longmire, S., Leduc, L., Jones, M.M., et al. The hemodynamic effects of intubation during nitroglycerin infusion in severe preeclampsia. *Am. J. Obstet. Gynecol.* 164:551, 1991.

Plumer, M.H., and Rottman, R. How anesthesiologists practice obstetric anesthesia. *Reg. Anesth.* 21:49, 1996.

Poulton, T.J., and James, F.M. III. Reply to correspondence. *Anesthesiology* 51:475, 1979.

Ramsay, B., de Belder, A., Campbell, S., et al. A nitric oxide donor improves uterine artery diastolic blood flow in normal early pregnancy and in women at high risk of pre-eclampsia. *Eur. J. Clin. Invest.* 24:76, 1994.

Redick, L.F., Livingston, E., and Bell, E. Sublingual aerosol nitroglycerin for uterine relaxation in attempted external version. *Am. J. Obstet. Gynecol.* 176:497, 1997.

Robertson, R.M., and Robertson, D. Drugs used for the treatment of myocardial ischemia. Chapter 32 in *Goodman and Gilman's The*

Pharmacological Basis of Therapeutics (9th ed.), J.G. Hardman and L.E. Limbird, eds. New York: McGraw-Hill, 1996. Pp. 760–767.

Snyder, S.W., Wheeler, A.S., and James, F.M. The use of nitroglycerin to control severe hypertension of pregnancy during cesarean section. *Anesthesiology* 51:563, 1979.

Wessén, A., Elowsson, P., Axemo, P., et al. The use of intravenous nitroglycerin for emergency cervico-uterine relaxation. *Acta Anaesthesiol. Scand.* 39:847, 1995.

Writer, W.D.R., et al. Intracranial effects of nitroglycerin—an obstetrical hazard? *Anesthesiology* 53:S309, 1980.

Nonsteroidal Antiinflammatory Drugs: Diclofenac (Cataflam®, Voltaren®), Etodolac (Lodine®), Fenoprofen (Nalfon®), Flurbiprofen (Ansaid®), Ibuprofen (Advil®, Motrin®, Nuprin®, Rufen®), Ketorolac (Toradol®), Ketoprofen (Orudis®), Meclofenamate (Meclomen®), Mefenamic Acid (Ponstel®), Nambumetone (Relafen®), Naproxen (Anaprox®, Naprosyn®), Oxaprozin (Daypro®), Piroxicam (Feldene®), Tolmetin (Tolectin®)

INDICATIONS AND RECOMMENDATIONS

The use of nonsteroidal antiinflammatory drugs (NSAIDs) should be avoided during pregnancy, if possible, especially in the last trimester. If the administration of one of these drugs becomes necessary, as for the treatment of a chronic inflammatory state, ibuprofen appears to be the safest agent to use. In nonpregnant patients, NSAIDs are used in the treatment of various inflammatory states including osteoarthritis, rheumatoid arthritis, and dysmenorrhea.

SPECIAL CONSIDERATIONS IN PREGNANCY

Naproxen, diclofenac, and mefenamic acid treatment during pregnancy induced cleft palate in varying frequencies in the offspring of mice. Thus far, no teratogenic effects have been documented in humans.

All of the NSAIDs studied to date, including ibuprofen and naproxen, have been shown to cross the placenta; it must be assumed that all agents of this class have similar potential. NSAIDs act to inhibit cyclooxygenase and thus reduce the synthesis of prostaglandins; therefore, they all have the potential to cause adverse effects during pregnancy. They are known to prolong pregnancy and labor and to increase maternal blood loss. In the fetus and neonate, they can constrict and possibly close the ductus arteriosus, produce pulmonary hypertension, cause hemostatic abnormalities, reduce fetal renal output, and cause oligohydramnios.

Thus far, only naproxen use has been associated with these types of fetal hemodynamic problems. Hypoxemia due to persistent pulmonary hypertension, low prostaglandin E levels, premature closure of the ductus arteriosus, increased bilirubin levels, and abnormalities in blood clotting and renal function have been anecdotally reported to occur in infants born to mothers who received naproxen to delay delivery.

Most studies describing the use of NSAIDs during pregnancy report on their use as tocolytic agents. In this setting, ibuprofen, naproxen, and ketoprofen have been associated with constricting the ductus arteriosus and reducing fetal urine output, causing a decreased volume of amniotic fluid. There is evidence that both of these effects are reversible after discontinuation of the drug.

Reports of NSAID use during the first two trimesters are few. One report of 44 pregnant women with chronic inflammatory disease found that those who used NSAIDs in standard doses during pregnancy had no differences in pregnancy outcome, duration of labor, complications at delivery, or neonatal health when compared to controls who did not take NSAIDs. Specifically, the authors noted no sign of renal impairment, pulmonary hypertension, or premature closure of the ductus arteriosus in the newborns. Of the 44 treated patients, 23 took naproxen, 8 took ibuprofen, and the others took either indomethacin, ketoprofen, piroxicam, or aspirin; all were told to discontinue treatment during the last 4 weeks of pregnancy. Although the numbers of pregnancies studied is small, this is evidence that NSAID use during pregnancy (except at term) in patients with rheumatic disease may not adversely effect the neonate.

Maternal use of piroxicam for 15 days around the 26th week of gestation has been associated with fetal renal maldevelopment and oligohydramnios in the newborn. The renal anomalies seen were hypothesized to be due to reduction of renal blood flow caused by piroxicam.

Ketorolac, the only NSAID approved for parenteral use, has been used to treat the pain of labor. When compared to meperidine, ketorolac was found to have inferior analgesic properties, but it caused less maternal drowsiness and neonatal depression. One report of ketorolac given during labor documented significant inhibition of neonatal platelet function and recommended that the drug be used with caution in patients whose newborns are at risk for hemostatic problems. The manufacturer states that ketorolac is contraindicated for use during labor and delivery because it may cause inhibition of contractions and possible fetal effects.

When no alternative is available, ibuprofen, which has a short half-life and whose effects have been relatively well studied, should be used at the maximally tolerated dosage interval. Treatment should be discontinued in the third trimester.

All NSAIDs thus far studied appear to be minimally excreted in breast milk. The American Academy of Pediatrics considers ibuprofen, ketorolac, mefenamic acid, naproxen, tolmetin, and piroxicam to be compatible with breast-feeding.

DOSAGE

Each of these drugs has its own individual recommended dosing regimen. The following are the recommending dosage ranges for rheumatoid arthritis for some commonly used NSAIDs.

Drug	Daily dosage range for rheumatoid arthritis
Diclofenac	150–200 mg in 3–4 divided doses
Fenoprofen	1.2–2.4 g in 3–4 divided doses
Ibuprofen	1.2–3.2 g in 4 divided doses
Ketoprofen	150–300 mg in 3–4 divided doses
Meclofenamate	200–400 mg in 3–4 divided doses
Naproxen	500 mg–1.2 g in 2 divided doses
Piroxicam	20 mg qd
Tolmetin	1.2–1.8 g in 3–4 divided doses

ADVERSE EFFECTS

The most common adverse effects of NSAID use is gastric or intestinal irritation manifested as nausea, vomiting, diarrhea, and ulceration. Such irritation may lead to bleeding, ulceration, and perforation at any time with or without warning symptoms. NSAIDs may also cause acute renal insufficiency, interstitial nephritis, and renal papillary necrosis. Platelet function may be affected but is usually of shorter duration and quantitatively lesser effect than that seen with aspirin.

MECHANISM OF ACTION

The NSAIDs inhibit the activity of cyclooxygenase, the first enzyme in the prostaglandin synthesis pathway. Due to this common mechanism of action, they produce a similar array of therapeutic actions as well as adverse reactions.

ABSORPTION AND BIOTRANSFORMATION

NSAIDs are rapidly and almost completely absorbed from the gastrointestinal tract. Their elimination depends largely on hepatic biotransformation; metabolites are excreted in the urine. Nabumetone is an inactive prodrug converted by the liver to active metabolites.

RECOMMENDED READING

Brocks, D.R., and Jamali, F. Clinical pharmacokinetics of ketorolac tromethamine (published erratum appears in *Clin. Pharmacokinet.* 24:270, 1993). *Clin. Pharmacokinet.* 23:415, 1992.

Insel, P.A. Analgesic-antipyretic and antiinflammatory agents and drugs employed in the treatment of gout. Chapter 27 in *Goodman and Gilman's The Pharmacological Basis of Therapeutics* (9th ed.), J.G. Hardman and L.E. Limbird, eds. New York: McGraw-Hill, 1996. Pp. 617–642.

Kaplan, B.S., et al. Renal failure in the neonate associated with in utero exposure to non-steroidal anti-inflammatory agents. *Pediatr. Nephrol.* 8:700, 1994.

MacKenzie, I.Z., Graf, A.K., and Mitchell, M.D. Prostaglandins in the fetal circulation following maternal ingestion of a prostaglandin synthetase inhibitor during mid-pregnancy. *Int. J. Gynaecol. Obstet.* 23:455, 1985.

Menahem, S. Administration of prostaglandin inhibitors to the mother; the potential risk to the fetus and neonate with duct-dependent circulation. *Reprod. Fertil. Dev.* 3:489, 1991.

Montenegro, M.A., and Palomino, H. Induction of cleft palate in mice by inhibitors of prostaglandin synthesis. *J. Craniofac. Genet. Dev. Biol.* 10:83, 1990.

Nelson, J.L., and Ostensen, M. Pregnancy and rheumatoid arthritis. *Rheum. Dis. Clin. North Am.* 23:195, 1997.

Ostensen, M., and Ostensen, H. Safety of nonsteroidal antiinflammatory drugs in pregnant patients with rheumatic disease. *J. Rheumatol.* 23:1045, 1996.

Ostensen, M. Optimization of antirheumatic drug treatment in pregnancy. *Clin. Pharmacokinet.* 27:486, 1994.

Rudolph, A.M. The effects of non-steroidal antiinflammatory compounds on fetal circulation and pulmonary function. *Obstet. Gynecol.* 58:63S, 1981.

Townsend, R.J., et al. Excretion of ibuprofen into breast milk. *Am. J. Obstet. Gynecol.* 149:184, 1984.

Voyer, L.E., Drut, R., and Mendez, J.H. Fetal renal maldevelopment with oligohydamnios following maternal use of piroxicam. *Pediatr. Nephrol.* 8:592, 1994.

Walker, J.J., et al. A comparative study of intramuscular ketorolac and pethidine in labour pain. *Eur. J. Obstet. Gynecol. Reprod. Biol.* 46:87, 1992.

Wilkinson, A.R., Aynsley-Green, A., and Mitchell, M.P. Persistent pulmonary hypertension and abnormal prostaglandin E levels in preterm infants after maternal treatment with naproxen. *Arch. Dis. Child.* 54:942, 1979.

Witter, R.E. Clinical pharmacokinetics in the treatment of rheumatoid arthritis in pregnancy. *Clin. Pharmacokinet.* 25:444, 1993.

Norepinephrine, Levarterenol (Levophed®)

INDICATIONS AND RECOMMENDATIONS

The use of norepinephrine in pregnancy is controversial, and if used at all, it should be restricted to life-threatening situations. It is an adrenergic agent that has a preponderance of alpha activity and is used to treat shock. An increased frequency of uterine contractions has been noticed with its use. In addition, the uterine vasculature, thought to be maximally dilated during pregnancy, reacts to adrenergic stimulus solely by contracting. Radial arteries obtained from human myometrium at the time of cesarean section demonstrate a greater sensitivity to the vasoconstrictor activity of norepinephrine than similar arteries obtained from nonpregnant uteri. Such a decrease in uterine blood flow may adversely affect the fetus. Peripheral administration may cause vasoconstriction leading to local ischemia. Therefore if possible it should be administered into a large, preferably central vein. Should an adrenergic agent be required to treat hypotension associated with conduction anesthesia during pregnancy, ephedrine is the drug of choice. In other situations in which a vasopressor is needed to treat life-threatening hypotension, safer agents, such as dopamine or dobutamine, are the drugs of choice.

RECOMMENDED READING

Hoffman, B.B., and Lefkowitz, R.J. Catecholamines, sympathomimetic drugs, and adrenergic receptor antagonists. Chapter 10 in *Goodman and Gilman's The Pharmacological Basis of Therapeutics* (9th ed.), J.G. Hardman and L.E. Limbird, eds. New York: McGraw-Hill, 1996. Pp. 209–210.

Smith, N.T., and Corbascio, A. The use and misuse of pressor agents. *Anesthesiology* 33:58, 1970.

Steele, S.C., Warren, A.Y., and Johnson, I.R. Effect of the vascular endothelium on norepinephrine induced contractions in uterine radial arteries form the nonpregnant and pregnant human uterus. *Am. J. Obstet. Gynecol.* 168:1623, 1993.

Nystatin (Mycostatin®, Nilstat®)

INDICATIONS AND RECOMMENDATIONS

Nystatin is safe to use during pregnancy for the treatment of *Candida* infections of the skin, mucous membranes, and intestinal tract. It should not be applied vaginally when membranes have ruptured.

SPECIAL CONSIDERATIONS IN PREGNANCY

Because nystatin is effectively contained at the site of application, it is safe to use during pregnancy. Its use has not been associated with an increased incidence of spontaneous abortion or teratogenesis.

DOSAGE

Oral (available in 500,000 unit tablets for intestinal fungal infections): 0.5–1.0 million units tid; continue for 48 hours after clinical cure to prevent relapse.

Oral (available in 100,000 units/ml suspension for thrush): 400,000–600,000 units qid; retain in mouth as long as possible, continue for at least 2 days after symptoms have subsided.

Topical (available in 100,000 unit/g cream and powder for cutaneous or mucocutaneous candidiasis): Apply liberally bid-tid; continue applications for 1 week after clinical cure.

Vaginal (available in 100,000-unit vaginal tablets for vulvovaginal candidiasis): 100,000–200,000 units via applicator placed daily high in the vagina for 2 weeks.

ADVERSE EFFECTS

Untoward effects of nystatin are uncommon. Oral doses of more than 5 million units/day have caused nausea and gastrointestinal upset.

MECHANISM OF ACTION

Nystatin probably acts by binding to fungal cell membranes and creating a change in permeability of the membrane. This change allows leakage of essential small molecules out of the cell.

ABSORPTION AND BIOTRANSFORMATION

Nystatin is poorly absorbed from intact skin and mucous membranes. Absorption from the gastrointestinal tract is negligible and results in no detectable blood levels at recommended dosages.

RECOMMENDED READING

Bennett, J.E. Antimicrobial agents: antifungal agents. Chapter 49 in *Goodman and Gilman's The Pharmacological Basis of Therapeutics* (9th ed.), J.G. Hardman and L.E. Limbird, eds. New York: McGraw-Hill, 1996. P. 1188.

Ernest, J.M. Topical antifungal drugs. *Obstet. Gynecol. Clin. North Am.* 19:587, 1992.

Omeprazole (Prilosec®)

INDICATIONS AND RECOMMENDATIONS

Omeprazole is safe to use during pregnancy only when given as an adjunct to anesthesia prior to cesarean section. In a nonpregnant patient, omeprazole is used for the treatment duodenal ulcer, gastroesophageal reflux disease, and pathologic hypersecretory conditions.

SPECIAL CONSIDERATIONS IN PREGNANCY

Omeprazole is known to cross the human placenta. The experience with omeprazole use during pregnancy is contradictory. In one patient who took omeprazole 10 mg qd for esophageal reflux throughout two pregnancies, one pregnancy was terminated because the fetus was anencephalic, and the second pregnancy was also terminated because the fetus had severe talipes. Other women, however, have taken omeprazole throughout pregnancy for Zollinger-Ellison syndrome without adverse fetal effects. Because of the lack of any further data regarding the use of omeprazole early in pregnancy, the drug should be avoided.

Omeprazole has been used successfully to increase gastric pH and decrease gastric volume in women undergoing cesarean section. Although early studies using oral omeprazole indicate that it may be ineffective in maintaining gastric pH, subsequent studies using the intravenous route indicate that the drug can raise gastric pH higher than rantidine and, with metoclopramide, can significantly reduce gastric volume. Its use in this setting has not been associated with adverse fetal effects.

DOSAGE

The dosage usually given prior to cesarean section was 40 mg IV administered at the time of the decision to operate, at least 30 minutes prior to surgery.

ADVERSE EFFECTS

Omeprazole usually causes few adverse effects. Its use is associated with nausea, diarrhea, headache, dizziness, and somnolence. Skin rash and transient increase in hepatic enzymes are occasionally seen.

MECHANISM OF ACTION

Omeprazole is a prodrug that when activated by a low pH environment binds irreversibly to the proton pump of the parietal cell, inhibiting secretion of hydrogen ions into the gastric lumen. With chronic use, it can reduce daily production of acid by more than 95%.

ABSORPTION AND BIOTRANSFORMATION

Orally administered, omeprazole is rapidly but variably absorbed depending on the dose and the gastric pH. It is formulated as an enteric-coded granule because it is acid-labile. It is extensively bound to plasma proteins. Its plasma half-life is 30–90 minutes. Most of the drug is metabolized with the metabolites being excreted in the urine.

RECOMMENDED READING

Brunton, L.L. Agents for control of gastric acidity and treatment of peptic ulcers. Chapter 37 in *Goodman and Gilman's The Pharmacological Basis of Therapeutics* (9th ed.). J.G. Hardman and L.E. Limbird, eds. New York: McGraw-Hill, 1996. Pp. 907–909.

Harper, M.A., et al. Successful pregnancy in association with Zollinger-Ellison syndrome. *Am. J. Obstet. Gynecol.* 173:863, 1995.

Moore, J., et al. Effect of single dose omeprazole on intragastric acidity and volume during obstetric anesthesia. *Anaesthesia* 44: 559, 1989.

Orr, D.A., et al. Effects of omeprazole with and without metoclopramide, in elective anaesthesia. *Anaesthesia* 48:114, 1993.

Rocke, D.A., et al. Intravenous administration of the proton pump inhibitor omeprazole reduces the risk of acid aspiration at emergency cesarean section. *Anesth. Analg.* 78:1093, 1994.

Stuart, J.C., et al. Acid aspiration prophylaxis for emergency caesarean section. *Anaesthesia* 51:415, 1996.

Tripathi, A., et al. A comparison of intravenous rantidine and omeprazole on gastric volume and pH in women undergoing emergency caesarean section. *Can. J. Anaesth.* 42:797, 1995.

Tsirogitis, M., et al. Potential effects of omeprazole in pregnancy. *Hum. Reprod.* 10:2177, 1995.

Ondansetron (Zofran®)

INDICATIONS AND RECOMMENDATIONS

Ondansetron is an antiemetic agent that is particularly effective in treating nausea accompanying cancer chemotherapy and radiation. It has also been used with success as an intraoperative antiemetic in patients undergoing cesarean section under epidural anesthesia. Others have used this drug in managing refractory cases of hyperemesis gravidarum. There is little information available regarding pregnancy risks, including the potential for human teratology. Ondansetron is considerably more expensive than other antiemetics. The use of ondansetron during pregnancy should be limited to situations where other, better characterized alternatives are not effective, such as cancer chemotherapy and severe hyperemesis resistant to other antiemetics.

SPECIAL CONSIDERATIONS IN PREGNANCY

Animal teratology studies conducted by the manufacturer revealed no apparent harm to the fetuses at intravenous dosages up to 4 mg/kg/day. However, no data regarding potential human effects are available. There are three published case reports of ondansetron's use in the treatment of severe, and otherwise resistant, hyperemesis gravidarum at various stages of pregnancy, but always after 11 weeks. The drug was considered an alternative to parenteral nutrition and appeared to be quite successful. In a randomized trial of intravenous ondansetron versus promethazine for severe hyperemesis, Sullivan and co-workers were unable to find any measurable advantage with respect to relief of nausea, weight gain, days of hospitalization, or number of doses of medication required. There was clearly less sedation with ondansetron than with promethazine. The gestational age at treatment averaged 11 ± 2.7 weeks, so that an unknown number of patients received the drug during organogenesis. Pregnancy outcomes, including malformation rates, were not mentioned in this small series.

A randomized double-blind trial found that prophylactic intravenous ondansetron, administered after clamping of the umbilical cord, was as effective as droperidol, and significantly more effective than placebo, at preventing nausea and vomiting during cesarean section under epidural anesthesia. Ondansetron has also been reported to be effective in treating postoperative pruritus in two patients whose cesarean sections were performed using spinal morphine.

DOSAGE

Ondansetron can be administered intravenously or orally. There are two usual intravenous regimens for prevention of chemotherapy-induced nausea and vomiting. One consists of a single 32-mg dose infused over 15 minutes, beginning about 30 minutes before the start of chemotherapy. The other is the use of three doses of 0.15 mg/kg each, administered over 15 minutes, beginning about 30 minutes before the start of chemotherapy, and then again at 4 and 8 hours after the first dose. The usual dose for postoperative nausea and vomiting is 4 mg given over at least 30 seconds, and preferably over 2–5 minutes. In the randomized trial of treating hyperemesis gravidarum with ondansetron, the dose was 10 mg in 50 ml of compatible intravenous fluid given over 30 minutes. The case reports of its use for intractable hyperemesis both described dosages of 8 mg IV 3 times a day, in one case for 14 days and in the other for only 24 hours followed by oral dosing. The usual oral dose is 8 mg twice a day.

ADVERSE EFFECTS

Adverse effects have been rare. In view of the fact that the drug is generally used for cancer patients receiving chemotherapy, it may be difficult to distinguish adverse drug effects from effects of the underlying disease or its treatment. Although headache, constipation, dizziness, musculoskeletal pain, sedation, shivering, malaise, injection site reactions, and urinary retention were all reported by the manufacturer in 3% or more of patients receiving ondansetron, the rates of these events were not different from those seen in the patients receiving placebo. Similarly, liver function abnormalities have been reported but could not be ascribed to ondansetron rather than the cancers or the chemotherapeutic agents.

MECHANISM OF ACTION

Ondansetron specifically antagonizes the effect of serotonin on the 5-hydroxytryptamine (5-HT$_3$) receptors in the gastrointestinal tract, and probably also in the chemoreceptor trigger zone and the solitary tract nucleus. It is not a dopamine receptor antagonist.

ABSORPTION AND BIOTRANSFORMATION

The oral bioavailability of ondansetron is approximately 60%, and blood levels are attained 30–60 minutes after oral dosing. The plasma half-life is 3–4 hours, and the drug is metabolized by the liver. There are gender differences in pharmacokinetics, with women showing greater and more rapid absorption than men, as well as slower clearance. The clinical importance of these differences is not known, and the manufacturer makes no specific recommendations for different dosing schedules in men and women.

RECOMMENDED READING

Crighton, I.M., Hobbs, G.J., and Reid, M.F. Ondansetron for the treatment of pruritus after spinal opioids. *Anaesthesia* 51:199, 1996.

Glaxo Wellcome Oncology/HIV Company. Zofran (ondansetron hydrochloride). Entry in *Physicians Desk Reference* (52nd ed.). Montvale, NJ: Medical Economics, 1998. Pp. 1177–1183.

Guikontes, E., Spantideas, A., and Diakakis, J. Ondansetron and hyperemesis gravidarum. *Lancet* 340:1223, 1992.

Pan, P.H. Intraoperative antiemetic efficacy of prophylactic ondansetron versus droperidol for cesarean section patients under epidural anesthesia. *Anesth. Analg.* 83:982, 1996.

Sullivan, C.A., Johnson, C.A., Roach, H., et al. A pilot study of intravenous ondansetron for hyperemesis gravidarum. *Am. J. Obstet. Gynecol.* 174:1565, 1996.

Tincello, D.G., and Johnstone, M.J. Treatment of hyperemesis gravidarum with the 5-HT$_3$ antagonist ondansetron (Zofran). *Postgrad. Med. J.* 72:688, 1996.

World, M.J. Ondansetron and hyperemesis gravidarum. *Lancet* 341:185, 1993.

Paraldehyde (Paral®)

INDICATIONS AND RECOMMENDATIONS

Paraldehyde is relatively contraindicated during pregnancy because other therapeutic agents are preferable. It is a short-acting sedative-hypnotic used in the treatment of abstinence (from alcohol) phenomena and other psychiatric states characterized by excitement. It has also been used in the emergency treatment of various types of seizures.

Because of numerous reports of death from paraldehyde intoxication, and because of the tendency of the drug to become contaminated by corrosive decomposition products, it has been replaced by other drugs in most situations. Paraldehyde readily crosses the placenta and depression of the fetus has been reported with its use. It is recommended that agents such as magnesium sulfate, used for the prevention of convulsions in preeclampsia, and phenothiazine drugs, used as psychotherapeutic agents, be administered instead of paraldehyde.

RECOMMENDED READING

Hobbs, W.R., Rall, T.W., and Verdoorn, T.A. Hypnotics and sedatives; ethanol. Chapter 17 in *Goodman and Gilman's The Pharmacological Basis of Therapeutics* (9th ed.), J.G. Hardman and L.E. Limbird, eds. New York: McGraw-Hill, 1996. Pp. 380–381.

Kittel, J. Paraldehyde toxicity. *Hosp. Pharm.* 8:8, 1973.

Konje, J.C., et al. Presentation and management of eclampsia. *Int. J. Gynaecol. Obstet.* 38:31, 1992.

Penicillamine (Cuprimine®, Depen®)

INDICATIONS AND RECOMMENDATIONS

Penicillamine (dimethylcysteine), a chelating agent, may be used during pregnancy in patients with Wilson's disease, although the dose should be kept at or below 500 mg/day if possible. Because other forms of therapy are available, case reports of congenital cutis laxa and growth retardation make the use of this drug during pregnancy controversial in patients with cystinuria and rheumatoid arthritis. Penicillamine is also used for the acute treatment of heavy metal poisoning.

SPECIAL CONSIDERATIONS IN PREGNANCY

Penicillamine crosses the placenta and is capable of inducing fetal resorptions and congenital anomalies in laboratory animals. The mechanism for this is believed to be through fetal deficiency of certain metals, including copper and zinc. However, these speculations have not been confirmed to date.

A large number of case reports of penicillamine exposure during pregnancy have been reported in the literature. At least five neonates were noted to have generalized loose skin (cutis laxa). Three had inguinal hernias. There is some suggestion that the effect of penicillamine on the offspring might be dose-related, since one mother took 900 mg/day and the other three took 1.5–2.0 g/day throughout pregnancy. This has led to recommendations to reduce the dosage if possible.

If cutis laxa is related to penicillamine therapy, the case reports suggest that it is no more common than approximately 3% of exposures. It is problematic to make such an estimate in view of a lack of appropriate denominator figures; however, since normal outcomes are less apt to be reported than are abnormal ones, it is unlikely that the true incidence is higher than 3%. Reports of elevated serum copper levels in two affected offspring of mothers with Wilson's disease suggest that the cause may not be related to copper depletion; other heavy metals may be depleted by this therapy, and some investigators believe that zinc deficiency may be at fault. Whether zinc supplementation would be helpful has not been established.

Continued treatment with penicillamine is necessary to prevent recrudescence of Wilson's disease. The effects of this disorder can be life threatening, and it is thus reasonable to continue treatment during pregnancy, although at reduced dosage if possible. There are case reports of fulminant hepatic failure in untreated Wilson's disease during pregnancy, and of copper deposition in the placenta and high copper levels in the fetus in another untreated case. In cystinuria, the major problem is urinary calculus formation. High fluid intake and alkalinization may help prevent stones from forming. In patients who form stones despite these therapeutic interventions, penicillamine may be continued. The physician and patient must decide together whether the fetal risk outweighs the maternal benefit of this drug in a particular case. When the patient has rheumatoid arthritis, numerous other agents may be used. Thus, the physician is faced with a choice between the risk of fetal hemorrhage (salicylates), possible teratogenicity (gold), maternal adverse effects (corticosteroids), and so forth.

Penicillamine interferes with collagen formation and may delay wound healing. It is for this reason that reduction in dosage is recommended during the last 6 weeks of pregnancy.

No data have been found regarding breast milk excretion or the safety of breast-feeding for women taking penicillamine.

DOSAGE

Penicillamine is available as 250 mg tablets and capsules. For Wilson's disease, the patient is maintained on a low-copper diet and the drug is begun at 250–2000 mg/day (depending on the patient's tolerance of side effects). The dose is titrated against urinary copper excretion, the goal being to maintain negative copper balance. It is rarely necessary to prescribe more than 2 g/day. During pregnancy, the dosage should be as low as is compatible with maintenance of negative copper balance.

For cystinuria, the drug is initiated at 250 mg/day and increased to the point at which urinary cystine excretion is below 100 mg/day; 2 g/day is a common dose. Patients with cystinuria should also be instructed to drink enough water to maintain the urinary specific gravity below 1.010, take enough alkali to maintain the urinary pH at 7.5, and maintain a diet low in methionine.

When penicillamine is used to treat rheumatoid arthritis, it is usually initiated at a dose of 250 mg/day and increased in

250 mg/day increments every 2–3 months to achieve a therapeutic effect. Usual maintenance doses are 500–750 mg/day.

Penicillamine should be taken on an empty stomach (at least 1 hour after the last meal and before the next meal) to ensure appropriate absorption and to minimize gastrointestinal side effects.

ADVERSE EFFECTS

Allergic reactions have been reported in 5% of patients who take penicillamine, and these most often appear early in the course of therapy. They include fever, rashes, leukopenia, eosinophilia, and thrombocytopenia. For this reason, complete blood counts (including platelets) should be performed every 2 weeks during the first 6 months of therapy, and monthly thereafter. If allergic manifestations develop in a patient with Wilson's disease or one with cystinuria who has formed stones despite a high fluid intake and alkalinization, it may be necessary to desensitize the patient and resume therapy because alternative forms of treatment are not available.

Other adverse effects include gastrointestinal disturbance (anorexia, nausea, vomiting, abdominal pain), seen in 17% of patients, decreased taste sensation, proteinuria, tinnitus, optic neuritis, myasthenia gravis, and a variety of other problems. The development of insulin antibodies accompanied by severe hypoglycemia has been reported in two patients with rheumatoid arthritis who were treated with penicillamine.

It should be emphasized that penicillamine has many side effects and that these problems occur in a high proportion of individuals who take the drug. It is only for conditions that are serious and not amenable to other forms of treatment that penicillamine is appropriate.

MECHANISM OF ACTION

Penicillamine is prepared by hydrolysis of penicillin. It is an effective chelator of copper, mercury, zinc, and lead, leading to an increased urinary excretion of these metals. In Wilson's disease, in which ceruloplasmin, the copper-carrying plasma protein, is deficient, copper builds up in various tissues. Penicillamine increases copper excretion. In patients with cystinuria, large amounts of cystine appear in the urine. Cystine (a disulfide composed of two cysteine molecules) is relatively insoluble and forms renal stones, especially in acid urine. Penicillamine forms a disulfide with cysteine, which is considerably more soluble than cystine, thus lowering the potential for stone formation. The mechanism of penicillamine's action against rheumatoid arthritis is not understood at present.

ABSORPTION AND BIOTRANSFORMATION

Penicillamine is rapidly absorbed after oral dosing, with peak plasma levels being achieved at approximately 130 minutes. Absorption is decreased by concomitant intake of foods, antacids, and iron. Plasma half-life is 60.7 ± 8.2 minutes. Approximately 20% of an oral dose is excreted in the urine within 24 hours, and 50% appears in the stool.

RECOMMENDED READING

Albukerk, J.N. Wilson's disease and pregnancy. A case report. *Fertil. Steril.* 24:494, 1973.

Arbisser, A.I., Scott, C.I., Jr., and Howell, R.R. Mannosidosis and maternal penicillamine therapy. *Lancet* 1:312, 1976.

Benson, E.A., Healey, L.A., and Barron, E.J. Insulin antibodies in patients receiving penicillamine. *Am. J. Med.* 78:857, 1985.

Endres, W. d-Penicillamine in pregnancy—to ban or not to ban? *Klin. Wochenschr.* 59:535, 1981.

Fukuda, K., et al. Pregnancy and delivery in penicillamine treated patients with Wilson's disease. *Tohoku J. Exp. Med.* 123:270, 1977.

Gregory, M.C., and Mansell, M.A. Pregnancy and cystinuria. *Lancet* 2:1158, 1983.

Harpey, J.P., et al. Cutis laxa and low serum zinc after antenatal exposure to penicillamine. *Lancet* 2:858, 1983.

Keen, C.L., Lonnerdal, B., and Hurley, L.S. Drug-induced copper deficiency: a model for copper deficiency teratogenicity. *Teratology* 28:155, 1983.

Klaassen, C.D. Heavy metals and heavy-metal antagonists. Chapter 66 in *Goodman and Gilman's The Pharmacological Basis of Therapeutics* (9th ed.), J.G. Hardman and L.E. Limbird, eds. New York: McGraw-Hill, 1996. Pp 1667–1668.

Laver, M., and Fairley, K.F. d-Penicillamine treatment in pregnancy. *Lancet* 1:1019, 1971.

Linares, A., et al. Reversible cutis laxa due to maternal d-penicillamine treatment. *Lancet* 2:43, 1979.

Lyle, W.H. Penicillamine in pregnancy. *Lancet* 1:606, 1978.

Marecek, Z., and Graf, M. Pregnancy in penicillamine-treated patients with Wilson's disease. *N. Engl. J. Med.* 295:841, 1976.

Mjolnerod, O.K., et al. Congenital connective-tissue defect probably due to d-penicillamine treatment in pregnancy. *Lancet* 1:673, 1971.

Nunns, D., Hawthorne, B., Goulding, P., et al. Wilson's disease in pregnancy. *Eur. J. Obstet. Gynecol.* 62:141, 1995.

Oga, M., Matsui, N., Anai, T., et al. Copper disposition of the fetus and placenta in a patient with untreated Wilson's disease. *Am. J. Obstet. Gynecol.* 169:196, 1993.

Scheinberg, I.H., and Sternlieb, I. Pregnancy in penicillamine-treated patients with Wilson's disease. *N. Engl. J. Med.* 293:1300, 1975.

Shimono, N., Ishibashi, H., Ikematsu, H., et al. Fulminant hepatic failure during perinatal period in a pregnant woman with Wilson's disease. *Gastroenterologia Japonica* 26:69–73, 1991.

Solomon, L., et al. Neonatal abnormalities associated with d-penicillamine treatment during pregnancy. *N. Engl. J. Med.* 296:54, 1977.

Toaff, R., et al. Hepatolenticular degeneration (Wilson's disease) and pregnancy. *Obstet. Gynecol. Surv.* 32:497, 1977.

Walshe, J.M. Pregnancy in Wilson's disease. *Q. J. Med.* (new series) 181:73, 1977.

Penicillins: Amoxicillin (Amoxil®, Larotid®), Ampicillin (Omnipen®, Polycillin®), Bacampicillin (Spectrobid®), Carbenicillin (Geocillin®), Cloxacillin (Cloxapen®, Tegopen®), Dicloxacillin (Dycill®, Dynapen®), Methicillin (Staphcillin®), Mezlocillin (Mezlin®), Nafcillin (Nafcil®, Unipen®), Oxacillin (Bactocill®, Prostaphlin®), Penicillin G, Penicillin V, Piperacillin (Pipracil®), Ticarcillin (Ticar®), Amoxicillin and Potassium Clavulanate (Augmentin®), Ampicillin and Sulbactam (Unasyn®), Piperacillin and Tazobactam (Zosyn®), Ticarcillin and Clavulanate Potassium (Timentin®)

INDICATIONS AND RECOMMENDATIONS

Penicillins are safe to use during pregnancy in nonallergic patients. These compounds are among the most effective and least toxic antimicrobials available. The family consists of natural and semisynthetic compounds that have differing spectra and pharmacologic properties. There is a paucity of clinical experience with the more recently released penicillins (e.g., piperacillin, mezlocillin, and bacampicillin). These newer drugs should, therefore, be considered only when another, better studied antibiotic cannot be used.

The lactamase inhibitors—sulbactam, clavulanic acid, and tazobactam—are combined with individual penicillins to increase their efficacy against resistant organisms. Amoxicillin combined with potassium clavulanate and ampicillin combined with sulbactam appear to be safe for the treatment of preterm premature rupture of the membranes.

SPECIAL CONSIDERATIONS IN PREGNANCY

Penicillin G and most of the other penicillins appear in the amniotic fluid and fetal blood and tissues. There is no evidence that any of these agents is teratogenic.

Plasma levels of several of the penicillins (i.e., ampicillin, penicillin G, penicillin V, and piperacillin) as well as sulbactam have been shown to be lower in pregnant patients than in nonpregnant women receiving equivalent dosages. Their volumes of distribution and plasma clearances are higher and their half-lives shorter during pregnancy. In order to maintain adequate blood and tissue levels, therefore, it is recommended that these agents be prescribed at a higher dosage or a more frequent dosing interval. While the trend may be similar for other penicillins, further studies must be undertaken to determine the pharmacokinetics of each agent.

In in vitro testing, ticarillin and clavulanic acid have been shown to achieve relatively low fetal levels at therapeutic maternal concentrations. Therefore, other agents with similar activities but superior transfer should be used for the treatment of intrauterine infections.

While amoxicillin plus clavulanate and ampicillin plus sulbactam have been used with success to treat preterm premature rupture of the membranes and to prevent infection in infants exposed to antenatal steroids, their efficacy in these situations has not been proven. The lactamase inhibitors, however, do not appear to be detrimental to fetus or mother when used near term.

Penicillins appear in breast milk and may cause diarrhea and candidiasis in the nursing infant. Sulbactam is excreted into breast milk in very small quantities. The maximum exposure to a nursing infant has been calculated to be approximately 0.7 mg/kg/day.

DOSAGE

Dosage Chart for Penicillins

Drug	Route	Dose[a]	Interval
Penicillin G	IM	600,000–1.2 million units	q12–24h
	IV	1–5 million units	q4–6h
Penicillin V	PO	250–500 mg	q6h
Methicillin	IM/IV	1–2 g	q4–6h
Nafcillin	PO	250–1000 mg	q4–6h
	IM/IV	500 mg	q4–6h
Oxacillin	PO	500 mg	q4–6h
	IM/IV	250–1000 mg	q4–6h
Cloxacillin	PO	250–500 mg	q6h
Dicloxacillin	PO	125–250 mg	q6h
Ampicillin	PO	250–1000 mg	q6h
	IM/IV	500–2000 mg	q4–6h
Amoxicillin	PO	250–500 mg	q8h
Carbenicillin	PO[b]	382–764 mg	q6h
Ticarillin	IM/IV	1–3 g	q4–6h
Mezlocillin	IM/IV	2–4 g	q6h
Piperacillin	IM/IV	3–4 g	q4–6h
Bacampicillin	PO	400–800 mg	q6h
Ampicillin and[c] sulbactam	IV/IM	1.5 g–3 g	q6h
Piperacillin and[c] tazobactam	IV	3.375 g	q6h

Drug	Route	Dose[a]	Interval
Amoxicillin and[d] clavulanate	PO	500 mg	q12h
Ticarillin and[c] clavulanate	IV	3.1 g	q4–6h

[a]Dosage may require reduction in the face of renal impairment.
[b]For treatment of urinary tract infections only.
[c]Dose expressed as total Ampicillin & sulbactam, piperacillin & tazobactam, or ticarillin & clavulanate.
[d]Dose expressed as amoxicillin only.

ADVERSE EFFECTS

The penicillins are reported to be among the most common causes of drug allergy. The severity of allergic reactions ranges from a mild rash to anaphylaxis. The most common side effects of orally administered penicillins are nausea, vomiting, epigastric distress, diarrhea, and black hairy tongue. Penicillins are irritating to the central and peripheral nervous systems, especially at very high dosages and in patients with impaired renal function. As parenteral formulations may contain large quantities of sodium or potassium, electrolyte imbalances may occur with intravenous therapy. Candidal vaginitis is a common sequel to penicillin therapy, presumably because of suppression of normal vaginal flora. Interstitial nephritis has been associated primarily with methicillin, whereas oxacillin has been implicated as the cause of a reversible hepatotoxicity and neutropenia.

MECHANISM OF ACTION

This group of antibiotics acts by interfering with cell wall synthesis. They are therefore more effective when organisms are actively dividing. In general, the penicillins are active against gram-positive cocci and bacilli and some gram-negative bacilli; some have a broader spectrum and are active against many gram-negative bacilli. No penicillin is active against viruses, mycobacteria, plasmodia, fungi, or rickettsiae.

The lactamase inhibitors—clavulanic acid, sulbactam, and tazobactam—are molecules that combine with certain lactamases to inactivate them, thus preventing the destruction of lactam antibiotics, including penicillins. Although they are poor antibiotics alone, the lactamase inhibitors increase the efficacy of penicillins against lactamase-producing strains of *Staphylococcus, Haemophilus influenzae, Escherichia coli,* and other aerobic gram-negative bacilli. They do not increase a penicillin's activity against *Pseudomonas* species.

ABSORPTION AND BIOTRANSFORMATION

The penicillins are variably absorbed from the gastrointestinal tract and are widely distributed throughout the body. They diffuse into ascitic fluid and attain high concentrations in lungs, intestine, and liver. The penicillins are concentrated in bile. Only small amounts diffuse into cerebrospinal fluid, with penetration being greater through inflamed meninges. Penicillins are bound to plasma proteins to varying degrees; the free drug appears to be the active form. Most penicillins are primarily excreted unchanged in the urine, with only small amounts being inactivated by the liver. The latter mode of elimination assumes more importance in the presence of renal failure. The half-lives of the penicillins are in general short, ranging from 30 to 90 minutes. In an anuric patient, half-lives may be as high as 10 hours. Concomitant administration of probenecid increases and prolongs serum penicillin levels by competitively inhibiting renal tubular secretion and thus slowing the rate of penicillin elimination.

RECOMMENDED READING

Adamkin, D.H., Marshall, E., and Weiner, L.B. The placental transfer of ampicillin. *Am. J. Perinatol.* 1:310, 1984.

Adlercreutz, H., et al. Effect of ampicillin administration on plasma, conjugated and unconjugated estrogen, and progesterone levels in pregnancy. *Am. J. Obstet. Gynecol.* 128:266, 1977.

Campbell, B.A., and Cox, S.M. The penicillins. *Obstet. Gynecol. Clin. North Am.* 19:435, 1992.

Chamberlain, A., et al. Pharmacokinetics of ampicillin and sulbactam in pregnancy. *Am. J. Obstet. Gynecol.* 168:667, 1993.

Cox, S.M., et al. Randomized investigation of antimicrobials for the prevention of preterm birth. *Am. J. Obstet. Gynecol.* 174:206, 1996.

Duff, P. Antibiotic selection in obstetric patients. *Infect. Dis. Clin. North Am.* 11:1–12, 1997.

Garland, S.M., and O'Reilly, M.A. The risks and benefits of antimicrobial therapy in pregnancy. *Drug Safety* 13:188, 1995.

Heikkila, A., and Erkkola, R. Review of beta-lactam antibiotics in pregnancy. The need for adjustment of dosage schedules. *Clin. Pharmacokinet.* 27:49–62, 1994.

Landers, D.V., Green, M.D., and Sweet, R.L. Antibiotic use during pregnancy and the postpartum period. *Clin. Obstet. Gynecol.* 26:391, 1983.

Lovett, S.M. A prospective, double-blind randomized, controlled clinical trial of ampicillin-sulbactam for preterm premature rupture of membranes in women receiving antenatal corticosteroid therapy. *Am. J. Obstet. Gynecol.* 176:1030, 1997.

Mandell, G.L., and Petri, Jr., W.A. Antimicrobial agents: penicillins, cephalosporins, and other β-lactam antibiotics. Chapter 44 in *Goodman and Gilman's The Pharmacological Basis of Therapeutics* (9th ed.), J.G. Hardman and L.E. Limbird, eds. New York: McGraw-Hill, 1996. Pp. 1073–1089.

Philipson, A. Pharmacokinetics of ampicillin during pregnancy. *J. Infect. Dis.* 136:370, 1977.

Ray, J.G. Lues-lues: maternal and fetal considerations of syphilis. *Obstet. Gynecol.* Survey 50:845, 1995.

Wright, A.J., and Wilkowski, C.J. The penicillins. *Mayo Clin. Proc.* 58:21, 1983.

Pentamidine (Pentam®)

Pentamidine isethionate is an aromatic diamidine agent that is used intramuscularly to treat a number of protozoan infections, such as trypanosomiasis and leishmaniasis. However, its most important use in the United States is in the prophylaxis and treatment of mild to moderate *Pneumocystis carinii* pneumonia (PCP), a very common opportunistic infection in AIDS patients. When used for prophylaxis the drug is administered as an aerosolized spray. Presumably, there would be little systemic absorption through the lungs and thus little potential for fetal exposure. Although trimethoprim-sulfamethoxazole is more commonly used for PCP prophylaxis and appears to be safe in pregnancy, pentamidine may also be used for this purpose. The use of intravenous or intramuscular pentamidine to treat PCP during pregnancy should be avoided if possible, because of unknown but potential fetal risks and the availability of other forms of treatment. However, when other alternatives are not practical or effective, consideration should be given to counseling the patient appropriately and using intravenous pentamidine for severe disease in patients with $pO_2 < 70$ torr.

SPECIAL CONSIDERATIONS IN PREGNANCY

In studies of laboratory rats, intravenous pentamidine was transferred to the fetus in significant amounts. Doses similar to those used to treat humans resulted in increased pregnancy resorptions compared to placebo. In studies utilizing the isolated perfused human placenta, however, little transfer of pentamidine could be detected.

Pentamidine has not been demonstrated to be teratogenic in animals or humans, but data addressing this issue are scant. Because pentamidine has a high affinity for lung tissue, minimal blood levels result from use of aerosolized spray.

The American College of Obstetricians and Gynecologists suggests that prophylaxis is indicated in pregnant patients with CD4 cell levels less than 200/mm^3 and those with symptoms, with the first-line drug being trimethoprim-sulfamethoxazole. This organization recommends intravenous pentamidine as an alternative treatment for those with severe disease.

DOSAGE

The usual parenteral dose of pentamidine is 4 mg/kg daily for 14 days. Lower doses may produce less toxicity and have similar efficacy. The dose of aerosolized pentamidine recommended for prophylaxis against PCP is 300 mg every 4 weeks administered by nebulizer over 30–45 minutes.

ADVERSE EFFECTS

When pentamidine is administered intravenously or intramuscularly, side effects are quite common. Rapid intravenous administration may be accompanied by a sudden fall in blood pressure, breathlessness, tachycardia, dizziness, fainting, headache, and/or vomiting. Other significant side effects of pentamidine include pancreatitis, hyperglycemia, hypoglycemia, skin rashes, thrombophlebitis, thrombocytopenia, anemia, neutropenia, liver enzyme elevation, and nephrotoxicity. Inhaled aerosolized pentamidine may be associated with cough and bronchospasm.

MECHANISM OF ACTION

The mechanism of action of pentamidine is not entirely clear, but proposals have included folic acid antagonism, interference with glycolysis, and inhibition of nucleic acid synthesis.

ABSORPTION AND BIOTRANSFORMATION

Pentamidine is well absorbed after parenteral administration and has a plasma half-life of approximately 6 hours. However, the drug tends to accumulate in tissues and may be detectable in the urine 6 weeks after a 13-day course. Aerosol inhalation of pentamidine leads to accumulation of the drug in lung tissues and little systemic absorption.

RECOMMENDED READING

American College of Obstetricians and Gynecologists. *Human Immunodeficiency Virus Infections in Pregnancy.* ACOG Educational Bulletin #232. Washington, DC: ACOG, 1997.

Connelly, R.T., and Lourwood, D.L. Pneumocystis carinii pneumonia prophylaxis during pregnancy. *Pharmacotherapy* 14:424, 1994.

Conover, B., Goldsmith, J.C., Buehler, B.A., et al. Aerosolized pentamidine and pregnancy. *Ann. Intern. Med.* 109:927, 1988.

Fortunato, S.J., and Bawdon, R.E. Determination of pentamidine transfer in the in vitro perfused human cotyledon with high-performance liquid chromatography. *Am. J. Obstet. Gynecol.* 160:759, 1989.

Harstad, T.W., Little, B.B., Bawdon, R.E., et al. Embryofetal effects of pentamidine isethionate administered to pregnant Sprague-Dawley rats. *Am. J. Obstet. Gynecol.* 163:912, 1990.

Little, B.B., Harstad, T.H., Bawdon, R.E., et al. Pharmacokinetics of pentamidine in Sprague-Dawley rats in late pregnancy. *Am. J. Obstet. Gynecol.* 164:927, 1991.

Minkoff, H.L., and Moreno, J.D. Drug prophylaxis for human immunodeficiency virus-infected pregnant women: ethical considerations. *Am. J. Obstet. Gynecol.* 163:111, 1990.

Minkoff, H. Human immunodeficiency virus infections in pregnancy. Chapter 1 in *Current Obstetric Medicine,* Vol. 4, R.V. Lee, P.R. Garner, W.M. Barron, and D.R. Coustan, eds. St. Louis: CV Mosby, 1996. Pp. 1–18.

Tracy, J.W., and Webster, L.T., Jr. Drugs used in the chemotherapy of protozoal infections. Chapter 41 in *Goodman and Gilman's The Pharmacological Basis of Therapeutics* (9th ed.), J.G. Hardman and L.E. Limbird, eds. New York: McGraw-Hill, 1996. Pp. 999–1001.

Phenazopyridine (Pyridium®)

INDICATIONS AND RECOMMENDATIONS

Phenazopyridine is relatively contraindicated in pregnancy because other therapeutic agents are preferable. It is an azo dye that exhibits an analgesic action on the urinary tract. It is used only to alleviate the symptoms of lower urinary tract mucosal irritation, including burning, urgency, and frequency. It is not a urinary tract antiseptic. Phenazopyridine is known to cross the placenta and can reach levels of 13 μg/ml in amniotic fluid. It has been used in some obstetric patients without reported adverse fetal effects. Because it is indicated only for symptomatic treatment, it is best to treat the underlying cause of the irritation rather than to administer a drug with unknown fetal effect.

RECOMMENDED READING

Heinonen, O.P., Slone, D., and Shapiro, S. *Birth Defects and Drugs in Pregnancy.* Littleton, MA: PSG, 1977. Pp. 299–308.

Myer, B.A., Gonik, B., and Creasy, R.K. Evaluation of phenazopyridine hydrochloride as a tool in the diagnosis of premature rupture of the membranes. *Am. J. Perinatol.* 8:297, 1991.

Phenazopyridine and phenazopyridine hydrochloride. *I.A.R.C. Monogr. Eval. Carcinog. Risk Chem. Hum.* 24:163, 1980.

Phencyclidine (Angel Dust, PCP)

INDICATIONS AND RECOMMENDATIONS

Phencyclidine, originally developed as an anesthetic agent but now widely used as a street drug, is contraindicated in pregnancy. It is administered by smoking, snorting, swallowing, or injecting, and may also be absorbed through the skin. Acute effects of phencyclidine use include euphoria, dizziness, ataxia, dysarthria, nystagmus, and psychosis. Deaths have been reported and have been attributed to convulsions, cardiac and respiratory arrest, or hypertensive crisis. There are no known indications for phencyclidine use, and there is both animal and anecdotal human evidence suggesting possible teratogenicity, but solid data are lacking. Phencyclidine crosses the placenta, with fetal concentrations approximately twice maternal levels. The placenta is also capable of phencyclidine biotransformation. Neonatal jitteriness and hypertonicity, poor attention span, and depressed reflexes have been reported after chronic maternal phencyclidine use; this presumed behavioral teratogenesis was long-lasting. Animal studies suggest that phencyclidine is concentrated in breast milk at as much as 10 times maternal blood levels. One survey in an urban population reports a 0.8% incidence of phencyclidine use during pregnancy.

RECOMMENDED READING

Glantz, J.C., and Woods, J.R., Jr. Cocaine, heroin and phencyclidine: obstetric perspectives. *Clin. Obstet. Gynecol.* 36(2):279, 1993.

Golden, N.L., Sokol, R.J., and Rubin, I.L. Angel dust: possible effects on the fetus. *Pediatrics* 65:18, 1980.

Golden, N.L., et al. Phencyclidine use during pregnancy. *Am. J. Obstet. Gynecol.* 148:254, 1984.

Golden, N.L., Kuhnert, B.R., Sokol, R.J., et al: Neonatal manifestations of maternal phencyclidine exposure. *J. Perinat. Med.* 15: 185, 1987.

Nicholas, J.M., Lipshitz, J., and Schreiber, E.C. Phencyclidine: its transfer across the placenta as well as into breast milk. *Am. J. Obstet. Gynecol.* 143:143, 1982.

Rayburn, W.F., Holsztynska, E.F., and Domino, E.F. Phencyclidine: biotransformation by the human placenta. *Am. J. Obstet. Gynecol.* 148:111, 1984.

Strauss, A.A., Modanlou, H.D., and Bosu, S.K. Neonatal manifestations of maternal phencyclidine (PCP) abuse. *Pediatrics* 68:550, 1981.

Phenobarbital

INDICATIONS AND RECOMMENDATIONS

The epileptic gravida can be reassured that most pregnant women with epilepsy have a successful pregnancy outcome, although there is an increased risk of congenital malformations (2–3 times that seen in the normal population). It is unclear as to whether this increase is due to the disease itself or the medications given to help control the disease. Whenever possible, a single medication for control of seizures is preferable to multiple drug regimens. Phenobarbital can be administered to pregnant women for the treatment of status epilepticus, generalized tonic-clonic and simple partial seizures. It is only minimally effective against complex partial seizures and not useful in the treatment of absence seizures. It is not recommended for the stimulation of fetal hepatic enzymes. Phenobarbital has also been used in an attempt to prevent/minimize intracranial hemorrhage. Some studies indicate a reduction in moderate and severe intracranial hemorrhage in infants born at less than 35 weeks or weighing less than 1250 g, but the results of the most recent placebo-controlled trial with more than 600 women involved indicate that antenatal administration of phenobarbital does not decrease the risk of intracranial hemorrhage or early death in preterm infants.

SPECIAL CONSIDERATIONS IN PREGNANCY

Phenobarbital rapidly crosses the placenta. It has been implicated as a possible teratogen causing cleft lip, congenital heart disease, microcephaly, and decreased intellectual performance. Thus far, the data are not conclusive.

Phenobarbital induces the production of fetal liver enzymes, including the glucuronyl transferase needed for bilirubin conjugation and excretion, and consequently has been recommended for both the prevention and treatment of neonatal hyperbilirubinemia. Enzyme induction is also associated with an increased rate of steroid metabolism and altered vitamin D metabolism. Neonatal hypocalcemia has been reported. Coagulopathies resulting from a decrease in vitamin K-dependent clotting factors have been seen in neonates after ingestion of phenobarbital by the mother. This tendency can be reversed by administration of vitamin K_1 (10 mg/day) to the mother during the last month of the pregnancy. Withdrawal symptoms are commonly seen in neonates whose mothers have taken 90–120 mg phenobarbital daily for at least 12 weeks before delivery.

Maternally ingested phenobarbital is present in breast milk. The milk/plasma ratio is sufficiently high that the ingested neonatal dose may reach 2–4 mg/day. The American Academy of Pediatrics recommends that phenobarbital be used with caution during lactation. The WHO Working Group on Drugs and Human Lactation considers phenobarbital use during breast-feeding to be unsafe.

DOSAGE

In the treatment of epilepsy, the usual adult maintenance dose of phenobarbital is 60–200 mg (orally or parenterally) once daily. The therapeutic plasma concentration is 10–25 µg/ml. Dosage requirements may increase during pregnancy as a result of the fall in drug concentration seen in 60% to 85% of patients. This decline in concentration is not associated with an increased incidence of seizures in most patients, and at least one study has shown that drug level monitoring did not improve seizure control in pregnancy.

ADVERSE EFFECTS

Side effects include sedation, paradoxic irritability or hyperactivity in children, and confusion in the elderly. Nystagmus and ataxia are seen at excessive dosages. Megaloblastic anemia and osteomalacia have been associated with long-term phenobarbital therapy. Rare idiosyncratic reactions include scarlatiniform or morbilliform rashes, exfoliative dermatitis, agranulocytosis, and hepatitis. One study found that individuals exposed to phenobarbital in utero had lower verbal IQ scores than unexposed controls. Phenobarbital enhances the cytochrome P_{450} system, which may lead to increased degradation of steroid hormones. Increased degradation of the steroid hormones in birth control pills may allow ovulation. All anticonvulsants interfere with folic acid metabolism. Periconceptional and first-trimester folic acid supplementation (0.4 mg/day) is recommended in women on maintenance phenobarbital therapy.

MECHANISM OF ACTION

Phenobarbital increases the seizure threshold and limits the spread of seizure activity. These effects may be due to an augmented response to γ-aminobutyric acid (GABA), an inhibitory synaptic transmitter, without an increased level of this compound in the brain.

Barbiturates depress the activity of all excitable tissue, with the central nervous system being the most sensitive. There is little effect on skeletal, cardiac, or smooth muscle at therapeutic dosages. By its combination with cytochrome P_{450} and induction of hepatic microsomal enzymes, phenobarbital alters the metabolism of other drugs.

ABSORPTION AND BIOTRANSFORMATION

Phenobarbital is well absorbed through the small intestine and from intramuscular injection sites. Approximately 40% to 60% of the drug is protein-bound. From 10% to 25% is excreted unchanged in the urine; this process is enhanced by alkalization and diuresis. The liver microsomal oxidizing system metabolizes the remaining drug, after which metabolites are excreted by the kidney. The half-life in adults is 2–6 days; it is longer in neonates and shorter in children.

RECOMMENDED READING

Committee on Drugs, American Academy of Pediatrics. The transfer of drugs and other chemicals into human breast milk. *Pediatrics* 93:137, 1994.

Friis, B., and Sardemann, H. Neonatal hypocalcemia after intrauterine exposure to anticonvulsant drugs. *Arch. Dis. Child.* 52: 239, 1977.

Lander, C.M., and Eadie, M.J. Plasma antiepileptic drug concentrations during pregnancy. *Epilepsia* 32:257, 1991

McNamara, J.O. Drugs effective in the therapy of the epilepsies. Chapter 20 in *Goodman and Gilman's The Pharmacological Basis of Therapeutics* (9th ed.), J.G. Hardman and L.E. Limbird, eds. New York: McGraw-Hill, 1996. Pp. 471–472.

Reinisch, J.M., Sanders, S.A., Mortensen, E.L., and Rubin, D.B. In utero exposure to phenobarbital and intelligence deficits in adult men. *J.A.M.A.* 274:1518, 1995

Seizure Disorders in Pregnancy. American College of Obstetricians and Gynecologists Educational Bulletin #231, December 1996.

Shankaran, S., Cepeda, E., Muran, G., et al. Antenatal phenobarbital therapy and neonatal outcome. I: Effect on intracranial hemorrhage. *Pediatrics* 99:751, 1997.

Shankaran, S., Papile, L.A., Wright, L., et al. The effect of antenatal phenobarbital therapy on neonatal intracranial hemorrhage in preterm infants. *N. Engl. J. Med.* 337, 1997

The WHO Working Group, and Bennet, P.N., eds. *Drugs and Human Lactation.* Amsterdam: Elsevier Science, 1988. Pp. 329–330.

Wilder, B.J., and Bruni, J. *Seizure Disorders: A Pharmacological Approach to Treatment.* New York: Raven Press, 1981.

Woodbury, D.M., Penry, J.K., and Pippenger, C.L. *Antiepileptic Drugs* (2nd ed.). New York: Raven Press, 1982.

Phenols (Over-the-Counter)

INDICATIONS AND RECOMMENDATIONS

Phenols may be used safely during pregnancy in over-the-counter preparations containing dilute solutions. They should not be used in a strength greater than a 2% aqueous solution or on broken skin.

These drugs are used as an antiseptic in mouthwashes as well as in dermatologic and anorectal preparations. Hexylresorcinol is the phenol most commonly used in mouthwashes. Thymol, while used in mouthwashes, is more frequently employed as a remedy for acne, hemorrhoids, and tinea pedis. Phenols have also been used alone or in combination with calamine lotion as an antipruritic agent. Phenol is found in many throat lozenges, where it acts as a topical anesthetic.

SPECIAL CONSIDERATIONS IN PREGNANCY

No unusual maternal effects have been described during pregnancy, and no mutagenic or teratogenic effects have been reported. Convulsions, hepatic toxicity, and bone marrow depression are possible problems if toxic levels were to reach the fetus.

DOSAGE

Hexylresorcinol is used in a 1:1000 concentration in mouthwashes. The various phenols are utilized in different concentrations, with all being absorbed to some degree.

ADVERSE EFFECTS

Significant skin penetration may occur when phenols are applied topically in solutions that are stronger than 2% aqueous or 4% in glycerin. This can result in tissue necrosis and systemic absorption. Erythema associated with some sloughing may occur. Cardiovascular effects include myocardial depression with secondary hypotension. Central nervous system action includes hypothermia. Ulceration of the stomach may occur if phenols are taken orally.

MECHANISM OF ACTION

Phenols are bacteriostatic as a 0.2% solution, bactericidal as a 1% solution, and fungicidal at 1.3% or greater. They combine with skin proteins to form a toxic substance. Phenol also acts as a topical anesthetic. These drugs are more effective in an acid media, at higher temperatures, and in aqueous solution.

ABSORPTION AND BIOTRANSFORMATION

After being absorbed, about 80% is excreted by the kidney either unchanged or as a glucuronide. The remainder is oxidized to hydroquinone and pyrocatechol.

RECOMMENDED READING

Nelson, M.M., and Forfar, J.O. Associations between drugs administered during pregnancy and congenital abnormalities of the fetus. *Br. Med. J.* 1:523, 1971.

Schenkel, B., and Vorherr, H. Non-prescription drugs during pregnancy: potential teratogenic and toxic effects upon embryo and fetus. *J. Reprod. Med.* 12:27, 1974.

Phenothiazines: Chlorpromazine (Thorazine®), Fluphenazine (Prolixin®), Perphenazine (Trilafon®), Prochlorperazine (Compazine®), Promethazine (Phenergan®), Thioridazine (Mellaril®), Trifluoperazine (Stelazine®)

INDICATIONS AND RECOMMENDATIONS

The use of phenothiazines during pregnancy should be limited to treatment of psychotic patients who require continued medication or for severe nausea and vomiting. They are also used in the treatment of anxiety and restlessness, but safer alternatives are available. Phenothiazines have also been used to diminish fetal erythroblastosis with inconclusive results.

SPECIAL CONSIDERATIONS IN PREGNANCY

Based on sheep and human studies, phenothiazines may pose a threat of maternal hypotension and consequent uteroplacental insufficiency. Phenothiazines may also amplify fetal response to umbilical cord compression. There have been five reported cases of shock after the administration of phenothiazines to patients with pheochromocytomas, including one pregnant woman.

The Collaborative Perinatal Study evaluated 1309 children exposed to phenothiazines during the first 4 months in utero. The overall rates of congenital malformations were similar among these exposed children and the 48,973 unexposed offspring without apparent dose effect. A statistically significantly higher rate of malformations (3.5% among exposed and 1.6% among controls) among phenothiazine-exposed individuals was identified in a prospective French study of first trimester exposure among 315 women. However, this observation has not been repeated and may simply reflect the large number of comparisons made. Case reports of five infants have questioned an association of prochlorperazine to variable types of limb defects but this association has not been observed in large prospective cohort studies. In summary, reports of birth defects in phenothiazine exposed infants do not show a pattern of phenothiazine-associated defects and cohort studies show no consistent increase in any type of defect or increase in the overall rate of birth defects compared to usually observed populational rates.

Anecdotally, infants born to mothers who received phenothiazines during pregnancy have been reported to suffer from extrapyramidal effects lasting up to 6 months, but a significant increase in symptomatic infants has not been associated with its use in cohort studies. Case reports have also noted jaundice, mild sedation followed by motor excitement, agitation, hypertonicity, depression, and chromosomal abnormalities in infants. Neonatal fever, ileus, and episodic cyanosis have also been associated with maternal use of phenothiazines. However, these conditions have not been shown to be more prevalent in cohort studies of drug use in pregnancy.

Several studies have documented the presence of phenothiazines in the breast milk of nursing mothers, but with a single exception, all state that no adverse effects have been noted in either the mother or the infant. A study of chlorpromazine in four nursing mothers documented maternal plasma levels of 16–52 ng/ml, milk levels of 7–98 ng/ml (two were greater than corresponding maternal plasma levels), and one neonatal plasma level of 7 ng/ml measured in the case with the highest milk level. One infant demonstrated drowsiness. The Committee on Drugs of the American Academy of Pediatrics has concluded that chlorpromazine's effect on breast-fed infants' neurologic function is unknown but may be of concern.

DOSAGE

Phenothiazine dosage should be individualized according to the severity of the condition, the patient's age, and the clinical response. It should be administered in divided doses during the first few weeks of therapy, but thereafter may be administered in a once- daily or twice-daily regimen. Fluphenazine is also available in injectable forms that may be administered every 2 weeks.

As an antiemetic, prochlorperazine may be given as an oral tablet, 5 or 10 mg q4–6h, or as a rectal suppository, 25 mg q12h. The intramuscular dose is 5–10 mg q6h. Promethazine is given orally, rectally, or intramuscularly, 12.5–25.0 mg q4–6h.

Dosage range of phenothiazines for psychosis[a]

Drug	Usual daily dosage range PO or IM (mg)	Maximum daily dose (mg)
Chlorpromazine	50–800	2000
Fluphenazine	2.5–20.0	40
Perphenazine	8–24	64
Thioridazine[b]	50–600	800
Trifluoperazine	2–15	64

[a]Prochlorperazine and promethazine are discussed in more detail in the text.
[b]Only given orally.

ADVERSE EFFECTS

Side effects of phenothiazines include drowsiness, postural hypotension, and anticholinergic effects, including dry mouth, constipation, mydriasis and cycloplegia, urinary retention, and tachycardia, but tolerance usually develops. Because phenothiazines depress the mechanism for heat regulation they may cause hyperthermia or hypothermia, depending on ambient temperature. Parkinsonism, dystonia, lowered convulsive threshold, photosensitivity, and blood dyscrasias have also been noted occasionally with their use.

MECHANISM OF ACTION

Effects of phenothiazines may be due to blockade of dopamine receptors and dopamine release in the caudate nucleus, and to inhibition of the dopamine activation of adenyl cyclase. In the brainstem, the inflow of stimuli to the reticular formation is selectively decreased. Most phenothiazine derivatives exert a depressant action on the chemoreceptor trigger zone, thereby suppressing emesis due to conditions in which this center is stimulated.

ABSORPTION AND BIOTRANSFORMATION

The phenothiazines are generally rapidly absorbed from the gastrointestinal tract and from parenteral injection sites, and readily cross the placenta. They are highly soluble and strongly bound to plasma proteins. Inactivation occurs largely through oxidation by hepatic microsomal enzymes.

RECOMMENDED READING

Ananth, J. Side effects in the neonate from psychotropic agents excreted through breast-feeding. *Am. J. Psychiatry* 135:801, 1977.

Baldessarini, R.J. Drugs and the treatment of psychiatric disorders. Chapter 18 in *Goodman and Gilman's The Pharmacological Basis of Therapeutics* (9th ed.), J.G. Hardman and L.E. Limbird, eds. New York: McGraw-Hill, 1996. Pp. 400–420.

Cleary, M.F. Fluphenazine decanoate during pregnancy. *Am. J. Psychiatry* 134:7, 1977.

Committee on Drugs of the American Academy of Pediatrics. The transfer of drugs and other chemicals into human milk. *Pediatrics* 93:137, 1994.

Cottle, M.K.W., Van Petten, G.R., and van Muyden, P. Maternal and fetal cardiovascular indices during fetal hypoxia due to cord compression in chronically cannulated sheep: II. Responses to promazine. *Am. J. Obstet. Gynecol.* 146:686, 1983.

Montiminy, M., and Teres, D. Shock after phenothiazine administration in a pregnant patient with a pheochromocytoma. *J. Reprod. Med.* 28:159, 1983.

McElhatton, P.R. The use of phenothiazines during pregnancy and lactation. *Reprod. Toxicol.* 6:475, 1992.

Rumeau-Rouquette, C., Goujard, J., and Huel, G. Possible teratogenic effect of phenothiazines in human beings. *Teratology* 15:57, 1977.

Slone, D., et al. Antenatal exposure to the phenothiazines in relation to congenital malformations, perinatal mortality rate, birth weight, and intelligence quotient score. *Am. J. Obstet. Gynecol.* 128:486, 1977.

Stenchever, M.A. Promethazine hydrochloride: Use in patients with Rh isoimmunization. *Am. J. Obstet. Gynecol.* 130:665, 1978.

Wiles, D.H., Orr, M.W., and Kolakowska, T. Chlorpromazine levels in plasma and milk of nursing mothers. *Br. J. Clin. Pharmacol.* 5:272, 1978.

Phenoxybenzamine (Dibenzyline®)

INDICATIONS AND RECOMMENDATIONS

The use of phenoxybenzamine during pregnancy should be limited to the treatment of hypertension due to pheochromocytoma. Acute hypertensive crises associated with pheochromocytoma, however, should be controlled with intravenous phentolamine. Phenoxybenzamine then becomes the drug of choice for oral maintenance therapy. Control of blood pressure during cesarean section or during surgery to remove the tumor should also be maintained with intravenous phentolamine.

SPECIAL CONSIDERATIONS IN PREGNANCY

Untreated pheochromocytoma during pregnancy has been associated with maternal and fetal mortality rates of up to 48% and 47%, respectively. It is presumed that most of these deaths were due to maternal cardiovascular problems that led to fetal anoxia. Phenoxybenzamine has been used successfully in all three trimesters of pregnancy for the treatment of hypertension secondary to pheochromocytoma without serious adverse effect on the neonate. One case report associates a maternal/fetal plasma concentration ratio of 1.6 after prolonged maternal therapy with neonatal respiratory depression and transient hypotension at term. Reported clinical experience and pediatric follow-up is very limited, however, suggesting caution in its use during pregnancy.

One case of premature rupture of the membranes following 3 days of phenoxybenzamine therapy in the 26th week of pregnancy has been reported. The subsequent hypertensive crisis was controlled by phentolamine. A 640-g infant was born 21 hours later and died shortly thereafter. One instance of maternal and fetal tachycardia after parenteral administration of phenoxybenzamine has been reported. The child was normal at follow-up 8 years later.

DOSAGE

Only the oral form of phenoxybenzamine is currently available for use in the United States. The usual oral dose for treatment of pheochromocytoma is an initial dose of 10 mg twice daily 1–3 weeks prior to surgery. This can then be raised by 10-mg increments every second day until the desired response is obtained.

ADVERSE EFFECTS

The most frequently noticed side effects are due to α-adrenergic blockade and vary with the degree of blockade. These include postural hypotension, reflex tachycardia, miosis, and nasal congestion. Sedation, nausea, and vomiting are also seen. Patients with hypovolemia may suffer from a sharp fall in blood pressure when this drug is administered. Because pregnancy is often associated with postural hypotension, care in observing this effect is warranted.

MECHANISM OF ACTION

Phenoxybenzamine produces α-adrenergic blockade by establishing stable bonds at receptor sites, thus reducing the total population of available α receptors and decreasing responses mediated by their excessive stimulation. β-Adrenergic stimulation is consequently unopposed. Vasodilatation in various vascular beds depends in part on the degrees of α-adrenergic and β-adrenergic control.

Normal subjects who are standing and receive phenoxybenzamine slowly by the intravenous route show little change in blood pressure, although diastolic values tend to fall; in normal recumbent subjects, however, a precipitous fall in blood pressure occurs. Cerebral and coronary vascular resistance is not altered greatly. Hypertension due to excessive catecholamine production in patients with pheochromocytoma can be controlled by the oral administration of phenoxybenzamine.

ABSORPTION AND BIOTRANSFORMATION

From 20% to 30% of an oral dose of phenoxybenzamine is absorbed from the gastrointestinal tract. The drug is primarily excreted in the urine, with 50% being eliminated in the first 12 hours and 80% being eliminated in 24 hours.

RECOMMENDED READING

Brenner, W.E., et al. Pheochromocytoma: Serial studies during pregnancy. *Am. J. Obstet. Gynecol.* 113:779, 1972.

Hoffman, B.B., and Lefkowitz, R.J. Catecholamines, sympathomimetic drugs, and adrenergic receptor antagonists. Chapter 10 in *Goodman and Gilman's The Pharmacological Basis of Therapeutics* (9th ed.), J.G. Hardman and L.E. Limbird, eds. New York: McGraw-Hill, 1996. Pp. 225–229.

Griffith, M.I., et al. Successful control of pheochromocytoma in pregnancy. *J.A.M.A.* 229:437,1974.

Leak, D., et al. Management of pheochromocytoma during pregnancy. *Can. Med. Assoc. J.* 116:371, 1977.

Maughan, G.B., Shabanah, E.H., and Toth, A. Experiments with pharmacologic sympatholysis in the gravid. *Am. J. Obstet. Gynecol.* 97:764, 1967.

Santeiro, M.L., Stromquist, C., and Wyble, L. Phenoxybenzamine placental transfer during the third trimester. *Ann. Pharmacother.* 30(11): 1249, 1996.

Phensuximide (Milontin®)

INDICATIONS AND RECOMMENDATIONS

Phensuximide is contraindicated for use during pregnancy because other therapeutic agents are preferable. This drug is one of the succinimide group of anticonvulsants used in the treatment of absence seizures. It was the first of these compounds to be introduced for therapy, but low efficacy and toxic effects have relegated it to a secondary role. Experience with phensuximide in pregnancy is limited. In three cases in which other antiepileptic medications were also administered, fetal abnormalities including ambiguous genitalia, inguinal hernia, and pyloric stenosis were reported. When therapy for absence seizures is indicated during pregnancy, ethosuximide is the drug of choice.

RECOMMENDED READING

Annegers, J.F., et al. Do anticonvulsants have a teratogenic effect? *Arch. Neurol.* 31:364, 1974.

Fabro, S., and Brown, N.A. Teratogenic potential of anticonvulsants. *N. Engl. J. Med.* 300:1280, 1979.

Fedrick, J. Epilepsy and pregnancy: a report from the Oxford record linkage study. *Br. Med. J.* 2:442, 1973.

Heinonen, O.P., Slone, D., and Shapiro, S. *Birth Defects and Drugs in Pregnancy.* Littleton, MA: PSG, 1977. Pp. 358–359.

McMullin, G.P. Teratogenic effects of anticonvulsants. *Br. Med. J.* 2:430, 1971.

McNamara, J.O. Drugs effective in the treatment of the epilepsies. Chapter 20 in *Goodman and Gilman's The Pharmacological Basis of Therapeutics* (9th ed.), J.G. Hardman and L.E. Limbird, eds. New York: McGraw-Hill, 1996. Pp. 475–476.

National Institutes of Health. Anticonvulsants found to have teratogenic potential. *J.A.M.A.* 241:36, 1981.

Phentolamine (Regitine®)

INDICATIONS AND RECOMMENDATIONS

The use of phentolamine during pregnancy should be limited to the treatment of acute hypertensive episodes in patients with pheochromocytoma and for the immediate preoperative and intraoperative management of such a patient undergoing cesarean section for delivery of the infant and removal of the tumor. Both mother and fetus should be monitored carefully during the procedure.

SPECIAL CONSIDERATIONS IN PREGNANCY

Phentolamine should not be used as a diagnostic or chronic therapeutic agent for pheochromocytoma in the pregnant patient because its use may cause maternal hypotension and result in fetal hypoxia. Safer diagnostic tests, such as bioassays and chemical assays for catecholamines, are available.

Phenoxybenzamine is the agent of choice for preoperative management of pheochromocytoma. Phentolamine, however, is given intravenously for the control of hypertension during delivery or tumor removal. One case of a baby born with "jitters" following treatment of the mother with phentolamine and guanethidine has been reported, although other cases have been reported with no observed perinatal effects.

Human teratogenicity studies are lacking. Studies of rodents given 20–30 times the therapeutic human dose did not demonstrate birth defects. Phentolamine may have tocolytic effects on uterine muscle.

DOSAGE

For use in preoperative reduction of elevated blood pressure, 5 mg IV or IM is given 1–2 hours before surgery and repeated if necessary. During surgery, 5 mg may be administered intravenously to prevent or control paroxysms of hypertension, tachycardia, or other effects of epinephrine intoxication. The 5-mg dose is also used for treatment of acute hypertensive crises and may be repeated as necessary. Blood pressure should be monitored frequently for 10 minutes after injection. Norepinephrine may be used to reverse hypotension.

ADVERSE EFFECTS

The primary side effects of phentolamine are caused by gastrointestinal and cardiac stimulation. Gastrointestinal symptoms include pain, nausea, vomiting, diarrhea, and exacerbation of peptic ulcer. Cardiac stimulation may lead to tachycardia, angina, and cardiac arrhythmias, especially after parenteral administration. Death due to hypoglycemia has been observed with chronic overdosage.

MECHANISM OF ACTION

Phentolamine is a moderately effective α-adrenergic blocker; vasodilatation produced at dosages usually used in adults, however, results primarily from its direct effect on vascular smooth muscle. Only high dosages produce characteristic α-adrenergic blockade. The drug increases circulatory catecholamines in normal patients.

Clinical manifestations of pheochromocytoma result from the secretion of catecholamines. Vasodilatation produced by phentolamine causes a fall in blood pressure, especially in patients with pheochromocytoma. The hypotension may be potentially severe in such patients.

ABSORPTION AND BIOTRANSFORMATION

Phentolamine is absorbed after oral administration, but the drug is less than 20% as active when given orally than when given by parenteral administration. Approximately 10% of an intravenous dose is recovered unchanged in the urine. The fate of the remaining drug is unknown.

RECOMMENDED READING

Brenner, W.E., et al. Pheochromocytoma: serial studies during pregnancy. *Am. J. Obstet. Gynecol.* 113:779, 1972.

Griffith, M.I., et al. Successful control of pheochromocytoma in pregnancy. *J.A.M.A.* 229:437, 1974.

Leak, D., Carroll, J.J., and Robinson, D.C. Management of pheochromocytoma during pregnancy. *Can. Med. Assoc. J.* 116: 371, 1977.

Maughan, G.B., Shabanah, E.H., and Toth, A. Experiments with pharmacologic sympatholysis in the gravid. *Am. J. Obstet. Gynecol.* 97:764, 1967.

Phenylbutazone (Butazolidin®)

INDICATIONS AND RECOMMENDATIONS

The use of phenylbutazone should be limited to a 4-day course of treatment for an attack of acute gouty arthritis. Gout is uncommon in women and rarely seen before menopause. If treatment of an acute attack becomes necessary during pregnancy, a short course of phenylbutazone is preferable to the use of colchicine or allopurinol. Monitoring of blood counts, serum electrolytes, and fluid balance is mandatory. This drug is a potent antiinflammatory agent, a poor analgesic, and a weak antipyretic agent. It is contraindicated for the treatment of rheumatoid arthritis and allied disorders during pregnancy because aspirin or corticosteroids are preferable therapeutic agents.

SPECIAL CONSIDERATIONS IN PREGNANCY

Phenylbutazone causes marked sodium and water retention accompanied by decreased urinary output and increased plasma volume up to 50%. Since plasma volume in pregnancy is already expanded, cardiac decompensation could result from the administration of this drug. In addition, phenylbutazone, a prostaglandin synthetase inhibitor, could theoretically cause constriction of the ductus arteriosus in utero and may reduce fetal urine output with secondary oligohydramnios and can inhibit labor and prolong pregnancy (see "Nonsteroidal Antiinflammatory Agents"). Observation of amniotic fluid volume before and during use of this or other nonsteroidal antiinflammatory drugs may be helpful but the utility of Doppler monitoring of fetal ductal velocity in this circumstance has not been established.

The risk of teratogenesis in humans is unknown. The package insert states that animal studies, though inconclusive thus far, exhibit evidence of embryotoxicity. Phenylbutazone has been reported in breast milk in small amounts, but is not considered a contraindication to breast-feeding.

DOSAGE

The recommended dose to be used for an attack of gouty arthritis is 200 mg PO qid for the first day followed by 100 mg PO tid for 3 additional days.

ADVERSE EFFECTS

Side effects are noted in 10% to 45% of patients who take phenylbutazone and include nausea, vomiting, epigastric discomfort, skin rashes, diarrhea, vertigo, insomnia, euphoria, nervousness, and edema. Drug-related complications include peptic ulceration, serum sickness–like hypersensitivity reactions, hepatitis, nephritis, and bone marrow suppression. Phenylbutazone administration increases the risk of bleeding in patients taking warfarin derivatives. Because of its toxicity potential its use has been largely replace by other NSAIDs.

MECHANISM OF ACTION

The mechanism of action of the antiinflammatory effects of phenylbutazone is not known. Like the salicylates, this drug inhibits the biosynthesis of prostaglandins, uncouples oxidative phosphorylation, and inhibits the adenosine triphosphate (ATP)–dependent biosynthesis of mucopolysaccharide sulfates in cartilage. The uricosuric effect results from diminished tubular reabsorption of uric acid. Sodium and chloride retention also results from a direct effect on the renal tubules. The excretion of potassium is not changed. Phenylbutazone reduces iodine uptake by the thyroid gland by a direct action that inhibits the synthesis of organic iodine compounds.

Other antiinflammatory drugs, oral anticoagulants, oral hypoglycemic agents, sulfonamides, and some other drugs may be displaced from binding proteins by phenylbutazone. This can result in an increased pharmacologic or toxic effect of the displaced drug.

ABSORPTION AND BIOTRANSFORMATION

Phenylbutazone is rapidly absorbed from the gastrointestinal tract, and peak levels are reached in 2 hours. The drug is 98% bound to plasma proteins, and the serum half-life is 50–100 hours.

Phenylbutazone is almost entirely metabolized in the liver. Oxyphenbutazone, one of the two metabolites, has pharmacologic and toxic properties similar to those of the parent compound. Both phenylbutazone and oxyphenbutazone are slowly excreted in the urine since binding to plasma proteins limits their glomerular filtration. Because of their slow metabolism and excretion, these compounds may accumulate in considerable quantities during long-term administration.

RECOMMENDED READING

Committee on Drugs, American Academy of Pediatrics. The transfer of drugs and other chemicals into human breast milk. *Pediatrics* 93: 137, 1994.

Goldfinger, S.E. Treatment of gout. *N. Engl. J. Med.* 285:1303, 1971.

Insel, P.A. Analgesic-antipyretic and antiinflammatory agents and drugs employed in the treatment of gout. Chapter 27 in *Goodman and Gilman's The Pharmacological Basis of Therapeutics* (9th ed.), J.G. Hardman and L.E. Limbird, eds. New York: McGraw-Hill, 1996. Pp. 642–643.

Phosphodiesterase III inhibitors: Amrinone (Inocor®), Milrinone (Primacor®)

INDICATIONS AND RECOMMENDATIONS

Both amrinone and milrinone, phosphodiesterase III inhibitors, are used as short-term vasodilators in advanced congestive cardiac failure. Because of the potential for teratogenicity and the availability of alternate drugs, amrinone should be avoided during the first trimester of pregnancy. In limited rodent studies milrinone was not found to be teratogenic, but its chemical similarity to amrinone suggests that it too should be avoided if alternative drugs are available.

SPECIAL CONSIDERATIONS IN PREGNANCY

Amrinone is teratogenic, producing skeletal and gross external malformations in rabbits but not in other rodents. Few data are available regarding teratogenicity of milrinone; there have been no findings of teratogenic effect at doses of 5 mg/kg/day (less than with clinical use in humans). However, its structural similarity with amrinone suggests that it should be avoided in the first trimester. In one baboon study uterine blood flow was not affected by maternal amrinone infusion though it did cause external iliac artery dilatation. Use of milrinone in ewes and baboons was not observed to disturb fetal cardiovascular homeostasis or acid–base balance. In one reported case of amrinone use during pregnancy complicated by severe congestive heart failure, a 2 µg/kg/min infusion rate produced maternal ventricular ectopy limiting dosage. Fetal/neonatal blood levels of milrinone have been observed to be about 25% of those in maternal plasma.

DOSAGE

Amrinone is given as a loading bolus injection of 0.5 µg/kg, followed by a 2 to 20 µg/kg/min infusion. The loading dose of milrinone is usually 50 µg/kg, followed by a 0.25–1.0 µg/kg/min infusion.

ADVERSE EFFECTS

Compared to either digoxin or placebo, a randomized trial has found no increased efficacy of amrinone but an increase in cardiac arrhythmias. Other observations have noted an increase in hypotension and syncope.

MECHANISM OF ACTION

Both drugs are bipyridine derivative inhibitors of type III cyclic AMP phosphodiesterase, which acts to reduce peripheral vascular resistance, reduce preload pressure, increase cardiac contraction force and rate of myocardial relaxation. However, milrinone, is preferred because of its increased specificity for PDE III isoenzymes, shorter half-life, and fewer side effects, including thrombocytopenia. Because of increased cardiac morbidity and mortality among patients randomized to oral therapy with this class of drugs, its use is limited to short-term duration, usually in combination with other intravenous drugs.

ABSORPTION AND BIOTRANSFORMATION

Amrinone has a half-life of 2–4 hours and milrinone of 0.5–1.0 hours depending on individual rates of acetylation. Clearance is decreased in congestive heart failure and uremia. Thirty-five percent to 49% is bound in plasma. Toxicity is common at plasma concentrations higher than 2.5 µg/ml.

RECOMMENDED READING

Atkinson, B.D., Fishburne, J.L., Jr., Hales, K.A., Levy, G.H., and Rayburn, W.F. Placental transfer of milrinone in the nonhuman primate (baboon). *Am. J. Obstet. Gynecol.* 174:895, 1996.

DiBianco, R., Shabetai, R., Kostuk, W., Moran, J., Schlant, R.C., and Wright, R. for the Milrinone Trial Group. A comparison of oral milrinone, digoxin, and their combination in the treatment of patients with chronic heart failure. *N. Engl. J. Med.* 320:677, 1989.

Fishburne, J.L.,Jr., Dormer, K.J., Payne, G.G., Gill, P.S., Ashrafzadeh, A.R., and Rossavik, I.K. Effects of amrinone and dopamine on uterine blood flow and vascular responses in the gravid baboon. *Am. J. Obstet. Gynecol.* 158:829, 1988.

Jelsema R.D., Bhatia, R.K., and Ganguly, S. Use of intravenous amrinone in the short-term management of refractory heart failure in pregnancy. *Obstet. Gynecol.*78:935, 1991

Kelly, R.A., and Smith, T.W. Pharmacological treatment of heart failure. Chapter 34 in *Goodman and Gilman's The Pharmacological Basis of Therapeutics* (9th ed.), J.G. Hardman and L.E. Limbird, eds. New York: McGraw-Hill, 1996. Pp. 829–834.

Ono, C., Ishitobi, H., Iwama, A., Fujiwara, M., and Shibata, M. Reproductive and developmental toxicity studies in rats and rabbits given milrinone (YM018) intravenously. *Oyo Yakuri* 46:305, 1993.

Santos, A.C., Baumann, A.L., Wlody, D., Pederson, H., Morishima, H.O., and Finster, M. The maternal and fetal effects of milrinone and dopamine in normotensive pregnant ewes. *Am. J. Obstet. Gynecol.* 166:257, 1992.

Piperazine (Antepar®)

INDICATIONS AND RECOMMENDATIONS

Piperazine is relatively contraindicated in pregnancy. Usually considered to be a second-line drug, it is an oral antiparasitic agent that is highly effective against *Ascaris lumbricoides* and *Enterobius vermicularis* infections. It paralyzes the parasite by blocking the response of the neuromuscular junction to acetylcholine, allowing the worm to be expelled by peristalsis. There is little information available regarding piperazine's use in pregnancy. In the Collaborative Perinatal Project there were only three cases of piperazine exposure reported, with no malformations found. There is a single case report of hand and foot anomalies in an exposed neonate. Piperazine is known to be absorbed into the maternal bloodstream, with 15% to 75% recoverable in the urine as active drug and metabolite, and may, therefore, have adverse effects on the fetus. A piperazine derivative, bisheteroypiperazine, is being tested as a nonnucleoside reverse transcriptase inhibitor for HIV-1 infections, and was demonstrated to cross the placenta freely. As the infections for which piperazine is commonly used are not life threatening and because treatment can safely be postponed, it is best to defer treatment until after delivery.

RECOMMENDED READING

Heinonen, O.P., Lone, D., and Shapiro, S. *Birth Defects and Drugs in Pregnancy*. Boston: PSG, 1977. P. 299.

Meyer, H.H., and Brenner, P. Spalthand- und spaltfussmissbildung als eine mögliche teratogene nebenwirkung des anthelminticums piperazin? *Internist* 29:217, 1988.

Roberts, S., Bawdon, R., Sobhi, S., et al. The maternal-fetal transfer of bisheteroypiperazine (U-87201-E) in the ex vivo human placenta. *Am. J. Obstet. Gynecol.* 172:88, 1995.

Tracy, J.W., and Webster, L.T., Jr. Drugs used in the chemotherapy of helminthiasis. Chapter 42 in *Goodman and Gilman's The Pharmacological Basis of Therapeutics* (9th ed.), J.G. Hardman and L.E. Limbird, eds. New York: McGraw-Hill, 1996. P. 1020.

Villar, M.A., and Sibai, B.M. Nematode infections: is it wise to withhold medical treatment during pregnancy? *Am. J. Obstet. Gynecol.* 166:549, 1992.

Potassium Chloride, Oral (Kaochlor®, Kaon-Cl®, K-Lor®, Klotrix®, K-Lyte/Cl®, K-Tab®, Micro-K®, Slow-K®)

INDICATIONS AND RECOMMENDATIONS

Oral potassium chloride is safe to use during pregnancy. It is indicated for treatment or prophylaxis of potassium deficiency. Serum potassium levels should be followed when this compound is administered. It may be necessary to prescribe potassium chloride when a pregnant woman is taking thiazide diuretics for control of hypertension.

SPECIAL CONSIDERATIONS IN PREGNANCY

Fetal potassium levels are dependent on maternal potassium levels. Fetal bradycardia due to heart block has been reported in association with hypokalemia in the mother.

DOSAGE

The usual dose is 16–24 mEq/day for prevention of hypokalemia and 40–100 mEq/day or more for treatment of potassium depletion. Oral potassium should be taken with a full glass of water or orange juice. Measurement of serial serum potassium levels should be used to monitor efficacy of therapy. The chloride salt of potassium should be given because failure to replace chloride will enhance the potassium loss in metabolic alkalosis.

Potassium chloride is available in a variety of dosage forms, including liquids of 10% (20 mEq/15 ml) and 20% (40 mEq/15 ml) strengths; powders providing 15, 20, and 25 mEq/dose; and wax matrix tablets in 8 or 10 mEq strengths. In addition there is a gelatin capsule containing 8 mEq potassium chloride embedded in polymer-coated crystalline particles. Although enteric-coated tablets are available, their use is not recommended as they are associated with an increased incidence of intestinal ulceration.

ADVERSE EFFECTS

Side effects of excessive oral potassium supplementation include vomiting, diarrhea, nausea, and abdominal discomfort. Toxicity is more likely to occur in conditions such as oliguria, azotemia, acute dehydration, and untreated Addison's disease. Manifestations of toxicity include paresthesias of the extremities, flaccid paralysis, listlessness, mental confusion, weakness, and decrease in blood pressure. Electrocardiographic changes include loss of the P wave, widening of the QRS complex, ST segment changes, and tall peaked T waves.

MECHANISM OF ACTION

The mechanisms of action of potassium on skeletal, cardiac, and smooth muscle, and its renal and metabolic effects, are beyond the scope of this book. The reader is referred to a current textbook of physiology.

Causes of potassium deficiency include diarrhea, vomiting, decreased intake, increased renal excretion (as in diuresis, acidosis, or adrenocortical hyperactivity), increased cellular uptake (as in treatment of diabetic ketoacidosis), persistent alkalosis, and familial periodic paralysis.

RECOMMENDED READING

Klotrix and other slow-release potassium tablets. *Med. Lett. Drugs Ther.* 23:1, 1981.
Micro-K potassium therapy. *Med. Lett. Drugs Ther.* 24:71, 1982.

Potassium Iodide

INDICATIONS AND RECOMMENDATIONS

The prolonged use of potassium iodide, or any iodide, is contraindicated during pregnancy and lactation due to the effect of iodide on the fetal thyroid gland. Potassium iodide is used in antifungal and expectorant medications, and its use in chronic, large daily doses is contraindicated. A short course of potassium iodide in the treatment of thyroid storm, or prior to maternal thyroid surgery, does not carry this risk to the fetus.

Administration of large daily doses of this agent to pregnant rats results in a decrease in pup number, various malformations, and behavioral abnormalities in the pups. Iodide readily crosses the placenta to the fetus. Prolonged use, or use close to term, can cause fetal/neonatal goiter, with consequences such as tracheal compression and death. Iodide is concentrated in breast milk. The average iodide content of breast milk was recently assessed and is considerably higher than previously reported. The higher levels are probably due to dietary iodide supplements, such as in salt, bread, and cow's milk. The significance to the nursing infant of higher levels of iodide is unknown. However, the American Academy of Pediatrics, although recognizing the potential effect on the infant's thyroid function, considers the agents to be compatible with breast-feeding.

RECOMMENDED READING

Carswell, F., Kerr, M.M., and Hutchison, J.H. Congenital goiter and hypothyroidism produced by maternal ingestion of iodides. *Lancet* 1:1241, 1970.
Committee on Drugs, American Academy of Pediatrics. The transfer of drugs and other chemicals into human milk. *Pediatrics* 93:137, 1994.

Gushurt, C.A., Mueller, J.A., Green, J.A., and Sedor, F. Breast milk iodide: reassessment in the 1980s. *Pediatrics* 73:354, 1984.

Lee, J.Y., Shoji, S., and Satow, Y. Developmental toxicity of potassium iodide in rats. *Teratology* 40: 676, 1989.

Mehta, P.S., Mehta, S. J., and Vorherr, H. Congenital iodide goiter and hypothyroidism: a review. *Obstet. Gynecol. Surv.* 38:237, 1983.

Postellon, D.C., and Aronow, R. Iodine in mother's milk. *J.A.M.A.* 247, 1982.

Vorhees C.V., et al. Developmental toxicity and psychotoxicity of potassium iodide in rats: a case for the inclusion of behavior in toxicological assessment. *Food Cosmet. Toxicol.* 22:963, 1984.

Prazosin (Minipress®), Doxazosin (Cardura®), Terazosin (Hytrin®)

INDICATIONS AND RECOMMENDATIONS

Prazosin is a quinazoline derivative that is relatively contraindicated in pregnancy because other drugs that seem to be equally effective have been studied far more extensively. It is used for the control of mild to moderate hypertension. Doxazosin and terazosin are closely related compounds with longer durations of action. However, there is no reported experience with these agents in pregnancy.

SPECIAL CONSIDERATIONS IN PREGNANCY

Experience with prazosin in pregnant women is quite limited. In a series of 22 hypertensive gravidas with new onset hypertension, treatment with prazosin was for 5–95 days, with mean prolongation of pregnancy of 24 days. There were 4 fetal deaths, and 18 live births, half with intrauterine growth retardation. Twelve patients required addition of a second agent to control hypertension. Blood pressure control was satisfactory in 24 of 25 gravidas with severe chronic hypertension, but only 6 of 19 gravidas with preeclampsia with a combination of prazosin and oxprenolol.

One study of eight hypertensive women unresponsive to β-adrenergic blockade in the third trimester revealed that prazosin satisfactorily lowered both supine and standing blood pressure in six of the eight. The median prolongation of pregnancy in these cases was 22 days. Neonatal outcome was satisfactory, and all the infants were judged to have been developing normally at the time of the report. Pharmacokinetic analysis of these patients revealed that maternal absorption of the drug was delayed and its half-life prolonged when compared to healthy male control subjects of similar age.

A case of intrauterine demise with cleft palate, shortened digits, and ischemic kidneys born to a mother taking prazosin from the first trimester has been reported. In fetal sheep, prazosin causes a decrease in breathing movements. The clinical significance of these findings is uncertain.

Until more is known about long-term fetal and neonatal effects as well as the drug's disposition in breast milk, more standard agents such as methyldopa, beta blockers, or hydralazine should be used in hypertensive obstetric patients.

DOSAGE

The initial dose of 1 mg is usually taken at bedtime to avoid the syncope that may occur with the first dose. Usual starting dose is 1 mg 2–3 times per day. The maximum recommended dose is 20 mg/day.

ADVERSE EFFECTS

The major side effect of prazosin is a marked postural hypotension and syncope that may occur with the first dose, or with a rapid increase in dosage or addition of a second antihypertensive agent. This effect can be avoided by taking the initial dose at bedtime and increasing the dose slowly. Occasionally, postural hypotension is longstanding and may limit therapy. There are few other side effects, which are nonspecific, such as headache, nausea, and dizziness.

MECHANISM OF ACTION

Prazosin is a highly selective specific antagonist of α_1-adrenoreceptors. It functions as an antagonist to the constrictor actions of α-adrenergic catecholamines on arterial and venous smooth muscle, and has little direct vasodilator activity. It is also a potent phosphodiesterase inhibitor and has some ganglionic blocking and anticholinergic activity. Since prazosin reduces peripheral vascular resistance without secondary reflex tachycardia, probably secondary to central suppression of sympathetic outflow, it rarely causes palpitations or tachycardia. There has been increased interest in this agent recently because in theory the decrease in sympathetic stimulation may improve lipid profile and decrease vascular smooth muscle hypertrophy.

ABSORPTION AND BIOTRANSFORMATION

Prazosin is well absorbed orally, with a bioavailability of 44% to 70%. Peak concentrations are achieved 1–3 hours after an oral dose. It is tightly bound to plasma proteins and is metabolized in the liver. The plasma half-life is 2–4 hours, with a duration of action of 4–6 hours.

RECOMMENDED READING

Dommisse, J., Davey, D.A., and Roos, P.J. Prazosin and oxprenolol therapy in pregnancy hypertension. *S. Afr. Med. J.* 64:233, 1983.

Giussani, D.A., Moore, P.J., Bennet, L., Spencer, J.A.D., and Hanson, M.A. α_1 and α_2 adrenoreceptor actions of phentolamine and prazosin on breathing movements in fetal sheep in utero. *J. Physiol.* 486:249, 1995.

Hoffman B.B., and Lefkowitz, R.J. Catecholamines, sympathomimetic drugs, and adrenergic receptor agonists. Chapter 10 in *Goodman and Gilman's The Pharmacological Basis of Therapeutics* (9th ed.), J.G. Hardman and L.E. Limbird, eds. New York: McGraw-Hill, 1996. Pp. 229–231.

Hurst, J.A., Houlston, R.S., Roberts, A., Gould, S.J., and Tingey, W.G. Transverse limb deficiency, facial clefting and hypoxic renal damage: an association with treatment of maternal hypertension? *Clin. Dysmorph.* 4:359, 1995.

Lubbe, W.F., and Hodge, J.V. Combined α and adrenoceptor antagonism with prazosin and oxprenolol in control of severe hypertension in pregnancy. *N. Z. Med. J.* 94:169, 1981.

Rubin, P.C., Butters, L., Low, R.A., and Reid, J.L. Clinical pharmacological studies with prazosin during pregnancy complicated by hypertension. *Br. J. Clin. Pharmacol.* 16:543, 1983.

Vincent, J., Meredith, P.A., Reid, J.L., Elliot, H.L., and Rubin, P.C. Clinical pharmacokinetics of prazosin—1985. *Clin. Pharmacokinet.* 10:144, 1985.

Primaquine Phosphate

INDICATIONS AND RECOMMENDATIONS

The use of primaquine phosphate during pregnancy is relatively contraindicated because of the possibility of hemolysis in the fetus with glucose 6-phosphate dehydrogenase (G6PD) deficiency. Primaquine, an 8-aminoquinoline derivative, is highly active against the primary exoerythrocytic forms of *Plasmodium vivax* and *Plasmodium falciparum.* It disrupts the parasite's mitochondria, creating major changes in its metabolic processes. In nonpregnant patients, primaquine is recommended specifically for the radical cure of vivax malaria, the prevention of relapse in vivax malaria, or after the termination of chloroquine phosphate suppressive therapy in an area where vivax malaria is endemic.

Its major side effect in the large majority of people is mild to moderate epigastric distress or, with larger dosages, mild anemia or cyanosis due to methemoglobinemia and leukocytosis. In susceptible patients whose red blood cells are deficient in G6PD, however, even small dosages of primaquine can be associated with severe hemolytic anemia. All patients with possible G6PD deficiency should be tested for adequate enzyme levels prior to implementation of therapy.

The effects of primaquine on the pregnant woman or fetus have not been studied. Chloroquine, a related 4-aminoquinoline derivative, is known to cross the placenta. Because it is not possible to know whether the fetus has G6PD deficiency in utero, it is best to avoid prescribing primaquine during pregnancy. When radical cure or terminal prophylaxis is indicated, the pregnant patient should receive chloroquine once weekly until delivery. Primaquine may be given after delivery.

RECOMMENDED READING

Bruce-Chawatt, L.J. Malaria and pregnancy. *Br. Med. J.* 286:1457, 1983.

Centers for Disease Control. *Health information for international travel* 1996–1997. Atlanta: Public Health Service, 1997.

Centers for Disease Control. Prophylaxis during pregnancy. Health Information for International Travel 1996–97. Yellow Book Online: http://www.cdc.gov/travel/yellowbk/.

Tracy, J.W., and Webster, L.T., Jr. Drugs used in the chemotherapy of protozoal infections: malaria. Chapter 40 in *Goodman and Gilman's The Pharmacological Basis of Therapeutics* (9th ed.), J.G. Hardman and L.E. Limbird, eds. New York: McGraw-Hill, 1996. Pp. 977–978.

Primidone (Mysoline®)

INDICATIONS AND RECOMMENDATIONS

The use of primidone, a congener of phenobarbital, during pregnancy should be limited to the treatment of those women who require chronic anticonvulsant therapy. It is used alone or in combination with other anticonvulsants for the treatment of generalized tonic-clonic, simple partial, or complex partial seizures. Primidone may be given to breast-feeding mothers, but the nursing infants should be observed for drowsiness.

SPECIAL CONSIDERATIONS IN PREGNANCY

Primidone crosses the placenta, and it has been cited as a possible cause of birth anomalies. Reported incidents in past years, however, have been inconclusive in the light of the practice of multidrug therapy of epilepsy.

Offspring of pregnant mice receiving 25–150 mg/kg/day of primidone exhibited a high incidence of palatal defects, including full-length and submucosal clefts. No strong dose dependence was found in association with the abnormalities. The mice demonstrated the same metabolites as those found in humans. Administered doses were not much larger, on an mg/kg basis, than those used in humans.

The most commonly reported human fetal anomalies ascribed to primidone include cardiac malformations, nail or phalangeal hypoplasia, craniofacial anomalies (hypertelorism, epicanthal folds, and a broad, depressed nasal bridge), growth retardation, and delayed development. In some of these reports primidone was the only drug used by the mother during pregnancy, but in others it was one of the several agents prescribed. The latter fact is important because many of these anomalies are similar to those reported in newborns who were exposed to phenytoin in utero.

In addition to the gross defects found at birth, a withdrawal-like syndrome has been reported in some otherwise normal infants born to mothers who received daily doses of primidone. In two reports, the infants were tremulous and irritable for 3 days, cord blood contained 8 µg/ml primidone, and the drug could be detected in the infants' urine for 10–11 days. In another report, tremulousness was also associated with neonatal hypocalcemia, which was refractory to therapy for 2 weeks. Hypoprothrombinemia has been reported in infants of mothers who received a combination of primidone and phenobarbital. It is not conclusive that primidone alone can decrease prothrombin levels, but because primidone is metabolized to phenobarbital, it is possible. The condition usually responds to vitamin K therapy.

The manufacturers recommend that mothers taking primidone discontinue nursing if the infant appears unusually drowsy.

DOSAGE

The usual adult oral dose is 500–1500 mg/day given in divided doses. The dosage is adjusted on the basis of therapeutic results as well as the primidone and phenobarbital concentrations. The relationship between dosage and plasma concentrations is complex; both plasma primidone levels and phenobarbital levels should be measured. Primidone levels of 8–12 µg/ml and phenobarbital levels of 15–35 µg/ml are optimal. Increases in dosage must be undertaken slowly to minimize adverse effects, particularly if the patient has not been treated previously.

ADVERSE EFFECTS

The side effects of primidone are similar to those of phenobarbital and include sedation, vertigo, dizziness, ataxia, diplopia, nystagmus, megaloblastic anemia, and possible osteomalacia. Idiosyncratic reactions include skin rashes, leukopenia, thrombocytopenia, lymphadenopathy, and a systemic lupus erythematosus–like syndrome.

MECHANISM OF ACTION

The mechanism of action of primidone is complex due to the presence of two active metabolites, phenobarbital and phenylethylmalonamide (PEMA), in addition to the drug itself. In rat studies, PEMA has been shown to raise the thresholds for myoclonic jerks and clonic-tonic seizures induced by hexafluorodiethyl ether. In studies of electroconvulsion in both humans and animals, primidone appears more selective than phenobarbital alone in controlling certain phases of seizure activity. (See "Phenobarbital" for its actions.)

Primidone is useful in the control of generalized tonic-clonic, simple partial, or complex partial seizures. It can be used alone, particularly in the treatment of complex partial seizures, or in combination with other anticonvulsants, such as phenytoin, carbamazepine, or ethosuximide. Because primidone is metabolized to phenobarbital, these two drugs are rarely used in combination.

ABSORPTION AND BIOTRANSFORMATION

The drug is rapidly absorbed through the gastrointestinal tract and is metabolized in the liver to phenobarbital and PEMA, both of which are active compounds. Pregnancy does not consistently alter primidone pharmacokinetics although its rate of metabolism to phenobarbital may be decreased. It is not known if this decreased conversion is associated with a clinically important change in drug activity. Primidone's plasma half-life is 7–9 hours. Whereas PEMA appears within 24 hours and has a half-life of 24–48 hours, phenobarbital is measurable after 24–96 hours and has a half-life of 48–120 hours. Steady-state plasma levels of primidone are achieved within 2–4 days of initiating therapy or dosage adjustment. In children, more than 90% of the drug is excreted by the kidneys as both unaltered primidone and its active metabolites.

RECOMMENDED READING

AAP Committee on Drugs in collaboration with the ACOG Committee on Obstetrics: Maternal and Fetal Medicine. *Anticonvulsants and pregnancy.* January 1979.

Committee on Drugs, American Academy of Pediatrics. The transfer of drugs and other chemicals into human breast milk. *Pediatrics* 93: 137, 1994.

Czeizel, A.E., Bod, J., and Halasz, P. Evaluation of anticonvulsant drugs during pregnancy in a population-based Hungarian study. *Eur. J. Epidemol.* 8:122, 1992.

Linchout, D., Meinardi, H., Meijer, J.W., Nau, H. Antiepileptic drugs and teratogenesis in two consecutive cohorts: changes in prescription policy paralleled by changes in pattern of malformations. *Neurology* 42, S94–110, 1992.

Lindhout, D., Omtzigt, J.G. Pregnancy and the risk of teratogenicity. *Epilepsia* 4, S41–8, 1992.

McNamara, J.O. Drugs effective in the therapy of the epilepsies. Chapter 20 in *Goodman and Gilman's The Pharmacological Basis of Therapeutics* (9th ed.), J.G. Hardman and L.E. Limbird, eds. New York: McGraw-Hill, 1996. Pp. 472–473.

Mynre, S.A., and Williams, R. Teratogenic effects associated with maternal primidone therapy. *J. Pediatr.* 99:160, 1981.

Rating, G., et al. Teratogenic and pharmacokinetic studies of primidone during pregnancy and in the offspring of epileptic women. *Acta Paediatr. Scand.* 71:301, 1982.

Rudd, N.L., and Freedom, R.M. A possible primidone embryopathy. *J. Pediatr.* 94:835, 1979.

Schardein, J.L. *Chemically Induced Birth Defects,* 2nd ed., New York, Marcel-Dekker, Inc., 1993, Pp. 169–173.

Wilder, B.J., and Bruni, J. *Seizure Disorders: A Pharmacologic Approach to Treatment.* New York: Raven, 1981.

Woodbury, D.M., Penry, J.K., and Pippenger, C.E. *Antiepileptic Drugs* (2nd ed.). New York: Raven, 1982.

Probenecid (Benemid®)

INDICATIONS AND RECOMMENDATIONS

The use of probenecid during pregnancy should be limited to the treatment of gout or potentially symptomatic hyperuricemia. Because it has no analgesic or antiinflammatory activity, it is of no value in the treatment of acute attacks of gout; phenylbutazone may be used in these instances. Probenecid is also commonly given before the administration of penicillin or ampicillin, especially in the treatment of gonorrheal infections, to increase blood levels of the antibiotics by inhibiting their renal excretion. It seems judicious to avoid using two drugs in pregnancy if one will suffice, particularly because alternative single drugs are safe and effective.

SPECIAL CONSIDERATIONS IN PREGNANCY

Probenecid is known to cross the placental barrier. With the exception of the death of one neonate not definitely related to probenecid therapy, the drug has been used in pregnancy without adverse effect to mother or child, including no detectable increase in the incidence of labor complications, prematurity, or low birth weight.

DOSAGE

Therapy for gout should not be started until 2–3 weeks after an acute attack. The usual dose is 250 mg bid for 1 week followed by 500 mg bid. Daily dosage may be increased every 4 weeks by increments of 500 mg to a maximum of 2–3 g.

ADVERSE EFFECTS

Frequently reported side effects include headache, anorexia, nausea, and vomiting. Dizziness, flushing, sore gums, urinary frequency, and anemia have also been reported. Probenecid therapy may exacerbate and prolong inflammation during the acute phase of gout. The frequency of attacks may also be increased during the first 6–12 weeks of therapy.

MECHANISM OF ACTION

Renal transport of organic acids is influenced by probenecid therapy. It is a competitive inhibitor to active reabsorption of uric acid at the proximal convoluted tubule. Urinary excretion of uric acid is therefore increased and serum urate levels are reduced. Subtherapeutic dosages may inhibit renal secretion of uric acid.

By decreasing serum urate levels, probenecid prevents or reduces chronic joint changes and tophi formation. It eventually reduces the frequency of attacks and may improve renal function in gouty patients. Serum urate levels usually reach a minimum within a few days after therapy is begun.

At the proximal and distal tubules, probenecid competitively inhibits secretion of many weak organic acids such as the penicillins. Plasma levels of acidic drugs primarily eliminated by tubular secretion can be substantially increased.

ABSORPTION AND BIOTRANSFORMATION

Probenecid is rapidly and completely absorbed from the gastrointestinal tract. After oral administration of 2 g, plasma half-life ranges from 4–17 hours and decreases as the dose decreases. Approximately 75% of the drug is bound to plasma proteins. Probenecid is metabolized in the liver.

RECOMMENDED READING

American Hospital Formulary Service. *Drug Information, 1996.* Monograph on Probenecid. G.K. McEvoy, ed. Bethesda: American Society of Health-System Pharmacists, Inc. Pp. 1941–1944.

Cavenee, M.R., et al. Treatment of gonorrhea in pregnancy. *Obstet. Gynecol.* 8133–8138, 1993.

Lee, F.I., and Loeffler, F.E. Gout and pregnancy. *J. Obstet. Gynaecol. Br. Commonw.* 69:299, 1962.

Mandell G.L., and Petri, W.A., Jr. Antimicrobial agents. Chapter 48 in *Goodman and Gilman's The Pharmacological Basis of Therapeutics* (9th ed.), J.G. Hardman and L.E. Limbird, eds. New York: McGraw-Hill, 1996. Pp. 1159–1161.

Stoll, B.J., et al. Treated maternal gonorrhea without adverse effect on outcome of pregnancy. *South. Med. J.* 75:1236, 1982.

Procainamide (Pronestylt)

INDICATIONS AND RECOMMENDATIONS

The use of procainamide in pregnancy should be limited to the treatment of mothers and fetuses with cardiac arrhythmias that are unresponsive to safer antiarrhythmic agents. Quinidine, with its similar electrophysiologic effects, is preferred during pregnancy because it has been studied more extensively.

SPECIAL CONSIDERATIONS IN PREGNANCY

Successful procainamide cardioversion of a supraventricular tachycardia in a 24-week-old fetus has been reported. Digoxin and propranolol had been given initially but no response was obtained. After procainamide was administered, temporary fetal cardioversion occurred within 1 hour. The authors suggest that fetal blood, which is slightly more acidic than that of the mother, may trap procainamide and limit back-diffusion. However, a synergistic effect among digoxin, propranolol, and procainamide cannot be excluded. Therefore, until more is learned about procainamide's pharmacokinetics in pregnancy, other more familiar agents should be used in initial attempts at treating fetal arrhythmias. Several other reports describing the successful use of procainamide to treat fetal arrhythmias during the second and third trimester have been published; no adverse outcomes have been reported.

The American Academy of Pediatrics has listed procainamide as compatible with breast feeding. Long-term effects are not known, however, regarding the development of lupus-like syndromes in the neonate.

DOSAGE

The intravenous loading dose of procainamide is 6–12 mg/kg administered at 0.2–0.5 mg/kg/min. The maintenance dose should continue at 2–6 mg/min. Alternatively, the oral loading dose is 500–1000 mg, with a maintenance dose of 350–1000 mg q3–6h. The therapeutic range of plasma levels is 4–8 g/ml.

ADVERSE EFFECTS

The use of procainamide is often accompanied by prolongation of the QRS interval on electrocardiogram and by hypotension. Ventricular tachycardia and heart block may be seen with toxic doses (blood levels greater than 12 g/ml). Other side effects include nausea, as well as bone marrow aplasia (0.2% of patients). Besides these electrophysiologic side effects, chronic administration of procainamide is associated with a systemic lupus erythematosus–like syndrome. Most patients receiving long-term therapy develop a positive antinuclear antibody titer, although a few show a complete lupus syndrome. In a well-controlled age- and sex-matched study to characterize the autoimmune phenomena in patients receiving procainamide, there was a significant increase in the frequency of positive direct antiglobulin (Coombs) tests in those patients receiving the drug. The mechanism of red cell sensitization appears to be the production of red cell autoantibody, which is indistinguishable from that seen in warm autoimmune hemolytic anemia.

MECHANISM OF ACTION

Class IA antiarrhythmics, such as procainamide, lengthen the refractory period by blocking sodium channels; conduction is slowed in the AV node as well as accessory pathways. Automaticity is therefore decreased.

ABSORPTION AND BIOTRANSFORMATION

Procainamide is rapidly and almost completely absorbed from the gastrointestinal tract. Maximal plasma concentration after oral administration occurs at about 60 minutes, and at 15–60 minutes after intramuscular administration. Procainamide has a half-life of 2.5–5.0 hours in patients with normal renal function. It is acetylated in the liver to n-acetylprocainamide (NAPA), a compound that also possesses antiarrhythmic activity. The rate of acetylation of procainamide is genetically determined and varies among individuals. The half-life of NAPA is 6–10 hours in patients with normal renal function. The total amount of unchanged procainamide excreted in the urine varies from 40% to 70% and depends on acetylator phenotype. Both procainamide and NAPA cross the placenta. However, reports have been conflicting regarding the maternal/fetal serum component. Pharmacokinetics may be altered in pregnancy such that dosage adjustment may be required postpartum in women taking procainamide for maternal arrhythmias.

RECOMMENDED READING

Allen, N.M., and Page, R.L. Procainamide administration during pregnancy. *Clin. Pharmacol.* 12:58, 1993.

American Academy of Pediatrics, Committe on Drugs. The transfer of drugs and other chemicals into human milk. *Pediatrics* 93:137, 1994.

Avery, G.S. *Drug Treatment: Principles and Practice of Clinical Pharmacology and Therapeutics.* Sydney, Australia: Adis, 1976.

Gwen, B.D., et al. Procainamide cardioversion of fetal supraventricular tachycardia. *Am. J. Cardiol.* 53:1460, 1984.

Kleinman, S., et al. Positive direct antiglobulin tests and immune hemolytic anemia in patients receiving procainamide. *N. Engl. J. Med.* 311:809, 1984.

Roden, D.M. Antiarrhythmic drugs. Chapter 35 in *Goodman and Gilman's The Pharmacological Basis of Therapeutics* (9th ed.), J.G. Hardman and L.E. Limbird, eds. New York: McGraw-Hill, 1996. Pp. 868–869.

Progestins

NATURAL PROGESTERONE AND ITS ESTERS (DELALUTIN®, PROVERA®)

Indications and Recommendations

The use of progesterone and its esters, 17-hydroxyprogesterone, medroxyprogesterone acetate (Provera), and 17-hydroxyprogesterone caproate (Delalutin), during pregnancy is controversial, and if used at all, they should be restricted to very specific situations.

Natural progesterone can probably be given safely during pregnancy for the treatment of an inadequate luteal phase, and along with its esters for the prevention of premature delivery. The efficacy of these agents is still open to question, however. There is no convincing evidence that progesterone in any form is useful in the management of threatened abortion or habitual abortion except in the specific case of inadequate luteal phase syndrome.

Natural progesterone and its esters are commonly used in assisted reproductive technologies in order to approximate the normal hormonal milieu and maintain an induced pregnancy during the first trimester.

Special Considerations in Pregnancy

The effectiveness of progestins in preventing premature delivery remains controversial. Their use in preventing abortion (other than in the case of inadequate luteal phase) is unproved. Even in the case of inadequate luteal phase, significant benefit from the use of progesterone suppositories or oral dehydroprogesterone has not been shown.

At least two random, prospective, double-blind studies have investigated the benefits of administering 17-hydroxyprogesterone caproate prophylactically to a group of women with histories of premature delivery. The groups receiving this hormone exhibited a significantly lower prematurity rate than the placebo-treated control groups. The rationale for this therapy is based on the hypothesis that labor is at least partially a result of low or falling progesterone levels. In a randomized, double-blind trial of the same drug administered to gravidas at high risk for prematurity only on the basis of their status as an active duty military population, Hauth et al. were unable to demonstrate any improvement in outcome.

The use of natural progestins and their esterified derivatives during pregnancy has been associated with limb anomalies, but the literature is unclear as to whether any causal relationship exists. When 1608 newborns whose mothers were treated with progestins (generally medroxyprogesterone acetate) for first-trimester bleeding were compared with 1146 whose mothers bled during the first trimester but were not treated with progestins, the incidence of major congenital abnormalities was similar in both groups (6.3% versus 7.2%). It may be that the previously reported increased anomaly rate was related not to the progestins but to the bleeding for which progestins were administered.

Although decreased lactation was noted when higher dose progestational contraceptives were prescribed in the past, there appears to be no adverse effect with current low-dose formulations. The Committee on Drugs of the American Academy of Pediatrics considers progesterone to be usually compatible with breast-feeding.

Dosage

In the maintenance of pregnancy with a luteal phase defect, the usual recommendation is to give progesterone vaginal suppositories, 25 mg bid, until the 12th week, or progesterone in oil, 150 mg IM every other day, until the 12th week. In the study mentioned previously in which 17-hydroxyprogesterone caproate was given to prevent premature labor, the dose was 250 mg IM every week from the 18th to 37th week of gestation.

Adverse Effects

Side effects of progesterone include weight gain and occasional episodes of depression. Because plasma progesterone levels are generally quite high in pregnancy, the addition of exogenous hormone should not cause noticeable side effects.

Mechanism of Action

Naturally occurring progesterone works at the intracellular level to produce many physiologic changes, among which is smooth muscle relaxation. This effect on the uterine musculature is probably critical for the maintenance of pregnancy. Exogenously administered progesterone may supplement that produced by the corpus luteum in early pregnancy and is therefore useful in the management of an inadequate luteal phase. In the absence of this condition, the prevailing evidence is that progestins are not useful in preventing first-trimester abortion.

Absorption and Biotransformation

These drugs are generally given parenterally and hydrolyzed in the liver to pregnanediol and its derivatives that are excreted in the urine. Natural progesterone can be absorbed vaginally from suppositories. The progestins are secreted in breast milk at a concentration of 1% to 10% of their blood levels.

SYNTHETIC 19-NORTESTOSTERONE DERIVATIVES

Indications and Recommendations

Progestins derived from 19-nortestosterone are contraindicated during pregnancy. They are used as oral contraceptive agents and, in the past, as pregnancy tests. These compounds have also been utilized in attempts to prevent abortion or premature delivery, or both. They are contraindicated because of reported associations between their use and cardiac anomalies, limb reduction defects, and masculinization of the female fetus. If progestin therapy is believed to be necessary during pregnancy, natural progesterone and its esters may be associated with less risk to the fetus.

If 19-nortestosterone-derived progestins are taken inadvertently during the first trimester, the patient should be told of the potential adverse sequelae. Although incidence figures are not available, the risk to the fetus appears to be small and elective termination of the pregnancy does not seem to be warranted.

RECOMMENDED READING

Aarskog, D. Maternal progestins as a possible cause of hypospadias. *N. Engl. J. Med.* 300:75, 1979.

Chez, R.A. Proceedings of the symposium on progesterone, progestins, and fetal development. *Fertil. Steril.* 30:16, 1978.

Committee on Drugs of the American Academy of Pediatrics. The transfer of drugs and other chemicals into human milk. *Pediatrics* 93:137, 1994.

Ferre, F., et al. Oral administration of micronized natural progesterone in late human pregnancy. *Am. J. Obstet. Gynecol.* 148:26, 1984.

Hauth, J.C., Gilstrap, L.C. III, Brekken, A.L., et al. The efficacy of 17α-hydroxyprogesterone caproate on pregnancy outcome in an active-duty military population. *Am. J. Obstet. Gynecol.* 146:187, 1983.

Hill, L.M., Johnson, C.E., and Lee, R.A. Prophylactic use of hydroxyprogesterone caproate in abdominal surgery during pregnancy. *Obstet. Gynecol.* 46:287, 1975.

Johnson, J.W.C., et al. Efficacy of 17 alpha-hydroxyprogesterone caproate in the prevention of premature labor. *N. Engl. J. Med.* 293:675, 1975.

Karamardian, L.M., and Grimes, D.A. Luteal phase deficiency: effect of treatment on pregnancy rates. *Am. J. Obstet. Gynecol.* 167:1391, 1992.

Katz, Z., et al. Teratogenicity of progestogens given during the first trimester of pregnancy. *Obstet. Gynecol.* 65:775, 1985.

Keith, L., and Berger, G.S. The relationship between congenital defects and the use of exogenous progestational "contraceptive" hormones during pregnancy: a 20-year review. *Int. J. Gynecol. Obstet.* 15:115, 1977.

Lawrence, R.A. *Breastfeeding* (4th ed.). St. Louis: C.V. Mosby, 1994. Pp. 588–590.

Linn, S., Schoenbaum, S.C., Monson, R.R., et al. Lack of association between contraceptive usage and congenital malformations in offspring. *Am. J. Obstet. Gynecol.* 147:923, 1983.

Nora, J.J., et al. Exogenous progestogen and estrogen implicated in birth defects. *J.A.M.A.* 240:837, 1978.

Williams, C.L., and Stancel, G.M. Estrogens and progestins. Chapter 57 in *Goodman and Gilman's The Pharmacological Basis of Therapeutics* (9th ed.), J.G. Hardman and L.E. Limbird, eds. New York: McGraw-Hill, 1996. Pp. 1426–1430.

Yemini, M., Borenstein, R., Dreazen, E., et al. Prevention of premature labor by 17 α-hydroxyprogesterone caproate. *Am. J. Obstet. Gynecol.* 151:574, 1985.

Propoxyphene (Darvon®, Dolene®)

INDICATIONS AND RECOMMENDATIONS

The use of propoxyphene is relatively contraindicated in pregnancy because other therapeutic agents are preferable. Propoxyphene is a synthetic analgesic that is structurally related to methadone. Its pharmacologic actions are similar to those of other narcotic analgesics; however, its clinical effects are no greater than those of aspirin or codeine. Chronic use can produce primarily psychological but, with high dosages, also physical dependence. It is estimated that the incidence of propoxyphene abuse is equivalent to that of codeine. As with other narcotic analgesics, propoxyphene use during pregnancy has been associated with neonatal withdrawal syndromes. Because of its limited analgesic activity, it should not be used to treat minor pain in the pregnant woman. Acetaminophen is the drug of choice in these situations.

RECOMMENDED READING

Reisine, T., and Pasternak, G. Opioid analgesics and antagonists. Chapter 23 in *Goodman and Gilman's The Pharmacological Basis of Therapeutics* (9th ed.), J.G. Hardman and L.E. Limbird, eds. New York: McGraw-Hill, 1996. Pp. 521–555.

Ringrose, C.A.D. The hazard of neurotropic drugs in the fertile years. *Can. Med. Assoc. J.* 106:1058, 1972.

Tyson, H.R. Neonatal withdrawal symptoms associated with maternal use of propoxyphene hydrochloride (Darvon). *J. Pediatrics* 85:684, 1974.

Protamine Sulfate

INDICATIONS AND RECOMMENDATIONS

The use of protamine sulfate during pregnancy should be limited to the treatment of excessive anticoagulation due to an overdose of heparin. In this instance, the risk of maternal hemorrhage outweighs consideration of direct toxicity to the fetus.

SPECIAL CONSIDERATIONS IN PREGNANCY

There is a single case report of a neonate born with severe respiratory and cardiac depression, whose mother had received 25 mg of protamine intravenously just prior to delivery. Because there were no other obvious causes, and the cord umbilical blood gases showed no acidemia or hypercarbia, it was assumed that the maternally administered protamine was responsible for the neonatal depression. Protamine is a low molecular weight species that would be expected to traverse the placenta with ease.

DOSAGE

Each milligram of protamine sulfate neutralizes approximately 100 units of heparin. It should be given intravenously at a rate of no more than 50 mg over a 10-minute period. Protamine itself possesses anticoagulant properties, and it is therefore unwise to give more than 100 mg over a short period unless there is certain knowledge of a larger requirement. This will avoid "overneutralization" of the heparin. Because of the rapid clearance of heparin, proportionately less protamine should be administered when more than a half-hour has passed following administration of the former.

ADVERSE EFFECTS

Hypotension, the most common side effect of protamine, is usually associated with infusion at rates greater than 50 mg/10 min. Bradycardia, dyspnea, and transitory flushing may also be associated with rapid infusion. Allergic reactions have been reported after protamine administration to persons allergic to fish, and particularly to individuals with diabetes who have been exposed to protamine-insulin and have serum antiprotamine IgE and IgG antibodies.

MECHANISM OF ACTION

The protamines are simple, low molecular weight, strongly basic proteins found in the sperm of certain fish, including salmon. They are capable of combining with the strongly acidic heparin to form a stable salt with loss of anticoagulant activity. They also can combine with insulin to retard its absorption. The protamine–heparin complex is excreted in the kidney.

RECOMMENDED READING

Caplan, S.N., and Berkman, E.M. Protamine sulfate and fish allergy (letter). *N. Engl. J. Med.* 295:172, 1976.

Goldstein, A., Aronow, L., and Kalman, S.M. *Principles of Drug Action.* New York: Harper and Row, 1968.

Majerus, P.W., Broze, G.J., Jr., Miletich, J.P., and Tollefsen, D.M. Anticoagulant, thrombolytic, and antiplatelet drugs. Chapter 54 in *Goodman and Gilman's The Pharmacological Basis of Therapeutics* (9th ed.), J.G. Hardman and L.E. Limbird, eds. New York: McGraw-Hill, 1996. P. 1346.

Weiss, M.E., Nyhan, D., Peng, Z., et al. Association of protamine IgE and IgG antibodies with life-threatening reactions to intravenous protamine. *N. Engl. J. Med.* 320:886, 1989.

Wittmaack, F.M., Greer, F.R., and FitzSimmons, J. Neonatal depression after a protamine sulfate injection. *J. Reprod. Med.* 39:655, 1994.

Pseudoephrine

INDICATIONS AND RECOMMENDATIONS

The use of pseudoephedrine in pregnancy should be limited to the treatment of allergic rhinitis and upper respiratory tract infection when symptomatic relief is not afforded by other non-medicinal treatments. Neither pseudoephedrine nor ephedrine significantly elevates blood pressure when given orally or topically in standard decongestant dosages, but they may cause cardiac stimulation and a redistribution of blood flow.

SPECIAL CONSIDERATIONS IN PREGNANCY

Pseudoephedrine is a sympathomimetic agent that is a common component of many proprietary compounds containing antihistamines and other ingredients. Although sympathomimetic amines are teratogenic in some animal species, human teratogenicity has never been proved.

The Collaborative Perinatal Project found an association between first-trimester sympathomimetic use and certain minor malformations such as inguinal hernia and clubfoot. Although these data do not serve as a specific indictment against the administration of pseudoephedrine in pregnancy, judicious use of this agent and other sympathomimetics is warranted. In 1992, Werler, et al. reported on a possible association between first-trimester use of pseudoephedrine and gastroschisis, with a relative risk of 3.2 (95% confidence interval 1.3–7.7). This study was limited by the use of maternal recall, as well as a lack of information regarding the effects of drug dosage, timing, and duration in addition to intercurrent illness. Studies in third-trimester patients have included a case report of transient fetal tachycardia in association with use of long-acting pseudoephedrine (120 mg) at 39 weeks gestation. No adverse neonatal outcome was noted. Blood flow velocities in the uterine and fetal circulations were studied in 12 third-trimester patients after a single dose (60 mg) of pseudoephedrine and no significant changes were found.

DOSAGE

The usual oral dose of pseudoephedrine is 30–60 mg q4–6h for decongestion of mucous membranes.

ADVERSE EFFECTS

Adverse effects include blanching of mucous membranes and "rebound" congestion when applied topically, dryness of mucous membranes, and occasional tachycardia and palpitations. These effects are usually mild and self-limited.

MECHANISM OF ACTION

Pseudoephedrine is predominantly an α-adrenergic stimulant that produces vasoconstriction in hyperemic nasal mucosa as well as in other vascular beds. Pseudoephedrine is a stereoisomer of ephedrine that produces less tachycardia, hypertension, or stimulation of the central nervous system.

ABSORPTION AND BIOTRANSFORMATION

Pseudoephedrine is well absorbed when given orally. Most of the drug is metabolized by deamination and conjugation. Both metabolites and unchanged drug are excreted in the urine.

BREAST-FEEDING

Pseudoephedrine is excreted in breast milk. It is considered by the American Academy of Pediatrics to be safe for use by nursing mothers.

RECOMMENDED READING

American Academy of Pediatrics, Committee on Drugs. The transfer of drugs and other chemicals into human milk. *Pediatrics* 93: 137, 1994.

Anastasio, G.D., and Harston, P.R. Fetal tachycardia associated with maternal use of pseudoephedrine, an over-the-counter oral decongestant. *J. Am. Bd. Fam. Pract.* 5:527, 1992.

Heinonen, O.P., Slone, D., and Shapiro, S. *Birth Defects and Drugs in Pregnancy.* Littleton, MA: PSG, 1977. Pp. 345–356, 439.

Hoffman B.B., Lefkowitz R.J. Catecholamines, sympathomimetic drugs, and adrenergic receptor antagonists. Chapter 10 in *Goodman and Gilman's The Pharmacological Basis of Therapeutics* (9th ed.), J.G. Hardman and L.E. Limbird, eds. New York: McGraw-Hill, 1996. Pp. 221–224.

Shepard, T.H. *Catalog of Teratogenetic Drugs* (3rd ed.). Baltimore: Johns Hopkins University Press, 1980. Pp. 134–135.

Smith, C.V., and Rayburn, W.F., Anderson, J.C., et al. Effect of a single dose of oral pseudoephedrine on uterine and fetal doppler blood flow. *Obstet. Gynecol.* 76:803, 1990.

Werler, M.M., Mitchell, A.A., and Shapiro, S. First trimester maternal medication use in relation to gastroschisis. *Teratology* 45:361, 1992.

Pyrantel Pamoate (Antiminth®)

INDICATIONS AND RECOMMENDATIONS

The use of pyrantel pamoate during pregnancy should be limited to treatment of infections due to susceptible helminths when the mother's well-being is compromised. It is a broad-spectrum antihelminthic agent useful in the treatment of hookworm, roundworm, pinworm, and (investigationally) *Trichostrongylus* infections. Because most parasitic infections are not life threatening, it is safest to defer therapy until after delivery. Examples of infections that might be treated include a chronic hookworm infection that has produced a significant anemia and heavy roundworm infection with potential for intestinal obstruction.

SPECIAL CONSIDERATIONS IN PREGNANCY

Teratogenicity has not been described in animals, but no human data are available.

DOSAGE

For hookworm *(Ancyclostoma duodenale* or *Necator americanus)*, roundworm *(Ascaris lumbricoides)*, and *Trichostrongylus* species, 11 mg/kg (up to a maximum of 1 g) is given as a single oral dose. For pinworm *(Enterobius vermicularis)*, the same dosage is given and repeated in 2 weeks.

Pyrantel pamoate is available as a suspension containing 50mg base/ml.

ADVERSE EFFECTS

Pyrantel has caused complete neuromuscular blockade in animals given the drug parenterally. Oral dosages in humans are relatively free of side effects, with the exception of occasional gastrointestinal disturbance, headache, dizziness, rash, or fever.

MECHANISM OF ACTION

Pyrantel is a depolarizing neuromuscular blocking agent that paralyzes the worm, allowing it to be eliminated in the feces. Pyrantel pamoate is 1000 times more effective than piperazine, a hyperpolarizing agent, for *A. lumbricoides* infections. Pyrantel and piperazine are mutually antagonistic and should not be used together.

ABSORPTION AND BIOTRANSFORMATION

Pyrantel is poorly absorbed from the gastrointestinal tract, with less than 15% of the parent compound or its metabolites recovered in the urine.

RECOMMENDED READING

LaPorte, V.D., and Gibbs, R.S. Acute pancreatitis in pregnancy with *Ascaris* infestation. *Obstet. Gynecol.* 49 (Suppl 1):84S, 1977.

Pitts, N.E., and Migliardi, J.R. Antiminth (pyrantel pamoate). *Clin. Pediatr.* 13:87, 1974.

Tracy, J.W., and Webster, L.T., Jr. Drugs used in the chemotherapy of helminthiasis. Chapter 42 in *Goodman and Gilman's The Pharmacological Basis of Therapeutics* (9th ed.)., J.G. Hardman and L.E. Limbird, eds. New York: McGraw-Hill, 1996. P. 1022.

Quinidine (Cardioquin®, Quinaglute®)

INDICATIONS AND RECOMMENDATIONS

Quinidine is safe to use during pregnancy. It is an antiarrhythmic agent used in both atrial and ventricular arrhythmias. It may be administered to pregnant women if it is believed to be the drug of choice for the particular arrhythmia encountered.

SPECIAL CONSIDERATIONS IN PREGNANCY

Although quinine, a stereoisomer of quinidine, appears to have oxytocic properties and is reported to be an abortifacient, the oxytocic properties of quinidine itself are considered to be insignificant. Quinidine has been used in place of quinine to treat severe falciparum malaria in pregnancy, in order to avoid the oxytocic effect of quinine.

Therapeutic levels of quinidine have been demonstrated to suppress plasma pseudocholinesterase activity in pregnant women by 60% to 70%, leading to a recommendation for caution when succinylcholine or ester-type local anesthetics are used in such patients.

Quinidine has been shown to cross the placenta, with levels in the fetus being slightly lower than those in the mother. Neonatal thrombocytopenia has been reported. Although eighth nerve damage has also been reported, it was associated with much higher dosages than are ordinarily used.

DOSAGE

The usual maintenance dose of quinidine sulfate or quinidine gluconate is 200–300 mg PO q6h, or 300–600 mg PO q8–12h if the sustained release forms are used. Serum levels should be monitored, the therapeutic range being 2–5 µg/ml. Intravenous administration of quinidine should only be undertaken in hospitalized patients who can have continuous electrocardiographic monitoring. Quinidine treatment reduces the clearance of digitalis glycosides, a clinically important effect because the two drugs are often prescribed together. Quinidine also inhibits the enzyme cytochrome P_{450} 2D6, which is responsible for metabolism of many drugs such as β-adrenergic blockers. Codeine, which is metabolized to morphine by that enzyme, is less effective as an analgesic agent in patients taking quinidine. Phenobarbital and phenytoin may induce enzymes responsible for quinidine metabolism, leading to greater doses being necessary to achieve the desired quinidine effect.

ADVERSE EFFECTS

The most common toxic effects of quinidine are gastrointestinal. Cardiac effects include acceleration of existing atrial arrhythmias and ventricular tachycardia. Idiosyncratic reactions, such as angioedema and vascular collapse, may occur more commonly than with many other drugs.

MECHANISM OF ACTION

Quinidine is a sodium channel blocker that also blocks multiple cardiac potassium currents. When it is given, QRS duration increases from about 10% to 20%. The QT interval is prolonged variably up to 25%. Quinidine increases the threshold for electrical excitation, decreases automaticity, and decreases the conduction velocity in cardiac tissue. Other actions include vagal blockade and an increase in the effective refractory period. Quinidine therapy is effective in the prevention or abolition of such cardiac arrhythmias as atrial fibrillation, atrial flutter, paroxysmal supraventricular and ventricular tachycardia, and premature systoles. Quinidine also acts as an α-adrenergic blocker and vagal inhibitor, which is why intravenous administration may cause hypotension and tachycardia.

ABSORPTION AND BIOTRANSFORMATION

Quinidine salts are nearly completely absorbed after oral administration, with maximal effects occurring in 1–3 hours. Quinidine is 70% to 95% bound to plasma proteins, primarily albumin. It is metabolized in the liver, mainly to 2-hydroxyquinidine. However, another metabolite, 3-hydroxyquinidine, is biologically active, and there has been at least one case report of a pregnant woman being treated with quinidine for fetal supraventricular tachycardia who experienced toxicity due to high levels of this metabolite despite midtherapeutic plasma levels of quinidine. Within 24 hours, 10% to 50% of the administered drug is excreted unchanged in the urine.

An in vitro study comparing protein binding in blood obtained from three groups of infants of different ages disclosed that the binding of quinidine is diminished in neonates and young infants. This, of course, may result in enhanced drug activity. Analysis of 6 cord blood samples obtained at delivery, 8 samples from infants aged 8–18 months, and 12 samples from children over the age of 2 demonstrated free quinidine levels of 39.2%, 24.4%, and 16.6%, respectively.

RECOMMENDED READING

Hill, L.M., and Malkasian, G.D. The use of quinidine sulfate throughout pregnancy. *Obstet. Gynecol.* 54:366, 1979.

Kambam, J.R., Franks, J.J., and Smith, B.E. Inhibitory effect of quinidine on plasma pseudocholinesterase activity in pregnant women. *Am. J. Obstet. Gynecol.* 157:897, 1987.

Killeen, A.A., and Bowers, L.D. Fetal supraventricular tachycardia treated with high-dose quinidine: toxicity associated with marked elevation of the metabolite, 3(S)-3-hydroxyquinidine. *Obstet. Gynecol.* 70:445, 1987.

Pickoff, A.S., et al. Age-related differences in the protein binding of quinidine. *Dev. Pharmacol. Ther.* 3:108, 1981.

Roden, D.M. Antiarrhythmic drugs. Chapter 35 in *Goodman and Gilman's The Pharmacological Basis of Therapeutics* (9th ed.)., J.G. Hardman and L.E. Limbird, eds. New York: McGraw-Hill, 1996. Pp. 869–871.

Wong, R.D., Murthy, A.R., and Mathisen, G.E. Treatment of severe falciparum malaria during pregnancy with quinidine and exchange transfusion. *Am. J. Med.* 92:561, 1992.

Quinine

INDICATIONS AND RECOMMENDATIONS

The use of quinine during pregnancy should be limited to the treatment of attacks of chloroquine-resistant falciparum malaria. In this situation, the risk of teratogenicity and adverse pregnancy outcome is outweighed by that of congenital malaria. Its use is not warranted in the treatment of leg cramps in light of its oxytocic and possible teratogenic effects. Special counseling may be required because of quinine's availability without a prescription.

SPECIAL CONSIDERATIONS IN PREGNANCY

Quinine is known to have an oxytocic action in the pregnant woman. The nongravid human uterus is only slightly influenced, but as pregnancy proceeds, the oxytocic action of quinine becomes more noticeable. Toxic amounts of the drug may cause abortion. However, a number of case series from various parts of the world suggest that patients critically ill with malaria may have better pregnancy outcomes with quinine treatment than if allowed to remain untreated.

Quinine crosses the placental barrier and causes toxicity in the fetus. Congenital anomalies of the eye and deafness have been attributed to quinine use during pregnancy.

DOSAGE

The dose of quinine given in the treatment of uncomplicated attacks of falciparum malaria is 650 mg tid for 10–14 days. It should be given in conjunction with pyrimethamine, sulfadiazine, or (in the nonpregnant patient) tetracycline. When parenteral therapy is necessary for severe infections, quinidine sulfate (an optical isomer of quinine) is generally recommended, with an intravenous loading dose of 10 mg/kg followed by a continuous infusion of 0.02 mg/kg/min until oral treatment can be initiated. Quinidine has more severe cardiovascular side effects (but less oxytocic effect) than does quinine, and so the patient needs constant blood pressure and ECG monitoring while receiving this drug intravenously.

ADVERSE EFFECTS

Therapeutic dosages of quinine can produce cinchonism, a syndrome that includes tinnitus, headache, nausea, and visual disturbances. The acute treatment of falciparum malaria with quinine is often accompanied by maternal hypoglycemia. With continued treatment or large dosages, dermatologic, gastrointestinal, central nervous system, and cardiovascular symptoms may become prominent. Hematologic side effects are rare and include hemolytic anemia; hypoprothrombinemia, which can be reversed by vitamin K; and thrombocytopenia.

MECHANISM OF ACTION

Quinine has been described as a general protoplasmic poison affecting many enzyme systems. Its exact mechanism of action as an antimalarial is unknown. Quinine has analgesic activity and is a poor antipyretic. It exhibits cardiovascular effects similar to its isomer quinidine, oxytocic activity in late pregnancy, and curare-like effects on skeletal muscle.

ABSORPTION AND BIOTRANSFORMATION

Quinine is readily absorbed from the gastrointestinal tract. Peak levels are seen 1–3 hours after an oral dose. Approximately 70% of plasma quinine is bound to proteins. It is cleared primarily by the liver, with less than 5% of the dose excreted unchanged in the urine.

RECOMMENDED READING

Dannenberg, A.L., Dorfman, S.F., and Johnson, J. Use of quinine for self-induced abortion. *South. Med. J.* 76:846, 1983.

Davis, T.M.E., Suputtamongkol, Y., Spencer, J.L., et al. Glucose turnover in pregnant women with acute malaria. *Clin. Sci.* 86:83, 1994.

Heinonen, O.P., Slone, O., and Shapiro, S. (eds.). *Birth Defects and Drugs in Pregnancy.* Littleton, MA: PSG, 1977. Pp. 299–302, 313.

Jose, R., Kekre, A.N., George, S.S., et al. Falciparum malaria in pregnancy. *Aust. N.Z. J. Obstet. Gynaecol.* 35:99, 1995.

Lewis, R., Lauerson, N.H., and Birnbaum, S. Malaria associated with pregnancy. *Obstet. Gynecol.* 42:696, 1973.

Looareesuwan, S., White, N.J., Silamut, K., et al. Quinine and severe falciparum malaria in late pregnancy. *Acta Leidensia* 55:115, 1987.

Siroty, R.R. Purpura on the rocks-with a twist. *J.A.M.A.* 235:2521, 1976.

Tracy, J.W., and Webster, L.T., Jr. Drugs used in the chemotherapy of protozoal infections. Chapter 40 in *Goodman and Gilman's The Pharmacological Basis of Therapeutics* (9th ed.), J.G. Hardman and L.E. Limbird, eds. New York: McGraw-Hill, 1996. Pp. 965–981.

Ribavirin (Virazole®)

INDICATIONS AND RECOMMENDATIONS

Ribavirin is contraindicated in pregnancy. This antiviral drug is administered by inhalation to infants and young children with severe lower respiratory tract infections due to respiratory syncytial virus (RSV).

Ribavirin has been found to be teratogenic, causing malformations of skull, palate, eye, jaw, skeleton, and gastrointestinal tract, or embryocidal in nearly every animal species in which it has been tested. There are no data regarding its use in the pregnant woman.

Because ribavirin is administered by inhalation, health care workers who are pregnant or attempting to conceive should avoid exposure to aerosolized ribavirin.

RECOMMENDED READING

Centers for Disease Control. Assessing exposures of health care personnel to aerosols of ribavirin: california. *M.M.W.R.* 37:560, 1988.

Watts, D.H. Antiviral agents. *Obstet. Gynecol. Clin. North Am.* 19:563, 1992.

Rifampin (Rifadin®, Rimactane®)

INDICATIONS AND RECOMMENDATIONS

The use of rifampin in pregnancy should be limited to cases of maternal tuberculosis in which the use of a third drug is necessary. It should be avoided in the treatment of nonmycobacterial infections for which other, safer antibiotic therapy is available.

SPECIAL CONSIDERATIONS IN PREGNANCY

Experience with the use of rifampin in pregnancy is limited. It is known to cross the placenta and to cause malformations in both rats and mice. Although some reports indicate that rifampin is not teratogenic in humans, others suggest that rifampin use during pregnancy may be associated with complications. Collected case reports involving gestational exposure to rifampin include almost 300 births. The incidence of malformations was approximately 4%, not significantly greater than the expected rate in the general population. However, the data are difficult to evaluate because rifampin is often used in combination with other antitubercular agents.

Prenatal exposure to rifampin may increase the likelihood of hemorrhagic disease in the newborn. Prophylactic vitamin K has been recommended as a preventative measure.

DOSAGE

The usual dose given for chemotherapy of tuberculosis is 600 mg given once daily.

ADVERSE EFFECTS

The most common side effects are rash, fever, and nausea and vomiting. Intermittent, high-dose administration is often associated with more frequent reactions including a flu-like syndrome, thrombocytopenia, and, rarely, acute reversible renal failure sometimes appearing with concomitant hepatic failure. Subclinical hepatitis is also seen, whereas clinical hepatitis is rare.

MECHANISM OF ACTION

Rifampin inhibits the action of DNA-dependent RNA polymerase in mycobacteria and other microorganisms, thus inhibiting RNA synthesis.

ABSORPTION AND BIOTRANSFORMATION

Rifampin is well absorbed from the gastrointestinal tract, but absorption may be delayed by food or by such drugs as aminosalicylic acid. First-pass hepatic extraction is substantial. The primary pathway of elimination is deacetylation in the liver to a partially active metabolite that undergoes extensive enterohepatic circulation. About 50% to 60% of a dose is eventually excreted in the feces. The half-life is 1.5–5.0 hours and is increased by liver disease or biliary obstruction.

RECOMMENDED READING

Eggermont E., et al. Hemorrhagic disease of the newborn in the offspring of rifampin and isoniazid treated mothers. *Acta Paediatr. Belg.* 29:87, 1976.

Good, J.T., et al. Tuberculosis in association with pregnancy. *Am. J. Obstet. Gynecol.* 140:492, 1981.

Mandell, G.L., and Petri, W.J., Jr. Antimicrobial agents. Chapter 48 in *Goodman and Gilman's The Pharmacological Basis of Therapeutics* (9th ed.), J.G. Hardman and L.E. Limbird, eds. New York: McGraw-Hill, 1996. Pp. 1159–1161.

Scheinhorn, D.J., and Angelillo, V.A. Antituberculosis therapy in pregnancy: risks to the fetus. *West. J. Med.* 127:195, 1977.

Snider, D.E., et al. Treatment of tuberculosis during pregnancy. *Am. Rev. Resp. Dis.* 122:65, 1980.

Stein, J.S.M., and Stainton-Ellis, D.M. Rifampicin in pregnancy (letter). *Lancet* 2:604, 1977.

Warkany, J. Antituberculous drugs. *Teratology* 20:133, 1979.

Ritodrine (Yutopar®)

INDICATIONS AND RECOMMENDATIONS

Ritodrine is the first and only β-adrenergic drug approved by the Food and Drug Administration (FDA) for use as a tocolytic agent. It is a β_2-adrenergic agonist that primarily acts on myometrial receptors.

Ritodrine's major usefulness is in the treatment of premature labor that is not due to an obvious cause. Premature labor accompanied by chorioamnionitis, fetal death, severe preeclampsia, life-threatening maternal complications, or severe third-trimester bleeding should be allowed to continue and is thus a contraindication to the use of a tocolytic agent. Women with cardiac disease may be adversely affected by the cardiovascular effects of ritodrine and diabetic control may be compromised by its effects on carbohydrate metabolism. Finally, great care must be exercised when ritodrine is used in combination with glucocorticoids because of the possibility of causing pulmonary edema.

There exists an ongoing controversy regarding the efficacy of ritodrine, and indeed of all tocolytic agents, in preventing preterm delivery. A small randomized trial published in 1986 found that ritodrine was effective in delaying delivery for 24 hours, but not in modifying the ultimate perinatal consequences of preterm labor. In 1992, the Canadian Preterm Labor Investigators Group published the results of a larger randomized, double-blind, placebo-controlled trial of ritodrine in preterm labor. Again, although ritodrine-treated patients were significantly less likely to deliver within 48 hours (21% versus 35%, $p < 0.001$) and perhaps 1 week (38% versus 47%, $p < 0.05$), differences in delivery before 30 weeks and before 37 weeks were not significant, nor were neonatal mortality or morbidities. Based on annual sales of ritodrine, Leveno et al. estimated that between 1983 and 1986 approximately 116,000 cases of preterm labor per year were treated with ritodrine, with no effect on the number of low birth weight or very low birth weight infants born during those years, compared to the years prior to FDA approval of ritodrine in 1980. A number of meta-analyses have reached similar conclusions about the efficacy of ritodrine and other tocolytic agents. Perhaps the greatest proven benefit from ritodrine should be considered the delay of delivery for 48 hours in order to administer glucocorticoids to enhance fetal pulmonic maturation.

SPECIAL CONSIDERATIONS IN PREGNANCY

Ritodrine decreases the intensity and frequency of uterine contractions in women with spontaneous or induced labor. It has been found to be more effective than either placebo or ethanol for this purpose. Prospective clinical trials comparing ritodrine with other selective β_2 agonists and with other tocolytic agents are numerous, and the results tend to be equivocal. There is no clear evidence of superior efficacy of one β-mimetic over another. Ritodrine appears to be equally efficacious to other tocolytics, but drugs such as nifedipine and indomethacin appear to have fewer maternal side effects. The incidence of maternal cardiovascular side effects with ritodrine is reported to be lower than with less selective β_2 agonists such as isoxsuprine.

Ritodrine is not indicated for use in the first half of pregnancy. Nevertheless, to date there are no reports of teratogenesis in humans associated with the use of this drug during embryogenesis. Ritodrine crosses the placenta but cord concentrations are lower than concomitant maternal values. Long-term follow-up study of children exposed to this drug in utero have thus far shown no adverse effects.

Uterine and placental blood flow are increased in women taking ritodrine, and fetal tachycardia may occur after maternal administration. It has also been shown to increase maternal and fetal serum glucose concentrations, as well as maternal insulin levels. Because neonatal hypoglycemia has been observed with maternal administration of ritodrine, infants who were exposed to this drug in utero should have their blood sugars carefully monitored. Diabetic mothers who take this drug may need increased dosages of insulin to maintain adequate glucose control.

In a retrospective analysis of data from a large multicenter preterm birth prevention trial, neonatal periventricular and intraventricular hemorrhage have been reported to occur more frequently in prematurely delivered offspring of mothers who received β-mimetic tocolysis. Another retrospective study failed to detect such a difference.

No data exist concerning the secretion of ritodrine in breast milk, but as it is not indicated for use after delivery and the half-life is quite short, it is unlikely that ritodrine administered antenatally would cause significant problems in the nursing infant.

DOSAGE

Ritodrine is administered intravenously by constant infusion. According to the manufacturer, the recommended starting dose is 100 μg/min. This should be increased in 50 μg/min increments every 10 minutes until a dose that provides satisfactory tocolytic action has been reached or the maternal heart rate reaches 130 beats/min or more. If tocolysis has been accomplished, this dose is maintained for 24–48 hours. Maternal cardiovascular side effects may be a limiting factor, and maternal tachycardia may necessitate lowering the dose or discontinuing the drug. The maximal recommended infusion rate is 350 μg/min.

Based on pharmacokinetic data in laboring women, Caritis et al. have recommended starting at a lower infusion rate of 50 μg/min, in order to reduce the likelihood of side effects in women with low clearance rates. In addition, they point out that an occasional patient may require infusion rates higher than 350 μg/min, in order to reach plasma concentrations around 90 ng/ml, which these authors believe to be therapeutic. They caution that rates exceeding 350 μg/min should only be given when the maternal pulse is not rapid and there is no evidence of abruptio placentae or chorioamnionitis. Once labor is inhibited, these authors suggest beginning reduction of the infusion rate after 1 hour, rather than after 12–24 hours as the manufacturer recommends. While the rate of reduction and ultimate maintenance rate are not as well supported by data, Caritis et al. generally reduce the infusion rate by 50 μg/min every 30 minutes until a maintenance rate of 150 μg/min has been reached.

Holleboom et al. have devised a model for initiating ritodrine treatment that appears to be distinctly different from the Caritis model. The initial infusion rate is 200 μg/min and the dose is increased by 200 μg/min every 2 hours until uterine quiescence is achieved, up to a maximum of 600 μg/min. The dose is then cut back based on a table that takes into account the rapidity with which tocolysis was achieved, and maintained at that level for 48 hours, then discontinued. When this regimen was compared in 203 patients in preterm labor, in a randomized trial, with the standard approach recommended by the manufacturer, success was similar in both groups. Side effects were better tolerated in the former group.

Although ritodrine is approved only for intravenous use in the United States, it has been given intramuscularly, in a dose of 5–10 mg every 2 hours for three doses, with success.

Although the manufacturer originally recommended switching patients to oral ritodrine after 12–24 hours of intravenous therapy, plasma concentrations attained with oral maintenance are extremely low, and a meta-analysis has failed to support a role for oral therapy with β-mimetics once preterm labor has been stopped.

ADVERSE EFFECTS

In trials in the United States, intravenous ritodrine was associated with palpitations in 33% of patients; tremor, nausea, vomiting, headache, or erythema in 10% to 15%; and nervousness, restlessness, emotional upset, or anxiety in 5% to 6%. Cardiac symptoms including chest pain or tightness and arrhythmias were reported in 1% to 2% of patients. Other infrequently reported maternal effects included anaphylactic shock, rash, epigastric distress, ileus, bloating, constipation, diarrhea, dyspnea, hyperventilation, sweating, and weakness. Agranulocytosis, cutaneous vasculitis, and vulvar edema have also been reported.

Maternal cardiac arrhythmias are due to ritodrine's chronotropic activity, and these include premature ventricular contractions as well as supraventricular tachycardias. This drug also increases stroke volume and, therefore, systolic pressure. Peripheral vascular resistance, on the other hand, is decreased, and this reduces diastolic pressure and consequently widens the pulse pressure. Maternal myocardial ischemia and corresponding electrocardiographic changes have been noted in women being treated with ritodrine. Some, but not all, of these patients were symptomatic. The changes usually reverted to normal when therapy was discontinued. ST segment depression has also been found to occur with increased frequency when laboring patients receive ritodrine, but cardiac enzymes generally remained within normal limits. Transient arrhythmias have been reported in newborns exposed to this drug in utero.

Ritodrine may cause hyperglycemia, and possibly metabolic acidosis in poorly controlled diabetic women. In addition, the drug may cause hyperlactacidemia with secondary metabolic acidosis. Transient hypokalemia develops in most patients during ritodrine therapy. This is generally believed to be secondary to the hyperglycemia and hyperinsulinemia that drive serum potassium into the cells. Because there is no loss of potassium from the body, serum levels quickly return to baseline values after ritodrine is discontinued. When present, the hypokalemia is usually asymptomatic and rarely requires treatment.

Pulmonary edema has been reported with the use of ritodrine alone or in combination with glucocorticoids, but the incidence is higher with combined therapy. Pulmonary edema is also more likely to occur when ritodrine is administered to women with twin gestations. Whenever this drug is given, care should be taken to avoid iatrogenic fluid overloading. The manufacturer recommends administering ritodrine in 5% dextrose in water rather than in salt-containing solutions in order to minimize the likelihood of pulmonary edema.

Abnormal liver enzymes have also been reported, affecting 2 in 101 singleton pregnancies and 2 in 22 multiple pregnancies in one series.

MECHANISM OF ACTION

Ritodrine is a sympathomimetic agent with predominantly β_2 activity. It is believed that such agents stimulate adenyl cyclase, the enzyme that catalyzes the conversion of adenosine triphosphate to cyclic AMP. Increased intracellular concentrations of cyclic AMP cause relaxation of the uterine musculature. Studies comparing the effects of ritodrine, terbutaline, magnesium sulfate, and nifedipine on isolated human myometrial strips from laboring patients found no clear differences in tocolytic potency.

ABSORPTION AND BIOTRANSFORMATION

Orally administered ritodrine is rapidly absorbed in the gastrointestinal tract. Bioavailability of an oral dose is approximately 30%. The drug is conjugated in the liver, with a plasma half-life of 1.32 hours. Ninety percent of the drug may be recovered from the urine within 24 hours of administration.

RECOMMENDED READING

American College of Obstetricians and Gynecologists. Preterm labor. ACOG Technical Bulletin #206, Washington, DC, 1995.

Barden, T.P., Peter, J.B., and Merkatz, I.R. Ritodrine hydrochloride: a beta-mimetic agent for use in preterm labor. *Obstet. Gynecol.* 56:1, 1980.

Benedetti, T.J. Maternal complications of parenteral beta-sympathomimetic therapy for premature labor. *Am. J. Obstet. Gynecol.* 145:1, 1983.

Benedetti, T.J., Gonik, B., Hayashi, R.H., et al. A multicenter evaluation of intramuscular ritodrine hydrochloride as initial parenteral therapy for preterm labor management. *J. Perinatol.* 14: 403–407. 1994.

Besinger, R.E., Niebyl, J.R., Keyes, W.G., et al. Randomized comparative trial of indomethacin and ritodrine for the long-term treatment of preterm labor. *Am. J. Obstet. Gynecol.* 164:981–988, 1991.

Bieniarz, J., Ivankovich, A., and Scommegna, A. Cardiac output during ritodrine treatment in premature labor. *Am. J. Obstet. Gynecol.* 118:910, 1974.

Bosnyak, S., Baron, J.M., and Schreiber, J. Acute cutaneous vasculitis associated with prolonged intravenous ritodrine hydrochloride therapy. *Am. J. Obstet. Gynecol.* 165:427, 1991.

Brettes, J.P., Renand, R., and Gandar, R. A double-blind investigation into the effects of ritodrine on uterine blood flow during the third trimester of pregnancy. *Am. J. Obstet. Gynecol.* 124:164, 1976.

Brittain, C., Carlson, J.W., Gehlbach, D.L., et al. A case report of massive vulvar edema during tocolysis of preterm labor. *Am. J. Obstet. Gynecol.* 165:420, 1991.

Canadian Preterm Labor Investigators Group. Treatment of preterm labor with the beta-adrenergic agonist ritodrine. *N. Engl. J. Med.* 327:308, 1992.

Caritis, S.N., Venkataramanan, R., Darby, M.J., et al. Pharmacokinetics of ritodrine administered intravenously: recommendations for changes in the current regimen. *Am. J. Obstet. Gynecol.* 162:429, 1990.

Caritis, S.N., Venkataramanan, R., Cotroneo, M., et al. Pharmacokinetics and pharmacodynamics of ritodrine after intramuscular administration to pregnant women. *Am. J. Obstet. Gynecol.* 162: 1215, 1990.

DeArcos, F., Gratacós, E., Palacio, M., et al. Toxic hepatitis: a rare complication associated with the use of ritodrine during pregnancy. *Acta Obstet. Gynecol. Scand.* 75:340, 1996.

Faidley, C.K., Dix, P.M., and Morgan, M.A. Electrocardiographic abnormalities during ritodrine administration. *South. Med. J.* 83:503, 1990

Ferguson, J.E., II, Dyson, D.C., Schutz, T., et al. A comparison of tocolysis with nifedipine or ritodrine: analysis of efficacy and maternal, fetal, and neonatal outcome. *Am. J. Obstet. Gynecol.* 163:105, 1990.

Groome, L.J., Goldenberg, R.J., Cliver, S.P., et al. Neonatal periventricular-intraventricular hemorrhage after maternal-sympathomimetic tocolysis. *Am. J. Obstet. Gynecol.* 167:873, 1992.

Hadi, H.A., and Albazzaz, S.J. Cardiac isoenzymes and electrocardiographic changes during ritodrine tocolysis. *Am. J. Obstet. Gynecol.* 161:318, 1989.

Higby, K., Xenakis, E.M.-J., and Pauerstein, C.J. Do tocolytic agents stop preterm labor? A critical and comprehensive review of efficacy and safety. *Am. J. Obstet. Gynecol.* 168:1247, 1993.

Holleboom, C.A.G., Merkus, J.M.W.M., van Elferen, L.W.M., et al. Randomized comparison between a loading and incremental dose model for ritodrine administration in preterm labor. *Br. J. Obstet. Gynaecol.* 103:695, 1996.

Hosenpud, J.D., Morton, M.J., and O'Grady, J.P. Cardiac stimulation during ritodrine hydrochloride tocolytic therapy. *Obstet. Gynecol.* 62:52, 1983.

Humphrey, M., et al. The effect of intravenous ritodrine on the acid–base status of the fetus during the second stage of labor. *Br. J. Obstet. Gynaecol.* 82:234, 1975.

Ikushima, Y., Kobayashi, H., Imaishi, K., et al. Ritodrine-induced agranulocytosis. *Arch. Gynecol. Obstet.* 248:53–54, 1990.

King, J.F., Grant, A., Keirse, M.J.N.C., et al. Betamimetics in preterm labour: an overview of the randomized controlled trials. *Br. J. Obstet. Gynaecol.* 95:211, 1988.

Kupferminc, M., Lessing, J.B., Yaron, Y., et al. Nifedipine versus ritodrine for suppression of preterm labour. *Br. J. Obstet. Gynaecol.* 100:1090, 1993.

Leveno, K.J., Guzick, D.S., Hankins, G.D.V., et al. Single-centre randomized trial of ritodrine hydrochloride for preterm labor. *Lancet* 1:1293, 1986.

Macones, G.A., Berlin, M., and Berlin, J.A. Efficacy of oral beta-agonist maintenance therapy in preterm labor: a meta-analysis. *Obstet. Gynecol.* 85:313–317, 1995.

Nochimson, D.J., et al. The effects of ritodrine hydrochloride on uterine activity and the cardiovascular system. *Am. J. Obstet. Gynecol.* 118:523, 1974.

Özcan, T., Turan, C., Ekici, E., et al. Ritodrine tocolysis and neonatal intraventricular-periventricular hemorrhage. *Gynecol. Obstet. Invest.* 39:60–62, 1995.

Philipsen, T., Eriksen, P.S., and Lynggård, F. Pulmonary edema following ritodrine-saline infusion in premature labor. *Obstet. Gynecol.* 58:304, 1981.

Saade, G.R., Taskin, O., Belfort, M.A., et al. In vitro comparison of four tocolytic agents, alone and in combination. *Obstet. Gynecol.* 84:374, 1994.

Schiff, E., Sivan, E., Terry, S., et al. Currently recommended oral regimens for ritodrine tocolysis result in extremely low plasma levels. *Am. J. Obstet. Gynecol.* 169:1059, 1993.

Shen, O., Lavie, O., Grisaru, S., et al. Elevated liver enzyme concentrations during ritodrine therapy. *Acta Obstet. Gynecol. Scand.* 75:183, 1996.

Wesselius-DeCasparis, A., et al. Results of a double-blind, multicentric study with ritodrine in premature labor. *Br. Med. J.* 3:144, 1971.

Wilkins, I.A., Lynch, L., Mehalek, K.E., et al. Efficacy and side effects of magnesium sulfate and ritodrine as tocolytic agents. *Am. J. Obstet. Gynecol.* 159:685, 1988.

Salicylates: Acetylsalicylic Acid (Aspirin), Sodium Salicylate

INDICATIONS AND RECOMMENDATIONS

The usual therapeutic doses of salicylates should be avoided, especially in the later stages of pregnancy. Full-dose salicylate use near term has been associated with prolonged labor, an increased blood loss during delivery, and neonatal bleeding problems.

Salicylates may be used as antiinflammatory agents in the treatment of various forms of arthritis but should be considered as second-line analgesic and antipyretic drugs because acetaminophen is an effective and potentially less toxic substitute. Long-term salicylate therapy may be necessary for treating arthritis during pregnancy. If so, patients should be counseled about potential adverse maternal and fetal effects.

Patients who take large doses of salicylates during pregnancy may have prolonged gestations. Any patient receiving such therapy whose pregnancy exceeds 42 weeks from her last menstrual period should be followed closely to rule out the postmaturity syndrome.

Because of the availability of salicylates in combination over-the-counter agents, those women who use these drugs as self-medications should be identified antenatally, advised of the potential adverse effects, and encouraged to stop. Because of possible fetal sequelae, full-dose salicylates should not be used for their antiplatelet aggregation effect during pregnancy. Should anticoagulation be needed, heparin is the agent of choice.

On the other hand, low-dose aspirin is widely used as part of the treatment of lupus anticoagulant and other phospholipid antibody syndromes. In addition, a number of randomized trials have evaluated the efficacy of low-dose aspirin as prophylaxis against preeclampsia and intrauterine growth restriction in low-risk and high-risk populations. On the whole, the studies of low-risk women have been somewhat disappointing, with the magnitude of effect in reducing the risk of preeclampsia being less than was anticipated by enthusiasts.

SPECIAL CONSIDERATIONS IN PREGNANCY

Prolongation of the maternal bleeding time can occur after ingestion of only one 325-mg aspirin tablet, whereas 650 mg, the usual dose, has been shown to double the mean bleeding time for 4–7 days. Although this would be of most concern in the third trimester, the possibility of spontaneous abortion, premature labor, and placental hemorrhage makes bleeding diatheses a potential problem at any time during pregnancy. Daily aspirin dosages of 3 g during the last months of pregnancy have been associated with increased length of gestation, prolonged labor, and increased blood loss during labor.

Potential fetal problems include increased bleeding time secondary to platelet dysfunction, and jaundice (due to competition with bilirubin for albumin binding). Impaired platelet function was found in 10 of 10 tested neonates whose mothers took usual-dose aspirin within a week of delivery. In a case-control study, evidence of impaired hemostasis was found in the majority of neonates whose mothers had taken usual dose aspirin within 5 days of delivery, with an apparent time-related gradient with longer dose-to-delivery intervals. Continuous administration of large doses to the pregnant woman has been associated with decreased birth weights and increased incidence of stillbirths, premature closure of the ductus arteriosus, and intracranial hemorrhage. The incidence of cephalhematoma and melena is reportedly increased in neonates exposed to salicylates in utero. Various severe birth defects have been anecdotally reported in the offspring of salicylate users, but no cause-and-effect relationship has been established. One case-control surveillance study of 1381 infants with structural cardiac defects and 6966 infants with other malformations found no significant associations between first-trimester aspirin use and any or all cardiac defects.

The above considerations apply to individuals taking usual-dose aspirin, whereas low-dose aspirin (generally less than 150 mg/day and most commonly 60–80 mg) does not appear to be associated with most of the above problems. Aspirin in low dosage preferentially decreases thromboxane, but not prostacyclin, levels in the mother and, to some extent, the fetus. Thromboxane is associated with platelet adhesiveness, whereas prostacyclin causes vasodilatation. In 1986, Wallenburg et al. demonstrated in a small randomized trial that 60 mg/day of aspirin administered to women at high risk for preeclampsia on the basis of increased angiotensin II sensitivity decreased the likelihood of hypertensive disorders from 52% to 9%. In 1989, another small randomized trial in Israel found that 100 mg/day of aspirin reduced the rate of hypertensive disorders of pregnancy from 36% to 12%, and of preeclampsia from 23% to 3%, in women identified as being at high risk because of positive rollover tests. In that same year, the EPREDA randomized trial in France found that 150 mg/day of aspirin reduced the likelihood of fetal growth restriction in a high-risk group from 26% to 13%. Two years later the Italian Study of Aspirin in Pregnancy reported a large randomized trial of over 1000 patients judged to be at moderate risk for intrauterine growth retardation (IUGR) and found that

50 mg/day of aspirin had no effect on the likelihood of IUGR (19% versus 18%) or pregnancy-induced hypertension (19% versus 15%). Although this study was criticized because it included both prophylaxis and treatment groups (i.e., those with early signs of pregnancy induced hypertension or growth restriction), there was no effect observed in either group. In that same year, two randomized, placebo-controlled studies of patients at relatively low risk for preeclampsia were published. Both enrolled nulliparous women prior to the third trimester and used 60 mg/day of aspirin. The Alabama study of 604 subjects found that preeclampsia occurred in 1.7% of treated subjects and 5.6% of controls ($p = 0.009$). The multicenter NICHD Network Study of 2985 subjects reported that preeclampsia occurred in 4.6% of treated subjects and 6.3% of controls ($p = 0.05$). Although both studies showed a statistically significant reduction in preeclampsia, the magnitude of the reduction did not appear to justify widespread aspirin administration to gravidas not at high risk of pre-eclampsia. When the CLASP study of 9634 moderate-risk women in 16 countries was published the following year, again using 60 mg of aspirin/day versus placebo, and found no significant protection against preeclampsia (6.7% versus 7.6%), it became even clearer that the benefits of aspirin could be expected to accrue primarily to those at high risk for this disorder. Similarly, there was no apparent protective effect against IUGR. Surprisingly, preterm delivery was significantly lower in subjects assigned to aspirin therapy (17% versus 19%, $p = 0.03$). However, the magnitude of this difference was unimpressive. Although abruptio placentae occurred in 0.7% of patients on aspirin and only 0.1% of those on placebo ($p = 0.01$) in the NICHD study, a subsequent meta-analysis by the authors of the Alabama study found no difference in the incidence of abruptio in the 11 published randomized trials including almost 15,000 subjects (1.7% versus 1.4%). Finally, a single small randomized trial failed to find a significant protective effect of aspirin on the clinical course of women who already have mild pregnancy-induced hypertension. It thus appears that low-dose aspirin should be reserved for prophylaxis of preeclampsia or IUGR in patients at particularly high risk. Most authorities recommend beginning this treatment by the middle of the second trimester.

DOSAGE

The usual analgesic-antipyretic dose for aspirin or sodium salicylate is 162–650 mg q4h. Higher doses, 3–6 g/day, are often used for severe arthritis. Low-dose aspirin is usually given as 60–80 mg/day.

ADVERSE EFFECTS

Side effects of acetylsalicylic acid are numerous; they include nausea and vomiting, gastrointestinal irritation, and occult bleeding. Acute hemorrhage from gastric erosion is a rare occurrence. Iron deficiency anemia may occur with long-term use. Large dosages may prolong prothrombin time; a single analgesic dose may suppress platelet aggregation and lead to prolonged bleeding time.

Mild chronic salicylate intoxication (salicylism) consists chiefly of headache, dizziness, ringing in the ears, difficulty in hearing, blurred vision, and nausea and vomiting. Severe central nervous system disturbances (including restlessness, incoherent speech, tremor, delirium, and even convulsions, coma, and toxic encephalopathy) are associated with more severe intoxication. Initial hyperventilation may lead to respiratory alkalosis, but increased oxygen consumption and renal damage eventually produce a metabolic acidosis.

The NICHD study of low-dose aspirin to prevent preeclampsia found no incidence of bleeding related to epidural anesthesia among 451 women assigned to low-dose aspirin therapy, despite a higher mean bleeding time measured in 149 aspirin-treated patients compared to 154 controls (6.99 versus 5.99 minutes, $p = 0.004$). The Alabama study reported no decrease in fetal urine output or amniotic fluid volume with low-dose aspirin treatment.

MECHANISM OF ACTION

Salicylates act peripherally by inhibiting prostaglandin synthesis in inflamed tissues. Pain receptors are thereby rendered insensitive to mechanical or chemical stimulation. Salicylates inhibit histamine release, render neutrophils unresponsive to chemotactic stimuli, and interfere with granulocyte adherence. At the high dosages used for arthritis therapy, they interfere with formation of antigen–antibody complexes and suppress lymphocyte function. The antipyretic action of salicylates is mediated via hypothalamic centers and may be due to inhibition of prostaglandin E release. Because acetylsalicylic acid preparations irreversibly reduce platelet aggregation by inhibiting the release of platelet adenosine diphosphate (ADP), they are sometimes prescribed as mild anticoagulants.

Physiologic effects include relief of low-intensity pain, antipyresis, antiinflammatory action, decreased urinary excretion of urates with low dosages, and increased urate excretion with high dosages.

As mentioned above, low-dose aspirin is believed to act by inhibiting the release of thromboxane, but not prostacyclin, from platelets and vessel walls. Interestingly, in the Alabama study of low-dose aspirin for prevention of preeclampsia, patients experiencing a twofold or greater fall in serum thromboxane had less preeclampsia and prematurity.

ABSORPTION AND BIOTRANSFORMATION

Acetylsalicylic acid and sodium salicylate are the most commonly available salicylates. Oral administration results in rapid absorption from the stomach and upper small intestine. Therapeutic effects are observed 20–30 minutes after ingestion. Although absorption is fastest at low pH, solubility increases with rising pH such that "buffering" agents have little effect on absorption. Rectal administration is unreliable.

The absorbed drug is distributed to all tissues of the body, including cerebrospinal fluid. About 50% to 90% of salicylates are bound to serum albumin. Salicylates are metabolized in the liver to four main metabolites. Excretion of free drug and metabolites is mainly renal, and free drug excretion increases with alkalinization of the urine. The apparent half-life of salicylates is dependent on the serum concentration and ranges from 2 to 22 hours.

RECOMMENDED READING

CLASP (Collaborative Low-Dose Aspirin Study in Pregnancy) Collaborative Group. CLASP: a randomised trial of low-dose aspirin for the prevention and treatment of pre-eclampsia among 9364 pregnant women. *Lancet* 343:619, 1994.

Collins, E. Maternal and fetal effects of acetaminophen and salicylates in pregnancy. *Obstet. Gynecol.* 58:57S, 1981.

Collins, E., and Turner, C. Maternal effects of regular salicylate ingestion in pregnancy. *Lancet* 2:335, 1975.

Corby, D.G., Schulman, I. The effects of antenatal drug admninistration on aggregation of platelets of newborn infants. *Pediatr. Pharmacol. Ther.* 79:307, 1971.

Hauth, J.C., Goldenberg, R.L., Parker, C.R., Jr., et al. Low-dose aspirin therapy to prevent preeclampsia. *Am. J. Obstet. Gynecol.* 168:1083, 1993.

Hauth, J.C., Goldenberg, R.L., Parker, C.R., Jr., et al. Low-dose aspirin: lack of association with an increase in abruptio placentae or perinatal mortality. *Obstet. Gynecol.* 85:1055, 1995.

Hauth, J.C., Goldenberg, R.L., Parker, C.R., Jr., et al. Maternal serum thromboxane B_2 reduction versus pregnancy outcome in a low-dose aspirin trial. *Am. J. Obstet. Gynecol.* 173:578, 1995.

Italian Study of Aspirin in Pregnancy. Low-dose aspirin in prevention and treatment of intrauterine growth retardation and pregnancy-induced hypertension. *Lancet* 341:396, 1993.

Maher, J.E., Owen, J., Hauth, J., et al: The effect of low-dose aspirin on fetal urine output and amniotic flouid volume. *Am. J. Obstet. Gynecol.* 169:885, 1993.

Niederhoff, H., and Zahradnik, H. Analgesics during pregnancy. *Am. J. Med.* 75:117, 1983.

Rudolph, A.M. The effects of non-steroidal anti-inflammatory compounds on fetal circulation and pulmonary function. *Obstet. Gynecol.* 58:63S, 1981.

Rumack, C.M., et al. Neonatal intracranial hemorrhage and maternal use of aspirin. *Obstet. Gynecol.* 58:52S, 1981.

Schiff, E., Peleg, E., Goldenberg, M., et al. The use of aspirin to prevent pregnancy-induced hypertension and lower the ratio of thromboxane A_2 to prostacyclin in relatively high risk pregnancies. *N. Engl. J. Med.* 321:351, 1989.

Schiff, E., Barkai, G., Ben-Baruch, G., et al. Low-dose aspirin does not influence the clinical course of women with mild pregnancy-induced hypertension. *Obstet. Gynecol.* 76:742–744, 1990.

Sibai, B.M., Caritis, S.N., Thom, E., et al. Prevention of preeclampsia with low-dose aspirin in healthy, nulliparous pregnant women. *N. Engl. J. Med.* 329:1213, 1993.

Sibai, B.M., Caritis, S.N., Thom, E., et al. Low-dose aspirin in nulliparous women: safety of continuous epidural block and correlation between bleeding time and maternal-neonatal complications. *Am. J. Obstet. Gynecol.* 172:1553, 1995.

Stuart, M.J., Gross, S.J., Elrad, H., et al. Effects of acetylsalicylic acid ingestion on maternal and neonatal hemostasis. *N. Engl. J. Med.* 307:909, 1982.

Uzan, S., Beaufils, M., Breart, G., et al. Prevention of fetal growth retardation with low-dose aspirin: findings of the EPREDA trial. *Lancet* 337:1427, 1991.

Wallenburg, H.C.S., Dekker, G.A., Makovitz, J.W., et al. Low-dose aspirin prevents pregnancy-induced hypertension and pre-eclampsia in angiotensin-sensitive primigravidae. *Lancet* 1:1, 1986.

Werler, M.M., Mitchell, A.A., and Shapiro, S. The relation of aspirin use during the first trimester of pregnancy to congenital cardiac defects. *N. Engl. J. Med.* 321:1639, 1989.

Ylikorkala, O., Mäkilä, U.-M., Kääpä, P., et al. Maternal ingestion of acetylsalicylic acid inhibits fetal and neonatal prostacyclin and thromboxane in humans. *Am. J. Obstet. Gynecol.* 155: 345, 1986.

Scopolamine

INDICATIONS AND RECOMMENDATIONS

Parenteral scopolamine administration is contraindicated during pregnancy, especially when delivery is thought to be imminent. This drug is an anticholinergic agent used as a pre-anesthetic to decrease salivary and bronchial secretions and produce amnesia. When given to laboring patients, it may cause restlessness, hallucinations, or excitement.

Scopolamine readily crosses the placenta within 15 minutes of maternal administration. A prospective study of 309 infants exposed to scopolamine in the first trimester found no association with fetal malformations. One report suggests that it may induce fetal tachycardia, decrease beat-to-beat variability, and mask decelerations in heart rate. Another report describes neonatal fever, tachycardia, and lethargy in an infant born to a mother who was treated with six doses of parenteral scopolamine along with meperidine and levallorphan tartrate during labor. Scopolamine toxicity was suspected and within 15 minutes of administration of 0.1 mg IM physostigmine, the neonatal heart rate fell from 200 to 140 beats/min. The remainder of the infant's symptoms resolved completely over the following few hours. No reports of adverse effects in breast-feeding infants secondary to maternal scopalomine use has been reported.

The use of scopolamine in over-the-counter medications is discussed under "Belladonna Alkaloids."

RECOMMENDED READING

Ayromlooi, J., Tobias, M., and Berg, P. The effects of scopolamine and ancillary analgesics upon the fetal heart rate recording. *J. Reprod. Med.* 25:323, 1980.

Brown, J.H., and Taylor, P. Muscarinic receptor agonists and antagonists. Chapter 7 in *Goodman and Gilman's The Pharmacological*

Basis of Therapeutics (9th ed.), J.G. Hardman and L.E. Limbird, eds. New York: McGraw-Hill, 1996. Pp. 146–160.

Evens, R.P., and Leopold, J.C. Scopolamine toxicity in a newborn. *Pediatrics* 66:329, 1980.

Heinonen, O.P., Slone, D., and Shapiro, S. *Birth Defects and Drugs in Pregnancy.* Littleton, MA: PSG, 1977.

McDonald, J.S. Preanesthetic and intrapartal medications. *Clin. Obstet. Gynecol.* 20:447, 1977.

Serotonin Reuptake Inhibitors and Atypical Antidepressants Fluoxetine (Prozac®), Setraline (Zoloft®), Paroxetine (Paxil®), Bupropion (Wellbutrin®), Trazodone (Desyrel®)

INDICATIONS AND RECOMMENDATIONS

Serious depression in pregnancy and the puerperium occurs in 10% to 15% of gravidas. Many patients can be managed through counseling and other nonpharmacologic interventions; others might benefit from pharmacologic therapy, yet this has frequently been withheld due to fear of fetal and neonatal effects. While data are very limited for most of these newer antidepressants, there is adequate evidence at this time that fluoxetine does not have teratogenic effects and is therefore a good choice for treatment of depression in early pregnancy. A 1998 prospective study of fluvoxamine paroxetine and sertraline also failed to demonstrate teratogenicity. There are conflicting results regarding neonatal effects. Therefore, recommendations regarding use in the third trimester must be tempered pending future research. While there is more information regarding fluoxetine in pregnancy than other serotonin reuptake inhibitors, the half-life is extremely prolonged. Therefore if the patient wishes to remain on medication for most of the third trimester and discontinue shortly before delivery, setraline may be a better choice. Data regarding the use of the atypical antidepressants (trazodone and bupropion) in pregnancy are very limited and other agents with more safety information are available. Therefore, they cannot be recommended for use in pregnancy at this time. Other indications for use of the serotonin uptake inhibitors are panic disorders and obsessive-compulsive disorders.

SPECIAL CONSIDERATIONS IN PREGNANCY

Overall, animal studies regarding teratogenicity of the serotonin reuptake inhibitors are reassuring. There is one study demonstrating craniofacial and neural abnormalities in vitro in mice embryo culture, presumably due to interference with serotonin uptake into differentiating cells. However, these findings were not duplicated in in vivo studies of oral administration of fluoxetine to gravid rats or rabbits. In humans, in two large reports, there is no increase in the number of major malformations with first-trimester exposure to fluoxetine. In a database maintained by the manufacturer, outcomes of 796 pregnancies identified prospectively involving first-trimester use of fluoxetine show no increase in spontaneous abortions, and a rate of major malformation of 5%, similar to the general population, with no clustering of particular abnormalities. In a report from the California Teratogen Registry of 228 women identified prospectively with fluoxetine exposure during pregnancy, there was no excess of spontaneous abortions, and the rate of major malformation was 5.5% versus 4.0% in a matched control group—not a significant difference. In this same cohort, of the 97 infants exposed to fluoxetine who were available for examination by the investigators, minor anomalies were identified significantly more often (15.5%) than in the 153 control infants (6.5%). A prospective controlled multicenter study in nine teratology information centers demonstrated no increase in major congenital malformations, miscarriages, stillbirths, or premature deliveries among 287 pregnancies exposed to newer serotonin reuptake inhibitors during the first trimester.

Several studies in animals have not demonstrated an effect of in utero exposure to fluoxetine on behavior in the neonatal or adult periods. At 28 days of life, there is no reduction in the number or affinity of serotonin receptors in the brain in rats exposed to fluoxetine in utero. However, in adult male rats there was a decreased receptor number as well as a decrease in the ACTH release response to serotonin agonists. However, levels of ACTH achieved were sufficient to saturate the adrenal ACTH receptors, so that the significance of this finding is uncertain. In humans, exposure to fluoxetine during the third trimester of pregnancy has been variously reported as having no effect on neonatal complications or increasing abnormal behaviors and findings such as jitteriness, tachypnea, hypoglycemia, hypothermia, poor tone, respiratory distress, and weak cry. However, in this later study, caregivers reporting the behaviors were not blinded to drug exposure and therefore may have been more likely to seek and record perceived abnormalities than in non-drug-exposed infants. In addition, an increased rate of preterm birth was noted in the group of patients receiving fluoxetine in the third trimester, in comparison to patients who discontinued drug earlier in pregnancy, and non-drug-exposed women. An alternate explanation to a direct drug effect for this finding is that women who required continued medication throughout the pregnancy suffered higher degrees of stress, a factor well documented to be associated with a higher risk of preterm birth. In a long-term follow-up study of 55 children exposed to fluoxetine in utero, there was no significant difference in IQ, language or behavioral development in comparison to control children.

There have been several case reports of possible neonatal withdrawal symptoms, one in a neonate whose mother received fluoxetine up to the time of delivery and another whose mother was lactating while receiving setraline, which was abruptly discontinued.

While animal studies of bupropion and trazodone suggest no teratogenicity, there are no published studies of use of these agents during human pregnancy.

DOSAGE

The usual starting dose of fluoxetine is 20 mg/day, with a maximum recommended dose of 80 mg/day. The elimination half-life of an acute administration is 1–3 days and of chronic administration is 4–6 days. Full drug effect is not seen until 4 weeks after initiation of therapy. Therefore, dosage changes should not occur at intervals of less than several weeks. The usual starting dose of setraline is 50 mg/day, with a maximum recommended dose of 200 mg/day. Dosage changes should not occur at intervals of less than 1 week. The usual starting dose of paroxetine is 20 mg/day with a recommended maximum dose of 50 mg. Dosage change in 10 mg/day increments should occur at intervals of at least 1 week.

ADVERSE EFFECTS

Common adverse effects of the serotonin uptake inhibitors include nausea, decreased appetite, somnolence, dizziness, insomnia, agitation, tremor, and diarrhea/loose stools. Serious adverse reactions are rare, even with accidental or deliberate overdosage. Deaths due to overdosage were associated with other drug ingestion. Seizures have been reported with overdosage.

MECHANISM OF ACTION

The mechanism of action of the serotonin reuptake inhibitors is presumed to be related to inhibition of CNS neuronal uptake of serotonin. Bupropion is a weak inhibitor of serotonin, norepinephrine, and dopamine uptake. While chemically unrelated to the serotonin reuptake inhibitors, trazodone appears to exert its action by inhibition of serotonin uptake as well.

ABSORPTION AND BIOTRANSFORMATION

Oral absorption of fluoxetine is high, with peak levels at 6–8 hours after ingestion. The drug is highly protein-bound and is metabolized in the liver to norfluoxetine, an active metabolite. Therefore the elimination half-life of the drug is very prolonged, with measurable drug or metabolite for weeks following cessation of ingestion. The drug is eventually excreted as inactive metabolites by the kidney. Oral absorption of setraline is high, with peak levels 4–8 hours after ingestion. Setraline undergoes extensive first-pass metabolism to weakly active metabolites. Therefore, the elimination half-life is much shorter than fluoxetine, about 24 hours. The drug is highly protein-bound. Both fluoxetine and setraline are excreted in breast milk. However, as they are highly protein-bound, the dose absorbed by the neonate should be minimal. Studies of neonatal serum levels, as well as platelet levels of serotonin, suggest that this is the case.

RECOMMENDED READING

Byrd, R.A., and Markham, J.K. Developmental toxicology studies of fluoxetine hydrochloride administered orally to rats and rabbits. *Fund. Appl. Toxicol.* 22:511, 1994.

Cabrera, T.M., and Battaglia, G. Delayed decreases in brain 5-hydroxytryptamine 2A/2C receptor density and function in male rat progeny following prenatal fluoxetine. *J. Pharmacol. Exp. Ther.* 269:637, 1994.

Chambers, C.D., Johnson, K.A., Dick, L.M., Felix, R.J., and Jones, K.L. Birth outcomes in pregnant women taking fluoxetine [see comments]. *N. Engl. J. Med.* 335:1010, 1996.

Epperson, C.N., Anderson, G.M., and McDougle, C.J. Sertraline and breast-feeding. *N. Engl. J. Med.* 336:1189, 1997.

Goldstein, D.J. Effects of third trimester fluoxetine exposure on the newborn. *J. Clin. Psychopharmacol.* 15:417, 1995.

Goldstein, D.J., Corbin, L.A., and Sundell, K.L. Effects of first trimester fluoxetine exposure on the newborn. *Am. J. Obstet. Gynecol.* 89:713, 1997.

Kulin, N.A., Pastuszak, A., Sage, S.R., et al. Pregnancy outcome following maternal use of the new selective serotonin reuptake inhibitors. *J.A.M.A.* 279:609, 1998.

Nulman, I., Rovet, J., Stewart, D.E., et al. Neurodevelopment of children exposed in utero to antidepressant drugs. *N. Engl. J. Med.* 336:258, 1997.

Pastuszak, A., Schick-Boschetto, B., Feldkamp, M., et al. Pregnancy outcome following first trimester exposure to fluoxetine. *J.A.M.A.* 269:2246, 1993.

Shuey, D.L., Sadler, T.W., and Lauder, J.M. Serotonin as a regulator of craniofacial morphogenesis: site specific malformations following exposure to serotonin uptake inhibitors. *Teratology* 46:367, 1992.

Vorhees, C.V., Acuff-Smith, K.D., Schilling, M.A., Fisher, J.E., Moran, M.S., Buelke-Sam, J. A developmental neurotoxicity evaluation of the effects of prenatal exposure to fluoxetine in rats. *Fund. Appl. Toxicol.* 23:194–205, 1994.

Simethicone (Over-the-Counter) (Mylicon®, Silain®)

INDICATIONS AND RECOMMENDATIONS

Simethicone is safe to use during pregnancy. It is used for the relief of gaseous distention, bloating, or flatulence.

SPECIAL CONSIDERATIONS IN PREGNANCY

There are no special considerations related to pregnancy.

DOSAGE

The usual dose is 40–80 mg chewed thoroughly 3–4 times a day.

ADVERSE EFFECTS

One study in rats has demonstrated a significant reduction in the absorption of phenytoin when simethicone was administered.

MECHANISM OF ACTION

Simethicone is a mixture of silica gel and dimethylpolysiloxanes. Its defoaming action relieves flatulence by dispersing and preventing the formation of mucus-surrounded gas pockets in the gastrointestinal tract. Simethicone changes the surface tension of gas bubbles in the stomach and intestine, allowing them to coalesce. The gas is freed and is eliminated easily by belching or passing flatus.

ABSORPTION AND BIOTRANSFORMATION

Simethicone is not absorbed to any extent.

RECOMMENDED READING

McEinay, J.C., and D'Arcy, P.F. Interaction of phenytoin with antacid constituents and kaolin. *Proc. Br. Pharm. Soc.* 9:126P, 1980.

Schenkel, B., and Vorherr, H. Non-prescription drugs during pregnancy. Potential teratogenic and toxic effects upon embryo and fetus. *J. Reprod. Med.* 12:27, 1974.

Sodium Nitroprusside (Nipride®)

INDICATIONS AND RECOMMENDATIONS

The use of sodium nitroprusside during pregnancy is controversial. It is the most potent and predictably effective drug available for hypertensive emergencies, but it has not been studied enough to define its safety before delivery. Due to the relative hypovolemia in severe preeclampsia, extreme sensitivity to nitroprusside should be anticipated, and therefore the drug should be reserved for cases complicated by pulmonary edema where the venodilatory effects may be beneficial, or cases refractory to other agents used in hypertensive emergency such as hydralazine or labetalol. As the safety of prolonged fetal exposure to nitroprusside is unknown, it is recommended that nitroprusside be used to stabilize the mother and that delivery of the infant be performed quickly thereafter. Sodium nitroprusside has been used to effect deliberate hypotension during surgery for intracranial aneurysm during pregnancy.

SPECIAL CONSIDERATIONS IN PREGNANCY

No changes in umbilical or uterine blood flow have been observed in pregnant sheep when nitroprusside has been administered. In experiments with pregnant ewes, the administration of steadily increasing dosages of nitroprusside given to maintain a 20% reduction in mean arterial pressure was associated with marked accumulation of cyanide in the fetus. However, to maintain this degree of hypotension in normotensive ewes, extraordinarily large doses of nitroprusside, a mean of 25 µg/kg/min, were required in 5 of 8 ewes. Cyanide levels in the fetus were significantly higher than those in the mother and were associated with death in utero, but maternal death also occurred within 1 hour, due to cyanide toxicity. The placenta has therefore been shown to be readily permeable to the nitroprusside molecule and, at least in the sheep model, cyanide trapping seems to occur. This experiment may have limited applicability to clinical use of nitroprusside as toxic doses were used. In the three ewes requiring more typical doses to maintain hypotension, no adverse maternal or fetal effects were seen.

In other sheep studies, nitroprusside was given to treat hypertension induced with norepinephrine. In these studies, mean doses of 2.3 and 4 µg/kg/min were required to correct the hypertension, and nitroprusside partially corrected the deficit in uterine blood flow induced by norepinephrine. In either mother or fetus there was no acidosis and no toxic levels of cyanide.

Human data include five cases in which sodium nitroprusside was used to treat severe hypertension associated with cardiac failure and pulmonary edema during pregnancy. In these women, hypotensive effects were noted within 2 minutes of infusion and disappeared within 5 minutes of discontinuance of the drug. They were all monitored with pulmonary artery (Swan-Ganz) catheters. Duration of therapy prior to delivery was up to 15 hours. Using infusion rates of 0.013–3.9 µg/kg/min, beneficial maternal antihypertensive effects were seen in each of these women, whereas the maternal and fetal cyanide and thiocyanate levels remained negligible.

In a study of 10 patients with uncomplicated severe preeclampsia, invasive hemodynamic monitoring was performed and sodium nitroprusside was used for blood pressure control. Eight of ten women experienced an abrupt hypotensive episode with a mean dose of only 0.35 µg/kg/min. Fortunately, due to the short half-life of the drug, fetal distress requiring delivery did not occur as the drug was discontinued.

In a case series of nine antepartum patients with severe preeclampsia, aggressive plasma volume expansion with 1–3 liters of colloid, with CVP guidance, was performed prior to administration of nitroprusside. The author does not report hypotension in any case, although hemodynamic data are not presented. Therapy was restricted to a maximum of 6 hours prior to delivery, and no neonatal complications are reported.

There have been three case reports of nitroprusside to effect deliberate hypotension during cerebral aneurysm repair in pregnancy. All three cases occurred in the second trimester. One patient required nitroprusside for the first 48 postoperative hours to control chronic hypertension. All delivered healthy infants at term.

DOSAGE

Nitroprusside is light-sensitive and must be delivered in a system wrapped in a light-shielding material such as aluminum foil. Its onset of action is within 30 seconds and its duration of action is 3–5 minutes; therefore the dose is easily titrated to the individual patient's requirements. It must be given by infusion pump while the patient's blood pressure is being continuously monitored. The dose range is 0.25–8.0 µg/kg/min by constant intravenous infusion, with most nonpregnant patients responding to a dose of 0.25–1.5 µg/kg/min. As patients with severe preeclampsia are frequently volume-depleted, they may be exquisitely sensitive to this potent vasodilator. Therefore, it is recommended to begin therapy at the lowest dose of 0.25 µg/kg/min.

ADVERSE EFFECTS

Side effects are usually minimal, but administration of large doses, greater than 5 µg/kg/min can result in cyanide toxicity. Cyanide is liberated by direct combination of nitroprusside with sulfhydryl groups in red blood cells and tissue. Circulating cyanide is converted to thiocyanate in the liver, and the thiocyanate is excreted in the urine. Thiocyanate toxicity may occur when nitroprusside is administered for more than 24–48 hours, especially with decreased renal function. Principal manifestations of thiocyanate toxicity are fatigue, nausea, and anorexia followed by disorientation, psychotic behavior, and muscle spasm. Hypothyroidism has been reported following prolonged therapy.

The earliest manifestations of cyanide toxicity are tachyphylaxis to the hypotensive effect of nitroprusside and metabolic acidosis, which is seen with cyanide levels of approximately 3 μg/ml. Twice this concentration is considered to be lethal. When cyanide toxicity has been diagnosed, intravenous sodium nitrite may be administered at a dose of 5 mg/kg. This will increase the rate of methemoglobin formation and bind cyanide ions, but will also further compromise oxygen delivery to the fetus. Alternatively, hydroxocobalamin (vitamin B_{12a}) can be utilized to treat cyanide toxicity. This compound binds cyanide to form cyanocobalamin. It is administered at a rate of 12.5 mg q 30-minutes, up to a total dose of 100 mg. Cyanide toxicity can be prevented by administration of sodium thiosulfate to patients receiving unusually large doses of sodium nitroprusside.

MECHANISM OF ACTION

Nitroprusside is metabolized by smooth muscle cells to nitric oxide, a potent vasodilator of arterial and venous vessels.

Nitroprusside causes variable effects on cardiac output and heart rate. These effects are related to the preexisting state of cardiac performance and are secondary to reductions in peripheral resistance and venous tone. When there is left ventricular dysfunction secondary to severe afterload mismatch, then reduction of the afterload by arteriolar vasodilatation may improve cardiac output. When left ventricular function is normal, then the predominant effect will be to decrease preload by venous vasodilatation, and a decrease in cardiac output may occur. There are no demonstrable effects on the autonomic or central nervous system.

ABSORPTION AND BIOTRANSFORMATION

Sodium nitroprusside is a lipid-soluble, ferrocyanide compound of low molecular weight that does not bind to plasma proteins. As such, its physicochemical characteristics favor rapid and significant transplacental passage as well as potential entry into breast milk. It is metabolized to thiocyanate, which is excreted almost exclusively by the kidney. Its half-life is approximately 1 week in patients with normal renal function.

RECOMMENDED READING

Baker, A.B. Management of severe pregnancy induced hypertension, or gestosis, with sodium nitroprusside. *Anaesth. Intens. Care.* 18:361, 1990.

Ellis, S.C., Wheeler, A.S., James, F.M., Rose, J.C., Meis, P.J., et al. Fetal and maternal effects of sodium nitroprusside used to counteract hypertension in gravid ewes. *Am. J. Obstet. Gynecol.* 143:766, 1982.

Lewis, P.E., et al. Placental transfer and fetal toxicity of sodium nitroprusside. *Gynecol. Invest.* 8:46, 1977.

Naulty, J., Cefalo, R.C., and Lewis, P.E. Fetal toxicity of nitroprusside in the pregnant ewe. *Am. J. Obstet. Gynecol.* 139:708, 1981.

Oates, J.A. Antihypertensive agents and the drug therapy of hypertension. Chapter 33 in *Goodman and Gilman's The Pharmacological Basis of Therapeutics* (9th ed.), J.G. Hardman and L.E. Limbird, eds. New York: Macmillan, 1996. Pp. 797–799.

Rigg, D., and McDonogh, A. Use of sodium nitroprusside for deliberate hypotension during pregnancy. *Br. J. Anesth.* 53:985, 1985.

Shoemaker, C.T., and Meyers, M. Sodium nitroprusside for control of severe hypertensive disease of pregnancy: a case report and discussion of potential toxicity. *Am. J. Obstet. Gynecol.* 149:171, 1984.

Stempel, J.E., et al. Use of sodium nitroprusside in complications of gestational hypertension. *Obstet. Gynecol.* 60:533, 1982.

Wasserstrum, N. Nitroprusside in preeclampsia: circulatory distress and paradoxical bradycardia. *Hypertension* 18:79, 1991.

Wheeler, A.S., James, F.M., Meis, P.J., Rose, J.C., Fishburne, J.I., et al. Effects of nitroglycerin and nitroprusside on the uterine vasculature of gravid ewes. *Anesthesiology* 52:390, 1980.

Willoughby, J.S. Sodium nitroprusside, pregnancy and multiple intracranial aneurysms. Anaesth. Intens. Care 12:358, 1984.

Spectinomycin (Trobicin®)

INDICATIONS AND RECOMMENDATIONS

Spectinomycin may be used to treat gonorrhea in the pregnant patient allergic to β-lactam antibiotics, particularly because concern exists regarding the use of quinolones during pregnancy. Available reports do not suggest a threat to mother or fetus or additional reproductive effects. It should be remembered, however, that spectinomycin is not effective against syphilis or chlamydia. Spectinomycin has also been used in combination with other drugs in the treatment of postpartum endometritis.

ADVERSE EFFECTS

Untoward effects are unusual with a single intramuscular injection, although dizziness, nausea, insomnia, urticaria, chills, and fever have been reported.

MECHANISM OF ACTION

Spectinomycin selectively inhibits protein synthesis in gram-negative bacteria by binding to the 30S ribosomal subunit.

ABSORPTION AND BIOTRANSFORMATION

There is rapid absorption after intramuscular injection with peak serum levels occurring at 1 hour. Spectinomycin is not significantly bound to plasma proteins and the entire administered dose can be recovered in the urine within 48 hours.

RECOMMENDED READING

Cavenee, M.R., et al. Treatment of gonorrhea in pregnancy. *Obstet. Gynecol.* 81:33, 1993.

Filler, L., Shipley, C.F., Dennis, E.J., and Nelson, G.H. Post cesarean endometritis: a brief review and comparison of three antibiotic regimens. *J. South. Carol. Med. Assoc.* 88(6):291, 1992.

Kapusnik-Uner, J.E., Sande, M.A., and Chambers, H.F. Antimicrobial agents (continued). Chapter 47 in *Goodman and Gilman's The Pharmacological Basis of Therapeutics* (9th ed.), J.G. Hardman and L.E. Limbird, eds. New York: McGraw-Hill, 1996. P. 1143.

McCormack, W.M., and Finland, M. Spectinomycin. *Ann. Intern. Med.* 84:712, 1976.

Spermicides

INDICATIONS AND RECOMMENDATIONS

Spermicides are contraindicated during pregnancy because they are used only as contraceptive agents. Those in most common use include nonoxynol-9 and octoxynol. Although it is unlikely that an individual would knowingly use a spermicide when already pregnant, it is also true that any contraceptive technique may fail, and it is thus possible to continue to use a spermicide during early pregnancy, before the contraceptive failure has been detected.

There is controversy as to the potential risk to a fetus from accidental exposure to spermicides around the time of conception. In a 1981 publication, Jick, et al. reported a relative risk of 2.2 for major congenital anomalies among the offspring of 763 white women who had obtained a vaginal spermicide 600 or fewer days before delivery or abortion, compared to the offspring of 3902 white women who had not obtained a spermicide. In particular, limb reduction deformities, neoplasms, severe hypospadias, and chromosomal anomalies appeared to occur with increased frequency. This report was criticized for problems in ascertainment of actual spermicide use (thus, actual exposure of the fetus), for the absence of data regarding spermicide purchased outside of the health maintenance organization pharmacy involved, and for the extremely long time interval covered by 600 days between purchase and pregnancy outcomes. In addition, many critics found it significant that the incidence of these major birth defects was considerably lower among the unexposed pregnancies than would be predicted for the general population. The authors of this report considered it preliminary and suggested that further investigation would be appropriate.

In 1982, the original data from the Collaborative Perinatal Project were reanalyzed to investigate the relationship between spermicides and birth defects. Information about drug exposure was obtained by history taken before delivery. Among the 50,282 pregnant women enrolled, 462 mothers had used vaginal spermicides (other than phenylmercuric acetate, which is no longer available) during the first 16 weeks of pregnancy. Most of these mothers had also used spermicides during the month prior to conception. The relative risk for major malformations among the offspring of these spermicide users was 0.9, and they did not have an excess of the particular defects described in the Jick study. In that same year, Mills et al. reported a prospective study conducted at the Kaiser-Permanente Hospitals of northern California, in which all women registering for care over 3 years filled out a questionnaire at the first prenatal visit. Information about contraceptive use during each of the 12 months before conception was solicited. Of 34,660 women in the study, 3146 had used spermicides before, but not after, their last menstrual period, and 2282 had used spermicides after their last menstrual period. When the 3146 women who used spermicides only before the last menstrual period were compared with 13,148 women who had used other forms of contraception before the last menstrual period, the relative risk for malformations was 1.04. When the 2282 women who had used spermicides after the last menstrual period were compared with 2831 who had used other methods, the relative risk was 1.01. Thus, again, no increased risk was associated with spermicide use. Similarly, there was no increased risk for the particular anomalies described in the Jick study.

Authors of a 1985 publication reviewed the 10 studies in the literature at the time in which the relationship between spermicides and congenital malformations was explored, and concluded that the available evidence did not support an etiologic role for these agents. Subsequent case-control and prospective questionnaire studies also failed to find an association between spermicide use and Down syndrome, hypospadias, limb reduction defects, neoplasms, and neural tube defects. From a practical perspective, since most questions will center around patients who have inadvertently used spermicides while already pregnant, it is reasonable to advise such couples that the risk, if any, is quite small compared to the general population background rate for congenital anomalies, usually quoted as upward of 3%.

RECOMMENDED READING

Bracken, M.B. Spermicidal contraceptives and poor reproductive outcomes: the epidemiologic evidence against an association. *Am. J. Obstet. Gynecol.* 151:552, 1985.

Bracken, M.B., and Vita, K. Frequency of non-hormonal contraception around conception and association with congenital malformations in offspring. *Am. J. Epidemiol.* 117:281, 1983.

Cordero, J.F., and Layde, P.M. Vaginal spermicides, chromosomal abnormalities and limb reduction defects. *Fam. Plan. Persp.* 15:16, 1983.

Einarson, T.R., Koren, G., Mattice, D., et al. Maternal spermicide use and adverse reproductive outcomes: a meta-analysis. *Am. J. Obstet. Gynecol.* 162:655, 1990.

Jick, H., et al. Vaginal spermicides and congenital disorders. *J.A.M.A.* 245:1329, 1981.

Louik, C., Mitchell, A.A., Werler, M.M., et al. Maternal exposure to spermicides in relation to certain birth defects. *N. Engl. J. Med.* 317:474, 1987.

Mills, J.L., et al. Are spermicides teratogenic? *J.A.M.A.* 248:2148, 1982.

Oakley, G.P., Jr. Spermicides and birth defects. *J.A.M.A.* 247:2405, 1982.

Shapiro, S., et al. Birth defects and vaginal spermicides. *J.A.M.A.* 247:2381, 1982.

Warburton, D., Neugut, R.H., Lustenberger, A., et al. Lack of association between spermicide use and trisomy. *N. Engl. J. Med.* 317: 478–482, 1987.

Spironolactone (Aldactone®)

INDICATIONS AND RECOMMENDATIONS

Spironolactone is contraindicated during pregnancy. If diuretics are necessary at that time, a thiazide or furosemide is preferable. Serum potassium levels should be followed closely whenever pregnant women are given diuretics. If hypokalemia develops, oral potassium supplementation will effectively correct this problem. There is, therefore, no important advantage of spironolactone over these other agents, whose effects in pregnancy are better known.

Spironolactone is a competitive antagonist of aldosterone at receptor sites in the distal renal tubules. Aldosterone normally acts to augment renal tubular reabsorption of sodium and chloride and to increase the excretion of potassium. Spironolactone has been used for the treatment of primary and secondary hyperaldosteronism and low renin level hypertension.

It also has antiandrogenic effects, probably through competitive inhibition at the level of testosterone, dihydrotestosterone (DHT), and androstenedione receptors. The drug has therefore been used to treat idiopathic hirsutism in females, as well as prostate carcinoma and precocious puberty in males. Messina and co-workers have shown that daily administration of 40-mg doses of spironolactone to pregnant rats between 13th and 21st day of gestation produced anomalies of the external genitalia in male fetuses. The defects observed included reduction of the anogenital distance, urethral malformations, and altered prostate development. There have been two case reports of pregnancies in which spironolactone treatment of Bartter's syndrome was continued and there was no apparent adverse effect on masculine characteristics of male offspring.

The effects of this drug on uterine blood flow and the human fetus have not been well studied. Metabolic products may appear in breast milk. The Committee on Drugs of the American Academy of Pediatrics considers spironolactone to be compatible with breast-feeding.

RECOMMENDED READING

Committee on Drugs of the American Academy of Pediatrics. The transfer of drugs and other chemicals into human milk. *Pediatrics* 93:137, 1994.

Groves, T.D., and Corenblum, B. Spironolactone therapy during human pregnancy. *Am. J. Obstet. Gynecol.* 172:1655, 1995.

Jackson, E.K. Diuretics. Chapter 29 in *Goodman and Gilman's The Pharmacological Basis of Therapeutics* (9th ed.), J.G. Hardman and L.E. Limbird, eds. New York: McGraw-Hill, 1996. Pp. 706–709.

Messina, M., et al. Possible contraindications of spironolactone during pregnancy (letter). *J. Endocrinol. Invest.* 2:222, 1979.

Molinatti, G.M. Can the anti-androgenic effect of spironolactone contraindicate its use in pregnancy? *Minerva Ginecol.* 32:239, 1980.

Rigó, J. Jr., Gláz, E., Papp, Z.: Low or high doses of spironolactone for treatment of maternal Bartter s syndrome. *Am. J. Obstet. Gynecol.* 174:297, 1996.

Sulfonamides: Sulfadiazine, Sulfamethizole (Thiosulfil Forte ®), Sulfamethoxazole (Gantanol®), Sulfasalazine (Azulfidine®), Sulfisoxazole (Gantrisin ®)

INDICATIONS AND RECOMMENDATIONS

Sulfonamides are antibiotics with a wide range of bacteriostatic activity against both gram-positive and gram-negative organisms, including *Chlamydia trachomatis*. Strains of *Escherichia coli* may be resistant to sulfonamides. They are relatively contraindicated during the last 3 months of pregnancy because of the danger of kernicterus to the neonate. If premature delivery is anticipated, these agents should not be administered at any time during the third trimester. Sulfasalazine may be used to treat inflammatory bowel disease in pregnancy, because it is not absorbed systemically to any significant extent.

SPECIAL CONSIDERATIONS IN PREGNANCY

There are no unusual maternal effects of sulfonamides during pregnancy. Although sulfonamides are teratogenic in some animal species, the Collaborative Perinatal Project did not identify any significant association between the use of sulfonamides during human pregnancy and congenital malformations. In contrast, a retrospective study of in utero drug exposures in children with oral clefts found a significant increase following first- and second-trimester exposure to sulfonamides, but only in association with multiple malformations. These drugs cross the placenta rapidly and appear in amniotic fluid at a slower rate than in fetal blood. They compete with bilirubin for binding with albumin. In utero the fetus can clear free bilirubin through the placental circulation, but in the neonatal period this route of clearance no longer exists. In the neonate elevated levels of free bilirubin traverse the blood–brain barrier, where binding to the basal ganglia, with subsequent kernicterus, may occur. Premature infants may be particularly susceptible to hyperbilirubinemia. No cases of kernicterus have been reported after maternal ingestion of sulfonamides, although jaundice and hemolytic anemia have occurred. The recommendations are based on cases of kernicterus following neonatal administration of sulfonamides.

DOSAGE

The sulfonamide most commonly prescribed during pregnancy is sulfamethoxazole, generally in a dose of 800 mg combined with 160 mg trimethoprim (see cotrimoxazole). The recommended dosage for treatment of urinary tract infections is generally 10–14 days of one double-strength tablet of trimethoprim/sulfamethoxazole. In the prophylaxis of *Pneumocytis carinii*, a daily dose of trimethoprim-sulfamethoxazole is generally advised. The dosage of sulfasalazine for inflammatory bowel disease is 3–4 g daily in divided doses, followed by a maintenance dose of 2 g daily.

ADVERSE EFFECTS

Common side effects consist of allergic reactions that include rash, photosensitivity, and drug fever. Rarely, these drugs can cause hepatic damage; vasculitis, hemolytic anemia, especially in those with glucose 6-phosphate dehydrogenase (G6PD) deficiency; and other blood dyscrasias. The long-acting sulfonamides may be associated with the Stevens-Johnson syndrome and can increase the effects of oral anticoagulants and hydantoin anticonvulsants. Renal damage may occur as a result of crystalluria, the risk of which, however, may be diminished by maintaining a high urine output.

MECHANISM OF ACTION

The relative antibacterial differences in this group are insignificant and preferences for one agent over another are based on pharmacologic or toxicologic considerations. They are competitive inhibitors of dihydropteroate synthase, the enzyme required for the incorporation of *p*-aminobenzoic acid (PABA) into the precursor of folic acid. The sulfonamides are used primarily to treat urinary tract infections due to susceptible organisms. Other indications for their use include chancroid, trachoma, inclusion conjunctivitis, toxoplasmosis, and nocardiosis. Sulfasalazine is used in the treatment of ulcerative colitis and regional enteritis.

ABSORPTION AND BIOTRANSFORMATION

Sulfonamides, with the exception of sulfasalazine, are rapidly absorbed from the small intestine and stomach. They quickly bind to albumin and are distributed throughout all of the tissues of the body, with peak plasma levels in 2–6 hours. Fetal levels are approximately 70% to 90% of maternal levels. About 10% to 40% is metabolized by acetylation to the inactive form. Both free and acetylated metabolites are excreted in the urine.

BREAST-FEEDING

Sulfonamides appear in breast milk. Infants with G6PD deficiency might develop hemolytic anemia if nursed by mothers taking sulfonamides. Theoretically, the chance of kernicterus might also be increased in babies with an Rh or ABO incompatibility. Although they are considered generally compatible with breast-feeding, they are relatively contraindicated in premature infants or those with hyperbilirubinemia or concurrent illness.

RECOMMENDED READING

American Academy of Pediatrics, Committee on Drugs. The transfer of drugs and other chemicals into human milk. *Pediatrics* 93: 137, 1994.

Connelly, R.T., and Lourwood, D.L. *Pneumocystis carinii* pneumonia prophylaxis during pregnancy. *Pharmacotherapy* 14:424, 1994.

Handbook of Antimicrobial Therapy. The Medical Letter on Drugs and Therapeutics (rev. ed.). New Rochelle, NY: The Medical Letter, 1978.

Landers, D.V., Green, J.R., and Sweet, R.L. Antibiotic use during pregnancy and the postpartum period. *Clin. Obstet. Gynecol.* 26:391, 1983.

Mandell, G.L., and Petri, W.A., Jr. Sulfonamides, trimethoprim-sulfamethoxazole, quinolones, and agents for urinary tract infections. Chapter 44 *in Goodman and Gilman's The Pharmacological Basis of Therapeutics* (9th ed.), J.G. Hardman and L.E. Limbird, eds. New York: McGraw-Hill, 1996. Pp. 1057–1062.

Saxen, I. Associations between oral clefts and drugs taken during pregnancy. *Int. J. Epidemiol.* 4:37, 1975.

Sulfonylureas: Acetohexamide (Dymelor®), Chlorpropamide (Diabinese®), Glimepiride (Amaryl®), Glipizide (Glucotrol®), Glyburide (DiaBeta®, Glynase®, Micronase®), Tolazamide (Tolinase®), Tolbutamide (Orinase®)

INDICATIONS AND RECOMMENDATIONS

Sulfonylureas are relatively contraindicated during pregnancy because other therapeutic agents are preferable. These drugs are orally administered to lower the blood glucose in patients with mild type 2 diabetes whose hyperglycemia cannot be controlled by diet alone. Their mechanism of action includes stimulation of pancreatic beta cells with increased release of endogenous insulin, and a postulated effect on both hepatic and peripheral insulin sensitivity. By enhancing insulin secretion, sulfonylureas lower circulating glucose levels. In turn, this hypoglycemic effect may ameliorate the toxic effect of hyperglycemia on insulin action. Chlorpropamide is considered a first-generation sulfonylurea, whereas glimepiride, glyburide and glipizide are second-generation agents and are considerably more potent.

Some studies have shown increased perinatal mortality when pregnant diabetic patients were treated with sulfonylureas rather than insulin, whereas other series have not borne out this finding. There is evidence of teratogenicity in laboratory animals given high doses of some of the sulfonylureas, and case reports of birth defects among offspring of sulfonylurea-treated human pregnancies have been published. In one series of 20 gravidas with type 2 diabetes who took oral agents, primarily sulfonylureas, during early pregnancy, 50% of offspring manifested congenital malformations, compared to 15% of offspring of 40 control mothers with diabetes who did not take oral agents. Ear anomalies were particularly common. However, another series of patients with type 2 diabetes reported a 16% anomaly rate in 147 pregnncies exposed to oral agents during the first trimester, compared to 19% in 125 pregnancies treated with diet and 15% in 60 pregnancies treated with insulin. The primary determinant of malformations in that study appeared to be maternal glycemic control. It should be remembered that maternal diabetes itself is a powerful teratogen, and there are no well-controlled human studies implicating sulfonylureas in congenital malformations.

It is known that tolbutamide and chlorpropamide cross the placenta easily. Glyburide did not cross the placenta in an in vitro study of isolated human placental cotyledons. Since it is widely believed that fetal hyperinsulinemia is the primary cause of the various manifestations of diabetic fetopathy, it would be illogical to treat maternal diabetes with drugs that would be expected to stimulate fetal insulin secretion. Although a number of investigators have used oral hypoglycemic agents in series of diabetic pregnancies without obvious ill effects on the fetus or neonate, there have been a number of isolated case reports of prolonged neonatal hypoglycemia when the mothers were taking these drugs. A case of transient neonatal diabetes insipidus (as well as hypoglycemia) was reported in the offspring of a mother taking chlorpropamide.

It is recommended that sulfonylureas not be used during pregnancy because of the relative lack of data regarding their safety and efficacy. When diabetes is present during pregnancy, insulin is the drug of choice.

RECOMMENDED READING

Adam, P.A.J., and Schwartz, R. Diagnosis and treatment: Should oral hypoglycemic agents be used in pediatric and pregnant patients? *Pediatrics* 42:819, 1968.

Davis, S.N., and Granner, D.K. Insulin, oral hypoglycemic agents, and the pharmacology of the endocrine pancreas. Chapter 60 in *Goodman and Gilman's The Pharmacological Basis of Therapeutics* (9th ed.), J.G. Hardman and L.E. Limbird, eds. New York: McGraw-Hill, 1996. Pp. 1507–1510.

Douglas, C.P., and Richards, R. Use of chlorpropamide in the treatment of diabetes in pregnancy. *Diabetes* 16:60, 1967.

Elliott, B.D., Langer, O., Schenker, S., et al. Insignificant transfer of glyburide occurs across the human placenta. *Am. J. Obstet. Gynecol.* 165:807, 1991.

Kemball, M.L., et al. Neonatal hypoglycaemia in infants of diabetic mothers given sulphonylurea drugs in pregnancy. *Arch. Dis. Child.* 45:696, 1970.

Kolterman, O.G., et al. The acute and chronic effects of sulfonylurea therapy in type II diabetic subjects. *Diabetes* 33:346, 1984.

Notelovitz, M., and James, S. Tolbutamide-induced insulin release in pregnant diabetics. *Horm. Metab. Res.* 9:167, 1977.

Piacquadio, K., Hollingsworth, D.R., and Murphy, H. Effects of in-utero exposure to oral hypoglycemic drugs. *Lancet* 338:866, 1991.

Sutherland, H.W., et al. Evaluation of chlorpropamide in chemical diabetes diagnosed during pregnancy. *Br. Med. J.* 3:9, 1973.

Towner, D., Kjos, S., Leung, B., et al. Congenital malformations in pregnancies complicated by NIDDM. *Diabetes Care* 18:1446, 1995.

Uhrig, J.D., and Hurley, R.M. Chlorpropamide in pregnancy and transient neonatal diabetes insipidus. *Can. Med. Assoc. J.* 128:368, 1983.

Sumatriptan (Imitrex®)

Sumatriptan is relatively contraindicated in pregnancy because other therapeutic agents are preferable. Sumatriptan is a selective 5-HT$_1$ agonist effective against acute migraine attacks. In rats, it is transferred across the placenta and is concentrated up to 8 times plasma levels in milk. In vitro testing with the human placenta shows that approximately 15% of a single dose reaches the fetal compartment over 4 hours. Given the average half-life of 2 hours, the author of the latter study concluded that very little of the drug would cross from mother to fetus with a single dose. The actual effects of sumatriptan on a pregnancy and fetus have yet to be studied.

Although most patients with migraine headaches improve during pregnancy, headaches do occur and some women have their first attack during pregnancy. In these instances, nonpharmacologic treatment is the ideal solution, whereas analgesics such as acetaminophen and narcotics can be used on a limited basis. Preventative treatment and sumatriptan are last resorts.

RECOMMENDED READINGS

Dixon, C.M., et al. Disposition of sumatriptan in laboratory animals and humans. *Drug Metab. Disp.* 21:761, 1993.

Peroutka, S.J. Drugs effective in the therapy of migraine. Chapter 21 in *Goodman and Gilman's The Pharmacological Basis of Therapeutics* (9th ed.), J.G. Hardman and L.E. Limbird, eds. New York: McGraw-Hill, 1996. Pp. 496–498.

Schenker, S., et al. Sumatriptan (Imitrex) transport by the human placenta. *Proc. Soc. Exp. Biol. Med.* 210:213, 1995.

Silberstein, S.D. Migraine and pregnancy. *Neurol. Clin.* 15:209, 1997.

Sympathomimetics (Over-the-Counter): Ephedrine, Phenylephrine, Phenylpropanolamine

INDICATIONS AND RECOMMENDATIONS

Sympathomimetics are generally safe to use during pregnancy. Members of this group of drugs are used in expectorants, decongestants, cough and cold medications, antiasthmatic combinations, and ophthalmic decongestants and vasoconstrictors. As a general policy, it is wise to avoid all medications during the first trimester whenever possible. These drugs should therefore not be used indiscriminately for upper respiratory symptoms during the period of embryogenesis, but should be reserved for conditions that create significant maternal discomfort or that impact on hemodynamic homeostasis.

SPECIAL CONSIDERATIONS IN PREGNANCY

There are no maternal side effects of these drugs unique to pregnancy. These substances cross the placental and blood–brain barriers. Fetal central nervous system effects may include hyperactivity and fetal tachycardia following maternal ingestion. Despite the fact that sympathomimetics are generally safe to use during pregnancy, they should be avoided in patients with essential hypertension or toxemia because of their potential for elevating systemic blood pressure. They should also be avoided in situations in which there is poor fetal reserve because distress in utero could be precipitated.

The Collaborative Perinatal Project found no evidence of an increase in major or minor anomalies when ephedrine was taken in the first trimester. Phenylephrine and phenylpropanolamine were associated with a slight increase in the incidence of minor abnormalities such as clubfoot and inguinal hernia, as well as eye or ear deformities, when taken in the first trimester. It should be noted, however, that quite often more than one compound was used in the same preparation. Furthermore, it was impossible to determine whether viral infections were present and possibly responsible for the associations observed.

Ephedrine and phenylephrine are the preferred vasoconstrictors for the treatment of maternal hypotension following conduction anesthesia. They appear to act by direct stimulation of vascular α-adrenoceptors. Compared to metaraminol, ephedrine causes less uterine artery vasoconstriction while maintaining its vasoconstrictive properties in other vascular bed. Such observations suggest that uterine perfusion is better maintained during maternal systemic hypertension with ephedrine. One randomized trial of ephedrine and phenylephrine treatment of post–spinal anesthesia maternal hypotension found phenylephrine to be associated with lower fetal blood catecholamine levels and higher pH and base excess measures at delivery. But ephedrine may be more effective in preventing maternal hypotension in this circumstance than phenylephrine. A saltatory fetal heart rate pattern identified in 10 of 433 consecutive recordings was associated with ephedrine use in 6.

DOSAGE

The dosage varies with the preparation being used. This group of drugs is most effective when administered orally. Their onset of action is rapid, and they are effective for hours because of their resistance to inactivating enzymes. When bolus intravenous fluid infusion does not satisfactorily maintain maternal blood pressure after conduction anesthesia, 5–10 mg of bolus intravenous ephedrine or 40 µg of bolus intravenous phenylephrine is recommended.

ADVERSE EFFECTS

Side effects from sympathomimetics include insomnia, anxiety, headache, tremor, dizziness, palpitations, anorexia, nausea, vomiting, abdominal cramps, and diarrhea.

MECHANISM OF ACTION

The sympathomimetic drugs used in over-the-counter preparations are primarily noncatecholamines. They may act directly on effector cells or act indirectly by stimulating the release of norepinephrine from adrenergic nerve endings. The structure of each substance determines its predominant mode of action.

Ephedrine causes norepinephrine release and has α-receptor effects. It also has a direct effect on β-receptors in the bronchial tree, resulting in a relaxation of bronchospasm. Phenylephrine acts directly on α-receptors, especially in the heart; it has little effect on β-receptors. Ephedrine and phenylpropanolamine may cause an increase in systolic and diastolic blood pressures as well as cardiac output. They may also increase alertness, decrease fatigue, and cause mild mood elevation. Phenylephrine can elevate both systolic and diastolic blood pressures and increase circulation time and venous pressure. It may also be associated with a reflex bradycardia.

ABSORPTION AND BIOTRANSFORMATION

The sympathomimetics included in over-the-counter preparations are generally well absorbed from the gastrointestinal tract. Their metabolic pathways include hydroxylation, n-demethylation, deamination, and conjugation in the liver, followed by urinary excretion. They may also be excreted unchanged by the kidneys, with the amount depending on urinary pH.

RECOMMENDED READING

Catterall, W., and Mackie, K. Local anesthetics. Chapter 15 in *Goodman and Gilman's The Pharmacological Basis of Therapeutics* (9th ed.), J.G. Hardman and L.E. Limbird, eds. New York: McGraw-Hill, 1996. p. 344.

Hall, P.A., Bennett, A., Wilkes, M.P., and Lewis, M. Spinal anaesthesia for caesarean section: comparison of infusions of phenylephrine and ephedrine. *Br. J. Anaesth.* 73(4):471, 1994.

Heinonen, O.P., Slone, D., and Shapiro, S. *Birth Defects and Drugs in Pregnancy.* Littleton, MA: PSG, 1977. Pp. 345–356, 439.

Hoffman, B.B., and Lefkowitz, R.J. Catecholamines, sympathomimetic drugs, and adrenergic receptor antagonists. Chapter 10 in *Goodman and Gilman's The Pharmacological Basis of Therapeutics* (9th ed.), J.G. Hardman and L.E. Limbird, eds. New York: McGraw-Hill, 1996. Pp. 221–224.

Jick, H., Aselton, P., and Hunter, J.R. Phenylpropanolamine and cerebral hemorrhage. *Lancet* 1:1017, 1984.

LaPorta, R.F., Arthur, G.R., and Datta, S. Phenylephrine in treating maternal hypotension due to spinal anaesthesia for caesarean delivery: effects on neonatal catecholamine concentrations, acid–base status and Apgar scores. *Anaesthesiol. Scand.* 39(7): 901, 1995.

Lasagna, L. Phenylpropanolamine and blood pressure (letters). *J.A.M.A.* 253:2491, 1985.

Li, P., Tong, C., and Eisenach, J.C. Pregnancy and ephedrine increase the release of nitric oxide in ovine uterine arteries. *Anesth. Analges.* 82(2):288, 1996.

Nelson, M.M., and Forfar, J.O. Associations between drugs administered during pregnancy and congenital abnormalities of the fetus. *Br. Med. J.* 1:523, 1971.

Noble, R.E. Phenylpropanolamine and blood pressure. *Lancet* 1:1419, 1982.

O'Brien-Abel, N.E., and Benedetti, T.J. Saltatory fetal heart rate pattern. *J. Perinatol* 12(1):13, 1992.

Pentel, P. Toxicity of over-the-counter stimulants. *J.A.M.A.* 252: 1898, 1984.

Schenkel, B., and Vorherr, H. Non-prescription drugs during pregnancy: potential teratogenic and toxic effects upon embryo and fetus. *J. Reprod. Med.* 12:27, 1974.

Tong, C., and Eisenach, J.C. The vascular mechanism of ephedrine's beneficial effect on uterine perfusion during pregnancy. *Anesthesiology* 76(5):792, 1992.

Tetracyclines: Demeclocycline, Oxytetracycline, Tetracycline, Minocycline

INDICATIONS AND RECOMMENDATIONS

Tetracyclines are contraindicated during pregnancy. These broad-spectrum antibiotics act by inhibiting protein synthesis. Alternate antibiotic treatment is indicated.

Problems attributable to tetracycline use in pregnancy include (a) deposition in fetal teeth and bone; (b) potential maternal hepatotoxicity; and (c) congenital defects. Tetracyclines cross the placenta and administration in the second and third trimesters can cause staining of deciduous teeth and depression in bone growth, the latter particularly in long-term chronic use. Tetracycline use in larger dosages, typically intravenously, has been associated with hepatotoxicity in the form of acute fatty liver. Symptoms include jaundice, azotemia, acidosis, and irreversible shock. Fetal morbidity and mortality is a consequence of maternal pathology. The Collaborative Perinatal Project did not identify tetracycline as causative of major birth defects, although there are a number of case reports of abnormalities in newborns following maternal tetracycline use. Possible associations with minor defects were suggested, but the small number of cases does not permit the conclusion that tetracyclines are teratogenic. Therefore, inadvertent use in the first trimester would not prompt a recommendation for termination.

Tetracycline is excreted into breast milk in low concentrations. Serum levels of tetracycline in breast-fed infants are undetectable. The American Academy of Pediatrics considers tetracycline to be compatible with breast-feeding.

RECOMMENDED READING

Cohlan, S.Q. Drugs and pregnancy. *Prog. Clin. Biol. Res.* 44:77, 1980.

Committee on Drugs, American Academy of Pediatrics. The transfer of drugs and other chemicals into human breast milk. *Pediatrics* 93:137, 1994.

Corcoran, R., and Castles, J.M. Tetracycline for acne vulgaris and possible teratogenesis. *Br. Med. J.* 2:807, 1977.

Heinonen, O.P., et al. *Birth Defects and Drugs in Pregnancy.* Littleton, MA: PSG, 1977. Pp. 297–313.

Kline, A.H., et al. Transplacental effect of tetracyclines on teeth. *J.A.M.A.* 188:178, 1964.

Knowles, J.A. Drugs in milk. *Pediatr. Curr.* 21:28, 1972.

Rendle-Short, T.J. Tetracycline in teeth and bone. *Lancet* 1:1188, 1962.

Schultz, J.C., et al. Fatty liver disease after intravenous administration by tetracycline in high dosage. *N. Engl. J. Med.* 269:999, 1963.

Wenk, R.E., et al. Tetracycline associated fatty liver of pregnancy, including possible pregnancy risk after chronic dermatologic use of tetracycline. *J. Reprod. Med.* 26:135, 1981.

Wilson, W.R., and Cockerill, F.R. Tetracyclines, chloramphenicol, erythromycin and clindamycin. *Mayo Clin. Proc.* 58:92, 1983.

Theophylline and Aminophylline (Elixophyllin®, Slo-Phyllin®, Theo-Dur®, Thedair®)

INDICATIONS AND RECOMMENDATIONS

Theophylline is safe to use during pregnancy. This drug is a bronchodilator that is considered a third-line agent for asthma therapy, due to decreased effectiveness when compared with other agents, as well as a narrow therapeutic window. It may also be used as an adjunctive agent in the therapy of acute pulmonary edema and in some cases of Cheyne-Stokes respirations. Theophylline is a central nervous system stimulant and has been used to treat apnea in the premature infant.

Blood levels should be monitored in patients receiving theophylline by any route, but clinical response should be the main guide to therapy. When the drug is administered orally, peak and trough levels should be monitored. Patients given the drug intravenously should undergo cardiac monitoring.

Neonates exposed to theophylline in utero as well as those ingesting it in breast milk should be observed for evidence of toxicity or withdrawal. Breast-feeding women should nurse their infants just before taking the drug in order to decrease the quantity of drug passing over to the neonate.

SPECIAL CONSIDERATIONS IN PREGNANCY

In pregnant women and newborn infants, the binding affinity of plasma protein for many drugs is decreased. Since only the unbound drugs in plasma are generally considered to be pharmacologically active, an enhanced response may be obtained in pregnant women when compared to their nonpregnant counterparts at similar total plasma theophylline concentrations. On the other hand, because of a larger volume of distribution, pregnant women may require a higher dosage to reach a given plasma concentration. Theophylline clearance is significantly decreased in the third trimester versus the postpartum period, largely due to decreased hepatic metabolism.

Theophylline in the neonate is less protein-bound than in the adult, resulting in higher levels of free drug. When two mother–neonate pairs were investigated, cord serum theophylline levels were equal to, or slightly higher than, maternal levels at delivery. Neonatal theophylline levels remained near or within the therapeutic range for at least 18 hours after birth but fell to minimal levels at 30 hours. One of the two infants was noted to be jittery, but no other toxic effects were observed. In a second report, 12 newborns of asthmatic mothers were found to have cord blood theophylline levels similar to the levels in their mothers, with a few infants manifesting tachycardia and transient jitteriness. As in the previous report, neonatal heel-stick theophylline levels tended to be higher than maternal levels.

Theophylline appears to be mutagenic only in lower organisms. This may be due to the inability of those animals to demethylate this compound, a process that takes place readily in humans. A single case report describes chromosomal abnormalities in association with ingestion of theophylline by the mother, but this remains an isolated occurrence to date. The limited data available appear to support the impression that teratogenesis with theophylline is unlikely. While theophylline has not been clearly associated with malformations or stillbirth, a report of severe complex cardiovascular anomalies in three infants exposed to theophylline during pregnancy raises some question as to its safety. One study noted increased fetal breathing movements in association with maternal theophylline therapy, raising potential implications for interpretation of biophysical profile scores in this setting.

In a randomized trial of maternal aminophylline therapy (250 mg IM q12h for 3 days), 70 neonates of treated mothers who delivered before 34 weeks gestation were compared to 78 born to untreated control mothers. The infants of aminophylline-treated mothers had a significantly lower incidence of perinatal death and respiratory distress syndrome. Confirmatory studies are not available. Reports regarding the incidence of preeclampsia in mothers receiving theophylline therapy have been conflicting.

Toxicity can occur by transplacental passage of the drug or in breast-fed infants. Toxic levels have not been well defined and vary from one infant to another. Symptoms may include vomiting, feeding difficulties, jitteriness, tachycardia, cardiac arrhythmias, and transient hyperglycemia. Theophylline concentration in breast milk reaches its peak 1–3 hours after an oral dose. The milk concentration parallels the serum concentration at a mean milk/serum ratio of 0.73. The drug is not bound to protein in breast milk. Methylxanthines have been shown to decrease lipid synthesis in the developing brain. Follow-up to 27 months in infants exposed to theophylline has not identified any neurologic abnormalities. No long-term deficits have been noted in neonates treated with theophylline for apnea. The American Academy of Pediatrics considers theophylline and aminophylline to be compatible with breast-feeding.

DOSAGE

The therapeutic range for theophylline in plasma is 10–20 µg/ml in the nonpregnant woman. Lower levels may suffice during pregnancy. Dosages should be adjusted downward for patients with liver disease or congestive heart failure.

The only intravenous preparation available is aminophylline (theophylline ethylenediamine), which is 86% theophylline by weight. It has been recommended that in the treatment of status asthmaticus a loading dose of 6 mg/kg (based on total body weight) given over 20–40 minutes be followed by a maintenance infusion of 0.7 mg/kg/h aminophylline (equivalent to 0.6 mg/kg/h anhydrous theophylline) in nonsmokers and 1.0 mg/kg/h (equivalent to 0.85 mg/kg/h theophylline) in smokers. If the patient continues to have bronchospasm but no signs of toxicity, a further increase can be attempted if plasma levels are not in the therapeutic range. After a bolus dose of 3 mg/kg given over 20 minutes, the maintenance infusion rate may be increased to 1.3–1.5 mg/kg/h depending on the plasma level. If the patient has been taking theophylline orally in adequate amounts, half the loading dose described previously and the same maintenance dosage should be administered. If she has been taking the drug erratically, it is probably best to proceed as if she were not taking it at all. Theophylline must be infused slowly due to a risk of serious arrhythmias.

Oral theophylline is used for the long-term treatment of bronchospasm. Its use is now commonly reserved for patients with nocturnal symptoms or those with acute asthma who are unresponsive to sympathomimetic therapy. Plain, enteric-coated, and sustained release preparations are available. The use of enteric-coated preparations is not recommended as absorption is unpredictable. Plain theophylline or aminophylline tablets or liquids are usually taken q6h. Sustained release preparations have the advantage of an 8- to 12-hour dose interval but may be associated with significant variability between patients with respect to absorption.

Aminophylline can be given rectally as suppository but, the use of suppositories is not recommended as they tend to be absorbed erratically and can produce unpredictable and dangerous blood levels.

Theophylline clearance is increased by cigarette smoking, alcohol use, and medications such as phenytoin, rifampin, and barbiturates. Clearance may be decreased in association with cimetidine, ciprofloxacin, or erythromycin.

ADVERSE EFFECTS

Side effects and toxicity are related in most cases to plasma concentrations of the drug. They are usually of minor significance when the drug is maintained within the usual therapeutic range. Side effects include anorexia, nausea, vomiting, diuresis, and abdominal distention. Palpitations and sinus and atrial tachycardias may occur. Precordial pain and hypotension have been reported with rapid intravenous administration of aminophylline. Excitation, anxiety, insomnia, diaphoresis, tremor, and even convulsions may occur. The latter is a toxic phenomenon and is usually seen with plasma levels close to 60 µg/ml. Seizures generally do not occur at levels less than 25 µg/ml.

MECHANISM OF ACTION

The actions of theophylline and other methylxanthines are mediated primarily through inhibition of phosphodiesterase, the enzyme responsible for the degradation of cyclic AMP. There may be additional effects on intracellular calcium concentration, as well as antagonism of adenosine receptors. In vitro studies suggest an antiinflammatory effect.

The primary action of theophylline is to relax bronchiolar smooth muscle, especially during muscle spasm. It also sensitizes the respiratory center to carbon dioxide, causing an increase in both respiratory rate and minute volume. It has both inotropic and chronotropic effects on the myocardium and causes vasodilatation in the pulmonary, coronary, and systemic circulations. Cardiac output is increased and venous filling pressure is reduced. Urine production is increased. It also increases gastric secretion and decreases small and large bowel motility. In addition, catecholamine release may be stimulated. Aminophylline may have a tocolytic effect on the uterine smooth muscle.

ABSORPTION AND BIOTRANSFORMATION

Ninety percent of an oral dose reaches the circulation, and absorption is better in the fasting state. Peak concentrations are achieved between 1 and 3 hours after administration of uncoated tablets and in 30 minutes with elixir and solutions. Theophylline is metabolized by the liver and excreted in the urine. Sixty percent of the drug is bound to plasma proteins at therapeutic concentrations. It does not displace bilirubin from albumin. The half-life is usually 4–5 hours in adults but may be elevated in patients with liver disease, congestive failure, or pneumonia. Theophylline readily crosses the placenta. It is metabolized to caffeine in the fetal liver.

RECOMMENDED READING

Carter, B.L., Driscoll, C.E., and Smith, G.D. Theophylline clearance during pregnancy. *Obstet. Gynecol.* 68:555, 1986.

Committee on Drugs of the American Academy of Pediatrics. The transfer of drugs and other chemicals into human milk. *Pediatrics* 93:137, 1994.

Gardner, M.J., Schatz, M., Cousins, L., Zeiger, R., Middleton, E., and Jusko, W.J. Longitudinal effects of pregnancy on the pharmacokinetics of theophylline. *Eur. J. Clin. Pharmacol.* 31:289, 1987.

Hadjigeorgiou, E., et al. Antepartum aminophylline treatment for prevention of the respiratory distress syndrome in premature infants. *Am. J. Obstet. Gynecol.* 135:257, 1979.

Horowitz, D.A., Jablonski, W., and Mehta, K.A. Apnea associated with theophylline withdrawal in a term neonate. *Am. J. Dis. Child.* 136:73, 1982.

Ishikawa, M., Yoneyama, Y., Power, G.G., et al. Maternal theo-phylline administration and breathing movements in late-gesta-tion human fetuses. *Obstet. Gynecol.* 88:973, 1996.

Labovitz, E., and Specter, S. Placental theophylline transfer in pregnant asthmatics. *J.A.M.A.* 247:786, 1982.

McFadden, E.R., Jr., and Hejal, R. Asthma. *Lancet* 345:1215, 1995.

Park, J.M., Schmer, V., and Myers, T.L. Cardiovascular anomalies associated with prenatal exposure to theophylline. *Southern Med. J.* 83:1487, 1990.

Pollowitz, J.A. Theophylline therapy during pregnancy. *J.A.M.A.* 243:651, 1980.

Serafin, W.E. Drugs used in the treatment of asthma. Chapter 28 in *Goodman and Gilman's The Pharmacological Basis of Therapeu-tics* (9th ed.), J.G. Hardman and L.E. Limbird, eds. New York: Mc-Graw-Hill, 1996. Pp. 659–682.

Stentus-Aarniala, B., Riikonen, S., and Teramo, K. Slow-release theophylline in pregnant asthmatics. *Chest* 107:642, 1995.

Volpe, J.J. Effects of methylxanthines on lipid synthesis in develop-ing neural systems. *Semin. Perinatol.* 5:395, 1981.

Thioamides: Methimazole (Tapazole®), Propylthiouracil (PTU)

INDICATIONS AND RECOMMENDATIONS

The thioamides carbimazole, propylthiouracil (PTU), and me-thimazole are antithyroid drugs used in the treatment of hy-perthyroidism. Although these drugs cross the placenta and may cause fetal goiter, they are generally regarded as the treat-ment of choice for hyperthyroidism during pregnancy. They should be used in the lowest dosage compatible with treatment goals, and it is usually possible to reduce the dosage during the third trimester. There is currently no documented advantage to using totally suppressive dosages of these drugs combined with thyroid replacement therapy.

SPECIAL CONSIDERATIONS IN PREGNANCY

Because thioamides cross the placenta, fetal thyroid suppres-sion may result, with increased thyroid-stimulating hormone (TSH) levels resulting in stimulation of the fetal thyroid gland. This stimulation may rarely result in fetal goiter, which, in turn, can cause hyperextension of the fetal head leading to dys-tocia during labor. Modest doses of PTU (100–200 mg/day) given to 11 hyperthyroid mothers were associated with chemi-cal evidence of hypothyroidism (i.e., low T4 and reverse T3 lev-els, elevated TSH) in the offspring, compared to 40 control neo-nates. One of the newborns met the clinical criteria for hypothyroidism, but the condition lasted less than 2 weeks.

If a pregnant woman has autoimmune hyperthyroidism, thy-roid-stimulating immunoglobulin G (IgG) may cross the pla-centa and cause fetal and neonatal thyrotoxicosis. There has been a report of a case of fetal goiter secondary to maternal PTU treatment, in which the diagnosis was made by ultrasound but cordocentesis was performed in order to differentiate goiter caused by fetal hypothyroidism from goiter caused by fetal hyperthyroidism secondary to transplacental thyroid-stimulating IgG. Hypothyroidism was diagnosed and the fetus was successfully treated with intraamniotic injections of thyroxine.

If a patient with high levels of thyroid-stimulating IgG is treated with a thioamide, the resulting transient neonatal hypothyroidism may temporarily mask thyrotoxicosis until the effects of the thioamide have dissipated. Unfortunately, such a neonate may be discharged from the hospital before the thyrotoxicosis is manifested, with a resultant delay in diagnosis. Awareness of this problem will permit appropriate short-term follow-up studies to be scheduled.

In one long-term follow-up study, 18 children born to PTU-treated mothers were compared to 17 siblings born at a time when the mothers were not taking PTU. There were no differences in intellectual or motor function between the two groups. Similar findings were reported in another follow-up study of 31 exposed offspring and 25 unexposed siblings.

Intrauterine fetal therapy (PTU given to the mother) has been successfully used to prevent fetal hyperthyroidism and growth retardation in a patient with Hashimoto's thyroiditis. This woman was hypothyroid, but had high levels of thyroid-stimulating immunoglobulins diagnosed because of the previous delivery of a hyperthyroid growth-retarded baby. A number of cases of treated Graves' disease with normal maternal thyroid function but high levels of thyroid-stimulating IgG have been managed by giving PTU when there is fetal tachycardia or poor fetal growth. In the absence of such signs, some investigators recommend fetal blood sampling to make this diagnosis. In at least one reported case, recurrent fetal hydrops has been successfully reversed with this approach.

Both PTU and methimazole inhibit thyroid hormone synthesis but only the former blocks the conversion of T4 to T3. Furthermore, methimazole administration during pregnancy has been associated with a number of case reports of aplasia cutis in the offspring. In one such case, maternal serum α-fetoprotein (AFP) was elevated, presumably because of the break in the fetal integument. Investigators in Spain have questioned whether an increase in the number of neonates with aplasia cutis may be related to methimazole illegally added to animal feed in the region. For these reasons, PTU is the more widely used of the two drugs in obstetric patients. Nevertheless, in one case series of 99 patients treated with PTU in pregnancy and 36 treated with methimazole, results were equally good in both groups and there were no cases of neonatal scalp defects.

Although old data on thiouracil suggested that significant amounts of this compound appeared in breast milk, a subsequent report on nine mother–infant pairs showed breast milk concentrations of PTU 1.5 hours after the ingestion of 400 mg to be only 10% of maternal serum concentrations. The total amount of PTU appearing in breast milk during the 4 hours after maternal ingestion was 0.025% of the administered dose. No abnormalities in thyroid function tests were found in a suckling baby followed for 5 months, during which time the mother took 200–300 mg PTU daily. A group of Japanese investigators followed thyroid function in eight infants exposed to PTU both in utero and during breast-feeding. While cord blood T4 levels showed thyroid suppression at birth in all eight, they all recovered to normal thyroid function despite the mothers continuing to take PTU. Methimazole, on the other hand, has been found in approximately equal concentrations in breast milk and maternal serum, with 0.18% of the maternal dose appearing in the milk over 8 hours. Nevertheless, a study of 35 infants of lactating mothers taking methimazole showed normal thyroid function.

DOSAGE

Propylthiouracil is available in 50-mg tablets that can be broken in half. Methimazole is manufactured in 5- and 10-mg tablets. Carbimazole, available mainly in Europe, comes as 5- and 10-mg tablets. The usual starting dose is 100 mg PTU, or 5–10 mg methimazole, taken every 8 hours. Because PTU has such a short half-life, a single daily dose of 300 mg is usually not effective.

Although serum PTU levels of 3 µg/ml have been shown to halve thyroid function, it is currently impractical to monitor this drug by measurement of serum levels. Thus, its efficacy is titrated by the patient's clinical response and by measurement of serum thyroid hormone levels. It should be borne in mind that many symptoms are common to both hyperthyroidism and pregnancy, and that the total T4 level is increased during normal pregnancy due to increased protein binding. Thus, an estimate of the free thyroxine level is the most useful parameter to follow. The advent of highly sensitive assays for TSH has made it possible to more precisely evaluate hyperthyroidism in pregnancy, and this test is helpful in following the efficacy of thioamide medications. The goal of therapy should be maintenance of the free thyroxine level in the high-normal or slightly elevated range and the TSH in the normal range. It is sometimes necessary to use doses as high as 1000 mg/day PTU in order to achieve euthyroidism. Although the hyperthyroid patient may begin to feel improvement within a week of starting thioamide therapy, it may be as long as 4 weeks before a full effect has occurred, depending on the amount of colloid stored in the thyroid gland.

It is most practical to measure thyroid function monthly. Once the therapeutic goal has been attained, a reduction in the dose of PTU or methimazole should be instituted, usually down to 50–150 mg/day PTU (5–15 mg methimazole) after 4–6 weeks. Thyroid function should be monitored because hyperthyroidism often improves spontaneously during the third trimester and it is sometimes possible to eliminate treatment entirely. Recrudescence post partum should be anticipated.

ADVERSE EFFECTS

Frequently noted side effects (1% to 5% of patients) include fever, rash, urticaria, arthralgias, and arthritis, all apparently dose-related. Transient leukopenia (>4000/mm^3) occurs in up to 12% of adults and is benign. This leukopenia is not an antecedent of agranulocytosis and its occurrence does not necessitate stopping of the medication. The incidence of cross-sensitivity between

PTU and methimazole is approximately 50%, so although the appearance of any of these side effects may prompt substitution of the other thioamide, the unwanted sequelae may recur.

Both PTU and methimazole are associated with agranulocytosis in approximately 0.5% of patients. This potentially life-threatening complication almost always develops during the first 3 months of treatment and is characterized by fever, systemic toxicity, bacterial pharyngitis, and an absolute granulocyte count below 250/mm^3. Because the onset is sudden, routine monitoring of the white cell count is not helpful. When thioamides are discontinued, clinical improvement usually occurs over days to weeks, but fatalities have occurred. This complication tends to be seen most frequently in patients over 40 years of age, and seems to be dose-related for methimazole but not for PTU. Patients who take thioamides should be instructed to discontinue them if fever, pharyngitis, or other signs of infection develop, and to report this to their physician.

Drug-related toxic hepatitis has been associated with PTU and may occasionally be life threatening; this may have an immune basis. Cholestatic jaundice has been associated with methimazole. Vasculitis and a lupus-like syndrome have also been reported and should be treated with corticosteroids and discontinuation of the thioamide. The appearance of circulating antibodies to insulin or glucagon has been reported with methimazole. Extremely rare complications include aplastic anemia (PTU or methimazole), nephrotic syndrome (methimazole), loss of taste (methimazole), and hypoprothrombinemia (PTU).

MECHANISM OF ACTION

The thioamides act directly on the thyroid gland and also have systemic effects. Within the thyroid gland, these drugs inhibit thyroglobulin formation by diverting iodide away from tyrosine residues. They also inhibit the coupling of iodotyrosines to form iodothyronines. Furthermore, they may alter the structure of thyroglobulin and inhibit thyroglobulin synthesis, but these effects have not been proved. Systemically, PTU inhibits the conversion of T4 to T3, the more active thyroid hormone. There is also some evidence to support a role of these agents in altering the immune system, perhaps contributing to remission of immune thyroid disease.

ABSORPTION AND BIOTRANSFORMATION

The thioamides are well absorbed from the gastrointestinal tract, with peak serum levels reached 1–2 hours after dosing. The serum half-life of PTU is approximately 1 hour, whereas that of methimazole is approximately 5 hours. Hepatic and renal disease may prolong the half-life of these drugs.

Thioamides are concentrated by the thyroid gland within minutes of dosing, peak intrathyroid levels occurring in 1 hour. Intrathyroidal concentrations are about 100 times serum levels, unless high dosages are given, at which point the active transport system evidently becomes saturated.

The action of these drugs is relatively short, with a 100-mg dose of PTU beginning to wane within 2–3 hours. Methimazole has a longer half-life, but even with this agent a single dose of

10–25 mg is needed to obtain a therapeutic effect lasting 24 hours. Carbimazole is metabolized to methimazole.

The thioamides and their metabolites are excreted in the urine.

RECOMMENDED READING

Azizi, F. Effect of methimazole treatment of maternal thyrotoxicosis on thyroid function in breast-feeding infants. *J. Pediatrics* 128:855, 1996.

Burrow, G.N. Thyroid diseases, in *Medical Complications During Pregnancy* (4th ed.), G.N. Burrow and T.F. Ferris, eds. Philadelphia: W.B. Saunders, 1995. Pp. 155–187.

Burrow, G.N., et al. Children exposed in utero to propylthiouracil. Subsequent intellectual and physical development. *Am. J. Dis. Child.* 116:161, 1968.

Check, J.H., et al. Prenatal treatment of thyrotoxicosis to prevent intrauterine growth retardation. *Obstet. Gynecol.* 60:122, 1982.

Cheron, R.G., et al. Neonatal thyroid function after propylthiouracil for maternal Graves' disease. *N. Engl. J. Med.* 304:525, 1981.

Cooper, D.S. Antithyroid drugs. *N. Engl. J. Med.* 311:1353, 1984.

Cooper, D.S., et al. Methimazole pharmacology in man: studies using a newly developed radioimmunoassay for methimazole. *J. Clin. Endocrinol. Metab.* 58:473, 1984.

Eisenstein, Z., Weiss, M., Katz, Y., et al. Intellectual capacity of subjects exposed to methimazole or propylthiouracil in utero. *Eur. J. Pediatrics* 151:558, 1992.

Farine, D., Maidman, J., Rubin, S., et al. Elevated alpha-fetoprotein in pregnancy complicated by aplasia cutis after exposure to methimazole. *Obstet. Gynecol.* 71:996, 1988.

Hatjis, C.G. Diagnosis and successful treatment of fetal goitrous hyperthyroidism caused by maternal Graves disease. *Obstet. Gynecol.* 81:837, 1993.

Kampmann, J.P., et al. Propylthiouracil in human milk: revision of a dogma. *Lancet* 1:736, 1980.

Martinez-Frias, M.L., Cereijo, A., Rodriguez-Pinilla, E., et al. Methimazole in animal feed and congenital aplasia cutis. *Lancet* 339:742, 1992.

Momotani, N., Yamashita, R., Yoshimoto, M., et al. Recovery from hypothyroidism: evidence for the safety of breast-feeding while taking propylthiouracil. *Clin. Endocrinol.* 31:591, 1989.

Mujtaba, Q., and Burrow, G.N. Treatment of hyperthyroidism in pregnancy with propylthiouracil and methimazole. *Obstet. Gynecol.* 46:282, 1975.

Tegler, L., and Lindstrom, B. Antithyroid drugs in milk. *Lancet* 2:591, 1980.

Treadwell, M.C., Sherer, D.M., Sacks, A.J., et al. Successful treatment of recurrent non-immune hydrops secondary to fetal hyperthyroidism. *Obstet. Gynecol.* 87:838, 1996.

VanLoon, A.J., Derksen, J.T.M., Bos, A.F., et al. In utero diagnosis and treatment of fetal goitrous hypothyroidism, caused by maternal use of propylthiouracil. *Prenat. Diagn.* 15:599, 1995.

Vogt, T., Stolz, W., and Landthaler, M. Aplasia cutis congenita after exposure to methimazole: a causal relationship? *Br. J. Dermatol.* 133:994–996, 1995.

Wallace, C., Couch, R., and Ginsberg, J. Fetal thyrotoxicosis: a case report and recommendations for prediction, diagnosis, and treatment. *Thyroid* 5:125, 1995.

Wing, D.A., Millar, L.K., Koonings, P.P., et al. A comparison of propylthiouracil versus methimazole in the treatment of hyperthyroidism in pregnancy. *Am. J. Obstet. Gynecol.* 170:90, 1994.

Thrombolytic drugs: Streptokinase (Kabikinase®), Tissue Plasminogen Activator, Alteplase (Activase®), Urokinase (Abbokinase ®)

INDICATIONS AND RECOMMENDATIONS

The use of fibrinolytic or thrombolytic drugs during pregnancy should be limited to life-threatening thromboembolic conditions including massive, hemodynamically significant pulmonary embolus and intracardiac thrombosis (including prosthetic valve thrombosis). Their use is associated with hemorrhagic complications in mothers and may contribute to fetal loss.

SPECIAL CONSIDERATIONS IN PREGNANCY

Generally pregnancy is considered a relative contraindication to thrombolytic therapy. One review cites 172 case reports of such treatment during pregnancy with an associated hemorrhagic complication rate of 8.1%, a pregnancy loss rate of 5.8%, and a maternal mortality rate of 1.2%.

When administered during pregnancy, only small amounts of streptokinase cross the placenta. Maternal streptokinase antibodies do cross the placenta and these can produce passive sensitization in the neonate. Maternal treatment with streptokinase has not been associated with fibrinolytic effects in exposed fetuses, preterm rupture of membranes, preterm labor, or placental hemorrhage. First trimester exposure numbers are limited, but no malformations were reported.

DOSAGE

Streptokinase is given as a 250,000-unit bolus (2.5 mg) to overcome binding by antistreptococcal antibodies; thereafter, its half-life is 40–80 minutes. The tissue plasminogen activator (t-PA) dose used for coronary thrombolysis is 0.75 mg/kg body weight over 30 minutes (max. = 50 mg) followed by 0.5 mg/kg/h up to a subsequent accumulated dose of 35 mg.

ADVERSE EFFECTS

All thrombolytic drugs dissolve both pathologic thrombi and those at the site of vascular injury, thereby creating a significant risk of hemorrhage, the major complication associated with their use. These agents also may induce a systemic formation of plasmin that produces generalized fibrinolysis and destruction of coagulant factors V and VIII. Streptokinase is associated with allergic, including anaphylactic, reactions. In nonsurgical patients already receiving heparin therapy, the risk of serious hemorrhage is 2% to 4%. Contraindications to use include recent surgery, hypertension, and active bleeding, which limit its use in the postpartum patient.

MECHANISM OF ACTION

Plasmin, a nonspecific protease that dissolves fibrin, is converted from its inactive precursor, plasminogen, by t-PA, produced by endothelial cells. Plasminogen activator inhibitors (1 and 2) and α_2-antiplasmin act to prevent t-PA action except in the local milieu of thrombosis. Streptokinase forms a stable bond with plasminogen that renders it available for enzymatic cleavage to plasmin. It lacks fibrin specificity and may induce a systemic lytic state. Streptokinase–plasminogen complexes are not inhibited by α_2-antiplasmin. The t-PA, which can be produced by recombinant DNA technology (alteplase), selectively binds to bound plasminogen such that at physiologic concentrations no systemic formation of plasmin occurs. During therapy with t-PA, however, plasma levels are much higher and are capable of creating a systemic lytic state. Urokinase has the same mechanism of action as streptokinase and also lacks fibrin specificity.

ABSORPTION AND BIOTRANSFORMATION

t-PA is cleared by hepatic metabolism with a half-life of 5–10 minutes.

RECOMMENDED READING

Ludwig, H. Results of streptokinase therapy in deep venous thrombosis during pregnancy. *Postgrad. Med. J.* 49(Suppl 5):65, 1973.

Majerus, P.W., Broze, G.J. Jr., Tiletich, J.P., Tollefsen, D.M. Anticoagulant, thrombolytic, and antiplatelet drugs. Chapter 54 in *Goodman and Gilman's The Pharmacological Basis of Therapeutics* (9th ed.), J.G. Hardman and L.E. Limbird, eds. New York: McGraw-Hill, 1996. Pp. 1351–1353.

Markel, A., et al. The potential role of thrombolytic therapy in venous thrombosis. *Arch. Int. Med.* 152:1265, 1992.

Mazieka, P.K., Oakley, C.M. Massive pulmonary embolism in pregnancy treated with streptokinase and percutaneous catheter fragmentation. *Eur. Heart J.* 15:1281, 1994.

Pfeifer, G.W. Distribution and placental transfer of 131-I streptokinase. *Australas. Ann. Med.* 19(Suppl.):17, 1970.

Tissot, H., et al. Fibrinolytic treatment with urokinase and streptokinase for recurrent thrombosis in two valve protheses for the aortic and mitral valves during pregnancy. *J. Gynecol. Obstet. Biol. Reprod.* 20:1093, 1991.

Turrentine, M.A., et al. Use of thrombolytics for the treatment of thromboembolic disease during prenancy. *Obstet. Gynecol. Surv.* 50:534, 1995.

Witchitz, S., et al. Fibrinolytic treatment of thrombus on prosthetic heart valves. *Br. Heart J.* 44:545, 1980.

Tobacco

INDICATIONS AND RECOMMENDATIONS

The use of tobacco is contraindicated during pregnancy. This drug is the dried leaf of the *Nicotiana tabacum* plant and a widely used agent that is smoked by approximately 26% of American women of childbearing age. An estimated 19% to 30% of women smoke throughout pregnancy. Tobacco has no known therapeutic uses.

Cigarette smoking should be actively discouraged in anyone, but particularly in pregnant women. Even if a habituated person cannot stop smoking completely, there is good evidence to show that she should try to decrease her cigarette consumption to less than seven cigarettes per day. Smoking cessation during pregnancy has been demonstrated to decrease the likelihood of low birth weight, and a number of smoking cessation programs have been shown to be effective in helping pregnant smokers discontinue their tobacco intake. The use of the nicotine patch has been a helpful adjunct to smoking cessation programs, with increased abstinence rates demonstrated in a number of randomized trials. There has been controversy regarding the prescription of nicotine patch therapy during pregnancy because nicotine is clearly one of the major contributors to adverse outcome from smoking. However, nicotine is not the only contributor, and if smoking cessation cannot be accomplished in any other way, it may make sense to prescribe the nicotine patch to pregnant women. An ACOG technical bulletin suggests reserving the nicotine patch for individuals who cannot discontinue or decrease their smoking, and who smoke at least 20 cigarettes per day, since the circulating nicotine levels absorbed from the patch approximate this degree of exposure or less. A short-term study of six pregnant smokers using the patch found no measurable differences in fetal or maternal well-being over 6 hours. Salivary nicotine levels increased in a similar manner to those of nonpregnant patch users, but salivary levels of cotinine, a metabolic product of nicotine, were much lower than those observed in nonpregnant controls. When pregnant smokers are prescribed the transdermal nicotine patch, they should be informed of the risks, benefits, and uncertainties associated with this form of treatment.

Lactating women also should be discouraged from smoking and should smoke as little as possible if they cannot achieve complete abstinence.

SPECIAL CONSIDERATIONS IN PREGNANCY

Nicotine, carbon monoxide, and probably other components of cigarette smoke cross the placenta and appear in fetal blood in higher concentrations than in maternal blood. Nicotine is also present in amniotic fluid and placental tissues in higher concentrations than in maternal serum. Although there has not been a conclusive relationship demonstrated between maternal smoking and congenital anomalies, some studies have shown a significantly increased relative risk of isolated cleft lip and/or palate in the offspring of smokers, and the Jerusalem Perinatal

Study demonstrated an excess of minor anomalies among the offspring of smokers aged 35 years and over. A review of cytotrophoblasts from chorionic villus sampling of the placentas of 7 smokers and 14 nonsmokers showed a significantly increased frequency of sister chromatid exchanges, suggesting direct damage to placental DNA.

Evidence linking cigarette smoking to complications of pregnancy has continued to accumulate. Every investigator who has looked at the relationship of birth weight to cigarette smoking has confirmed that offspring of smoking mothers have lower birth weights than those of nonsmokers. Although the actual difference in birth weight is only in the range of a few hundred grams, each study has shown a statistically significant difference in these weights. Not only have smokers been shown to have smaller offspring than nonsmokers, but over 30 investigations have indicated that they also have twice the number of growth-retarded babies.

This effect of smoking appears to be dose-related, as well as related to the stage of pregnancy in which smoking occurs. If a woman stops smoking before the end of the fourth month of pregnancy, it is probable that her offspring will not differ significantly in weight from that of a nonsmoker. In a prospective clinical trial, smokers randomly assigned to a smoking cessation intervention program prior to the 18th week of gestation delivered babies who were, on average, 92 g heavier and 0.6 cm longer than those of control smokers. Women who smoke fewer than 7–10 cigarettes/day tend to have children whose birth weights do not differ significantly from those of nonsmokers. The direct causative factor in cigarette smoke that leads to decreased birth weight is not known, although animal studies show that prolonged exposure to elevated levels of carbon monoxide will cause lowering of birth weight.

Retrospective and prospective studies of the relationship between cigarette smoking and spontaneous abortions have been suggestive of, but not conclusive for, such an association. While many of these studies do not adequately control for confounding variables, those of Kline et al. and Hemminki and associates attempted to do so. The former study revealed a nearly twofold greater risk of spontaneous abortion in smokers, whereas the latter was unable to demonstrate a significant difference in abortion incidence between 2313 nonsmokers and 389 smokers.

Cigarette smoking is most obviously related to stillbirth in women with other complicating problems, including low socioeconomic status and poor obstetric history. In the United States, for example, black women have more stillbirths than white women, and cigarette smoking magnifies this difference. Animal studies have shown that nicotine and some other cigarette components may significantly increase the incidence of stillbirths.

In large studies from both Canada and England, the perinatal mortality for infants of smokers was significantly higher than that for infants of nonsmokers. The Canadian study showed a highly significant dose–response relationship. In addition, the British study demonstrated a significant relationship between smoking after the fourth month of pregnancy and increased perinatal mortality. Patients who gave up smoking by the fourth month were found to reduce the risk of perinatal mortality to that of nonsmokers. In addition, this study showed that smoking in patients of low socioeconomic status caused an even higher than expected increase in perinatal mortality. The same association has been made with regard to poor obstetric history combined with smoking.

A prospective epidemiologic study of 30,596 pregnant women in northern California demonstrated a significant association between maternal cigarette smoking and preterm birth. Potential confounding variables were controlled; thus, this effect is probably a real one. A study by Kleinman et al. suggested a dose response relationship.

Paradoxically, the perinatal mortality for infants under 2500 g born to smokers is less than that of nonsmokers. The reason seems to be that these infants are primarily small for gestational age rather than premature. However, for infants of comparable gestational age, the mortality is higher for the offspring of smokers than nonsmokers. In a collaborative randomized trial of antenatal steroid therapy for the prevention of respiratory distress syndrome, it was found that premature infants of smokers had a significantly lower incidence of respiratory distress syndrome when compared to infants of nonsmokers born at similar gestational ages. The investigators interpreted this finding as evidence of accelerated pulmonary maturation caused by chronic fetal stress produced by maternal smoking. Other studies have confirmed earlier fetal lung maturation with maternal cigarette smoking. Of course, this process may be stress-related and thus may not represent a positive influence on subsequent pulmonary function.

Several epidemiologic studies reveal a significant decrease in the incidence of preeclampsia in smokers. This appears to be inversely proportional to the amount the woman smokes. However, there are data to show that if a smoker does develop preeclampsia her infant is at higher risk than that of a preeclamptic nonsmoker. One possible mechanism is the inhibition of thromboxane production by nicotine.

Other obstetric complications associated with maternal smoking include abruptio placentae, placenta previa, and premature rupture of membranes (both preterm and term).

Nicotine is present in higher concentrations in breast milk than in maternal serum. However, in one study in which both breast milk and infant serum were analyzed, infant blood contained very little nicotine despite high breast milk levels. Nevertheless, several cases of nicotine poisoning in infants of mothers who smoke 20–40 cigarettes/day have been reported. In addition, smoking mothers expose their children to the dangers of passive smoking. In one longitudinal study of 1156 children, there was a 10% reduction in pulmonary function below expected levels among the 1- and 2-year-old children of smokers. Another long-term study showed a higher incidence of mild cognitive and behavioral abnormalities among children of smokers compared to children of nonsmokers.

ADVERSE EFFECTS

Among the many medical conditions clearly associated with ingestion of cigarette smoke are mucosal epitheliomas; lung cancer; cancers of the oropharyngeal cavity, esophagus, and larynx; emphysema; "smoker's respiratory syndrome"; coronary artery disease; cerebrovascular disease; cardiac arrhythmias; and peripheral vascular disease.

Nicotine has parasympathetic effects on the gastrointestinal tract, occasionally resulting in diarrhea and often leading to decreased intestinal motility. It can cause respiratory depression and arrest by its action of blocking the neuromuscular junction of respiratory muscles. Furthermore, a minor central nervous system (CNS) paralysis may occur. Other CNS effects such as tremors (at low dosages) and convulsions (at higher dosages) can be reversed with antiparkinsonian drugs, curariform drugs, adrenergic blockers, hypnotics, and anticonvulsants. Nicotine also has an antidiuretic effect mediated through release of antidiuretic hormone (ADH).

MECHANISM OF ACTION

Nearly 500 compounds have been isolated from tobacco smoke. These include several chemicals irritating to mucous membranes; polonium-210 and nickel, which have been implicated in lung cancer; and carbon monoxide, which makes up approximately 1% of cigarette smoke by volume. The major active component of tobacco, however, is nicotine, which averages 6–8 mg/cigarette. Approximately 90% of the nicotine in inhaled tobacco smoke is systemically absorbed.

Nicotine, a toxic substance that acts on a variety of neuroeffector junctions, has both stimulant and depressant phases of action. Its net effect therefore is the algebraic summation of those actions. These are usually dose-related and depend on time since ingestion. An initial stimulatory effect is usually followed by a depressant effect. This pattern occurs in all autonomic ganglia and is responsible for many if not most of the effects of nicotine.

In general, nicotine will increase heart rate and blood pressure and its cardiovascular effects parallel those of sympathetic stimulation. The sympathomimetic effects can be negated by catecholamine blockers, which implies that they are mediated through the adrenal glands and other catecholamine-releasing organs.

ABSORPTION AND BIOTRANSFORMATION

Nicotine, the major component of tobacco smoke, is absorbed from oral and gastrointestinal mucosa, the respiratory tract, and skin. Between 80% and 90% is detoxified by the liver, kidney, and lungs; the remainder plus the detoxification products are excreted through the kidney. This occurs most expeditiously in acidified urine. Nicotine is also excreted in the milk of lactating women in direct proportion to the amount of tobacco consumed. The milk may contain as much as 0.5 mg/L.

RECOMMENDED READING

American College of Obstetricians and Gynecologists. Smoking and reproductive health. *ACOG Tech. Bull.* No. 180, 1993.

Chelmow, D., Andrew, E., and Baker, E.R. Maternal cigarette smoking and placenta previa. *Obstet. Gynecol.* 87:703, 1996.

Curet, L.B., et al. Maternal smoking and respiratory distress syndrome. *Am. J. Obstet. Gynecol.* 147:446, 1983.

Dolan-Mullen, P., Ramirez, G., and Groff, J.Y. A meta-analysis of randomized trials of prenatal smoking cessation interventions. *Am. J. Obstet. Gynecol.* 171:1328, 1994.

Fiore, M.C., Smith, S.S., Jorenby, D.E., et al. The effectiveness of the nicotine patch for smoking cessation: a meta-analysis. *J.A.M.A.* 271:1940, 1994.

Handler, A.S., Mason, E.D., Rosenberg, D.L., et al. The relationship between exposure during pregnancy to cigarette smoking and cocaine use and placenta previa. *Am. J. Obstet. Gynecol.* 170:884, 1994.

Hemminki, K., Mutanen, P., and Saloniemi, I. Smoking and the occurrence of congenital malformations and spontaneous abortions: multivariate analysis. *Am. J. Obstet. Gynecol.* 145:61, 1983.

Khoury, M.J., Gomez-Farias, M., and Mulinare, J. Does maternal cigarette smoking during pregnancy cause cleft lip and palate in offspring? *Am. J. Dis. Child.* 143:333, 1989.

Kleinman, J.C., Pierre, M.B., Jr., Madans, J.H., et al. The effects of maternal smoking on fetal and infant mortality. *Am. J. Epidemiol.* 127:274, 1988.

Kline, J., Stein, Z.A., and Susser, M. Smoking: a risk factor for spontaneous abortion. *N. Engl. J. Med.* 297:793, 1977.

Klonoff-Cohen, H., Edelstein, S., and Savitz, D. Cigarette smoking and preeclampsia. *Obstet. Gynecol.* 81:541, 1993.

Li, C.Q., Windsor, R.A., Perkins, L., et al. The impact on infant birth weight and gestatioal age of cotinine-validated smoking reduction during pregnancy. *J.A.M.A.* 269:1519, 1993.

Lieberman, E., Torday, J., Barbieri, R., et al. Association of intrauterine cigarette smoke exposure with indices of fetal lung maturation. *Obstet. Gynecol.* 79:564, 1992.

Luck, W., and Nau, H. Exposure of the fetus, neonate, and nursed infant to nicotine and cotinine from maternal smoking. *N. Engl. J. Med.* 311:672, 1984.

Marcoux, S., Brisson, J., and Fabia, J. The effect of cigarette smoking on the risk of preeclampsia and gestational hypertension. *Am. J. Epidemiol.* 130:950, 1989.

Meyer, M.B., and Tonascia, J.A. Maternal smoking, pregnancy complications, and perinatal mortality. *Am. J. Obstet. Gynecol.* 128:494, 1977.

Naeye, R.L., and Peters, E.C. Mental development of children whose mothers smoked during pregnancy. *Obstet. Gynecol.* 64: 601, 1984.

Seidman, D.S., Ever-Hadani, P., and Gale, R. Effect of maternal smoking and age on congenital anomalies. *Obstet. Gynecol.* 76: 1046, 1990.

Sexton, M., and Hebel, J.R. A clinical trial of change in maternal smoking and its effect on birth weight. *J.A.M.A.* 251:911, 1984.

Shiono, P.H., et al. Smoking and drinking during pregnancy: their effects on preterm birth. *J.A.M.A.* 255:82, 1986.

Shulman. L.P., Elias, S., Tharapel, A.T., et al. Sister chromatid exchange frequency in directly prepared cytotrophoblasts: demonstration of in vivo deoxyribonucleic acid damage in pregnant women who smoke cigarettes. *Am. J. Obstet. Gynecol.* 165:1877, 1991.

Tager, I.B., et al. Longitudinal study of the effects of maternal smoking on pulmonary function in children. *N. Engl. J. Med.* 309: 699, 1983.

Williams, M.A., Mittendorf, R., Stubblefield, P.G., et al. Cigarettes, coffee and preterm premature rupture of the membranes. *Am. J. Epidemiol.* 135:895, 1992.

Wright, L.N., Thorp, J.M., Jr., Kuller, J.A., et al. Transdermal nicotine replacement in pregnancy: maternal pharmacokinetics and fetal effects. *Am. J. Obstet. Gynecol.* 176:1090, 1997.

Tolazoline (Priscoline®)

INDICATIONS AND RECOMMENDATIONS

Tolazoline is relatively contraindicated during pregnancy because other therapeutic agents are preferable. Tolazoline, like phentolamine, is an α-adrenergic blocker. In addition to its α-blocking effects, it has a variety of nonrelated sympathomimetic, parasympathomimetic, and histaminic actions. There are no clear-cut indications for its use during pregnancy.

Tolazoline produces vasodilatation and cardiac stimulation, which usually result in a rise in systemic blood pressure. It can produce tachycardia and arrhythmias. Although the drug has been used to treat neonates for pulmonary hypertension, little is known of its effects when administered during pregnancy. In one study, neonates given tolazoline showed complications of gastrointestinal hemorrhage, thrombocytopenia, and transient renal failure.

There are few documented indications for the use of tolazoline. The most favorable clinical responses have been described with early Raynaud's syndrome. However, because tolazoline has had limited use in pregnancy, it cannot be recommended. The intense renal vasoconstriction associated with its use suggests that fetal renal dysfunction and oligohydramnios might be expected and that amniotic fluid volume should be monitored if talazoline were used in pregnancy.

RECOMMENDED READING

Hoffman B.B., and Lefkowitz, R.J. Catecholamines, sympathomimetic drugs, and adrenergic receptor antagonists. Chapter 10 in *Goodman and Gilman's The Pharmacological Basis of Therapeutics* (9th ed.), J.G. Hardman and L.E. Limbird, eds. New York: McGraw-Hill, 1996. Pp. 228–229.

Goetzman, B.W., et al. Neonatal hypoxia and pulmonary vasospasm response to tolazoline. *J. Pediatrics* 89:617, 1976.

Tricyclic Antidepressants: Amitriptyline (Elavil®), Desipramine (Norpramin®), Doxepin (Sinequan®), Imipramine (Tofranil®), Nortriptyline (Aventyl®, Pamelor®), Protriptyline (Vivactil®)

INDICATIONS AND RECOMMENDATIONS

The use of tricyclic antidepressants during pregnancy should be limited to the treatment of those women who clearly require the medication for psychiatric indications, especially endogenous depression of abrupt onset. Reactive depression and depression accompanied by anxiety are less likely to be relieved by these drugs and therefore do not indicate their use during pregnancy. It does not appear that any member of this family of drugs is the agent of choice for use during pregnancy, although nortriptyline and desipramine may have fewer side effects.

SPECIAL CONSIDERATIONS IN PREGNANCY

Animal studies have shown that the tricyclic antidepressants cross the placenta. Congenital malformations, including limb reduction deformities, have been reported in infants whose mothers used tricyclic antidepressants during pregnancy, but a causal relationship has not been demonstrated. The Finnish Registry of Congenital Malformations contains 2784 cases of birth defects for the years 1964–1972, which were matched with an equal number of controls. Four of the mothers of malformed infants had taken tricyclics during the first trimester, as opposed to one of the control mothers. No increase in the incidence of birth defects occurred in the 41 exposed pregnancies reported by the Collaborative Perinatal Project. Neither was there an increased incidence of exposure to such drugs in utero among hundreds of children with limb reduction defects. Similarly, in an uncontrolled series from England, none of 81 mothers treated with imipramine, 50 mg tid, delivered babies with anomalies. In the Royal College of General Practitioners' survey of 10,000 pregnancies in 1964, none of the 47 fetuses exposed to tricyclic antidepressants in utero had congenital malformations. A study of 689 women taking antidepressant therapy during pregnancy (283 exposures to tricyclic antidepressants) found no increase in congenital malformations or adverse pregnancy outcome when compared with European population statistics.

Studies in rodents have demonstrated biochemical alterations in the brains of offspring exposed to desipramine in utero. Behavioral abnormalities in the perinatal period have also been described in rats exposed to tricyclic antidepressant agents ante partum. There are limited data in humans. Two follow-up studies in children at 2½–3 years of age exposed to tricyclic antidepressants prior to birth revealed no evidence of developmental abnormalities. While these drugs do not appear to cause structural malformations in humans, their possible long-term effects on the developing central nervous system are less clear.

Fetal heart rate abnormalities (baseline tachycardia and increased accelerations) have been reported in a patient with imipramine overdose. Cases have been reported of infants born to women who received tricyclic antidepressants immediately before delivery who have suffered from heart failure, tachycardia, respiratory distress, cyanosis, colic, ileus, and urinary retention. Central nervous system effects, including myoclonus, tremors, hypotonia, irritability, and convulsions, have also been described following peripartum exposure. Withdrawal symptoms have been observed in infants whose mothers were treated with imipramine during the antenatal period. It is therefore prudent to limit the use of these medications in late gestation or to reduce dosages if possible.

Very small amounts of these drugs are excreted in breast milk. The WHO Working Group on Human Lactation has estimated that approximately 2% of the weight-adjusted maternal daily dose of nortriptyline will be passed through breast milk to a lactating infant. In general, such doses have not been shown to have an effect on the neonate. When serum samples from nursing infants whose mothers were taking tricyclics have been tested, levels of the drugs were not detectable. However, one study measured nortriptyline and its metabolites in the serum of seven nursing infants under 10 weeks of age and found evidence of one less active metabolite in two of the infants. Although limited by small numbers, the data suggest that tricyclic antidepressants are not associated with adverse effects in nursing infants, with one exception. Elevated levels of N-desmethyldoxepin, the chief metabolite of doxepin, have been detected in a lactating infant in association with sedation and respiratory depression. Preterm infants and those with hyperbilirubinemia may be at increased risk of adverse effects due to impaired drug metabolism. The American Academy of Pediatrics considers the effects of tricyclic antidepressants on breast-feeding infants to be unknown but may be of concern. It may be appropriate to consider obtaining serum levels in infants under 10 weeks of age.

DOSAGE

Dosages of the tricyclic antidepressants must be individualized. After an initial dose has been given, dosage is gradually increased over 1–2 weeks to the maintenance dosage that will provide maximal efficacy and minimal side effects. Table 4 details recommended dosages of these antidepressants. Dosage requirements may increase, particularly in the second half of gestation. In one study of eight women, the final dose required during pregnancy was 1.3–2 times greater than in the nonpregnant state. The increased dosages correlated with therapeutic serum levels.

**Table 4. Recommended dosages
of the tricyclic antidepressants**

Drug	Usual daily starting dose (mg)	Usual daily maintenance dosage range (mg)
Amitriptyline	50–75	75–300
Desipramine	50–75	75–300
Doxepin	50–75	75–300
Imipramine	50–75	75–300
Nortriptyline	75	40–100
Protriptyline	10	10–40

ADVERSE EFFECTS

Sedation is the most prominent initial effect of the tricyclic antidepressants, the magnitude of which depends on the individual agent. Other side effects include tachycardia and orthostatic hypotension. These agents have potent anticholinergic activity and commonly cause dry mouth, blurred vision, urinary retention, and constipation. Allergic reactions, inappropriate secretion of antidiuretic hormone, and galactorrhea are only encountered rarely. Toxicity due to acute overdosage is characterized by hyperpyrexia, hypertension, seizures, and coma. Occasionally, patients may undergo a transition from depression to a hypomanic or manic state. Problems with memory and concentration occur in approximately 10% of patients in the reproductive age group.

There are several important drug interactions that should be noted. Tricyclic antidepressant effects may be potentiated in the presence of phenytoin, aspirin, phenothiazines, and steroids. Conversely, their metabolism may be increased in the presence of barbiturates, some anticonvulsant medications, and cigarette smoking.

MECHANISM OF ACTION

The tricyclic antidepressants block the reuptake of neurotransmitters, including norepinephrine and serotonin, in adrenergic nerve endings. The resulting increased concentration of neurotransmitter at the receptor is postulated to be responsible for the therapeutic effects of these agents. Nortriptyline is a metabolite of amitriptyline, whereas desipramine is a metabolite of imipramine.

ABSORPTION AND BIOTRANSFORMATION

The tricyclic antidepressants are well absorbed from the gastrointestinal tract; they are metabolized in the liver. Plasma concentrations generally reach a peak within 2–8 hours, and the drugs are widely distributed due to their lipophilic properties. Half-lives are relatively long, enabling consideration of a once-daily bedtime dosage after therapeutic levels are reached. There is a great deal of individual variance in the response to a given dose, probably due to inherent differences in metabolism. Serum levels may not be reliable predictors of response in the absence of clinical correlation. The tricyclic antidepressants and their metabolites are excreted in urine and feces and are usually completely eliminated in 7–10 days.

RECOMMENDED READING

Altshuler, L.L., Cohen, L., Szuba, M.P., et al. Pharmacologic management of psychiatric illness during pregnancy: dilemmas and guidelines. *Am. J. Psychiatry.* 153:592, 1996.

American Academy of Pediatrics. The transfer of drugs and other chemicals into human milk. *Pediatrics* 93:137, 1994.

Bader, T.F., and Newman, K. Amitriptyline in human breast milk and the nursing infant's serum. *Am. J. Psychiatry* 137:855, 1980.

Baldessarini, R.J. Drugs and the treatment of psychiatric disorders. Chapter 19 in *Goodman and Gilman's The Pharmacological Ba-*

sis of Therapeutics (9th ed.), J.G. Hardman and L.E. Limbird, eds. New York: McGraw-Hill, 1996. Pp. 431–454.

Gimovsky, M.L., and Knee, D. Fetal heart rate monitoring casebook. *J. Perinatol.* 15:246, 1995.

Heinonen, O.P., Slone, D., and Shapiro, S. *Birth Defects and Drugs in Pregnancy.* Littleton, MA: PSG, 1977.

Kuller, J.A., Katz, V.L., McMahon, M.J., et al. Pharmacologic treatment of psychiatric disease in pregnancy and lactation: fetal and neonatal effects. *Obstet. Gynecol.* 87:789, 1996.

McElhatton, P.R., Garbis, H.M., Elefant, E., et al. The outcome of pregnancy in 689 women exposed to therapeutic doses of antidepressants. A collaborative study of the European network of teratology information services (ENTIS). *Reprod. Toxicol.* 10:285, 1996.

Miller, L.J. Psychiatric medication during pregnancy: understanding and minimizing risks. *Psychiatr. Ann.* 24:69, 1994.

Nulman, I., Rovet, J., Stewart, D.E., et al. Neurodevelopment of children exposed in utero to antidepressant drugs. *N. Engl. J. Med.* 336:258, 1997.

Wisner, K.L., Perel. J.M., and Findling, R.L. Antidepressant treatment during breast-feeing. *Am. J. Psychiatry* 153:1132, 1996.

Wisner, K.L., Perel, J.M., and Wheeler, S.B. Tricyclic dose requirements across pregnancy. *Am. J. Psychiatry* 150:1541, 1993.

Trimethadione (Tridione®)

Trimethadione is an anticonvulsant used in the treatment of petit mal epilepsy. It should be avoided during pregnancy because of its apparent association with a syndrome of abnormalities in offspring exposed to it. The fetal trimethadione syndrome consists of developmental delay, mental retardation, palatal defects, irregular teeth, speech disturbances, low-set ears, and V-shaped eyebrows. Analysis of 36 trimethadione-exposed pregnancies revealed 25 malformed offspring, for a congenital anomaly rate of 69%. Among other reported anomalies were growth restriction, cardiovascular and renal abnormalities. The preferred drug for control of petit mal epilepsy in pregnancy is ethosuximide.

RECOMMENDED READINGS

Dansky, L., et al. Major congenital malformations in the offspring of epileptic patients. Genetic and environmental risk factors. In *Epilepsy, Pregnancy and the Child.* Proceedings of a Workshop held in Berlin, September 1980. New York: Raven Press, 1981.

Fabro, S., and Brown N.A. Teratogenic potential of anticonvulsants. *N. Engl. J. Med.* 300:1280, 1979.

Feldman, G.L., et al. The fetal trimethadione syndrome. Report of an additional family and further delineation of this syndrome. *Am. J. Dis. Child.* 131:1389, 1977.

German, J., et al. Trimethadione and human teratogenesis. *Teratology* 3:349, 1970.

Nakane, Y., et al. Multi-institutional study on the teratogenicity and fetal toxicity of antiepileptic drugs: a report of a collaborative study group in Japan. *Epilepsia* 21:663, 1980.

National Institutes of Health. Anticonvulsants found to have teratogenic potential. *J.A.M.A.* 245:36, 1981.

Nichols, M.M. Fetal anomalies following maternal trimethadione ingestion. *J. Pediatrics* 82:885, 1973.

Rischbieth, R.J. Toxidone (trimethadione) embryopathy: case report with review of the literature. *Clin. Exp. Neurol.* 16:251, 1977.

Rosen, R.C., and Lightner, E.S. Phenotypic malformations in association with maternal trimethadione therapy. *J. Pediatrics* 92:240, 1978.

Zackai, E.H., et al. The fetal trimethadione syndrome. *J. Pediatrics* 87:280, 1975.

Zellweger, H. Anticonvulsants during pregnancy: a danger to the developing fetus? *Clin. Pediatrics* 13:338, 1974.

Trimethaphan (Arfonad®)

INDICATIONS AND RECOMMENDATIONS

Trimethaphan is relatively contraindicated in pregnancy as other therapeutic agents are preferable. It is a ganglionic blocker which prevents the interaction of acetylcholine with postganglionic receptors; this inhibits transmission of sympathetic and parasympathetic impulses. Its short-lived activity requires continuous infusion for a therapeutic, antihypertensive effect. However, decreased intravascular volume or any drug that inhibits sympathetic activity augments its antihypertensive action.

The antihypertensive effect of trimethaphan is accompanied by a decreased glomerular filtration rate. Side effects of its use include obstipation and urinary retention, and meconium ileus in the neonate. Trimethaphan use is limited to the occasion when other, more acceptable agents prove unsuccessful.

RECOMMENDED READING

Abdelwahab, W., Frishman, W., and Landau, A. Management of hypertensive urgencies and emergencies. *J. Clin. Pharmacol.* 35: 747, 1995.

Gutsche B.B., and Cheek, T.G. Anesthetic Considerations in Pre-eclampsia-Eclampsia in Anesthesia for Obstetrics (3rd ed.), S.M. Shnider and G. Levison, eds. Baltimore: Williams and Wilkins, 1993. Pp. 305–336.

Koch-Weser, J. Hypertensive emergencies. *N. Engl. J. Med.* 290:211, 1974.

Martin, J.D. A critical survey of drugs used in the treatment of hypertensive crises of pregnancy. *Med. J. Aust.* 2:252, 1974.

Trimethobenzamide (Tigan®)

INDICATIONS AND RECOMMENDATIONS

Trimethobenzamide is safe to use during pregnancy. The usual therapeutic dosages may be used for treatment of nausea and vomiting during pregnancy.

SPECIAL CONSIDERATIONS IN PREGNANCY

Large-scale prospective studies assessing the use of trimethobenzamide in pregnancy have failed to show an increased risk of malformation in the fetus at normal dosages.

DOSAGE

The usual adult oral dose of trimethobenzamide is 250 mg 3–4 times/day. The intramuscular and rectal dose is 200 mg 3–4 times/day.

ADVERSE EFFECTS

At recommended dosages, side effects are relatively uncommon; they include drowsiness and dizziness, and local irritation if the intramuscular or rectal route is used. Allergic skin eruptions, extrapyramidal symptoms, and convulsions have also been reported.

MECHANISM OF ACTION

The exact mechanism of action of trimethobenzamide as an antiemetic is obscure. It is a benzamide antagonist of dopamine receptors that has little prokinetic activity and modest antiemetic potency.

ABSORPTION AND BIOTRANSFORMATION

Trimethobenzamide is well absorbed after oral administration. Measurable blood levels may persist for as long as 24 hours. Within 72 hours, 30% to 50% of the administered dose is excreted unchanged in the urine. Trimethobenzamide may also be metabolized in the liver and its metabolites excreted in bile and urine.

RECOMMENDED READING

Brunton, L.L. Agents affecting gastrointestinal water flux and motility; emesis and antiemetics; bile acids and pancreatic enzymes. Chapter 38 in *Goodman and Gilman's The Pharmacological Basis of Therapeutics* (9th ed.), J.G. Hardman and L.E. Limbird, eds. New York: McGraw-Hill, 1996. P. 933.

Heinonen, D., Slone, D., and Shapiro, S., eds. *Birth Defects and Drugs in Pregnancy.* Littleton, MA: PSG, 1977. Pp. 323–330.

Milkovich, L., and van den Berg, B.J. An evaluation of the teratogenicity of certain antinauseant drugs. *Am. J. Obstet. Gynecol.* 125:244, 1976.

Troglitazone (Rezulin®)

Troglitazone is relatively contraindicated during pregnancy because other therapeutic agents, in particular insulin, are preferable. Troglitazone is used to treat type 2 diabetic patients who are not well controlled by modest doses of insulin. It is a thiazolidinedione derivative that acts by diminishing insulin resistance, possibly by increasing the number of glucose transporters. In a randomized trial of troglitazone in former gestational diabetic women with impaired glucose tolerance, the drug significantly improved insulin sensitivity and lowered insulin levels. Troglitazone was marketed in 1997. In the fall of that year the manufacturer reported an approximate 2% incidence of liver function abnormalities in patients taking the drug, with a few cases of serious hepatic disease and death. There is no information available regarding the use of troglitazone during pregnancy.

RECOMMENDED READING

Berkowitz, K., Peters, R., Kjos, S.L., et al. Effect of troglitazone on insulin sensitivity and pancreatic cell function in women at high risk for NIDDM. *Diabetes* 45:1572, 1996.

Medical Letter Inc. Troglitazone for non-insulin-dependent diabetes mellitus. *Med. Lett. Drugs Ther.* 39:49, 1997.

Ursodiol (Actigall®)

INDICATIONS AND RECOMMENDATIONS

The use of ursodiol (ursodeoxycholic acid) should be limited to the treatment of intrahepatic cholestasis of pregnancy (ICP) for which other, better studied therapies, such as cholestyramine, are ineffective. In the nonpregnant woman, ursodiol is used to dissolve gallstones. Gallstone dissolution requires many months of therapy; the use of ursodiol for this indication is not recommended during pregnancy.

SPECIAL CONSIDERATIONS IN PREGNANCY

Ursodiol is not teratogenic in animals and has not been associated with teratogenic effects in its limited use in humans.

ICP is a condition of unknown origin characterized by pruritis and abnormal liver function tests. It typically develops in the third trimester of pregnancy and subsides within a week of delivery. Whereas the prognosis for the mother is generally very good, it is associated with an increased risk of fetal distress, preterm delivery, and stillbirth. Several small-scale studies and case reports suggest that ursodiol therapy can provide significant improvement in maternal pruritis and laboratory values with no adverse fetal effect. In one series, three patients, each of whom had previously experienced a stillbirth or perinatal death associated with ICP, were treated with ursodiol late in pregnancy for severe pruritis, gross increase of serum bile acid, and deranged liver tests. All tolerated the treatment well with rapid clinical and biochemical improvement. Two infants were delivered by cesarean section and required oxygen therapy for several days before being discharged home. The other healthy infant was delivered vaginally.

DOSAGE

The usual dose is 8–10 mg/kg/day in 2–3 divided doses.

ADVERSE EFFECTS

The most common side effects are gastrointestinal, including abdominal pain, diarrhea, constipation, nausea, and vomiting.

It can also cause dizziness, headache, muscle and back pain, and respiratory symptoms.

MECHANISM OF ACTION

The exact mechanism of action of ursodiol in alleviating the symptoms and correcting the laboratory abnormalities of ICP is unknown. Ursodiol inhibits the absorption of dietary and biliary cholesterol and blunts the increase of hepatic cholesterol that would normally compensate for the reduced supply. It can also promote mobilization of cholesterol from gallstones by formation of a liquid-crystalline phase.

ABSORPTION AND BIOTRANSFORMATION

Ursodiol is a natural component of bile. As with naturally secreted bile acids, pharmacologic doses of ursodiol are absorbed well from the small bowel, reabsorbed in the ileum, and recycled via enterohepatic recirculation. Only small amounts appear in the systemic circulation and very small amounts are excreted in the urine. Any bile acids reaching the colon are eliminated in the feces.

RECOMMENDED READING

Davies, M.H., et al. Fetal mortality associated with cholestasis of pregnancy and the potential benefit of therapy with ursodeoxycholic acid. *Gut* 37:580, 1995.

Diaferia, A., et al. Ursodeoxycholic and acid therapy in pregnant women with cholestasis. *Int. J. Gynaecol. Obstet.* 52:133, 1996.

Floreani, A., et al. Ursodeoxycholic acid in intrahepatic cholestasis of pregnancy. *Br. J. Obstet. Gynaecol.* 101:64, 1994.

Reye, H. Review: intrahepatic cholestasis. A puzzling disorder of pregnancy. *J. Gastroenterol. Hepatol.* 12:211, 1997.

Valacyclovir (Valtrex®)

INDICATIONS AND RECOMMENDATIONS

Valacyclovir is contraindicated in pregnancy because other therapeutic agents are preferable. It is an antiviral agent indicated for the treatment of acute herpes zoster (shingles) and recurrent episodes of genital herpes. Shingles poses no threat to maternal or fetal health and need not be treated during pregnancy. Should treatment be necessary for recurrent episodes of genital herpes during pregnancy, acyclovir, for which there are more clinical data, would be the drug of choice.

RECOMMENDED READING

Hayden, F.G. Antimicrobial agents: antiviral agents. Chapter 50 in *Goodman and Gilman's The Pharmacological Basis of Therapeutics* (9th ed.), J.G. Hardman and L.E. Limbird, eds. New York: McGraw-Hill, 1996. Pp. 1193–1204.

Nelson, C.T., and Demmler, G.J. Cytomegalovirus infection in the pregnant mother, fetus, and newborn infant. *Clin. Perinatol.* 24: 151, 1997

Whitley, R.J., and Kimberlin, D.W. Treatment of viral infections during pregnancy and the neonatal period. *Clin. Perinatol.* 24: 267, 1997.

Valproic Acid (Depakene®)

INDICATIONS AND RECOMMENDATIONS

The use of valproic acid is relatively contraindicated during pregnancy because this agent is teratogenic and alternative agents that seem to be safer for the fetus are available. However, no anticonvulsant has been demonstrated to be totally safe for the fetus, and there may be fetal risks associated with maternal epilepsy itself. Valproic acid is used for the treatment of absence seizures, generalized seizures, and manic-depressive disorders.

Valproic acid readily crosses the placenta and is present in fetal serum at levels 1.4–2.4 times greater than maternal serum levels. Valproic acid–induced hepatotoxicity, which is dose-related, places fetuses at risk for liver damage. The neonate metabolizes the drug slowly and its plasma half-life is much longer than that of the adult.

From data collected at birth defects registries in several countries, an association between neural tube defects and exposure to valproic acid has emerged. Although this has yet to be confirmed in collaborative cohort studies, the estimated risk to exposed fetuses is 1% to 2%. An increased incidence of neonatal afibrinogenemia and fatal hemorrhage has also been reported in these fetuses although this is less well characterized. Finally, a fetal valproate syndrome has been described. Facial changes, including epicanthal folds connecting with an infraorbital crease, flat nasal bridge, small nose and mouth, and a long upper lip with a shallow philtrum, along with limb and heart defects and growth restriction, have been described.

The drug is found in very small quantities in breast milk, and breast-feeding is therefore considered safe.

RECOMMENDED READING

Clayton Smith, J., and Donni, D. Fetal valproate syndrome. *J. Med Genet.* 32:724, 1995.

Diliberti, J.H., et al. The fetal valproate syndrome. *Am J. Med. Genet.* 19:473, 1984.

Jager-Roman, E., et al. Fetal growth, major malformations and minor anomalies in infants born to women receiving valproic acid. *J. Pediatrics* 108:997, 1986.

Legius, E., et al. Sodium valproate, pregnancy and infantile fatal liver failure. *Lancet* 2:1518, 1987.

Lindhout, D., and Meinordi, H. Spina bifida and in-utero exposure to valproate. *Lancet* 2:396, 1984.

Majer, R.V., and Green, P.J. Neonatal afibrinogenemia due to sodium valproate. *Lancet* 2:740, 1987.

Markovitz, P.J., and Calabrese, J.R. Use of anticonvulsants for manic depression during pregnancy. *Psychosomatics* 31:118, 1990.

Nau, H., et al. Valproic acid and its metabolites: placental transfer, neonatal pharmacokinetics, transfer in a mother's milk, and clinical status in neonates of epileptic mothers. *J. Pharmacol. Exp. Ther.* 219:768, 1981.

Robert, E., and Rosa, F. Valproate and birth defects. *Lancet* 2:1142, 1983.

Vancomycin (Vancocin®)

INDICATIONS AND RECOMMENDATIONS

The use of intravenous vancomycin during pregnancy should be limited to the treatment of life-threatening infections in patients who are allergic to penicillin, or to treatment of serious staphylococcal infections caused by strains resistant to penicillinase-resistant penicillins or cephalosporins. Oral vancomycin may be used in the treatment of antibiotic-induced *Clostridium difficile* colitis.

SPECIAL CONSIDERATIONS IN PREGNANCY

Because of potential ototoxicity to the fetus, vancomycin should be used only when specifically indicated. The effect of vancomycin on hearing and renal function has been studied in 10 infants exposed during the second and third trimesters. One infant in the study group was noted to have an abnormal auditory brainstem response, which was believed to be a conduction defect, rather than a sensorineural one, and thus unrelated to the vancomycin exposure. Hearing tests at 12 months were normal. No renal function abnormalities were detected in any of the studied infants. No embryotoxicity has been documented in animals or humans. Vancomycin crosses the placenta, with a fetal/maternal concentration ratio of 0.76. One case report describes an acute maternal hypotensive episode, followed by transient fetal bradycardia, thought to be secondary to rapid infusion of vancomycin during labor.

Vancomycin is found in breast milk. As it is poorly absorbed from the gastrointestinal tract, systemic absorption in the newborn is probably limited. There are, however, theoretical risks of allergic reaction and/or modification of bowel flora.

DOSAGE

The usual intravenous dose is 2 g/day (approximately 30 mg/kg), divided into doses given q6–12h. The dose should be given in 100–200 ml of 5% dextrose in water over at least 60 minutes to reduce hypersensitivity reactions. If creatinine clearance is 50–80 ml/min, the dose should be given every 1–3 days. If the creatinine clearance is 10–50 ml/min, the dose is given every 3–10 days. If the creatinine clearance is less than 10 ml/min, only 1 g is given every 7 days. The targeted steady-state concentration in adults with normal renal function is 15 μg/ml, which can be achieved approximately 1 hour after a single 1-g dose. Increased doses may be needed during pregnancy, due to increased volume of distribution as well as clearance. In treatment of endocarditis, for example, it may be helpful to measure serum levels for dosage adjustment.

The oral dose for treatment of *C. difficile* colitis is 500 mg qid.

ADVERSE EFFECTS

The most common side effect of intravenous vancomycin is a histamine-like reaction occurring shortly after infusion and consisting of fever, chills, paresthesias, and erythema at the base of the neck and upper back. This reaction is minimized by administering the drug slowly in a large volume (100–200 ml) of fluid. Neurotoxicity is the most serious complication of vancomycin therapy. Damage to the auditory nerve, with possible deafness, is associated with serum levels of 60–80 µg/ml and is a problem primarily in patients with diminished renal function.

The nephrotoxicity previously ascribed to vancomycin use has been attributed to impurities found in earlier preparations. As purified preparations have become available, it is now uncommon, particularly when dosages are adjusted based on the patient's renal function.

MECHANISM OF ACTION

Vancomycin is a bactericidal antibiotic produced by *Streptococcus orientalis* that acts primarily by inhibiting cell wall synthesis. In addition, it has a small effect on inhibiting RNA synthesis in bacterial cytoplasmic membranes. At clinically achievable concentrations, vancomycin is only active against gram-positive organisms and is particularly useful against methicillin-resistant staphylococci. Synergism between vancomycin and an aminoglycoside (i.e., gentamicin, tobramycin) has been demonstrated with respect to *Staphylococcus aureus* and *Enterococcus.*

ABSORPTION AND BIOTRANSFORMATION

Vancomycin is almost negligibly absorbed from the gastrointestinal tract, achieving serum levels of less than 1 µg/ml in normal subjects and slightly higher levels in patients with inflammatory bowel disease. When administered intravenously to patients with normal renal function, its half-life is 4–8 hours, and it is almost completely excreted in the urine. In the presence of renal insufficiency, dangerously high blood concentrations may occur. Approximately 55% of the drug is protein-bound. Its clearance is linearly related to creatinine clearance.

RECOMMENDED READING

Bourget, P., Fernandez, H., Delouis, C., and Ribou, F. Transplacental passage of vancomycin during the second trimester of pregnancy. *Obstet. Gynecol.* 78:908, 1991.

Cunha, B.A., and Ristaccia, A.M. Clinical usefulness of vancomycin. *Clin. Pharmacol.* 2:417, 1983.

Kapusnik-Uner, J.E., Sande, M.A., and Chambers, H.F. Antimicrobial agents. Chapter 47 in *Goodman and Gilman's The Pharmacological Basis of Therapeutics* (9th ed.), J.G. Hardman and L.E. Limbird, eds. New York: McGraw-Hill, 1996. Pp. 1144–1146.

McHenry, M.C., and Gavan, T.L. Vancomycin. *Pediatr. Clin. North Am.* 30:31, 1983.

Reyes, M.P., Ostrea, E.M., Cabinian, A.E., Schmitt, C., and Rintelmann, W. Vancomycin during pregnancy: does it cause hearing loss or nephrotoxicity in the infant? *Am. J. Obstet. Gynecol.* 161:977, 1989.

Salzman, C., Weingold, A.B., and Simon, G.L. Increased dose requirements of vancomycin in a pregnant patient with endocarditis. *J. Infect. Dis.* 156:409, 1987.

Xanthines (Over-the-Counter): Caffeine, Theobromine, Theophylline

INDICATIONS AND RECOMMENDATIONS

Xanthines in the quantities present in coffee, tea, cocoa, and cola-flavored drinks are probably safe during pregnancy if consumed in moderation in the absence of peptic ulcer or hypertensive heart disease. In 1980, the Food and Drug Administration (FDA) cautioned pregnant women to avoid excessive caffeine intake. This warning was based on a study linking large dosages of caffeine (human equivalent of 20–24 cups of coffee daily), administered as a bolus via nasogastric tube to pregnant rats, with missing digits in the offspring. Teratogenicity has not been clearly associated with the ingestion of beverages containing xanthines during human pregnancy. Various pregnancy complications have been clearly associated with the ingestion of 300 mg/day or more of caffeine, the equivalent of three cups of coffee. The data are not as clear for lesser degrees of consumption, so it is not possible to make a clear recommendation regarding a so-called safe amount of caffeine.

It is recommended that nursing mothers limit their intake of coffee or tea to two cups per day or less.

One randomized, double-blind trial found that caffeine tablets (300 mg) were more effective than placebo at relieving postdural puncture headaches in postpartum patients.

SPECIAL CONSIDERATIONS IN PREGNANCY

The xanthines produce no unique effects in the mother during pregnancy. In pregnant sheep, slight reductions in uterine blood flow were demonstrated with intravenous infusion of 24–35 mg/kg caffeine (equivalent to more than 10 cups of coffee in the human). Maternal and fetal oxygenation and acid–base levels were unaffected. At lower dosages, the results were less clearcut. In a study of 20 third-trimester human pregnancies, Finnish investigators using xenon clearance methodology detected a slight decrease in intervillous blood flow after the ingestion of two cups of coffee. There were no changes in umbilical venous blood flow, maternal or fetal pulse rates, or maternal blood pressure, despite a doubling of maternal serum caffeine levels.

Human studies have demonstrated that caffeine elimination is significantly prolonged in pregnant women as compared to nonpregnant individuals, with the half-life increasing from 3 hours to approximately 10 hours in late pregnancy.

Caffeine has been shown to cross the placenta, with peak fetal levels approaching 75% of peak maternal levels. The fetus may be subject to stimulation of its central nervous system, skeletal musculature, or both, which could result in an increase in activity in utero. Fetal cardiac stimulation may cause tachycardia or premature contractions. In a study performed in Hungary, human fetal hearts were shown to increase in their contraction rates when exposed to caffeine in vitro.

Xanthines have caused chromosomal breakage in some microorganisms and in fruit flies. Breakages in human chromosomes, however, have only been observed with dosages far greater than those obtainable from drinking coffee or tea.

Three cases of hand anomalies in offspring of women who drank large amounts of coffee (8–25 cups/day) were collected in response to the FDA's warning stemming from the previously mentioned association with limb anomalies in rats. Unfortunately, no denominator information is available, so that these three cases may have occurred by chance in heavy coffee drinkers. An epidemiologic study of 12,205 pregnancies failed to uncover any association between caffeine consumption and malformations, low birth weight, or premature delivery after smoking and multiple other variables had been controlled. In a case-control study of 2030 malformed infants, caffeine ingestion during pregnancy was not associated with any of the defects being considered. However, only 22 infants with limb reduction defects were included in this study. Therefore, an association with caffeine ingestion could not be ruled out despite the similarity of these 22 mothers' caffeine habits to those of the control mothers.

A cross-sectional study of 1902 women interviewed at their first prenatal visit demonstrated a delay in conception related to caffeine consumption, with those taking more than 300 mg/day experiencing a 27% reduction in the likelihood of conception in any given menstrual cycle compared to non–caffeine users. A prospective cohort study of 3135 pregnant women demonstrated a significantly increased risk for late first-trimester and second-trimester spontaneous abortions (relative risk 1.73) among moderate to heavy caffeine users (more than 1.5 cups of coffee/day). A case-control study of 331 women with fetal loss, including spontaneous abortions and fetal deaths, showed a significant relationship with caffeine intake both before and during pregnancy, with a 22% increase in fetal loss rate for each 100 mg of coffee ingested daily during pregnancy. An analysis of data from the Diabetes in Early Pregnancy Study, a prospective cohort study, which included 431 women of whom 59 experienced spontaneous abortions, found no association between abortion and caffeine consumption in the first trimester. However, there were very few subjects who ingested more than 300 mg of caffeine/day, and not many who used over 200 mg/day. The authors pointed out that the lack of association could only be applied to moderate caffeine intake.

A number of studies have suggested that heavy caffeine users, who ingest in excess of 300 mg/day, are more likely to deliver low birth weight babies. Not all such studies are in agreement, however, and issues of confounding by other habits such as smoking have arisen. Nevertheless, most studies report a modest effect.

In a follow-up study of approximately 500 7-year-olds, no relation could be found between maternal caffeine consumption during pregnancy and infant development or IQ.

Caffeine reaches detectable levels in the blood of nursing infants. Jitteriness has been reported in an infant whose mother had a history of heavy caffeine use. Children and infants are more sensitive to the effects of xanthines than adults.

DOSAGE

Coffee and tea contain 60–150 mg caffeine per average cup. Nondietetic cola drinks contain 35–55 mg caffeine per 12-oz glass. Dietetic drinks in some cases contain unstated amounts of caffeine. Cocoa contains approximately 200 mg theobromine per cup. Tea contains theophylline in varying amounts.

ADVERSE EFFECTS

The fatal dose of caffeine is 10 g. It is quite unlikely that this amount will be ingested, however, because reactions usually begin after 1 g has been consumed. Central nervous system (CNS) side effects include restlessness and disturbed sleep patterns, tremor, tinnitus, and excitement, which may progress to delirium. Tachycardia and arrhythmias may occur. Other side effects include diuresis, dyspepsia, and nausea and vomiting. Theophylline may be fatal to adults, but only if administered intravenously. Children, however, have been fatally intoxicated by pharmacologic preparations of theophylline administered orally, rectally, or parenterally. In adults, theophylline may cause headaches, palpitations, nausea, and hypotension.

MECHANISM OF ACTION

The xanthines affect many systems in the body by increasing intracellular cyclic AMP, altering ionic calcium levels, and potentiating the action of catecholamines. CNS, respiratory, and skeletal muscle effects are greatest for caffeine, less for theophylline, and least for theobromine. Smooth muscle relaxation, coronary artery dilatation, myocardial stimulation, and diuresis, on the other hand, are related to theophylline, theobromine, and caffeine, in decreasing order of potency. Excitation of the CNS on all levels results from ingestion of 150–250 mg caffeine (1–2 cups of coffee). This is manifested by reduced drowsiness, increased motor activity, a reflex excitability, and awareness of sensory stimuli, as well as stimulation of respiratory, vasomotor, and vagal centers. Theophylline increases reflex excitability and the rate and depth of respirations.

The xanthines directly stimulate the myocardium and increase cardiac output. Heart rate may be slowed secondary to medullary vagal center stimulation but is increased with large dosages. Blood vessels are usually dilated by these agents, but there may be an increase in cerebrovascular resistance. Although bronchial and bile duct musculature are relaxed, there is an increase in the strength of skeletal muscle contraction. Glomerular filtration rate and renal blood flow are increased, with a resultant diuresis and increase in sodium and chloride excretion. Caffeine may increase the amount of gastric acid secretion and aggravate peptic ulcers. The xanthines also cause a slight increase in the basal metabolic rate and in higher concentrations stimulate lipolysis, glycogenolysis, and gluconeogenesis.

ABSORPTION AND BIOTRANSFORMATION

The xanthines are absorbed after oral, parenteral, or rectal administration. Because caffeine and theophylline have poor aqueous solubility, absorption from the gastrointestinal tract may be erratic, but when taken orally, their onset of action is usually within 30 minutes. The xanthines are metabolized by partial demethylation and oxidation, but about 10% is excreted unchanged in the urine.

RECOMMENDED READING

Anderson, P.O. Drugs in breast feeding: a review. *Drug Intell. Clin. Pharm.* 11:208, 1977.

Barr, H.M., and Streissguth, A.P. Caffeine use during pregnancy and child outcome: a 7-year prospective study. *Neurotoxicol. Teratol.* 13:441–448, 1991.

Camann, W.R., Murray, R.S., Mushlin, P.S., et al. Effects of oral caffeine on postdural puncture headache. *Anesth. Analg.* 70:181, 1990.

Conover, W.B., Key, T.C., and Resnik, R. Maternal cardiovascular response to caffeine infusion in the pregnant ewe. *Am. J. Obstet. Gynecol.* 145:534, 1983.

Devoe, L.D., Murray, C., Youssif, A., et al. Maternal caffeine consumption and fetal behavior in normal third-trimester pregnancy. *Am. J. Obstet. Gynecol.* 168:1105, 1993.

Eskenazi, B. Caffeine during pregnancy: grounds for concern? *J.A.M.A.* 270:2973, 1993.

Goyan, J.E. Food and Drug Administration News Release No. P80–36, September 4, 1980.

Hatch, E.E., and Bracken, M.B. Association of delayed conception with caffeine consumption. *Am. J. Epidemiol.* 138:1082, 1993.

Hinds, T.S., West, W.L., Knight, E.M., et al. The effect of caffeine on pregnancy outcome variables. *Nutr. Rev.* 54:203, 1996.

Infante-Rivard, C., Fernández, A., Gauthier, R., et al. Fetal loss associated with caffeine intake before and during pregnancy. *J.A.M.A.* 270:2940, 1993.

Jacobson, M.F., Goldman, A.S., and Syme, R.H. Coffee and birth defects. *Lancet* 1:1415, 1981.

Kirkinen, P., et al. The effect of caffeine on placental and fetal blood flow in human pregnancy. *Am. J. Obstet. Gynecol.* 147:939, 1983.

Knutti, R., Rothweiler, H., and Schlatter, C. Effect of pregnancy on the pharmacokinetics of caffeine. *Eur. J. Clin. Pharmacol.* 21:121, 1981.

Linn, S., et al. No association between coffee consumption and adverse outcomes of pregnancy. *N. Engl. J. Med.* 306:141, 1982.

Mills, J.L., Holmes, L.B., Aarons, J.H., et al. Moderate caffeine use and the risk of spontaneous abortion and intrauterine growth retardation. *J.A.M.A.* 269:593, 1993.

Morris, M.B., and Weinstein, L. Caffeine and the fetus: is trouble brewing? *Am. J. Obstet. Gynecol.* 140:607, 1981.

Narod, S.A., de Sanjosé, S., and Victora, C. Coffee during pregnancy: a reproductive hazard? *Am. J. Obstet. Gynecol.* 164:1109, 1991.

Parsons, W.D., and Pelletier, J.G. Delayed elimination of caffeine by women in the last 2 weeks of pregnancy. *Can. Med. Assoc. J.* 127:377, 1982.

Resch, B.A., and Papp, J.G. Effects of caffeine on the fetal heart. *Am. J. Obstet. Gynecol.* 146:231, 1983.

Rosenberg, L., et al. Selected birth defects in relation to caffeine-containing beverages. *J.A.M.A.* 247:1429, 1982.

Srisuphan, W., and Bracken, M.B. Caffeine consumption during pregnancy and association with late spontaneous abortion. *Am. J. Obstet. Gynecol.* 154:14, 1986.

Wilson, S.J., Ayromlooi, J., and Errick, J.K. Pharmacokinetic and hemodynamic effects of caffeine in the pregnant sheep. *Obstet. Gynecol.* 61:486, 1983.

Appendixes

Appendix A
Vitamins and Minerals

Vitamins

WATER-SOLUBLE VITAMINS

Folic Acid

Maternal folic acid deficiency during the first trimester of pregnancy is associated with an increased risk of fetal neural tube defects. Therefore, all women capable of bearing children should consume 0.4 mg of folate daily.

Folate and folic acid are nutrients required for amino and nucleic acid synthesis. Since the blockage of DNA synthesis is the major consequence of folate deficiency, the most rapidly dividing cells are those primarily affected. Bone marrow cells develop megaloblastic changes. The peripheral manifestation of this change is a macrocytic anemia, moderate leukopenia (with hypersegmented neutrophils), and thrombocytopenia.

Folates are present in large quantities in peanuts, liver, kidney, and green leafy vegetables. Cereal and dairy products contain low quantities. These folates are usually supplied as polyglutamates that are cleaved in the intestinal lumen. Only the monoglutamate form is absorbed into the bloodstream. Oral contraceptives and phenytoin may affect this metabolism and account, at least in part, for the alterations in folate levels when these medications are used.

Folic acid deficiency is rare except in malabsorption conditions, infancy, and pregnancy. The fetus can apparently extract some folate even in the presence of megaloblastic anemia in the mother. This extraction and possibly the reduced availability of folate produced by intestinal flora account for decompensation in pregnant women who have a long history of poor dietary intake.

Knowledge regarding the association between maternal folic acid levels and neural tube defects (NTDs) has been accumulating since the 1960s. Although numerous animal studies, case reports, retrospective analyses, and small-scale prospective studies seemed to indicate that folic acid played a part in the development of NTDs, convincing evidence was not available until the early 1990s. In a multinational, randomized, placebo-controlled, double-blind study of 1817 women with a previous pregnancy complicated by an NTD, folic acid 4 mg qd, taken for at least 14 days prior to the last menstrual period through week 12 of pregnancy, reduced the incidence of NTDs by 72%. Later studies in pregnant women who had no previously affected pregnancy indicated that lower doses, 0.4–0.8 mg/day taken 1 month before conception through 12 weeks gestation, could reduce the incidence of primary NTDs.

Because folate intake seems to be most important in the first trimester, the only way to ensure adequate folate for pregnancy is to recommend that all women of childbearing potential receive adequate intake. The Centers for Disease Control (CDC) currently recommends that all women who are capable of becoming pregnant consume 0.4 mg of folate per day. The CDC also recommends that women with a previous pregnancy complicated by NTD should take 4 mg of folic acid 3 months prior to conception through the twelfth week of gestation.

Prior to 1998, the average American consumed only about 0.2 mg of folate daily. Beginning of January 1, 1998, the FDA required the fortification of enriched flour with 0.14 mg of folic acid per 100 g of flour as a means of increasing the amount of folate in the diets of childbearing aged women without causing excessive intake among other population groups. Because of the potential risks associated with high doses of folate, patients must be educated about the fortification program and should be warned not to overconsume folate. The efficacy of this far-reaching public health program has yet to be determined.

High doses of folate can mask vitamin B_{12} deficiency by correcting its associated anemia. If vitamin B_{12} deficiency is undetected and untreated, irreversible neurologic damage can occur in the fetus. Therefore, daily consumption of folate should not exceed 1 mg except in special circumstances.

Commonly prescribed anticonvulsants, including phenobarbital, phenytoin, carbamazepine, and valproic acid, interfere with folic acid metabolism. Women taking these medications may develop folic acid deficiency. In addition, folic acid can increase hepatic microsomal enzyme activity and the clearance of anticonvulsants. Therefore, serum anticonvulsant levels should be monitored carefully after implementing folic acid supplementation. A 1 mg/day supplement for women taking anticonvulsants has been recommended.

The RDA for folate during pregnancy is 0.4 mg/day. During lactation, in order to replace folate loss in breast milk, the RDA is 280 µg/day for the first 6 months and 260 µg/day thereafter.

Thiamine (Vitamin B_1)

Thiamine is an essential coenzyme in carbohydrate metabolism. Dietary deficiency leads to beriberi, characterized by neurologic deficiencies and cardiovascular symptoms. Wernicke's encephalopathy and Korsakoff's psychosis are extreme neurologic manifestations of thiamine deficiency.

There have been several reports of Wernicke's encephalopathy complicating hyperemesis gravidarum that responded rapidly to thiamine therapy. Studies have revealed an increased requirement for thiamine during pregnancy if serum levels are to be maintained. The increased requirement appears early in pregnancy and remains constant throughout. In spite of increased maternal requirements, the fetus is able to achieve a higher serum level than the mother. One study has shown that maternal blood cell thiamine levels are considerably lower for infants with severe intrauterine growth retardation (IUGR) than for those with normal birth weights. The authors suggest thiamine supplementation, especially at the end of gestation, in cases with severe IUGR.

In view of these studies, the Recommended Dietary Allowance of thiamine in pregnancy is 0.4 mg greater than the 1.1 mg/day needed by a nonpregnant woman. Thiamine requirements also increase during lactation. The lactating woman secretes approximately 0.2 mg of thiamine/day in milk. To make up for the loss in milk and the increased energy consumption during lactation, an additional 0.5 mg daily is recommended throughout lactation.

Riboflavin (Vitamin B$_2$)

Riboflavin acts as a coenzyme required for the flavoproteins involved in oxidative metabolism. Moderate degrees of deficiency have caused fetal malformations in rodents. No association between deficiency and malformations in humans has been noted. Symptoms of riboflavin deficiency in humans include sore throat, stomatitis, glossitis, seborrheic dermatitis, and anemia.

Studies have revealed an increasing riboflavin requirement as pregnancy progresses. This has been clinically confirmed by the manifestations of deficiency (i.e., glossitis, angular stomatitis, cheilosis, and corneal vascularization) in the third trimester in mothers with low riboflavin intake. Despite symptoms in the mother, however, no influence on the outcome of pregnancy could be detected. This maternal–fetal discrepancy may be related to the active transport of riboflavin across the placenta. Cord levels have been reported to be as high as 4 times those in the mother's serum.

In view of these studies, the Recommended Dietary Allowance (RDA) during pregnancy includes an intake of 0.3 mg/day above the baseline of 1.3 mg/day. Riboflavin is excreted in breast milk and must be supplemented in the mother. The RDA for a lactating woman is an additional 0.5 mg for the first 6 months and 0.4 mg thereafter.

Niacin

Niacin is the generic name for nicotinic acid and nicotinamide. Niacin functions in coenzymes concerned with glycolysis, fat synthesis, and tissue respiration. In addition, nicotinic acid has its own independent pharmacology and is used in large doses to treat hyperlipoproteinemia.

Pellagra has been found to be associated with dietary deficiency of niacin and other vitamins in areas in which corn is the major source of protein. It is characterized by dermatitis, diarrhea, inflammation of the mucous membranes, and, in severe cases, dementia.

Some dietary tryphophan can be converted to niacin in a ratio of 60 mg tryphophan to 1 mg niacin. During pregnancy there is an increased conversion of tryphophan to niacin derivatives.

The Recommended Dietary Allowance (RDA) calls for an increased niacin intake during pregnancy of 2 mg niacin above the basal allowance of 15 mg (or its tryphophan equivalent). This accounts for the increased energy requirement of pregnancy. There have been no controlled studies regarding the influence of dietary deficiency during pregnancy. During lactation, the woman loses approximately 1 mg of niacin daily in

750 ml of milk. This loss plus the additional energy expenditure to support lactation accounts for the RDA of an additional 5 mg niacin (or its tryphophan equivalent) per day throughout lactation.

Vitamin B$_6$

Vitamin B$_6$ is a group of interrelated substances: pyridoxine, pyridoxamine, and pyridoxal. These chemicals are converted in the liver to pyridoxal phosphate and pyridoxamine phosphate, which are required as coenzymes in amino acid metabolism. A number of conditions have been related to B$_6$ deficiency; dietary deprivation can result in skin lesions, glossitis, seizures, anemia, and peripheral neuritis. The use of certain medications, such as penicillamine, isoniazid, and oral contraceptives, has been shown to affect the absorption or metabolism of vitamin B$_6$.

Serum levels of vitamin B$_6$ fall late in the first trimester and remain depressed throughout pregnancy. They rise to the normal values for nonpregnant women by the fourth postpartum day.

The placenta actively transports vitamin B$_6$, and levels in the fetus are 2–3 times higher than those in the mother, but they rise further with increases in the mother's levels. Umbilical vein levels are higher than those in the umbilical artery, indicating fetal utilization.

Attempts to normalize biochemical and excretion indices, as well as serum levels, in pregnant women have suggested that supplementation of 10–15 mg/day is needed. No controlled trials have suggested benefits to the mother or fetus by this type of supplementation. The use of megadose pyridoxine (2000–6000 mg/day) has been associated with a form of sensory neuropathy consisting of sensory ataxia and profound impairment of distal limb position and vibration sense in human adults.

Animal studies have shown that maternal vitamin B$_6$ deficiency during periods of brain development results in various neurochemical changes that manifest as tremors, irritability, abnormal motor function, and seizures. One study of Egyptian mothers and infants reported that poor maternal vitamin B$_6$ nutritional status was associated with more difficult consolability, shorter buildup to a crying state, and more irritable responses to aversive stimuli.

Administered in doses of between 25 and 75 mg/day, vitamin B$_6$ appears to be safe and effective in relieving the severity of nausea and vomiting of early pregnancy.

Pyridoxine in doses of 200–600 mg/day has been shown to be effective in reversing hyperprolactinemia in women with amenorrhea-galactorrhea syndromes and in suppressing postpartum lactation in normal individuals. For this reason, high dosages should not be taken by breast-feeding mothers.

The Recommended Dietary Allowance (RDA) includes an increase of 0.6 mg/day above the basal requirements of 1.6 mg/day. The RDA for the lactating woman is an additional 0.5 mg/day to account for vitamin B$_6$ loss in breast milk and increased maternal requirements.

Vitamin B$_{12}$

Vitamin B$_{12}$, which includes all cobalamides active in human beings, is present in all cells of mammalian tissue. Cyanocobalamin is the commercially available form of vitamin B$_{12}$ used in pharmaceuticals. It is essential in nucleic acid metabolism because of its role in allowing 5-methyltetrahydrofolate to return to the utilizable folate pool. Deficiency results in macrocytic, megaloblastic anemia as well as in neurologic dysfunction.

Humans depend on exogenous sources of vitamin B$_{12}$, primarily animal products. The average diet contains 5–15 g vitamin B$_{12}$ daily. Absorption via intrinsic factor is quite efficient, and dietary deficiency is very rare, except in strict vegetarians. Fetal vitamin B$_{12}$ demand appears to be high in the first 27 weeks of pregnancy when maternal-fetal erythropoiesis is at its maximum.

Average fetal demands of vitamin B$_{12}$ are approximately 0.1–0.2 µg/day. The fetus and placenta have been shown to concentrate vitamin B$_{12}$, and newborn serum levels are about 2 times maternal values. Breast-fed infants of mothers who are strict vegetarians are at risk for becoming profoundly deficient in vitamin B$_{12}$.

While normal maternal body stores are sufficient to meet the needs of pregnancy, the Recommended Dietary Allowance includes the addition of 0.2 µg/day during pregnancy above the basal requirement of 2 µg/day. The level of vitamin B$_{12}$ in breast milk approximates that of maternal serum. To replace maternal loss, an additional allowance of 0.6 µg/day is recommended throughout lactation.

Pantothenic Acid

Pantothenic acid is incorporated into coenzyme A, an integral link in the acetylation processes of intermediary metabolism. It is widely distributed in nature. Deficiency is manifested by symptoms of neuromuscular degeneration and adrenocortical insufficiency. Because of its ubiquitous nature, pantothenic acid deficiency has not been recognized in human beings consuming a normal diet.

Maternal pantothenic acid levels appear to fall during pregnancy, in part due to hemodilution. Placental transfer of pantothenic acid takes place via active transport mechanisms and newborn levels can be almost twice maternal levels.

Studies in pregnant women have shown that dietary pantothenic acid is often below the amount thought to be safe and adequate for adults and that a carefully chosen diet or pharmaceutical supplementation may be necessary.

There is no Recommended Dietary Allowance for pantothenic acid. The National Research Council found that ingestion of 4–7 mg daily should be safe and adequate for pregnant and lactating women as well as for nonpregnant adults.

Ascorbic Acid (Vitamin C)

Ascorbic acid is a cofactor in numerous hydroxylation and amidation reactions. It is required for synthesis of collagen, proteoglycans, and other tissue constituents, and is involved in the synthesis of epinephrine and the adrenal steroids. Humans and other primates, when deprived of vitamin C, develop scurvy, a potentially fatal disease characterized by weakening of collagen and impaired wound healing. Scurvy still occurs in infants who are fed only cow's milk and in malnourished and alcoholic adults.

Ascorbic acid levels decline progressively during pregnancy. Increased levels in the fetus appear to be due to "trapping." The placenta allows passive transfer of dehydroascorbic acid; conversion to the impermeable ascorbic acid in the fetus allows higher concentrations to accumulate. Although levels in the fetus are 2–3 times higher than those in the mother, congenital scurvy has occurred in children born to mothers with the disease. Preliminary studies show that plasma levels of reduced ascorbic acid are significantly decreased in mild and severe preeclampsia. It is hypothesized that patients with preeclampsia utilize antioxidant nutrients to a greater extent to counteract free-radical-mediated endothelial cell disturbances.

There is a theoretical risk that large amounts of ascorbic acid taken chronically during pregnancy could condition the fetus to large amounts of this substance and lead to the development of infantile scurvy despite a diet that contains adequate amounts of ascorbic acid. Therefore, large doses of vitamin C are not recommended during pregnancy.

The Recommended Dietary Allowance (RDA) for pregnant women includes an intake of 10 mg/day in addition to the usual allowance of 60 mg/day to offset maternal losses. The concentration of vitamin C in human milk varies. After accounting for such variations, the RDA is an extra 35 mg/day during the first 6 months of lactation and 30 mg/day thereafter.

FAT-SOLUBLE VITAMINS

Vitamin A

Dietary vitamin A is in the form of preformed vitamin A (retinol) and carotenoids, especially β-carotene. Carotenoids must be converted to retinol in order to be useful to the body. Retinol is required for growth and differentiation of epithelial tissue, bone growth, reproduction, embryonic development, and as an essential link in the conversion of light energy to nervous activity in the visual process. The chronic intake of large amounts of vitamin A (more than 50,000 units/day) has been associated with hypervitaminosis A, a syndrome that includes headache, dermatitis, nausea, stiff neck, elevated intracranial pressure, papilledema, and elevated serum glutamic oxaloacetic transaminase (SGOT) levels.

No effects on the fetus from low levels of vitamin A have been reported. Conversely, experiments in animals have shown that retinoids can be teratogenic. Retrospective studies and case reports in humans suggest a teratogenic effect for exposures to very high doses of vitamin A (more than 10,000 units/day). These findings relate to pre-formed vitamin A (retinol) and not to β-carotene, a vitamin A precursor. Animal studies indicated that high doses of β-carotene are neither toxic nor teratogenic. Based on these preliminary data and because there are few justifications for routine ingestion of supplemental doses of vitamin A in excess of 8000–10,000 units/day, fertile and pregnant women should avoid megadose vitamin A therapy. Isotretinoin, a vitamin A isomer, has been clearly associated with teratogenesis in humans. This drug is covered separately (see "Isotretinoin").

The Recommended Dietary Allowance for vitamin A during pregnancy is the same as that for the nonpregnant woman, 2700 IU of vitamin A or 800 retinol equivalents (RE). (1 RE is 1 µg of all *trans*-retinol, 6 µg of all *trans*-β-carotene, or 12 µg of other provitamin A carotenoids, based on their relative bioavailabilities.) To replace vitamin A lost in breast milk, lactating mothers should receive an extra 500 RE/day during the first 6 months of lactation and 400 RE/day thereafter.

Vitamin D

The physiologic importance of vitamin D resides in its regulatory role in calcium homeostasis. Vitamin D accelerates intestinal absorption of calcium against an electrochemical gradient and is required for proper bone formation. A deficiency results in rickets in children and osteomalacia in adults.

Vitamin D exists in two forms: D_2 (ergocalciferol) and D_3 (cholecalciferol). D_2 is synthetically produced by the ultraviolet irradiation of ergosterol in plants. D_3 is naturally formed in the skin by the exposure of 7-dehydrocholesterol to sunlight. Both forms are equally effective in humans. The primary active metabolite of vitamin D is calcitriol, 1,25-dihydroxyvitamin D, that is formed sequentially in the liver and kidney.

Biologically active calcitriol levels increase during pregnancy, as do levels of bound calcitriol and vitamin D–binding proteins. Calcitriol is transferred to the fetus from the maternal circulation and is also produced by the fetal kidney. Fetal calcitriol concentrations are persistently depressed, however, likely due to a relatively high fetal maternal calcium gradient (1.4:1). At birth, the infant's circulating calcium falls and calcitriol production is stimulated.

The importance of proper vitamin D intake during pregnancy has been documented by the finding of hypocalcemia, delayed bone ossification, and abnormal enamel formation with low 25-hydroxycholecalciferol levels in infants born to mothers with vitamin D deficiency.

Excessive levels of vitamin D intake may contribute to the production of severe maternal and neonatal hypercalcemia. This is especially hazardous with concomitant antacid ingestion. A syndrome of supravalvular aortic stenosis, as well as cranial and facial anomalies, has been reported in animal species and in humans exposed to large amounts of vitamin D in utero. For this reason, excessive dosages should not be ingested by pregnant women.

Because calcium is deposited in the growing fetus and secreted in small quantities in human milk, the Recommended Dietary Allowance (RDA) for both pregnant and lactating women is 10 µg (400 IU)/day, an increase of 5 µg from the RDA for women age 24 and over.

Vitamin E

The main function of vitamin E is as an antioxidant, preventing cellular membrane damage, subsequent neurologic manifestations, and anemia. Deficiency symptoms in humans are seen in premature, very-low- birth-weight infants and patients who do not absorb fat normally. Plasma levels of full-term newborns are about one-third those of adults, and lower levels are found in premature infants. Values in the mother rise during pregnancy in conjunction with rising plasma lipid levels to 60% above nonpregnant levels.

Recent studies have attempted to define the role of vitamin E in preeclampsia, fetal growth retardation, maternal infection, and birth weight. The data are conflicting as to whether vitamin E levels are elevated or depressed in preeclampsia. One case-control study did, however, document that patients with preeclampsia do not have a relative dietary deprivation of vitamin E.

The suggested Recommended Dietary Allowance for pregnant women is an intake of 10 mg/day, 2 mg above the recommendation for nonpregnant adults. Lactating women should take an extra 4 mg/day (total dose 12 mg) during the first 6 months, and an extra 3 mg/day (total dose 11 mg) thereafter.

Vitamin K

The synthesis of coagulation factors II, VII, IX, and X and proteins C and S requires the presence of vitamin K. This vitamin exists naturally as K_1 (phytonadione) and K_2 (a series of compounds, the menaquinones). The former is produced by plants, the latter by bacteria. Menadione, a fat-soluble synthetic product, has approximately twice the biological activity of the natural forms. Because intestinal bacteria produce vitamin K_2, dietary deficiency does not exist in the absence of suppression of gut flora.

Vitamin K does not pass readily from the maternal to fetal circulation. In addition, the newborn intestine contains few bacteria. Thus, the neonate is subject to hemorrhagic tendencies due to relative vitamin K deficiency as well as hepatic immaturity. Routine administration of vitamin K shortly after birth will help prevent neonatal morbidity and mortality related to this deficiency.

In an effort to influence coagulation in the early postnatal period, several investigators have given vitamin K prenatally. Oral administration of 10 mg vitamin K_1/day during the last 10–14 days of gestation has been shown to activate fetal vitamin K–responsive coagulation factors until at least the fifth day of life; and neonatal prothrombin times are significantly improved after maternal treatment with 5 mg/day administered orally for 12 days.

Maternal anticonvulsant therapy has been associated with an increased incidence of vitamin K deficiency in the newborn, but not in the mothers themselves. It is hypothesized that the anticonvulsants induce fetal microsomal enzymes which, in turn, increase the metabolism of vitamin K. High dose vitamin K (10 mg/day) administered throughout the last month of pregnancy to pregnant women on anticonvulsant therapy has been shown to increase fetal vitamin K levels and protect the newborn from bleeding tendencies.

Some investigators have studied the effect of maternally administered vitamin K on the incidence of intracranial hemorrhage (ICH) in the low birth weight infant. The studies performed to date are not consistent in their conclusions, finding either a decreased or an equal incidence of severe ICH as well as either improved or no difference in clotting parameters. As of now, there is no clear benefit to the use of vitamin K antenatally for the prevention of ICH in the premature infant.

Because vitamin K consumed in usual diets exceeds the Recommended Dietary Allowance (RDA) established for adult women, additional intake above the RDA of 65 mg is not necessary during pregnancy. Similarly, lactation imposes little additional need and no increase in the RDA is required. It is currently recommended that 0.5–1.0 mg vitamin K_1 be administered intramuscularly to the neonate immediately after birth.

Minerals

Iron

Iron deficiency is the most common cause of nutritional anemia in humans and the most prevalent nutrient deficiency problem of pregnancy. When severe, it manifests itself as a characteristic microcytic hypochromic anemia. Iron is also an essential component of myglobin, heme enzymes, and metalloflavoprotein enzymes. Iron deficiency, therefore, affects metabolism independent of its effect on oxygen delivery.

For adult, nonpregnant women, iron requirements are approximately 1.36 mg/day. About one-half of this iron is required to replace menstrual loss. During the first trimester of pregnancy, iron requirements decrease due to cessation of menses. At this time, iron stores may increase. However, iron requirements increase significantly beginning in the second trimester and reach their peak in the third trimester. More than 300 mg of iron is transferred to the fetus, placenta, and cord; and up to 600 mg can be incorporated into expanding maternal red cell mass. In addition, there is an average 320-mg external iron loss and blood loss at delivery. An average of 5.6 mg/day of absorbed iron is needed during the second and third trimesters of pregnancy, approximately 4.2 mg more than in the nonpregnant state.

There are few published data documenting severe morbidity from maternal iron deficiency anemia. Among postulated maternal risks are increased fatigue, decreased work performance, cardiovascular stress due to inadequate hemoglobin and low blood oxygen saturation, and poor tolerance to heavy blood loss at delivery. The postulated risks to the fetus relate to impaired delivery of hemoglobin and oxygen to the uterus, placenta, and developing fetus. Cross-sectional and longitudinal studies provide evidence that anemia during pregnancy may be associated with perinatal death, preterm birth, and low birth weight, but the data are unclear and further studies must be performed to quantify the risk, if any.

The U.S. Preventive Services Task Force (USPSTF) reviewed a large body of data to determine whether prenatal iron can reduce the incidence of obstetric complications, presumably by correcting hematologic indices. The data are inconclusive. Studies do show that iron supplements are effective in improving maternal hematologic indices; however, their effect on the hematologic status of the fetus is unclear, and there was limited evidence that iron supplementation can reduce the incidence of complications from iron deficiency or anemia. Recommendations regarding iron supplementation during pregnancy vary widely. The USPSTF concluded that the evidence was insufficient to recommend for or against routine iron supplementation. Other institutions and committees recommend that iron 30–120 mg/day be routinely administered to pregnant women. Still others strongly believe that iron supplementation is unnecessary.

The Recommended Daily Allowance (RDA) for pregnant women, to replace blood loss, allow expansion of maternal red cell mass, and provide iron to fetus and placenta, is an increase of 15 mg of iron/day over the 15 mg/day requirement for a nonpregnant woman. In order to provide this amount of iron, a woman eating a usual U.S. diet would require supplementation. Loss through lactation is approximately 0.15–0.3 mg/day, less than menstrual loss which is often absent during lactation. Thus, the RDA for a lactating woman is the same as for the nonpregnant woman, i.e., 15 mg/day.

Calcium

The body of the human adult contains approximately 1200 g calcium, 99% of which is present in bone. Bone calcium is complexed with phosphate as hydroxyapatite. The small amount of calcium outside of the skeletal structure is critically important to the regulation of many metabolic activities, including nerve and muscle function, hormonal actions, blood clotting, and cellular motility.

The level of calcium in the blood is controlled by complex hormonal and nutritional factors and is maintained in a narrow range. Only the free ionized calcium exerts physiologic effects and is hormonally governed.

The major influences on serum calcium concentration and phosphorus concentration are their solubility products, vitamin D intake and metabolism, and secretion of the hormones parathormone and calcitonin.

Parathormone, released in response to low or falling levels of ionized calcium, acts by increasing osteoclast activity, decreasing the renal tubular absorption of phosphate, and augmenting the action of vitamin D in facilitating calcium absorption. High serum levels of ionized calcium cause release of calcitonin, which inhibits release of calcium from bone. Vitamin D is essential for the active absorption of calcium from the gut as well as the proper synthesis of bone matrix.

During pregnancy, there is an obligatory transfer of approximately 30 g calcium to the fetus for mineralization of the skeleton. This transfer takes place primarily in the second and third trimesters. Changes in maternal calcium metabolism facilitate this transfer while protecting maternal bone and serum calcium levels. The substantial amount of calcium needed by the fetus is provided by increased maternal efficiency of calcium absorption, which doubles by the fifth or sixth month of gestation. The placenta actively transports calcium to the fetus. At full term, levels of parathormone in the fetus are low and calcitonin levels high, favoring bone formation.

Calcium has been used therapeutically to prevent maternal hypertension. Meta-analysis of 14 randomized trials involving 2459 women concluded that calcium supplementation reduced systolic and diastolic blood pressure and preeclampsia. However, in the most comprehensive, randomized, double blinded study completed to date, calcium was found to have an effect on the risk of preeclampsia. This multicenter study compared the incidence of preeclampsia in 4589 healthy nulliparous women, half of whom received 2 g of calcium carbonate daily and half of whom received placebo. Calcium supplementation did not prevent preeclampsia, pregnancy associated hypertension of adverse perinatal outcomes. Calcium supplementation during pregnancy has been associated with a lower incidence of preterm birth and low-birth-weight infants.

The calcium reserve in the mother's skeleton is quite high in comparison to the needs of the fetus. Although adequate fetal mineralization can occur without calcium supplementation, most authorities believe that the 30 g loss to the fetus should be replaced. The Recommended Dietary Allowance for calcium during pregnancy and lactation is 1200 mg/day. This amount of calcium can be obtained by drinking 1 quart of milk daily. This amount also provides adequate levels of vitamin D. For patients intolerant of milk, similar intake may be provided by means of calcium supplements.

Zinc

Zinc is essential as a cofactor for many human enzyme systems. Although the body contains relatively large amounts of zinc stored in bone, these supplies are not metabolically active. Dietary deficiency leads to loss of appetite, failure to grow, dermatitis, diarrhea, mental disturbances, and immune disorders. Gross zinc deficiency, seen in the Middle East, results in hypogonadism and dwarfism.

Mild zinc deficiency in the pregnant woman may be associated with significant maternal and fetal morbidity, including prolonged gestation, intrauterine growth restriction and inefficient labor. Maternal zinc deficiency has also been implicated as a causal factor in the pathogenesis of neural tube defects and congenital malformations. The risk of preterm delivery has also been reported to increase with zinc deficiency. Daily zinc supplementation in women with relatively low plasma zinc concentrations in early pregnancy has been associated with increased infant birth weight, decreased premature birth, and decreased prenatal death. Subnormal maternal serum zinc levels have been reported in the first trimester among women destined to develop preeclampsia and during labor in alcoholic women.

Congenital lesions of the central nervous system appear to be greater in geographic areas in which zinc deficiency exists. Some studies have revealed that zinc is an essential component of the bacterial inhibitory system of the amniotic fluid. There is some suggestion that dietary availability of zinc may alter the effectiveness of this system. A case report of four pregnant women given megadose (300 mg) zinc daily during the third trimester described three preterm live births and one stillbirth.

Total body zinc increases throughout pregnancy. Levels at full term are approximately 50% above those of nonpregnant women. Plasma and hair concentrations, however, fall during this period.

Despite the important implications of the above-mentioned observations, few data are available on the maintenance of homeostasis in the pregnant woman. The daily zinc content of the diet of an average American adult is 1025 mg. Metabolic studies have revealed that balance can be maintained with an intake of 8–10 mg daily in the nonpregnant state. The Recommended Dietary Allowance (RDA) is 15 mg/day during pregnancy, above basal recommendations of 12 mg/day for nonpregnant women. During the first 6 months of lactation, the RDA for zinc is 19 mg, calculated to replace zinc lost in breast milk. After 6 months, the RDA falls to 16 mg reflecting diminished average milk production in this period.

Chromium

Interest in chromium metabolism in pregnancy has centered around its role in glucose utilization. It is believed to play a physiological role as a cofactor for insulin. Chromium deficiency can be associated with decreased glucose tolerance, and its supplementation has ameliorated glucose intolerance in some clinical states. Some reports of chromium plasma and hair concentrations suggest that pregnancy may be associated with chromium depletion. Investigators have hypothesized that this depletion may potentiate the glucose intolerance of pregnancy.

There is no clear evidence that supplemental chromium is beneficial in improving glucose tolerance.

The Recommended Dietary Allowance (RDA) of chromium in adults is 50–200 μg/day. Not enough information is available to define an RDA for pregnant women.

Iodine

Iodine is required for the formation of the thyroid hormones thyroxine and triiodothyronine. Iodine deficiency leads to inadequate hormone production, excess thyroid-stimulating hormone secretion, and goiter formation. For nonpregnant adult women, the minimal requirement necessary to prevent goiter formation is approximately 1 μg/kg body weight. The most reliable source of iodine is through iodized salt, which contains 76 μg iodine/g. Since iodized salt is rarely used in commercially prepared foods, it is recommended that this preparation be used as added table salt.

Severe endemic iodine deficiency causes endemic cretinism, characterized by deaf-mutism, intellectual deficiency, rigid-spastic motor disorder, and, sometimes, hypothyroidism. Endemic cretinism is the world's most preventable cause of mental retardation. Endemic cretinism and neonatal hypothyroidism can best be prevented by iodine treatment prior to conception. Administration of iodine to pregnant women during the second trimester has improved the neurologic and psychological development of their children. However, treatment after the beginning of the third trimester was not associated with improved neurologic status.

It should be noted that pharmacologic dosages of iodides may cause goiter formation in the fetus. Rapid and sustained elevation of maternal serum iodine levels has been demonstrated after vaginal application of povidone-iodine solutions used to treat vaginitis.

The adult Recommended Dietary Allowance for iodine is 150 µg/day. It is suggested that pregnant and lactating women consume an extra 25 µg/day and 50 µg/day, respectively, to allow for fetal demands and loss via breast milk.

Copper

Copper is essential for all mammals. It is a component of certain proteins and enzymes, some of which are essential for the proper utilization of iron. In rare instances, copper dietary deficiency has occurred in humans, leading to anemia, neutropenia, and bone disease. In experimental animals with copper deficiencies, major anomalies have been produced as a result of defective crosslinking in elastin and collagen.

The fetus requires copper, which accumulates in certain fetal organs in much greater concentrations than are seen in adult tissue. The copper concentration in the fetal liver, for example, is 5–10 times that of an adult. Serum levels in the fetus rise throughout pregnancy. This may be related to elevated levels of estrogen because the increase of the two is coincident. Furthermore, exogenous estrogens raise serum levels of copper in nonpregnant women.

There is no Recommended Dietary Allowance for copper. Intake of 1.5–3 mg/day seems to maintain a homeostatic balance in adults.

RECOMMENDED READING

Allen, L.H. Pregnancy and iron deficiency: unresolved issues. *Nutrition Rev.* 55:91, 1997.

Allen, L.H. Vitamin B_{12} metabolism and status during pregnancy, lactation and infancy. *Adv. Exp. Med. Biol.* 352:173, 1994.

Brzezinski, A., Bromberg, Y.M., and Braun, K. Riboflavin excretion during pregnancy and early lactation. *J. Lab. Clin. Med.* 39:84, 1952.

Bucher, H.C., et al. Effect of calcium supplementation of pregnancy-induced hypertension and preeclampsia: a meta-analysis of randomized controlled trials. *J.A.M.A.* 275:1113, 1996.

Butterworth, C.E., Jr., and Bendich, A. Folic acid and the prevention of birth defects. *Annu. Rev. Nutr.* 16:73, 1996.

Cao, X.Y., et al. Timing of vulnerability of the brain to iodine deficiency in endemic cretinism. *N. Engl. J. Med.* 331:1739, 1994.

Centers for Disease Control and Prevention. Recommendations for the use of folic acid to reduce the number of cases of spina bifida and other neural tube defects. *M.M.W.R.* 41(RR 14):1, 1992.

Cleary, R.E., Lumeng, L., and Li, T. Maternal and fetal plasma levels of pyridoxal phosphate at term: adequacy of vitamin B_6 supplementation during pregnancy. *Am. J. Obstet. Gynecol.* 121:25, 1975.

Cochrane, W.A. Overnutrition in prenatal and neonatal life: A problem? *Can. Med. Assoc. J.* 93:893, 1965.

Cohenour, S.H., and Calloway, D.H. Blood, urine and dietary pantothenic acid levels of pregnant teenagers. *Am. J. Clin. Nutr.* 25:512, 1972.

Cornelissen, M., et al. Increased incidence of neonatal vitamin K deficiency resulting from maternal anticonvulsant therapy. *Am. J. Obstet. Gynecol.* 168:923, 1993.

Coursin, D.B., and Brown, V.C. Changes in vitamin B_6 during pregnancy. *Am. J. Obstet. Gynecol.* 82:1307, 1961.

Czeizel, A.E., and Dudas, I. Prevention of the first occurrence of neural-tube defects by periconceptional vitamin supplementation. *N. Eng. J. Med.* 327:1832, 1992.

Davidson, I.W., and Burt, R.L. Physiologic changes in plasma chromium of normal and pregnant women: effect of a glucose load. *Am. J. Obstet. Gynecol.* 116:601, 1973.

Davies, N.T., and Williams, R.B. Zinc balance during pregnancy and lactation. *Am. J. Clin. Nutr.* 30:300, 1977.

Dickson, R.C., Stubbs, T.M., and Lazarchick, J. Antenatal vitamin K therapy of the low-birth-weight infant. *Am. J. Obstet. Gynecol.* 170:85–9, 1994.

Dokumov, S.I. Serum copper and pregnancy. *Am. J. Obstet. Gynecol.* 101:217, 1968.

Flynn, A., et al. Zinc status of pregnant alcoholic women: a determinant of fetal outcome. *Lancet* 1:572, 1981.

Foukas, M.D. An antilactogenic effect of pyridoxine. *J. Obstet. Gynaecol. Br. Commw.* 80:718, 1973.

Friedman, W.F. Vitamin D and the supravalvular aortic stenosis syndrome. *Adv. Teratol.* 3:85, 1968.

Friedman, W.F., and Mills, L.F. The relationship between vitamin D and the craniofacial and dental anomalies of the supravalvular aortic stenosis syndrome. *Pediatrics* 43:12, 1969.

Gal, I., Sharman, I.M., and Pryse-Davies, J. Vitamin A in relation to human congenital malformations. *Adv. Teratol.* 5:143, 1972.

Haram, K., Thordarson, H., and Hervig, T. Calcium homeostasis in pregnancy and lactation. *Acta Obstet. Gynecolog. Scand.* 72:509, 1993.

Heinze, T., and Weber, W. Determination of thiamine (vitamin B_1) in maternal blood during normal pregnancies and pregnancies with intrauterine growth retardation. *Zeitschrift Ernahrungswissenschaft* 29:39, 1990.

Heller, S., Salkeld, R.M., and Korner, W.F. Riboflavin status in pregnancy. *Am. J. Clin. Nutr.* 27:1225, 1974.

Heller, S., Salkeld, R.M., and Korner, W.F. Vitamin B_1 status in pregnancy. *Am. J. Clin. Nutr.* 27:1221, 1974.

Hemminki, E., and Merilainen, J. Long-term follow-up of mothers and their infants in a randomized trial on iron prophylaxis during pregnancy. *Am. J. Obstet. Gynecol.* 173:205–209, 1995.

Higginbottom, M.C., Sweetman, L., and Nyhan, W.L. A syndrome of methylmalonic aciduria, homocystinuria, megaloblastic anemia and neurologic abnormalities in a vitamin B_{12}-deficient breastfed infant of a strict vegetarian. *N. Engl. J. Med.* 299:317, 1978.

Jain, S.K. and Wise, R. Relationship between elevated lipid peroxides, vitamin E deficiency and hypertension in preeclampsia. *Mol. Cell. Biol.* 151:33, 1995.

Jameson, S. Zinc status in pregnancy: the effect of zinc therapy on perinatal mortality, prematurity, and placental ablation. *Ann. N.Y. Acad. Sci.* 678:178, 1993.

Jovanovic-Peterson, L., and Peterson, C.M. Vitamin and mineral deficiencies which may predispose to glucose intolerance of pregnancy. *J. Am. Coll. Nutr.* 15:14, 1996.

Lavin, P.J.M., et al. Wernicke's encephalopathy: a predictable complication of hyperemesis gravidarum. *Obstet. Gynecol.* 62 (Suppl.): 13S, 1983.

Malone, J.M. Vitamin passage across the placenta. *Clin. Perinatol.* 2:295, 1975.

McCullough, A.L., et al. Vitamin B_6 status of Egyptian mothers: relation to infant behavior and maternal-infant interactions. *Am. J. Clin. Nutr.* 51:1067, 1990.

McIntosh, E.N. Treatment of women with the galactorrhea-amenorrhea syndrome with pyridoxine (vitamin B_6). *J. Clin. Endocrinol. Metab.* 42:1192, 1976.

Medical Research Council Vitamin Study Research Group. Prevention of neural tube defects: results of the Medical Research Council vitamin study. *Lancet* 338:131, 1991.

Menard, M.K. Vitamin and mineral supplement prior to and during pregnancy. *Obstet. Gynecol. Clin. North Am.* 24:479, 1997.

Mikhail, M.S., et al. Preeclampsia and antioxidant nutrients: decreased plasma levels of reduced ascorbic acid, alpha tocopherol, and beta-carotene in women with preeclampsia. *Am. J. Obstet. Gynecol.* 171:150, 1994.

Pitkin, R.M. Calcium metabolism in pregnancy: a review. *Am. J. Obstet. Gynecol.* 121:724, 1975.

Prasad, A.S. Zinc deficiency in women, infants and children. *J. Am. Coll. Nutr.* 15:113, 1996.

Recommended Daily Allowances (10th ed.). Washington, DC: National Academy Press, 1989.

Rhead, W.J., and Schrauzer, G.N. Risks of long-term ascorbic acid overdosage. *Nutr. Rev.* 29:2623, 1971.

Rosa, F.W., Wilk, A.L., and Kelsey, F.O. Teratogen update: vitamin A congeners. *Teratology* 33:355, 1986.

Rothman, K.J., et al. Teratogenicity of high vitamin A intake. *N. Engl. J. Med.* 333:1369, 1995.

Schaumburg, H., et al. Sensory neuropathy from pyridoxine abuse: a new megavitamin syndrome. *N. Engl. J. Med.* 309:445, 1983.

Schiff, E., et al. Dietary consumption and plasma concentrations of vitamin E in pregnancies complicated by preeclampsia. *Am. J. Obstet. Gynecol.* 75:1024, 1996.

Schlievert, P., Johnson, W., and Galask, R.P. Bacterial growth inhibition by the amniotic fluid: VII. The effect of zinc supplementation on bacterial inhibitory activity of amniotic fluids from gestation of 20 weeks. *Am. J. Obstet. Gynecol.* 127:603, 1977.

Sibai, B.M., et al. Risk factors associated with preeclampsia in healthy nulliparous women. The Calcium for Preeclampsia Prevention (CPEP) Study Group. *Am. J. Obstet. Gynecol.* 177:1003, 1997.

Song, W.O., Wyse, B.W., and Hansen, R.G. Pantothenic acid status of pregnant and lactating women. *J. Am. Diet. Assoc.* 85:192, 1985.

Specker, B.L. Do North American women need supplemental vitamin D during pregnancy or lactation? *Am. J. Clin. Nutr.* 59:484S, 1994.

Tamura, T., et al. Serum concentrations of zinc, folate, vitamins A and E, and proteins, and their relationships to pregnancy outcome. *Acta Obstet. Gynecol. Scand.* 165:63, 1997.

Thorp, J.A., et al. Combined antenatal vitamin K and phenobarbital therapy for preventing intracranial hemorrhage in newborns less than 34 weeks gestation. *Obstet.Gynecol.* 86:1, 1995.

Thorp, J.A., et al. Current concepts and controversies in the use of vitamin K. *Drugs* 49:376–387, 1995.

Tinkle, M. Folic acid and food fortification: implications for the primary care practitioner. *Nurse Practitioner* 22:105, 1997.

U.S. Preventive Services Task Force. Routine iron supplementation during pregnancy. Policy Statement. *J.A.M.A.* 270:284, 1993.

U.S. Preventive Services Task Force. Routine iron supplementation during pregnancy. Review Article. *J.A.M.A.* 270:2848, 1993.

Viteri, F.E. Iron supplementation for the control of iron deficiency in populations at risk. *Nutr. Rev.* 55:195, 1997.

Vorherr, H., et al. Vaginal absorption of povidone-iodine. *J.A.M.A.* 244:2628, 1980.

Zempleni, J., Link, G., and Bitsch, I. Intrauterine vitamin B_2 uptake of preterm and full-term infants. *Pediatr. Res.* 38:585, 1995.

Zimmerman, A.W., et al. Zinc transport in pregnancy. *Am. J. Obstet. Gynecol.* 149:523, 1984.

Appendix B
Antineoplastic Drugs

GENERAL BACKGROUND

Cancer is a leading cause of death in women of reproductive age. It is estimated that 1 in 1000 to 1 in 1500 pregnancies are complicated by a malignancy in the mother. The common malignancies associated with pregnancy are leukemia, lymphoma, melanoma, and breast cancer. For many of these conditions, the primary treatment involves cytotoxic chemotherapy. The use of these agents during pregnancy is associated with unique problems. Because the fetus is composed of rapidly dividing tissue, and because antineoplastic drugs are designed to inhibit the growth of rapidly dividing cells, it seems logical that the use of chemotherapeutic agents during pregnancy would be contraindicated. Similar to findings with other drugs in pregnancy, the highest risk for cytotoxic drug use is in the first trimester, with the risk of congenital malformations estimated to be 10%. This is especially true of the antimetabolite class of drugs. There is, however, a mounting body of evidence to suggest that the use of antineoplastic agents in the second and third trimesters of pregnancy is relatively safe. The largest reviews are published by Wiebe (1994), Doll (1988), Schapira and Chudley (1984), and Nicholson (1968). Because organogenesis occurs during the first trimester, administration of chemotherapy in the second and third trimesters should not produce fetal malformations as evidenced in the published literature. However, when chemotherapeutic agents are given in the second and third trimesters, low birth weight, intrauterine growth restriction, spontaneous abortion, and premature birth may be more likely. In addition, even without treatment, the underlying disease being treated could produce these effects on the pregnancy.

A woman presenting with a malignancy and a concomitant pregnancy presents physicians with a therapeutic dilemma. Although it is well established that cytotoxic drugs and/or irradiation during pregnancy may be detrimental to the fetus, delay or modification of cancer therapy may adversely affect maternal prognosis. Therefore, optimal treatment of a woman with malignancy and concurrent pregnancy requires an interdisciplinary approach to balance the effects of therapy and delivery on the maternal and fetal conditions. The multidisciplinary medical team should include perinatology, neonatology, gynecologic oncology, medical oncology, radiation oncology, nursing, and social services, as well as the patient and her family. The decision to initiate therapy is therefore a difficult one for all concerned and may be complicated by heightened emotions, ethical issues, and religious beliefs. Parents need to participate in the decision making process and need adequate information on which to base their decisions. It must be remembered that there are rarely right and wrong decisions in such a situation and ambivalence will inevitably accompany any choice. When chemotherapy is administered during pregnancy, delivery of the infant should be timed to avoid the chemotherapy nadir and its associated problems (e.g., bleeding disorders, infections).

This appendix is designed to provide information that may be helpful in making these management decisions. Although a comprehensive review of this subject is beyond the scope of this book, the most relevant body of knowledge and selected bibliography should be helpful to the reader.

RECOMMENDED READING

Beeley, L. Adverse effects of drugs in the first trimester of pregnancy. *Clin. Obstet. Gynaecol.* 13:177, 1986.

Caligiuri, M.A., and Mayer, R.J. Pregnancy and leukemia. *Semin. Oncol.* 16:388, 1989.

Catanzarite, V.A., and Ferguson, J.E. Acute leukemia and pregnancy. A review of management and outcome. *Obstet. Gynecol. Surv.* 39:663, 1981.

Doll, D.C., Ringenberg, Q.S., and Yarbro, J.W. Management of cancer during pregnancy. *Arch. Intern. Med.* 148:2058, 1988.

Fiorica, J.V. Special problems. Breast cancer and pregnancy. *Obstet. Gynecol. Clin. North Am.* 21(4):721, 1994.

Gershenson, D.M. Pregnancy in cancer survivors. *Curr. Obstet. Med.* 3:1, 1995.

Hoskins, W.J., Perez, C.A., and Young, R.C. *Principles and Practice of Gynecologic Oncology* (2nd ed.). Philadelphia: Lippincott-Raven Publishers, 1997.

Kawamura, S., Yoshiike, M., Shimoyama, T., Suzuki, Y., Itoh, J., Yamagata, K., Fukushima, K., Ogasawara, H., Saitoh, S., Tsushima, K., et al. Management of acute leukemia during pregnancy: from the results of a nationwide questionnaire survey and literature survey. *Tohoku J. Exp. Med.* 174(2):167, 1994.

Kim, W.Y., Webbe, T.W., and Akerley, W. A woman with a balanced autosomal translocation who received chemotherapy while pregnant. *Medicine and Health* / RI 79:396, 1996.

Nicholson, H.O. Cytotoxic drugs in pregnancy. *J. Obstet. Gynecol.* 75:307, 1968.

Perry, M.S., ed. *The Chemotherapy Source Book*. Baltimore: Williams and Wilkins, 1992.

Reichman, B.S., and Green, K.B. Breast cancer in young women: effect of chemotherapy on ovarian function, fertility, and birth defects. *Monogr. N.C.I.* 16:125, 1994.

Schapira, D.V., Chudley, A.E. Successful pregnancy following continuous treatment with combination chemotherapy before conception and throughout pregnancy. *Cancer* 54:800, 1984.

Sutcliffe, S.B. Treatment of neoplastic disease during pregnancy: maternal and fetal effects. *Clin. Invest. Med.* 8:333, 1985.

Wiebe, V.J., and Sipila, P.E. Pharmacology of antineoplastic agents in pregnancy. *Crit. Rev. Oncol. Hematol.* 16(2):75, 1994.

Zemlickis, D., Lishner, M., Degendorfer, P., Panzarella, T., Sutcliffe, S.B., and Koren, G. Fetal outcome after in utero exposure to cancer chemotherapy. *Arch. Intern. Med.* 152:573, 1992.

Altretamine (Hexalen®, hexamethylmelamine)

Altretamine is a synthetic *S*-triazine derivative with FDA approval for the treatment of persistent or recurrent ovarian carcinoma. The drug also exhibits antitumor activity against breast cancer, lymphoma, small cell carcinoma of the lung, endometrial and cervical carcinoma. The mechanism of action of altretamine is not completely understood. Although it bears structural similarity to, and cross-reactivity with, trimethylene melamine, a classic alkylating agent, evidence demonstrating altretamine as an alkylating agent is inconclusive. However, the clinical antitumor spectrum resembles that of an alkylating agent. It is believed that in the presence of liver enzymes the parent compound is demethylated and that the reactive intermediate and demethylated metabolites are the more cytotoxic compounds.

The drug is administered orally, is metabolized in the liver, and 90% of the metabolites can be recovered in the urine. The major side effects and toxicities include gastrointestinal disturbances, mild to moderate myelosuppression including granulocytopenia and thrombocytopenia, as well as a form of reversible peripheral neurotoxicity.

There are no known reports on the use of altretamine in pregnancy.

RECOMMENDED READING

Hoskins, W.J., Perez, C.A., and Young, R.C. *Principles and Practice of Gynecologic Oncology* (2nd ed.). Philadelphia: Lippincott-Raven Publishers, 1997.

Perry, M.S., ed. *The Chemotherapy Source Book*. Baltimore: Williams and Wilkins, 1992.

Bleomycin (Blenoxane®)

Bleomycin is a mixture of complex glycopeptides originally isolated from the fungus *Streptomyces verticillis*. The family of bleomycin glycopeptides have a relatively high molecular weight (about 1500) and are quantitated in units of cytotoxic activity (i.e., roughly 1 unit/mg polypeptide protein). Bleomycin is used in patients with advanced cervical and vulvar cancers as well as germ cell tumors of the ovary and testes. This agent also is active in the treatment of malignant pleural effusion associated with breast and ovarian carcinomas. Bleomycin becomes an active antitumor agent when complexed with ferrous iron, producing a potent oxidase. The molecule produces DNA strand breaks by oxygen free radicals. This unique mechanism of action is schedule-dependent and cell cycle–dependent for the G2 phase.

Bleomycin is eliminated predominately by renal excretion with more than 95% of the dose completely eliminated within 24 hours. Therefore, in patients with severe renal insufficiency the bleomycin dose should be reduced. The dose-limiting side effect of bleomycin is pulmonary toxicity, which occurs in approximately 10% of treated patients. Bleomycin-induced lung damage presents as pneumonitis with dry cough, dyspnea, rales, and may progress within weeks to pulmonary fibrosis. Bleomycin is nonmyelosuppressive. The primary acute side effects are mucocutaneous toxicities including mucositis. Fever, chills, and alopecia are common.

Although no direct data showing adverse effects from the use of this drug in pregnancy are available, it has been used as part of multiagent chemotherapy with good outcomes.

RECOMMENDED READING

Doll, D.C., Ringenberg, Q.S., and Yarbro, J.W. Management of cancer during pregnancy. *Arch. Intern. Med.* 148:2058, 1988.

Haerr, R.W., and Pratt, A.T. Multiagent chemotherapy for sarcoma diagnosed during pregnancy. *Cancer* 56:1028, 1985.

Hoskins, W.J., Perez, C.A., and Young, R.C. *Principles and Practice of Gynecologic Oncology* (2nd ed.). Philadelphia: Lippincott-Raven Publishers, 1997.

Nantel, S., Parboosingh, J., and Poon, M.C. Treatment of non-Hodgkin's lymphoma during pregnancy with MACOP-B chemotherapy. *Med. Pediatr. Oncol.* 18:143, 1990.

Rodriguez, J.M., and Haggag, M. VACOP-B chemotherapy for high grade non-Hodgkin's lymphoma in pregnancy. *Clin. Oncol.* 7(5): 319, 1995.

Wiebe, V.J., and Sipila, P.E.H. Pharmacology of antineoplastic agents in pregnancy. *Critical Reviews in Oncology/Hematology* 16: 75, 1994.

Busulfan (Myleran®)

Busulfan, an alkyl sulfate alkylating agent used in the treatment of chronic granulocytic leukemia, polycythemia vera, and primary thrombocytosis, acts by myelosuppression. At low dosages, selective depression of granulocyte and platelet production occurs. At high dosages, erythrocyte production is affected, and ultimately, pancytopenia may occur. Major toxic effects are related to both granulocytopenia and thrombocytopenia. Elevated urate levels can also occur, and patients are usually treated concomitantly with allopurinol. Nausea, vomiting, diarrhea, impotence, sterility, and amenorrhea have all been reported as occasional side effects. Rarely, generalized skin pigmentation, gynecomastia, cheilosis, glossitis, anhidrosis, and pulmonary fibrosis have occurred. The drug is extremely effective, inducing remission in 85% to 90% of patients with chronic granulocytic leukemia.

In animal studies, cleft palate, digital defects, eye defects, growth retardation, ovarian dysgenesis, and destruction of seminiferous tubules in male fetuses exposed to busulfan have been reported. Reports on nonpregnant laboratory animals and humans receiving busulfan have shown chromosomal changes in lymphocytes and bone marrow cells.

Human case reports are, as with most antineoplastic drugs, problematic because many patients were treated with multiple drug regimens. Literature reviews have turned up reports of 24 women treated with busulfan during the first trimester. Four of the offspring manifested congenital abnormalities, including multiple malformations, cleft palate, ocular defects, and liver anomalies, and one child had mosaic trisomy 21. Among patients treated after the first trimester of pregnancy, intrauterine growth restriction was common. Because the reported birth defects occur with use in the first trimester, there is no evidence to conclude that busulfan cannot be used safely later in pregnancy.

RECOMMENDED READING

Bhisey, A.N., Advani, S.H., and Khare, G. Cytogenetic anomalies in a child born to a mother receiving busulfan for chronic myeloid leukemia. *Ind. J. Cancer* 19:272, 1982.

Diamond, I., Anderson, M.M., and McCreadie, S.R. Transplacental passage of busulfan (Myleran) in a mother with leukemia. *Pediatrics* 25:85, 1960.

Doll, D.C., Ringenberg, Q.S., and Yarbro, J.W. Management of cancer during pregnancy. *Arch. Intern. Med.* 148:2058, 1988.

Glantz, J.C. Reproductive toxicology of alkylating agents. *Obstet. Gynecol. Surv.* 49:709, 1994.

Johnson, F.D. Pregnancy and concurrent chronic myelogenous leukemia. *Am. J. Obstet. Gynecol.* 112:640, 1972.

Nicholson, H.O. Cytotoxic drugs in pregnancy: Review of reported cases. *J. Obstet. Gynaecol. Br. Commonw.* 75:307, 1968.

Norhaya, M.R., Cheong, S.K., Hamidah, N.H., and Ainoon, O. Pregnancy in a patient receiving busulphan for chronic myeloid leukaemia. *Singapore Med. J.* 35:102, 1994.

Sokal. J.E., and Lesserman, E.M. Effects of cancer chemotherapy on the human fetus. *J.A.M.A.* 172:1765, 1960.

Sweet, D.L., and Kinzie, J. Consequences of radiotherapy and antineoplastic therapy for the fetus. *J. Reprod. Med.* 17:241, 1976.

Wiebe, V.J., and Sipila, P.E. Pharmacology of antineoplastic agents in pregnancy. *Crit. Rev. Oncol. Hematol.* 16:75, 1994.

Carboplatin (Paraplatin®)

Carboplatin is the first analog of cisplatin to become commercially available. It has demonstrated comparable activity to that of cisplatin. It is used in the treatment of advanced ovarian carcinoma as well as metastatic endometrial carcinoma, cervical carcinoma, and small cell carcinoma of the lung. There are also data suggesting activity in head and neck cancer, genitourinary cancers, and in certain pediatric brain tumors, specifically megaloblastoma.

Carboplatin and cisplatin share the same mechanism of action. Carboplatin binds to DNA, crosslinking the DNA and resulting in non–cell cycle–dependent cytotoxicity. Carboplatin is usually administered intravenously with short infusion times and is cleared by the kidneys through glomerular filtration. There is a significantly decreased risk of renal toxicity due to carboplatin in comparison to cisplatin; however, decreased renal function increases the risk of myelosuppression, which is the dose-limiting toxicity of carboplatin. The greatest myelosuppression is seen in platelet counts; however, granulocytopenia does occur. Nausea and vomiting are minimal with carboplatin and usually occur within 12 hours of administration. Peripheral neuropathy and ototoxicity are generally reported only by patients who have experienced these toxicities during prior cisplatin therapy, not with primary treatment.

One case report is found describing the use of carboplatin during pregnancy. In this case, carboplatin was given at 30 weeks gestation after two cycles of cisplatin for advanced ovarian cancer. Cisplatin was discontinued due to maternal ototoxicity. The infant, delivered at 36 weeks gestation, was normal at delivery and at 12 months of age.

RECOMMENDED READING

Canetta, R., Goodlow, J., Smaidone, L., Grogman, K., and Rozencweig, M. Pharmacologic characteristics of carboplatin: clinical experience in carboplatin in *Carboplatin, Current Perspectives and Future Directions.* P.A. Bunn, R. Canetta, R.F. Ozols, and M. Rozencweig, eds. Philadelphia: W.B. Saunders, 1990. Pp. 19–38.

Henderson, C.E., Elia, G., Garfinkel, D., Poirier, M.C., Shamkhani, H., and Runowicz, C.D. Platinum chemotherapy during pregnancy for serous cystadenocarcinoma of the ovary. *Gynecol. Oncol.* 49:92, 1993.

Hoskins, W.J., Perez, C.A., Young, R.C. *Principles and Practice of Gynecologic Oncology* (2nd ed.). Philadelphia: Lippincott-Raven Publishers, 1997.

Cisplatin (Platinol®)

Cisplatin has proven to be one of the most active antineoplastic agents in clinical use, with a broad spectrum of antitumor activity especially in gynecologic malignancies. Cisplatin is a prime drug in the treatment of advanced cancer of the ovary, cervix, endometrium, and vulva. The wide range of activity includes other genitourinary tumors, especially testicular carcinoma, bladder cancer, as well as lung cancer, osteogenic sarcoma, and many other malignancies. The mechanism of action of cisplatin is essentially that of an alkylating agent. The cisplatin binds directly to DNA, producing intrastructural crosslinks, and thereby inhibiting DNA synthesis. The activity is not cell cycle–dependent.

Cisplatin can be administered either intravenously or peritoneally. The predominant route of clearance of the drug (90%) is through the kidneys.

Dose-related nephrotoxicity is the major dose-limiting side effect of cisplatin. Adequate hydration and high urinary outputs can dramatically reduce the risk of nephrotoxicity. Other common side effects include nausea and vomiting that can be prolonged and/or delayed, ototoxicity manifested by high-frequency hearing loss, and peripheral neuropathies. This neurotoxicity is dose-dependent, usually seen with cumulative doses exceeding 300 mg/m², and may be irreversible. Myelosuppression infrequently occurs with standard doses.

Among males receiving cisplatin for testicular cancer, almost all become aspermic within the first two cycles of therapy, but recovery of normal sperm morphology, motility, and sperm counts occurs in 40% within 2 years. More than one-third of testicular cancer patients who received cisplatin therapy and desired to father children have successfully done so. Cisplatin is teratogenic in a number of animal species. These effects seem to occur early when the drug is given in pregnancy.

It is likely that the human fetus does sustain platinum drug exposure during pregnancy as cisplatin-DNA adducts have been demonstrated in fetal and maternal tissues in pregnant Patus monkeys and in an 8-week aborted fetus after three weekly cisplatin doses.

Experience with cisplatin in pregnancy is limited; however, there are increasing numbers of case reports of women treated during the second and third trimester of pregnancy with good outcomes. There are conflicting reports regarding the detection of cisplatin in human breast milk at the time of treatment.

RECOMMENDED READING

Ben-Baruch, G., Menczer, J., Goshen, R., Kaufman, B., Gorodetsky, R. Cisplatin excretion in human milk (letter). *J.N.C.I.* 84:451, 1992.

Bermas, B.L., Hill, J.A. Effects of immunosuppressive drugs during pregnancy, Arthritis & Rheum. 38:1722–32, 1995.

Christman, J.E., Teng, N.H., Leboric, G.S., et al. Delivery of a normal infant following cisplatin, vinblastine and bleomycin (PVB) chemotherapy for malignant teratoma of the ovary during pregnancy. *Gynecol. Oncol.* 37:292, 1990.

Diwan, B.A., Anderson, L.M., Ward, J.M., Henneman, J.R., and Rice, J.M. Transplacental carcinogenesis by cisplatin in F344/NCr rates: promotion of kidney tumors by postnatal administration of sodium barbital. *Toxicol. Appl. Pharmacol.* 132:115, 1995.

Egan, P.C., Costanza, M., Dadion, P., Egorin, M.J., and Bachur, N.R. Doxirubicin and cisplatin excretion into human milk. *Cancer Treat. Rep.* 69:1387, 1985.

Giacalone, P.L., Laffargue, F., Benos, P., Rousseau, O., and Hedon, B. Cis-platinum neoadjuvant chemotherapy in a pregnant woman with invasive carcinoma of the uterine cervix. *Br. J. Obstet. Gynaecol.* 103:932, 1996.

Giurgiovich, A.J., Diwan, B.A., Lee, K.B., Anderson, L.M., Rice, J.M., and Poirier, M.C. Cisplatin-DNA adduct formation in maternal and fetal rat tissues after transplacental cisplatin exposure. *Carcinogenesis* 17:1665, 1996.

Jacobs, A.J., et al. Oat cell carcinoma of the uterine cervix in a pregnant woman treated with cis-diamminedichloroplatinum. *Gynecol. Oncol.* 9:405, 1980.

Kiely, J.M. Clinical pharmacology (series on pharmacology in practice). 12. Antineoplastic agents. *Mayo Clin. Proc.* 56:384, 1981.

King, L.A., Nevin, P.C. Williams, P.P., and Carson L.F. Treatment of advanced epithelial ovarian carcinoma in pregnancy with cisplatin-based chemo. *Gynecol. Oncol.* 41:78, 1991.

Malfetano, J.H., and Goldkrand, J.W. Cis-platinum combination chemotherapy during pregnancy for advanced epithelial ovarian carcinoma. *Obstet. Gynecol.* 75:545, 1990.

Wiebe, V.J., and Sipila, P.E. Pharmacology of antineoplastic agents in pregnancy. *Crit. Rev. Oncol. Hematol.* 16:75, 1994.

Zemlickis, D., Klein, J., Moselhy, G., and Koren, G. Cisplatin protein binding in pregnancy and the neonatal period. *Med. Pediatr. Oncol.* 23:476, 1994.

Cyclophosphamide (Cytoxan®)

Cyclophosphamide is an alkylating agent, a nitrogen mustard derivative, that is one of the most commonly used antineoplastic preparations. It is most often part of multidrug combination therapy. Its spectrum of activity includes indolent lymphoma, intermediate and aggressive non-Hodgkin's lymphoma, small cell lung cancer, neuroblastoma, acute lymphoblastic leukemia in adults and children, Ewing's sarcoma, and breast, ovarian, and endometrial carcinoma.

Cyclophosphamide has also been used in the treatment of non-malignant diseases, primarily as an immunosuppressant therapy. It is the primary therapeutic agent in the treatment of Wegener's granulomatosis. There are also applications in rheumatic diseases including rheumatoid arthritis, polyarteritis nodosa, systemic necrotizing vasculitis, systemic lupus erythematosus, and other connective tissue disease. However, in each instance, the potential complications, including infections, risk of second malignancy, alopecia, hemorrhagic cystitis, and infertility, may outweigh the benefits of therapy.

Cyclophosphamide must be activated by the hepatic microsomal enzyme system to yield a direct cytotoxic metabolite. These active metabolites then cause interstrand DNA crosslinks and inhibit DNA replication. Myelosuppression, consisting primarily of leukopenia, is the usual dose-limiting toxic effect of cyclophosphamide. Significant thrombocytopenia can also occur at very high doses (more than 1.5 g/m^2). Acute sterile hemorrhagic cystitis is uncommon but occasionally can be dose limiting. Nausea and vomiting are common reactions but well controlled with antiemetic regimens. Alopecia, syndrome of inappropriate antidiuretic hormone (SIADH), interstitial pneumonitis, and pulmonary fibrosis, as well as gonadal failure in both men and women are other uncommon side effects. Second malignancies including bladder cancer, lymphoma, and leukemia have developed secondary to cyclophosphamide use.

As with all alkylating agents, drug-induced congenital abnormalities are possible. Cyclophosphamide is teratogenic in a number of animal models including mice, rats, and rabbits. In the literature, there were congenital abnormalities found in three of seven fetuses exposed during the first trimester of pregnancy. Analysis of most reported exposures are complicated by the multiple drugs or by concurrent use of cyclophosphamide with radiation. Exposure in the second or third trimester appears to be relatively benign, with the exception of possible intrauterine growth restriction. Cyclophosphamide has been demonstrated to cross the placenta and appear in amniotic fluid at term.

Cyclophosphamide has been shown to be present within human breast milk as evidenced by reversible leukopenia and thrombocytopenia in nursing infants.

RECOMMENDED READING

Amato, D., and Niblatt, J.S., Neutropenia from cyclophosphamide in breast milk. *Med. J. Aust.* 1: 383, 1997.

Blatt, J., Mulvihill, J.J., Ziegler, J.L., et al. Pregnancy outcome following cancer chemotherapy. *Am. J. Med.* 69:828, 1980.

Coates A. Cyclophosphamide in pregnancy. *Aust. N.Z. J. Obstet. Gynaecol.* 10:33, 1970.

D'Incalci, M., et al. Transplacental passage of cyclophosphamide. *Cancer Treat. Rep.* 66:1681, 1982.

Durodola, J.I. Administration of cyclophosphamide during late pregnancy and early lactation: a case report. *J. Natl. Med. Assoc.* 71:165, 1979.

Glantz, J.C. Reproductive toxicology of alkylating agents. *Obstet. Gynecol. Surv.* 49:709, 1994.

Greenberg, L.H., and Tanaka, K.R. Congenital anomalies probably induced by cyclophosphamide. *J.A.M.A.* 188:123, 1964.

Murray, C.L., et al. Multimodal cancer therapy for breast cancer in the first trimester of pregnancy. *J.A.M.A.* 252:2607, 1984.

Reichman, B.S., and Green, K.B. Breast cancer in young women: effect of chemotherapy on ovarian function, fertility, and birth defects. *Monogr. N.C.I.* 16:125, 1994.

Wiebe, V.J., and Sipila, P.E. Pharmacology of antineoplastic agents in pregnancy. *Crit. Rev. Oncol. Hematol.* 16:75, 1994.

Wiernik, P.H., and Duncan, J.H., Cyclophosphamide in human milk (letter). *Lancet* 1:912, 1971.

Cytosine Arabinoside (Cytarabine, Ara-C, Cytosar-U®)

Ara-C, an antimetabolite, is a pyrimidine analog believed to act by blocking nucleic acid polymerases, and possibly by incorporation into DNA and RNA. It is commonly used, either alone or in combination with other agents, to induce remission in acute leukemias. It also may be beneficial in Hodgkin's disease and other lymphomas. Toxic effects include myelosuppression, with leukopenia, thrombocytopenia, and anemia. Gastrointestinal disturbances, stomatitis, hepatic dysfunction, thrombophlebitis at injection sites, fever, and dermatitis have also been reported.

Animal studies have demonstrated the induction of facial clefts, skeletal defects, central nervous system anomalies, ear atresia, limb reduction defects, and renal changes with the administration of cytarabine during pregnancy.

Information about the effects of ara-c on the developing human fetus is limited to case reports. At least 12 cases with first-trimester exposure have been described, with 3 anomalous fetuses (1 with a trisomy, 1 with ear and limb anomalies, 1 with limb reduction defects) and 9 apparently normal conceptuses resulting. An additional 17 fetuses exposed in only the second and/or third trimester have been reported. Two of these pregnancies ended with fetal demise, another resulted in a trisomic abortus, and at least 4 delivered prematurely. The remaining 10 resulted in reportedly normal offspring. Most of these exposures during pregnancy were not to ara-c alone but to combinations of chemotherapeutic agents. In some cases, four or more different drugs were used.

Interestingly, two males taking this drug sired anomalous offspring, one with anencephaly and another with tetralogy of Fallot and syndactyly.

RECOMMENDED READING

Blatt, J., et al. Pregnancy outcome following cancer chemotherapy. *Am J. Med.* 69:828, 1980.

Caligiuri, M.A., and Mayer, R.J. Pregnancy and leukemia. *Semin. Oncol.* 16:388, 1989.

Gililland, J., and Weinstein, L. The effects of cancer chemotherapeutic agents on the developing fetus. *Obstet. Gynecol. Surv.* 38:6, 1983.

Krueger, J.A., Davis, R.B., and Field, C. Multiple-drug chemotherapy in the management of acute lymphocytic leukemia during pregnancy. *Obstet. Gynecol.* 48:324, 1976.

Manoharan, A., and Leyden, M.J. Acute non-lymphocytic leukaemia in the third trimester of pregnancy. *Aust. N.Z. J. Med.* 9:71, 1979.

Morgenstern, G. Cytarabine in pregnancy. Lancet 2:259, 1980.

Morishita, S., Imai, A., Kawabata, I., and Tamaya, T. Acute myelogenous leukemia in pregnancy: fetal blood sampling and early effects of chemotherapy. *Int. J. Gynaecol. Obstet.* 44:273, 1994.

Newcomb, M., et al. Acute leukemia in pregnancy: successful delivery after cytarabine and doxorubicin. *J.A.M.A.* 239:2691, 1978.

Nicholson, H.O. Cytotoxic drugs in pregnancy: review of reported cases. *J. Obstet. Gynecol. Br. Commw.* 75:307, 1968

Pawliger, D.F., McLean, F.W., and Noyes, W.D. Normal fetus after cytosine arabinoside therapy. *Ann. Intern. Med,* 74:1012, 1971.

Wagner, V.M., et al. Congenital abnormalities in baby born to cytarabine treated mother. *Lancet* 2:98, 1980.

Wiebe, V.J., and Sipila, P.E. Pharmacology of antineoplastic agents in pregnancy. *Crit. Rev. Oncol. Hematol.* 16:75, 1994.

Dactinomycin
(Actinomycin D, Cosmegen®)

Dactinomycin is an antitumor antibiotic isolated from *Streptomyces v. parvullus*. Present clinical indications for dactinomycin include childhood tumors, gestational trophoblastic neoplasms, germ cell tumors of the ovary, and testicular cancer. The childhood tumors for which good activity is described include Wilms' tumor, Ewing's sarcoma, and embryonal rhabdomyosarcoma.

Toxicities include severe bone marrow suppression, primarily leukopenia. Nausea, vomiting, alopecia, and mucositis are common. Hepatic function can be compromised with long-term therapy. All of these side effects are enhanced by concurrent radiation therapy. In addition, the phenomenon of radiation-recall dermatitis, consisting of cutaneous pain, erythema, blistering, or ulceration occurring in a previous radiation field within 3–7 days after treatment with an antitumor antibiotic, may occur. This phenomenon was first described in patients who received dactinomycin.

The mechanism of action is believed to be intercalation between DNA base pairs, thus resulting in inhibition of RNA and protein synthesis.

Because dactinomycin is extremely successful in the treatment of trophoblastic neoplasms, it would be expected to be quite dangerous when administered during pregnancy. Two case reports describe apparently normal offspring when dactinomycin was initiated in the second or third trimester. There are numerous descriptions of successful pregnancies subsequent to dactinomycin treatment.

RECOMMENDED READING

Rustin, G.J.S., et al. Pregnancy after cytotoxic chemotherapy for gestational trophoblastic tumours. *Br. Med. J.* 288:103, 1984.

Sweet, D.L., and Kinzie, J. Consequences of radiotherapy and antineoplastic therapy for the fetus. *J. Reprod. Med.* 17:241, 1976.

Weed, J.C., Roh, R.A., and Mendenhall, H.W. Recurrent endodermal sinus tumor during pregnancy. *Obstet. Gynecol.* 54:653, 1979.

Doxorubicin (Adriamycin®) and Daunorubicin (Cerubidine®)

Doxorubicin and daunorubicin are anthracycline antibiotics that are active in several types of cancers in women. Doxorubicin is the most commonly prescribed agent of the antitumor antibiotics.

Doxorubicin has a very broad spectrum of anticancer activity. In addition to the treatment of metastatic endometrial carcinoma, uterine sarcoma, germ cell and epithelial ovarian carcinoma, definite activity has been reported in the treatment of leukemias, Hodgkin's disease, non-Hodgkin's lymphomas, multiple myelomas, sarcomas, as well as carcinoma of the breast, bladder, and lung. It also has demonstrated activity against many other carcinomas. Daunorubicin is used in the treatment of leukemias.

The mechanism of action is not fully known. However, the anthracycline can intercalate among DNA base pairs, inhibiting the template activity of the nucleic acid. These compounds can also act as electron receptors from oxygen, giving rise to superoxide anion radicals that can directly damage DNA, RNA, lipids, and proteins.

The drugs, after short intravenous infusion or intravenous bolus injection, are rapidly distributed in body tissues, and about 75% of drug is bound to plasma proteins, principally albumin. Human tissues with high drug concentrations include liver, lymph nodes, muscle, bone, bone marrow, and skin. Pregnant patients with elevated bilirubin concentrations receiving anthracyclines are therefore at greater risk of anthracycline-induced fetal toxicities. Both are extensively metabolized and eliminated in the bile, feces, and urine. There is significant distribution of doxorubicin into human breast milk, and cumulative AUCs (areas under the concentration–time curve representing the total drug exposure integrated over time) measured in breast milk were greater than concurrent plasma AUC values. Doxorubicin, however, does not appear to consistently pass the placenta. Except for one study reporting low drug levels in placental blood of 0.78–1.19 nmol/g, and no drug in cord blood plasma, several other trials detected no drug in amniotic fluid after doxorubicin administration to pregnant patients.

The single acute dose-limiting toxicity of doxorubicin is bone marrow suppression, most commonly leukopenia. However, anemia and thrombocytopenia can also occur. Doxorubicin is most commonly known for its cardiotoxicity. Acute cardiac effects such as rare pericarditis/myocarditis syndrome or electrophysiologic aberrations occur during or immediately after infusion of the drug. These conduction abnormalities, which include T-wave flattening, ST depression, supraventricular tachyarrhythmias, and extrasystolic contractions, are generally transient. The more serious chronic cumulative dose-related cardiomyopathy results in a clinical syndrome identical to classic congestive heart failure. This cardiomyopathy is usually irreversible. Potential risk factors for cardiotoxicity include cumulative doses higher than 550 mg/m^2 (incidence with less than 500 mg/m^2 is less than 1%), prior mediastinal radiation, preexisting cardiovascular disease, or age greater than 70 years. Other toxic effects include marked alopecia in all hairy body areas. Stomatitis, nausea and vomiting, and hyperpigmentation of skin, especially the nail beds, may occur. The toxicities of daunorubicin are nearly identical to those of doxorubicin, with a lesser incidence of mucositis and lower incidence of colonic damage and perforation.

A variety of case reports have described the successful use of anthracyclines in combination therapy in all trimesters of pregnancy, with minimal fetal risk. The overall risk of teratogenicity appears minimal. A literature search revealed at least 4 cases exposed to doxorubicin during the first trimester and 16 during later pregnancy, with structurally normal fetuses resulting. A fetus exposed to doxorubicin, cyclophosphamide, and cobalt radiation therapy during the first trimester was born with imperforate anus and rectovaginal fistula at term. One anatomically normal fetus died in utero within 36 hours of the initiation of maternal chemotherapy with doxorubicin, vincristine, and prednisone. Twelve case reports of daunorubicin use in pregnancy, with one in first trimester, resulted in normal fetuses. One case of temporary bone marrow hyperplasia was reported, as was one fetal death after delivery for severe preeclampsia at 29 weeks gestation.

The American Academy of Pediatrics classifies doxorubicin, structurally related to mitoxantrone, as contraindicated during breast-feeding due to the potential for immunosuppression and an unknown effect on growth or association with carcinogenesis.

RECOMMENDED READING

Barni, S., Ardizzoia, A., Zanetta, G., Strocchi, E., Lissoni, P., and Tancini, G. Weekly doxorubicin chemotherapy for breast cancer in pregnancy. A case report. *Tumori* 78:349, 1992.

Committee on Drugs, American Academy of Pediatrics. The transfer of drugs and other chemicals into human milk. *Pediatrics* 93:137, 1994.

Doll, D.C., Ringenberg, Q.S., and Yarbro, J.W. Antineoplastic agents and pregnancy. *Semin. Oncol.* 16:337, 1989.

Egan, P.C., Costanza, M., Dadion, P., Egorin, M.J., and Bachur, N.R. Doxirubicin and cisplatin excretion into human milk. *Cancer Treat. Rep.* 69:1387, 1985.

Garcia, V., San Miguel, J., and Borrasca, A.L. Doxorubicin in the first trimester of pregnancy. *Ann. Intern. Med.* 94:547, 1981.

Gililland, J., and Weinstein, L. The effects of cancer chemotherapeutic agents on the developing fetus. *Obstet. Gynecol. Surv.* 38:6, 1983.

Karp, G.I., et al. Doxorubicin in pregnancy: possible transplacental passage. *Cancer Treat. Rep.* 67:773, 1983.

Karp, G.I., von Oeyen, P., Valone, F., et al. Doxorubicin in pregnancy: possible transplacental passage. *Cancer Treat. Rep.* 67: 773, 1983.

Morishita, S., Imai, A., Kawabata, I., and Tamaya, T. Acute myelogenous leukemia in pregnancy: fetal blood sampling and early effects of chemotherapy. *Int. J. Gynaecol. Obstet.* 44:273, 1994.

Murray, C.L., et al. Multimodal cancer therapy for breast cancer in the first trimester of pregnancy: a case report. *J.A.M.A.* 252:2607, 1984.

Roboz, J., et al. Does doxorubicin cross the placenta? *Lancet* 2:1382, 1979.

Thompson, D.J., et al. Teratogenicity of adriamycin and daunomycin in the rat and rabbit. *Teratology* 17:151, 1978.

Tobias, J.S., and Bloom, H.J.G. Doxorubicin in pregnancy. *Lancet* 1:776, 1980.

Turchii, J.J., and Villasu, C. Anthracyclines in the treatment of malignancy in pregnancy. *Cancer* 61:435, 1988.

Wiebe, V.J., and Sipila, P.E. Pharmacology of antineoplastic agents in pregnancy. *Crit. Rev. Oncol. Hematol.* 16:75, 1994.

Etoposide (VP-16, Vepesid®)

Etoposide is a semisynthetic epipodophyllotoxin derived from the root of podophyllum (the may apple plant or mandrake). Etoposide is most commonly used in the intravenous treatment of germ cell tumors of the ovary, refractory testicular carcinomas, and small cell lung carcinomas. It is also extremely active in non-Hodgkin's lymphomas, gestational trophoblastic tumors, and pediatric sarcomas, particularly Ewing's sarcoma.

Etoposide's activity is cell cycle–specific and maximal in the G2 phase. Etoposide produces protein-linked DNA strand breaks by inhibiting DNA topoisomerase II enzymes. Other postulated mechanisms of action include microsomal activation to reactive intermediates capable of generating oxygen free radicals. The drug is highly protein-bound, and renal excretion appears to account for approximately 30% of overall drug elimination.

The principle toxicity of etoposide is bone marrow suppression, predominately leukopenia. Other adverse effects include minor gastrointestinal complaints, nausea and vomiting, alopecia, headache, fever, and hypotension.

One case report of etoposide use in pregnancy for acute myeloid leukemia as part of combination multiagent therapy was found. The patient was treated at 25 weeks gestation. The infant delivered prematurely at 32 weeks gestation and suffered temporarily from anemia and neutropenia.

RECOMMENDED READING

Azuno, Y., Kaku, K., Fujita, N., Okubo, M., Kaneko, T., and Matsumoto, N. Mitoxantrone and etoposide in breast milk. *Am. J. Hematol.* 48:131, 1995.

Hoskins, W.J., Perez, C.A., and Young, R.C. *Principles and Practice of Gynecologic Oncology* (2nd ed.). Philadelphia: Lippincott-Raven Publishers, 1997.

Murray, N.A., Acolet, D., Deane, M., Price, J., and Roberts, I.A. Fetal marrow suppression after maternal chemotherapy for leukaemia. *Arch. Dis. Child. Fetal Neonat. Ed.* 71:209, 1994.

Pui, C.H., Ribeiro, R.C., Hancock, M.L., et al. Acute myeloid leukemia in children treated with epipodophylotoxins for acute lymphoblastic leukemia. *N. Engl. J. Med.* 325:1682, 1991.

5-Fluorouracil
(5-FU, Adrucil®, Efudex®)

5-Fluorouracil is an antimetabolite used for the palliative treatment of a number of solid tumors, including colorectal cancer, breast cancer, and gastric and pancreatic cancers. It appears to be an important component in cisplatin-based treatment of head and neck cancer. It has been used in a neoadjuvant fashion with cisplatin to treat cervical cancers as well as salvage therapy for advanced ovarian cancer. Topical 5-FU is used for the treatment of multiple actinic and solar keratoses as well as for persistent squamous cell dysplasias of the vagina and vulva and superficial basal cell carcinomas.

5-FU acts as a false pyrimidine, or antimetabolite, to ultimately inhibit the formation of the DNA-specific nucleoside base thymidine. 5-FU is cell cycle phase–specific with cytotoxic effects maximal in the S-phase.

Common side effects of systemic administration include stomatitis, esophagitis, and mild nausea and vomiting. Bone marrow suppression involves primarily granulocytopenia and thrombocytopenia. Other side effects include alopecia, dermatitis, photosensitivity, acute cerebellar syndrome, and rare cardiotoxicity. The most common side effect of topical 5-FU is local skin reaction.

5-Fluorouracil is considered to be teratogenic in animals and humans. Experience with this drug in human pregnancies is extremely limited. One case of second-trimester administration resulted in a normal fetus with reversible 5-FU toxicity in the neonate. A second case involved second- and third-trimester exposure along with cisplatin for cervical carcinoma without adverse effects. A third case involved first-trimester exposure along with exposure to 5 rads of radiation. The pregnancy was electively terminated at 16 weeks and the fetus was found to have multiple congenital abnormalities. A karyotype was not obtained in that case. In addition, two patients have been treated with topical 5-FU for human papillomavirus lesions (HPV), subsequently delivering healthy children.

RECOMMENDED READING

Gililland, J., and Weinstein, L. The effects of cancer chemotherapeutic agents on the developing fetus. *Obstet. Gynecol. Surv.* 38:6, 1983.

Stadler, H.E., and Knowles, J. Fluorouracil in pregnancy: Effect on the neonate. *J.A.M.A.* 217:214, 1971.

Stephens, J.D., et al. Multiple congenital anomalies in a fetus exposed to 5-fluorouracil during the first trimester. *Am. J. Obstet. Gynecol.* 136:747, 1980.

Ifosphamide (Ifex®)

Ifosphamide is a metabolically activated alkylating agent. Ifosphamide is commonly used for first-line therapy of advanced cervical cancer, second-line treatment for advanced ovarian carcinoma, testicular carcinoma, and in combination therapy for recurrent or refractory lymphoma. Ifosphamide is also active as a single agent or in combination for soft tissue sarcomas and has activity in other neoplasms such as pancreatic carcinoma, non–small cell lung cancer, and head and neck cancer. Like cyclophosphamide, it must first undergo hydroxylation by microsomal enzyme systems in the liver.

Urinary tract toxicity is a dose-limiting factor with ifosphamide. The clinical hallmark of hemorrhagic cystitis can be prevented with the coadministration of mesna and vigorous intravenous hydration during administration. Mesna is an agent, given concurrently with ifosphamide, that binds to the metabolite acrolein which is felt to be responsible for the hemorrhagic cystitis. The resulting nontoxic molecule is excreted in the urine. Alopecia and nausea and vomiting are common; however, hematologic toxicity is mainly moderate leukopenia. Lethargy and confusion are seen with high doses of ifosphamide as well as reports of seizures, ataxia, stupor, and weakness.

No reports of ifosphamide use in pregnancy could be found.

RECOMMENDED READING

Hoskins, W.J., Perez, C.A., and Young, R.C. *Principles and Practice of Gynecologic Oncology* (2nd ed.). Philadelphia: Lippincott-Raven Publishers, 1997.

Melphalan (Alkeran®)

Melphalan is a phenylalanine derivative of nitrogen mustard and acts as a bifunctional alkylating agent. Combination melphalan and prednisone remains standard therapy for multiple myeloma. Melphalan has also been historically used in the treatment of advanced ovarian cancer. The cytotoxicity appears to be related to the extent of the interstrand crosslinking with tumor cell DNA. Major side effects include bone marrow suppression, infrequent nausea and vomiting, and, rarely, skin rash and pulmonary toxicity. Acute nonlymphocytic leukemia has been reported in patients with multiple myeloma and ovarian cancer after prolonged melphalan therapy.

No specific reference to melphalan use in pregnancy could be found; however, other nitrogen mustard derivatives have been used with normal outcomes. Unilateral renal agenesis has been reported in two cases of chlorambucil use throughout pregnancy. Another case with multidrug therapy, including nitrogen mustard, resulted in abnormalities of both feet, right tibia, and cerebral hemorrhage.

RECOMMENDED READING

Glantz, J.C. Reproductive toxicology of alkylating agents. *Obstet. Gynecol. Surv.* 49:709, 1994.

Hoskins, W.J., Perez, C.A., and Young, R.C. *Principles and Practice of Gynecologic Oncology* (2nd ed.). Philadelphia: Lippincott-Raven Publishers, 1997.

6-Mercaptopurine (Purinethol®)

6-Mercaptopurine is a purine analog chemotherapeutic agent used primarily for the treatment of leukemia. It is administered alone or, more frequently, in combination with other agents in the treatment of acute lymphocytic, acute myeloblastic, and chronic myelogenous leukemias. It is also an immunosuppressive agent and has been used in the treatment of ulcerative colitis. In obstetric patients, it should only be given when a life-threatening condition exists.

The principal toxic effect of 6-mercaptopurine is bone marrow depression, although in general this develops more gradually than with folic acid antagonists. Other side effects include anorexia, nausea, vomiting, stomatitis, and diarrhea. Hyperuricemia is a common finding and can be treated with allopurinol. One-third of the patients develop jaundice, which resolves on discontinuation of therapy. Deaths have been reported from hepatic necrosis. Dermatologic manifestations can also occur.

This drug has severe teratogenic effects in animals. In humans, it is associated with an increased incidence of abortion and prematurity, but the precise risk of teratogenicity in the surviving offspring is not known.

A report by Gililland reviews 34 liveborn infants exposed in utero to 6-mercaptopurine, alone or in combination therapy. In this series, 15 fetuses were exposed in the first trimester and one of the liveborn infants was anomalous. That neonate had also been exposed to busulfan and radiation therapy and was born with bilateral microphthalmia, corneal opacities, and cleft palate. None of the 19 infants exposed after the first trimester had gross malformations. No long-term follow-up data were reported for any of these infants.

Increases in chromosomal aberrations were observed in peripheral lymphocytes of most of 14 nonpregnant patients with leukemia treated with 6-mercaptopurine in cumulative doses of between 0.2 and 1.1 g.

RECOMMENDED READING

Gililland, J., and Weinstein, L. The effects of cancer chemotherapeutic agents on the developing fetus. *Obstet. Gynecol. Surv.* 38:6, 1983.

Morishita, S., Imai, A., Kawabata, I., and Tamaya, T. Acute myelogenous leukemia in pregnancy: fetal blood sampling and early effects of chemotherapy. *Int. J. Gynaecol. Obstet.* 44:273, 1994.

Sokal, J.E., and Lesserman, E.M. Effects of cancer chemotherapy on the human fetus. *J.A.M.A.* 172:1765, 1960.

Methotrexate (Folex®)

Methotrexate is the most widely used antimetabolite in cancer chemotherapy. It is active in the first-line treatment of gestational trophoblastic disease, metastatic squamous cell carcinoma of the cervix as well as acute lymphoblastic leukemia, osteogenic sarcoma, non-Hodgkin's lymphoma, breast cancer, and squamous cell carcinoma of the head and neck. Nononcologic uses for methotrexate include management of psoriasis and severe rheumatoid arthritis. Most recently, methotrexate has become the primary agent used in the medical management of ectopic pregnancies.

Methotrexate is a folic acid antagonist that acts by inhibiting dehydrofolate reductase. This interferes with cellular DNA synthesis and cell division.

Methotrexate is widely distributed to body tissues and, in conventional doses, is excreted unchanged in the urine. Hematologic effects of methotrexate include leukopenia, thrombocytopenia, and anemia. Nausea, vomiting, and anorexia along with gingivitis, pharyngitis, stomatitis, and mucositis in the gastrointestinal tract may occur. Hepatotoxicity is most common in patients receiving high- dose therapy. Renal failure may occur in patients receiving methotrexate, especially in high doses. Other less common side effects include rashes, photosensitivity, alopecia, and blurred vision.

Use of folic acid antagonists during the first trimester results in craniofacial malformations in 20% to 30% of live births. Other abnormalities reported include tetralogy of Fallot, multiple hemangiomas, eczema, strabismus, and multiple congenital malformations. No anomalies have been reported when methotrexate was used after the first trimester but a significantly higher incidence of prematurity has been noted, as have been reports of pancytopenia, septicemia, and gastroenteritis. In most cases, multiple chemotherapeutic drugs were administered. No increased risk of congenital abnormalities has been noted in offspring of women exposed to methotrexate prior to pregnancy.

Because the drug is highly active against trophoblastic disease and has been associated with spontaneous abortion, fetal death, and congenital abnormalities when used in early pregnancy, it should only be used in obstetric patients who have a life-threatening condition for which it is the agent of choice.

RECOMMENDED READING

Baker, H. Some hazards of methotrexate treatment of psoriasis. *Trans. St. John's Hosp. Dermatol. Soc.* 56:111, 1970.

Doll, D.C., Ringenberg, Q.S., and Yarbro, J.W. Antineoplastic agents and pregnancy. *Semin. Oncol.* 16:337, 1989.

Feldkamp, M., and Carey, J.C. Clinical teratology counseling and consultation case report: low dose methotrexate exposure in the early weeks of pregnancy. *Teratology* 47:533, 1993.

Jolivet, J., et al. The pharmacology and clinical use of methotrexate. *N. Engl. J. Med.* 309:1094, 1983.

Pessy, W.H. Methotrexate and teratogenesis. *Arch. Dermatol.* 119:874, 1983.

Schottenfeld, D. Cancer risks of medical treatment. *CA* 32:258, 1982.

Mitomycin C (Mutamycin®)

The mitomycins are a family of antibiotics isolated from *Streptomyces caespitosus*. The drug has proven useful in first-line therapy of advanced cervical carcinoma, superficial bladder carcinoma, and as part of combination therapy for anal squamous cell carcinoma. It is also used for palliative treatment in recurrent ovarian, colon, breast, head and neck, and lung cancers.

The toxicities of mitomycin are substantial and unpredictable; most commonly delayed myelosuppression, especially leukopenia and thrombocytopenia, does occur. Bone marrow suppression is cumulative. Delayed nausea and vomiting and prolonged anorexia are common. The primary biochemical mechanism of action appears to be alkylation of DNA, producing crosslinking and DNA adduct formation halting DNA synthesis.

There are no reported cases of use of mitomycin during pregnancy.

RECOMMENDED READING

Hoskins, W.J., Perez, C.A., Young, R.C. Principles and Practice of Gynecologic Oncology (2nd ed.). Philadelphia: Lippincott-Raven Publishers, 1997.

Perry, M.S., ed. *The Chemotherapy Source Book*. Baltimore: Williams and Wilkins, 1992.

Mitoxantrone (Novantrone®)

Mitoxantrone is in the class of antitumor antibiotics and is approved for use in acute lymphocytic leukemia, acute nonlymphocytic leukemia, non-Hodgkin's lymphoma, and advanced ovarian carcinoma. It is also used in multiple leukemias, lymphomas, and solid tumors with palliative intent.

Mitoxantrone is believed to function by interacting with DNA via intercalation into the DNA helix. It has also been shown to inhibit the activity of enzyme DNA topoisomerase II, which leads to protein-associated double-strand breaks. Mitoxantrone is highly protein-bound and highest concentrations of the drug are found in the liver, pancreas, thyroid, spleen, heart, and bone marrow. Large amounts of the drug (up to 15% of the administered dose) may be retained in these organs for prolonged periods.

The dose-limiting side effect of mitoxantrone is myelosuppression, which can be manifested by pancytopenia but commonly involves only leukopenia. The most frequent reported acute toxicities are nausea, vomiting, and stomatitis, although fortunately these effects are usually mild. One major long-term dose-limiting side effect is cardiac toxicity, which ranges from electrocardiographic changes to severe congestive heart failure. This is typically associated with high cumulative doses of the drug.

Mitoxantrone administration to pregnant rats produced decreased fetal weight and retarded development of the fetal kidney. Although not teratogenic in rabbits, use of the drug was associated with an increased incidence of premature delivery. There are two case reports on the use of mitozantrone in human pregnancy, both during the second trimester. In the first report, a 26-year-old woman was treated for acute myeloblastic leukemia beginning at 20 weeks gestation initially with cytarabine and daunorubicin. After disease progression at 23 weeks, a second course with mitoxantrone and cytarabine induced complete remission. At approximately 28 weeks gestation, with normal fetal growth documented by weekly ultrasound, consolidation treatment with idarubicin and cytarabine was begun. The woman delivered a 2200- g stillborn infant. No apparent congenital malformations were observed; however, the author speculated that fetal death was secondary to the use of idarubicin.

In the second case, a 28-year-old woman with acute promyelocytic leukemia was treated with cytarabine, daunoribicin, and 6-mercaptopurine at 24 weeks gestation. Consolidation therapy with cytarabine and mitoxantrone preceded a cesarean section at 34 weeks gestation with delivery of a healthy 2960-g female infant now alive and well at 16 months of age.

Mitoxantrone is excreted in human breast milk. The woman in the second case noted above, after delivery, continued consolidation therapy with mitoxantrone, etoposide, and enocitabine (converted in vivo to cytarabine). She breast-fed her infant 21 days after drug administration against her physician's advisement and when mitoxantrone levels measured in the breast milk were still high (greater than 18 ng/ml). Again, the infant was doing well at 16 months of age. Although no adverse effects were observed in the above infant, the long term consequences of such exposure are unknown. Because of the long elimination time and the uncertainty over the potential toxicity, women who have been treated with this agent should not breast-feed.

RECOMMENDED READING

Azuno, Y., Keku, K., Fujita, N., Okubo, M, Kameko, T., and Matsumoto, N. Mitoxantrone and etoposide in breast milk. *Am. J. Hematol.* 48:131, 1995.

Product information. Novantrone. Immunex, 1996.

Paclitaxel (Taxol®)

Paclitaxel is an extremely important new drug used in the primary treatment for epithelial ovarian cancer and recurrent cancer of the breast, uterus, and other solid tumors. Paclitaxel is a diterpene plant product derived from the bark of the western Yew tree, *Taxus brevifolia*.

The mechanism of action of paclitaxel is that of a mitotic spindle poison. It promotes assembly of microtubules and stabilizes them, prevents depolymerization, and therefore prevents cellular replication.

Although initially plagued with hypersensitivity reactions during infusion, present infusion regimens and premedications have decreased the incidence of major hypersensitivity reactions to less than 3%. The major side effect of paclitaxel is myelosuppression, primarily neutropenia. Other common toxicities include alopecia, mild peripheral neuropathy, myalgia, and arthralgias. Asymptomatic bradycardia and arrhythmia are relatively common but are not indications for interruption of chemotherapy. Severe cardiac toxicity rarely occurs.

There are no published reports describing paclitaxel administration during pregnancy.

Reproductive and developmental toxicity studies of paclitaxel in rats have been performed. Various doses of paclitaxel in males and females prior to and during mating and through the first 7 days of gestation in females yielded decreased fertility indices in both sexes at the highest dose level of 1.0 mg/kg/day. All results at the lower levels, 0.3 mg/kg/day or less, were equivalent to the controls. When paclitaxel injections continued daily through gestation and post partum, no influence on prenatal development, learning ability, growth, or mental status of the offspring was detected. In addition, the reproductive performance of both male and female offspring were equivalent to that of the controls.

RECOMMENDED READING

Kai, S., Kohmura, H., Hiraiwa, E., Koizumi, S., Ishikawa, K., Kawano, S., Kuroyanagi, K., Hattori, N., Chikazawa, H., Kondoh, H., et al. Reproductive and developmental toxicity studies of paclitaxel. (I) Intravenous administration to rats prior to and in the early stage of pregnancy (Japanese). *J. Toxicol. Sci.* 19 (Suppl 1): 57, 1994.

Kai, S., Kohmura, H., Hiraiwa, E., Koizumi, S., Ishikawa, K., Kawano, S., Kuroyanagi, K., Hattori, N., Chikazawa, H., Kondoh, H., et al. Reproductive and developmental toxicity studies of paclitaxel (II). Intravenous administration to rats during the fetal organogenesis (Japanese). *J. Toxicol. Sci.* 19 (Suppl). 1:69, 1994.

Kai, S., Kohmura, H., Hiraiwa, E., Koizumi, S., Ishikawa, K., Kawano, S., Kuroyanagi, K., Hattori, N., Chikazawa, H., Kondoh, H., et al. Reproductive and developmental toxicity studies of paclitaxel. (III). Intravenous administration to rats during the perinatal and lactation periods (Japanese). *J. Toxicol. Sci.* 19 (Suppl 1):93, 1994.

Procarbazine (Matulane®)

Procarbazine is a synthetic methylhydrazine derivative originally conceived as a monoamine oxidase inhibitor. Although its exact mechanism of action is unknown, it appears to inhibit RNA, DNA, and protein synthesis. It may function as an antineoplastic agent by depolymerizing DNA through the liberation of hydrogen peroxide produced by autoxidation of the drug. Its major application has been in combination chemotherapy for Hodgkin's disease and other lymphomas.

Acute toxicity of procarbazine consists of nausea, vomiting, central nervous system depression, and a disulfiram-like reaction with alcohol. It is known to potentiate the action of the phenothiazine class of psychotherapeutic drugs. Delayed toxicity includes bone marrow depression, stomatitis, peripheral neuropathy, pneumonitis, and leukemia. The disposition of procarbazine in breast milk is not known.

Procarbazine is both mutagenic and carcinogenic in animals. In animal studies, single doses of procarbazine were lethal or teratogenic given on days 5–12 of gestation but had no effect given on days 14–17. Therefore, teratogenic effects are noted when the drug is given during the process of neurulation and early morphogenesis. Congenital malformations are described in case reports of four in five human fetuses exposed to procarbazine in the first trimester. There was no pattern of reproducible defects in these fetuses, whose mothers were also taking other chemotherapeutic agents (mechlorethamine, vinblastine, and vincristine). Two cases of procarbazine use in the second trimester reported no untoward results. In one case in which a mother mistakenly took 50 mg/day procarbazine orally for 30 days during the middle trimester of pregnancy, an apparently healthy, normal male infant was delivered at term. Even when used for short periods in standard dosages, procarbazine alone and in combination with other antineoplastic agents is known to produce reversible ovarian and testicular dysfunction.

RECOMMENDED READING

Daly, H., McCann, S.R., Hanratty, T.D., et al. Successful pregnancy during combination chemotherapy for Hodgkin's disease. *Acta Haematol.* 64:154, 1980.

Daw, E.G. Procarbazine in pregnancy. *Lancet* 2:984, 1970.

Garrett, M.J. Teratogenic effect of combination chemotherapy. *Ann. Intern. Med.* 80:667, 1974.

Johnson, S.A., Goldman, J.M., and Hawkins, D.F. Pregnancy after chemotherapy for Hodgkin's disease. *Lancet* 2:93, 1979.

Kiely, J.M. Clinical pharmacology (series on pharmacology in practice). 12. Antineoplastic agents. *Mayo Clin. Proc.* 56:384, 1981.

Lee, I.P., and Dixon, R.L. Mutagenicity, carcinogenicity and teratogenicity of procarbazine. *Mutat. Res.* 55:1, 1978.

Wells, J.H., Marshall, J.R., and Carbone, P.P. Procarbazine therapy for Hodgkin's disease in early pregnancy. *J.A.M.A.* 205:935, 1968.

Wiebe, V.J., and Sipila, P.E. Pharmacology of antineoplastic agents in pregnancy. *Crit. Rev. Oncol. Hematol.* 16:75, 1994.

Topotecan

Topotecan is a semisynthetic analog of camptothecin. The parent compound is derived from the bark of an Asian ornamental tree, *Camptotheca acuminata*.

Topotecan cytotoxicity results from the inhibition of topoisomerase I, an enzyme that relieves torsional strain during DNA replication. Campothecin analogs bind with and stabilize the transient DNA–topoisomerase complex, resulting in single-strand breakage and lethal DNA damage.

Topotecan is presently approved for use in recurrent ovarian carcinoma and is the subject of many clinical trials. An oral formulation is available and is presently under clinical trials.

Topotecan is predominantly cleared by the kidney, and hematologic toxicity is heightened in patients with moderate to severe renal insufficiency. A major dose-limiting toxicity of topotecan is neutropenia, which is generally brief and noncumulative. Non-hematologic side effects include mild nausea and vomiting, dose- related alopecia, and sometimes fever.

There is no reported experience of topotecan use in pregnancy at this time.

RECOMMENDED READING

Hoskins, W.J., Perez, C.A., and Young, R.C. *Principles and Practice of Gynecologic Oncology* (2nd ed.). Philadelphia: Lippincott-Raven Publishers, 1997.

Vinca alkaloids, Vincristine (Oncovin®) and Vinblastine (Velban®)

The vinca alkaloids are structurally complex organic bases, can be obtained as natural or semisynthetic, and are derived from the periwinkle plant. These drugs have played important roles in the development of curative therapy of Hodgkin's disease and non-Hodgkin's lymphomas, acute lymphoblastic leukemia, several pediatric solid tumors, and germ cell malignancies. Although structurally very similar, vincristine and vinblastine differ dramatically in their antitumor spectrum and clinical toxicities.

The vinca alkaloids bind to dimers of tubulin at sites that are distinctly different from other microtubule toxins. This binding results in disruption of the microtubular equilibrium and inhibits the assembly of microtubules. This is felt to lead to mitotic arrest within cancer cells.

Vincristine has a broad antineoplastic spectrum and is a component of combination chemotherapy for treatment of childhood and adult acute lymphocytic leukemias, Hodgkin's and non-Hodgkin's lymphomas, Wilms' tumor, Ewing's sarcoma, neuroblastoma, and rhabdomyosarcoma. Vincristine is also used in combination in treating multiple myeloma, sarcomas, breast and small cell lung carcinomas.

Peripheral neurotoxicity is the most frequent toxic effect of vincristine. This side effect is more common in patients over 40 years of age and related to cumulative doses. Gastrointestinal effects including constipation, paralytic ileus, abdominal cramps, and nausea and vomiting may occur. Bladder atony and acute urinary retention is possible as well as the syndrome of inappropriate antidiuretic hormone secretion (SIADH) and mild to moderate myelosuppression.

Vinblastine is used as a component in combination therapy for testicular carcinoma, Hodgkin's and non-Hodgkin's lymphomas, and germ cell tumors of the ovary. Toxicities of vinblastine are principally myelosuppression, particularly leukopenia. Gastrointestinal mucositis, pharyngitis, and stomatitis may occur more frequently than with vincristine. The neurologic effects, although similar to that seen with vincristine, are less common than with vincristine and usually occur in patients with prolonged therapy. Hypertension is the most common cardiovascular toxicity of vinblastine, and acute pulmonary edema has occurred with intravenous administration.

Vinblastine has been documented to be teratogenic in animal models; however, there has been only one reported abnormality in 14 women treated with vinblastine in the first trimester. Vincristine has been used in combination with other antineoplastic agents in over 30 cases during all trimesters of pregnancy, with favorable outcomes in most cases. These reports have established the relative safety of the use of these agents in pregnancy indicating that the human fetus may be less sensitive to the teratogenic effects of these agents than animals.

RECOMMENDED READING

Cohlan, S.W., and Kitay, D. The teratogenic effect of vincaleukoblastine in the pregnant rat. *J. Pediatrics* 66:541, 1965.

Doll, D.C., Ringenberg, Q.S., and Yarbro, J.W. Antineoplastic agents and pregnancy. *Semin. Oncol.* 16:337, 1989.

Rosenzweig, A.I., Crews, Q.E., and Hopwood, H.G. Vinblastine sulfate in Hodgkins disease in pregnancy. *Ann. Intern. Med.* 61:108, 1964.

Gross, Z., Rodriguez, J.J., and Stalnaker, B. Vincristine for refractory autoimmune thrombocytopenic purpura in pregnancy. *J. Reprod. Med.* 40:739, 1995.

Wiebe, V.J., and Sipila, P.E. Pharmacology of antineoplastic agents in pregnancy. *Crit. Rev. Oncol. Hematol.* 16:75, 1994.

Appendix C
Immunization of the Obstetric Patient

There are four types of immunobiologic agents commonly used in the United States. 1) Toxoids are preparations of chemically altered bacterial exotoxins. 2) Inactivated vaccines contain a suspension of heat-inactivated or chemically inactivated microorganisms or portions of microorganisms. 3) Live viral and bacterial vaccines are suspensions of viral or bacterial strains selected for their reduced virulence. Diminished virulence usually is produced by serial passages of the wild-type microorganism in tissue culture (attenuation). In all cases, although no significant illness is produced, the live viral or bacterial vaccine has sufficient antigenic properties in common with the infectious wild-type agent to stimulate protective immunity. 4) Immune globulin preparations are protein fractions of pooled human plasma containing antibodies that can produce transient, passive protection in the recipient. Specific immune globulins, which are produced from plasma of donors with very high antibody titers to a particular agent, are useful for protection against hepatitis B, rabies, tetanus, and varicella infections. Standard immune globulin is useful in providing protection against hepatitis A and measles. Bacterial polysaccharide immune globulin has been used for protection against *Haemophilus influenzae* type b, *Neisseria meningitidis,* and *Streptococcus pneumoniae.*

A systematic approach to vaccinating women of childbearing age is needed to ensure that every pregnant woman and her fetus are protected from preventable, serious diseases as well as from the possible risks that may accompany vaccination. Several factors should be weighed by the health care provider who is considering immunization for any adult female. Whenever possible, pregnant women should be immune to the diseases that pose the greatest and most common risks during pregnancy and for which there are effective vaccines. Accepted criteria for defining immunity vary by disease, and careful attention should be paid to prior illnesses, previous vaccination, and the results of past serologic tests ("Immunization during pregnancy." ACOG Tech. Bull. No. 160, October 1991).

Data on effectiveness are available for most of the agents listed in Table 5. Cholera vaccine is notable for the poor or transient immunity that it confers; influenza vaccine provides protection for about 1 year after its administration. Most other vaccines have been shown to produce long-lasting and probably permanent immunity for over 90% of those vaccinated.

Little information is available on the deleterious effects of most vaccines on a developing fetus. As of May 1982, rubella vaccine was probably the best-studied immunizing agent in this regard. A total of 111 women who were known to be susceptible and who received rubella vaccine shortly before becoming pregnant or early in pregnancy had been followed to term by the Immunization Division of the Centers for Disease Control (CDC). No infant had defects compatible with congenital rubella syndrome, although three had laboratory evidence of rubella virus infection. At that time, all three infants were developing normally. These data indicate that the risk of rubella vaccine to the fetus is negligible (an actual risk to date of 0%, with 95% confidence limits of 0 to 4%). Although the final decision rests with the patient and her physician, the Immunization Practices Advisory Committee of the CDC believes that rubella vaccination during pregnancy should not be a reason to routinely recommend interruption of pregnancy. Nevertheless, pregnancy is a contraindication to rubella vaccination, as well as to measles and mumps vaccination, because of the theoretical risk of damage to the fetus. In general, killed vaccines are safe. There is no evidence that they affect the fetus or increase the risk of abortion.

Live measles vaccine should not be given to the pregnant woman. Pooled immune globulin, however, usually will prevent or modify measles in the susceptible individual if given within 6 days after exposure. Conversely, pooled immune globulin has not been shown to prevent infection in a patient exposed to rubella or mumps. Pooled immune globulin is probably of little benefit, if any, for pregnant women exposed to rubella infection because subclinical infection, with attendant risk to the fetus, still may exist.

In summary, the use of immunizing agents during pregnancy should be limited to a few well-defined situations. Preferably, women should be protected from preventable diseases by vaccination before they become pregnant. Live virus vaccines, in particular, should not be given during pregnancy except when susceptibility and exposure are highly probable and the disease to be prevented poses a greater threat to the woman or fetus than does vaccination. An example would be giving yellow fever vaccine to a pregnant woman who will be living in an area in which yellow fever occurs.

In the United States the only immunizing agents recommended for routine administration during pregnancy are tetanus and diphtheria toxoids and, since 1997, influenza vaccine. The CDC now recommends influenza vaccine for women who will be in the second or third trimester of pregnancy during the influenza season. Measles, rubella, and mumps vaccine should be given to nonimmune women prior to pregnancy or in the immediate postpartum period. Pregnant women in the United States should receive primary vaccination against polio only when the risk of exposure is high. As with all adults, this should be done with inactivated polio virus vaccine (IPV) when available. Live attenuated oral polio virus vaccine (OPV) can be used if time does not allow the administration of at least two doses of IPV or if IPV is not available.

Varicella vaccine, which was introduced in 1996, is a live virus vaccine that is contraindicated in pregnancy.

RECOMMENDED READING

American College of Obstetricians and Gynecologists. Immunization during pregnancy. ACOG Tech. Bull. No. 160, October 1991.

Medical Letter, Inc: Varicella vaccine. *Med. Lett. Drugs. Ther.* 37:55, 1995.

U.S. Centers for Disease Control. Target groups for special vaccination programs. *M.M.W.R.* 46/RR-9: 5, April 25, 1997.

TABLE 5. Immunization During Pregnancy

Immunobiologic agent	Risk from disease to pregnant woman	Risk from disease to fetus or neonate	Type of immunizing agent	Risk from immunizing agent to fetus	Indications for immunization during pregnancy	Dose schedule*	Comments
			LIVE VIRUS VACCINES				
Measles	Significant morbidity, low mortality; not altered by pregnancy	Significant increase in abortion rate; may cause malformations	Live attenuated virus vaccine	None confirmed	Contraindicated (see immune globulins)	Single dose SC, preferably as measles–mumps–rubella[†]	Vaccination of susceptible women should be part of postpartum care
Mumps	Low morbidity and mortality; not altered by pregnancy	Probable increased rate of abortion in first trimester	Live attenuated virus vaccine	None confirmed	Contraindicated	Single dose SC, preferably as measles–mumps–rubella	Vaccination of susceptible women should be part of postpartum care

Poliomyelitis	No increased incidence in pregnancy, but may be more severe if it does occur	Anoxic fetal damage reported; 50% mortality in neonatal disease	Live attenuated virus (oral polio vaccine [OPV]) and enhanced-potency inactivated virus (e-IPV) vaccine‡	None confirmed	Not routinely recommended for women in U.S., except persons at increased risk of exposure	*Primary:* 2 doses of e-IPV SC at 4–8 week intervals and a 3rd dose 6–12 months after the 2nd dose. *Immediate protection:* 1 dose OPV orally (in outbreak setting)	Vaccine indicated for susceptible pregnant women traveling in endemic areas or in other high-risk situations
Rubella	Low morbidity and mortality; not altered by pregnancy	High rate of abortion and congenital rubella syndrome	Live attenuated virus vaccine	None confirmed	Contraindicated	Single dose SC, preferably as measles–mumps–rubella	Teratogenicity of vaccine is theoretic, not confirmed to date; vaccination of susceptible women should be part of postpartum care

Continued

TABLE 5. *Continued*

Immunobiologic agent	Risk from disease to pregnant woman	Risk from disease to fetus or neonate	Type of immunizing agent	Risk from immunizing agent to fetus	Indications for immunization during pregnancy	Dose schedule*	Comments
Yellow fever	Significant morbidity and mortality; not altered by pregnancy	Unknown	Live attenuated virus vaccine	Unknown	Contraindicated except if exposure is unavoidable	Single dose SC	Postponement of travel preferable to vaccination, if possible
			INACTIVATED VIRUS VACCINES				
Influenza	Possible increase in morbidity and mortality during epidemic of new antigenic strain	Possible increased abortion rate; no malformations confirmed	Inactivated virus vaccine	None confirmed	Women with serious underlying diseases; public health authorities to be consulted for current recommendation	One dose IM every year	

Rabies	Near 100% fatality; not altered by pregnancy	Determined by maternal disease	Killed virus vaccine	Unknown	Indications for prophylaxis not altered by pregnancy; each case considered individually	Public health authorities to be consulted for indications, dosage, and route of administration	
Hepatitis B	Possible increased severity during third trimester	Possible increase in abortion rate and prematurity; neonatal hepatitis can occur; high risk of newborn carrier state	Recombinant vaccine	None reported	Pre-and post-exposure for women at risk of infection	Three- or four-dose series IM	Used with hepatitis B immune globulin for some exposures; exposed newborn needs vaccination as soon as possible

Continued

TABLE 5. *Continued*

Immunobiologic agent	Risk from disease to pregnant woman	Risk from disease to fetus or neonate	Type of immunizing agent	Risk from immunizing agent to fetus	Indications for immunization during pregnancy	Dose schedule*	Comments
			INACTIVATED BACTERIAL VACCINES				
Cholera	Significant morbidity and mortality; more severe during third trimester	Increaed risk of fetal death during third-trimester maternal illness	Killed bacterial vaccine	None confirmed	Indications not altered by pregnancy; vaccination recommended only in unusual outbreak situations	Single dose SC or IM, depending on manufacturer's recommendations when indicated	
Plague	Significant morbidity and mortality; not altered by pregnancy	Determined by maternal disease	Killed bacterial vaccine	None reported	Selective vaccination of exposed persons	Public health authorities to be consulted for indications, dosage, and route of administration	

Continued

| Pneumococcus | No increased risk during pregnancy; no increase in severity of disease | Unknown | Polyvalent polysaccharide vaccine | No data available on use during pregnancy | Indications not altered by pregnancy; vaccine used only for high-risk individuals | In adults, 1 SC or IM dose only; consider repeat dose in 6 years for high-risk individuals |
| Typhoid | Significant morbidity and mortality; not altered by pregnancy | Unknown | Killed or live attenuated oral bacterial vaccine | None confirmed | Not recommended routinely except for close, continued exposure or travel to endemic areas | *Killed:* Primary: 2 injections SC at least 4 weeks apart. Booster: Single dose SC or ID (depending on type of product used) every 3 years. *Oral:* Primary: 4 doses on alternate days. Booster: Schedule not yet determined |

TABLE 5. *Continued*

Immunobiologic agent	Risk from disease to pregnant woman	Risk from disease to fetus or neonate	Type of immunizing agent	Risk from immunizing agent to fetus	Indications for immunization during pregnancy	Dose schedule*	Comments
			TOXOIDS				
Tetanus–diphtheria	Severe morbidity; tetanus mortality 30%, diphtheria mortality 10%; unaltered by pregnancy	Neonatal tetanus mortality 60%	Combined tetanus–diphtheria toxoids preferred: adult tetanus–diphtheria formulation	None confirmed	Lack of primary series, or no booster within past 10 years	*Primary:* 2 doses IM at 1–2-month interval with a 3rd dose 6–12 months after the 2nd. *Booster:* Single dose IM every 10 years, after completion of primary series	Updating of immune status should be part of antepartum care

SPECIFIC IMMUNE GLOBULINS

Hepatitis B	Possible increased severity during third trimester	Possible increase in abortion rate and prematurity; neonatal hepatitis can occur; high risk of carriage in newborn	Hepatitis B immune globulin	None reported	Postexposure prophylaxis	Depends on exposure; consult Immunization Practices Advisory Committee recommendations (IM)	Usually given with HBV vaccine; exposed newborn needs immediate postexposure prophylaxis
Rabies	Near 100% fatality; not altered by pregnancy	Determined by maternal disease	Rabies immune globulin	None reported	Postexposure prophylaxis	Half dose at injury site, half dose in deltoid	Used in conjunction with rabies killed virus vaccine
Tetanus	Severe morbidity; mortality 21%	Neonatal tetanus mortality 60%	Tetanus immune globulin	None reported	Postexposure prophylaxis	One dose IM	Used in conjunction with tetanus toxoid

Continued

TABLE 5. *Continued*

Immunobiologic agent	Risk from disease to pregnant woman	Risk from disease to fetus or neonate	Type of immunizing agent	Risk from immunizing agent to fetus	Indications for immunization during pregnancy	Dose schedule*	Comments
Varicella	Possible increase in severe varicella pneumonia	Can cause congenital varicella with increased mortality in neonatal period; very rarely causes congenital defects	Varicella-zoster immune globulin (obtained from the American Red Cross)	None reported	Can be considered for healthy pregnant women exposed to varicella to protect against maternal, not congenital, infection	One does IM within 96 hours of exposure	Indicated also for newborns of mothers who developed varicella within 4 days prior to delivery or 2 days following delivery; approx. 90–95% of adults are immune to varicella; not indicated for prevention of congenital varicella

STANDARD IMMUNE GLOBULINS

Hepatitis A	Possible increased severity during third trimester	Probable increase in abortion rate and prematurity; possible transmission to neonate at delivery if mother is incubating the virus or is acutely ill at that time	Standard immune globulin	None reported	Postexposure prophylaxis	0.02 ml/kg IM in one dose of immune globulin	Immune globulin should be given as soon as possible and within 2 weeks of exposure; infants born to mothers who are incubating the virus or are acutely ill at delivery should receive one dose of 0.5 ml as soon as possible after birth

Continued

TABLE 5. *Continued*

Immunobiologic agent	Risk from disease to pregnant woman	Risk from disease to fetus or neonate	Type of immunizing agent	Risk from immunizing agent to fetus	Indications for immunization during pregnancy	Dose schedule*	Comments
Measles	Significant morbidity, low mortality; not altered by pregnancy	Significant increase in abortion rate; may cause malformations	Standard immune globulin	None reported	Postexposure prophylaxis	0.25 ml/kg IM in one dose of immune globulin, up to 15 ml	Unclear it if prevents abortion; must be given within 6 days of exposure

*Abbreviations: SC = subcutaneously; PO = orally; IM = intramuscularly; ID = intradermally.
†Two doses necessary for adequate vaccination of students entering institutions of higher education, newly hired medical personnel, and international travelers.
‡Inactivated polio vaccine recommended for nonimmunized adults at increased risk.
From "Immunization During Pregnancy," ACOG. Technical Bulletin No. 160, Oct. 1991

Indexes

Drug Classification Index

Note: In the entries, 'Over-the-Counter' is represented by (OTC); in the page references, tables are represented by t

Generic and Trade Name Index

Note: In the entries, 'Over-the-Counter' is represented by (OTC); in the page references, tables are represented by t

500